Fetal Echocardiography

Fetal Echocardiography

Edited by

Darla B. Hess, MD
Associate Professor
Departments of Medicine and Obstetrics and Gynecology
University of Missouri—Columbia School of Medicine
Head, Adult Echocardiography Laboratory
Co-Director, Fetal Echocardiography Laboratory
Co-Director, Adult Congenital Heart Disease Clinic
University of Missouri—Columbia Medical Center
Columbia, Missouri

L. Wayne Hess, MD
Professor and Chairman
Department of Obstetrics and Gynecology
University of Missouri—Columbia School of Medicine
Co-Director, Fetal Echocardiography Laboratory
University of Missouri—Columbia Medical Center
Columbia, Missouri

With 39 Contributors

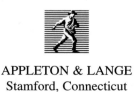

APPLETON & LANGE
Stamford, Connecticut

Notice: The authors and the publisher of this volume have taken care to make certain that the doses of drugs and schedules of treatment are correct and compatible with the standards generally accepted at the time of publication. Nevertheless, as new information becomes available, changes in treatment and in the use of drugs become necessary. The reader is advised to carefully consult the instruction and information material included in the package insert of each drug or therapeutic agent before administration. This advice is especially important when using, administering, or recommending new or infrequently used drugs. The authors and publisher disclaim all responsibility for any liability, loss, injury, or damage incurred as a consequence, directly or indirectly, of the use and application of any of the contents of this volume.

99 00 01 02 03 / 10 9 8 7 6 5 4 3 2 1

Prentice Hall International (UK) Limited, *London*
Prentice Hall of Australia Pty. Limited, *Sydney*
Prentice Hall of Canada, Inc., *Toronto*
Prentice Hall Hispanoamericana, S.A., *Mexico*
Prentice Hall of India Private Limited, *New Delhi*
Prentice Hall of Japan, Inc., *Tokyo*
Simon & Schuster Asia Pte. Ltd., *Singapore*
Editora Prentice Hall do Brasil Ltda., *Rio de Janeiro*
Prentice Hall, *Upper Saddle River, New Jersey*

Library of Congress Cataloging-in-Publication Data

Fetal echocardiography / edited by Darla B. Hess, L. Wayne Hess ; with
    39 contributors.
        p.   cm.
    ISBN 0-8385-2577-6 (case : alk. paper)
    1. Fetal heart—Ultrasonic imaging.   2. Fetal heart—
Abnormalities—Diagnosis.   3. Echocardiography.   4. Ultrasonic
cardiography.   5. Prenatal diagnosis.   6. Congenital heart disease—
Diagnosis.   I. Hess, Darla B.   II. Hess, L. Wayne.
    [DNLM: 1. Echocardiography.   2. Fetal Heart—Ultrasonography.
3. Heart Defects, Congenital—ultrasonography.   4. Ultrasonography,
Prenatal.   WG 141.5.E2 F419 1999]
RG628.3.E34F482   1999
618.3′26107543—dc21
DNLM/DLC
for Library of Congress   98-3614

Developmental Editor: Beth P. Broadhurst
Production Editor: Jeanmarie M. Roche
Production Service: Andover Publishing Services

PRINTED IN THE UNITED STATES OF AMERICA

ISBN 0-8385-2577-6
90000

9 780838 525777

Contents

Contributors

Kul B. Aggarwal, MD, MRCP(UK), FACC
Assistant Professor
Division of Cardiology
Department of Internal Medicine
University of Missouri—Columbia School of Medicine
Staff Physician
Division of Cardiology
Harry S. Truman Memorial Veterans Hospital
Columbia, Missouri
Chapter 10, "Fetal Cardiac Imaging"

Colin M. Bloor, MD
Distinguished Professor of Pathology
Director, Molecular Pathology Graduate Program
Department of Pathology
University of California at San Diego School of
    Medicine
La Jolla, California
Chapter 2, "Fetal and Neonatal Cardiac Anatomy"

Linda C. Buchheit, LPN, RDMS
Head Sonographer
Maternal-Fetal Medicine Division
Department of Obstetrics and Gynecology
University of Missouri—Columbia School of Medicine
Columbia, Missouri
Chapter 10, "Fetal Cardiac Imaging"

Guy A. Carter, MD
Associate Professor of Pediatric Cardiology
Department of Child Health
University of Missouri—Columbia School of Medicine
Columbia, Missouri
Chapter 14, "Congenital Cardiac Defects in the Fetus"
Chapter 17, "Interventional Cardiology in the Fetus"

Ramon A. Castillo, MD
Chairman
Department of Obstetrics and Gynecology
Baptist Medical Center
Jacksonville, Florida
Chapter 11, "Transvaginal Fetal Echocardiography in
    the First and Second Trimester"

Frank I. Clark, MD, JD
Associate Professor
Division of Neonatology
Department of Child Health
University of Missouri—Columbia School of Medicine
Columbia, Missouri
Chapter 23, "Legal Issues Associated with Fetal and
    Neonatal Cardiac Disease"

Joshua A. Copel, MD
Professor of Obstetrics and Gynecology
Head, Section of Maternal-Fetal Medicine
Department of Obstetrics and Gynecology
Yale University School of Medicine
Director of Obstetrics
Department of Obstetrics and Gynecology
Yale-New Haven Hospital
New Haven, Connecticut
Chapter 15, "Management of Fetal Cardiac
    Arrhythmias"

Tony L. Creazzo, PhD
Associate Professor
Institute of Molecular Medicine and Genetics
Developmental Biology Program
Medical College of Georgia School of Medicine
Augusta, Georgia
Chapter 3, "Fetal and Neonatal Cardiac Physiology"

Ronald W. Dudek, PhD
Professor
Department of Anatomy and Cell Biology
East Carolina University School of Medicine
Greenville, North Carolina
Chapter 1, "Cardiac Embryology"

Maria L. Evans, MD
Assistant Professor
Department of Pathology and Anatomical Services
University of Missouri—Columbia School of Medicine
Section Chief, Immediate Response Laboratory
Department of Pathology
University of Missouri—Columbia Hospitals and
    Clinics
Columbia, Missouri
Chapter 14, "Congenital Cardiac Defects in the Fetus"

Greg Flaker, MD
Professor of Medicine
Division of Cardiology
Department of Medicine
Head, Electrophysiology Laboratory
University of Missouri—Columbia School of Medicine
Columbia, Missouri
Chapter 10, "Fetal Cardiac Imaging"

John C. Fletcher, PhD
Professor of Biomedical Ethics
University of Virginia School of Medicine
Charlottesville, Virginia
Chapter 24, "Ethical Issues in Diagnosis and Treatment
    of Fetal and Neonatal Cardiac Disease"

Randall C. Floyd, MD
Assistant Professor
Director
Maternal-Fetal Medicine Division
Department of Obstetrics and Gynecology
University of Missouri—Columbia School of
    Medicine
Columbia, Missouri
Chapter 6, "The Etiology of Congenital Heart Disease"

Robert F. Fraser II, MD
Assistant Professor
Division of Maternal-Fetal Medicine
Department of Obstetrics and Gynecology
University of Missouri—Columbia School of
    Medicine
Columbia, Missouri
Chapter 4, "Using Doppler Ultrasound to Assess Fetal
    Circulation"

Alan H. Friedman, MD
Assistant Professor
Section of Pediatric Cardiology
Department of Pediatrics
Yale University School of Medicine
New Haven, Connecticut
Chapter 15, "Management of Fetal Cardiac Arrhythmias"

Alfredo González-Guayasamin, MD
Fifth Year Medical Student
Department of Obstetrics and Gynecology
Central University of Ecuador
Instituto Ecuatoriano de Seguridad Social
Quito, Ecuador
Chapter 22, "Fetal Imaging in Developing Countries"

Howard P. Gutgesell, MD
Professor
Head, Pediatric Cardiology
Department of Pediatrics
University of Virginia Health Sciences Center
Charlottesville, Virginia
Chapter 24, "Ethical Issues in Diagnosis and Treatment
    of Fetal and Neonatal Cardiac Disease"

Gina Harris, RNC, MS(N)
Women's Services
Perinatal Clinical Nurse Specialist
University of Missouri—Columbia Hospitals and Clinics
Columbia, Missouri
Chapter 13, "Operating a Fetal Echocardiography
    Laboratory"

Darla B. Hess, MD
Associate Professor
Departments of Medicine and Obstetrics and
    Gynecology
University of Missouri—Columbia School of Medicine
Head, Adult Echocardiography Laboratory
Co-Director, Fetal Echocardiography Laboratory
Co-Director, Adult Congenital Heart Disease Clinic
University of Missouri—Columbia Medical Center
Columbia, Missouri
Chapter 10, "Fetal Cardiac Imaging"
Chapter 14, "Congenital Cardiac Defects in the Fetus"

L. Wayne Hess, MD
Professor and Chairman
Department of Obstetrics and Gynecology
University of Missouri—Columbia School of Medicine
Co-Director, Fetal Echocardiography Laboratory
University of Missouri—Columbia Medical Center
Columbia, Missouri
Chapter 10, "Fetal Cardiac Imaging"
Chapter 14, "Congenital Cardiac Defects in the Fetus"

Elizabeth J.P. James, MD
Professor
Division of Neonatal/Perinatal Medicine
Department of Child Health and Obstetrics
University of Missouri—Columbia School of
    Medicine
Director of Neonatal/Perinatal Medicine; Division
    Chief
Division of Neonatal/Perinatal Medicine
Department of Child Health and Obstetrics
Children's Hospital at University of Missouri—
    Columbia Hospitals and Clinics
Columbia, Missouri
Chapter 16, "Early Stabilization and Medical
    Management for Congenital Cardiac Disease"

Alfredo Jose Jijón-Letort, MD
Associate Professor
Division of Obstetrics and Gynecology
Department of Medicine and Biology
Universidad Catolica del Ecuador y Universidad San
    Francisco de Quito
Medico Activo
Department of Obstetrics and Gynecology
Hospital Metropolitano
Quito, Ecuador
Chapter 22, "Fetal Imaging in Developing
    Countries"

Timothy R.B. Johnson, MD
Bates Professor and Chairman of Diseases of Women
    and Children
University of Michigan Medical School
Ann Arbor, Michigan
"Foreword"

Charles S. Kleinman, MD
Professor of Pediatrics, Diagnostic Imaging, and
    Obstetrics and Gynecology
Division of Pediatric Cardiology
Department of Pediatrics
Yale University School of Medicine
New Haven, Connecticut
Chapter 15, "Management of Fetal Cardiac
    Arrhythmias"

Noam Lazebnik, MD
Division Head
Maternal-Fetal Medicine
Henry Ford Hospital & Medical Centers
Detroit, Michigan
Chapter 7, "Recurrence Risks for Cardiac
    Malformations"

Cheryl L. Maslen, PhD
Assistant Professor
Division of Endocrinology, Diabetes, and Clinical
    Nutrition
Department of Medicine
Oregon Health Sciences University School of Medicine
Portland, Oregon
Chapter 20, "Prenatal Diagnosis of Congenital Heart
    Disease"

Michelle N. Meyer, AB
PhD Candidate in Religious Ethics
Division of Theology, Ethics, and Culture
Department of Religious Studies
University of Virginia
Research Assistant
Center for Biomedical Ethics
University of Virginia School of Medicine
Charlottesville, Virginia
Chapter 24, "Ethical Issues in Diagnosis and Treatment
    of Fetal and Neonatal Cardiac Disease"

John C. Morrison, MD
Professor and Chairman
Department of Obstetrics and Gynecology
University of Mississippi Medical Center
Jackson, Mississippi
"Foreword"

Susan B. Olson, PhD
Associate Professor
Department of Molecular and Medical Genetics
Oregon Health Sciences University School of Medicine
Portland, Oregon
Chapter 20, "Prenatal Diagnosis of Congenital Heart
    Disease"

William J. Ott, MD, FACOG
Associate Clinical Professor
Division of Maternal-Fetal Medicine
Department of Obstetrics and Gynecology
St. Louis University School of Medicine
Attending Perinatologist
Division of Maternal-Fetal Medicine
Department of Obstetrics and Gynecology
St. John's Mercy Medical Center
St. Louis, Missouri
Chapter 9, "Accuracy and Utilization of Fetal
    Echocardiography"

Kenneth G. Perry, Jr., MD
Associate Professor
Division of Maternal-Fetal Medicine
Department of Obstetrics and Gynecology
University of Mississippi School of Medicine
Jackson, Mississippi
Chapter 8, "Cardiac Defects and Extracardiac Anomalies"

Jeff Powers, PhD
Technical Staff
Advanced Technology Laboratories
Bothell, Washington
Chapter 25, "Digital Ultrasound Imaging: Current and
    Future Developments"

Mark D. Reller, MD
Professor and Chief
Division of Pediatric Cardiology
Department of Pediatrics
Oregon Health Sciences University School of
    Medicine
Portland, Oregon
Chapter 5, "Cardiac Function in the Late-Gestation
    Fetus"
Chapter 19, "Late Cardiac Physiology Following
    Palliative and Surgical Repair of Congenital Cardiac
    Defects"

Daniel A. Rightmire, MD, MS, RDMS, MBA
Associate Professor
Division of Maternal-Fetal Medicine
Department of Obstetrics and Gynecology
Southern Illinois University School of Medicine
Springfield, Illinois
Chapter 4, "Using Doppler Ultrasound to Assess Fetal
    Circulation"

William E. Roberts, MD
Associate Professor
Department of Obstetrics and Gynecology
University of Mississippi School of Medicine
Jackson, Mississippi
Chapter 8, "Cardiac Defects and Extracardiac
    Anomalies"

John W. Seeds, MD
Professor and Chairman
Department of Obstetrics and Gynecology
Medical College of Virginia Commonwealth
    University
Richmond, Virginia
Chapter 12, "Fetal Anatomic Imaging"

Robin D. Shaughnessy, MD
Fellow
Division of Cardiology
Department of Pediatrics
Oregon Health Sciences University School of Medicine
Portland, Oregon
Chapter 20, "Prenatal Diagnosis of Congenital Heart
    Disease"

Jacques Souquet, PhD
Chief Technology Officer
Senior Vice President, Product Generation
Advanced Technology Laboratories
Bothell, Washington
Chapter 25, "Digital Ultrasound Imaging: Current and
    Future Developments"

Kent L. Thornburg, PhD
Professor
Department of Physiology and Pharmacology
Oregon Health Sciences University School of Medicine
Portland, Oregon
Chapter 5, "Cardiac Function in the Late-Gestation Fetus"

Shaoqing Wang, MD
Director
Department of Diagnostic Ultrasound
Xi'an First Hospital
Director, Clinical Ultrasound Laboratory
Deputy Director, The Consultation Center of
    Ultrasonic Specialists of Xi'an
Xi'an, Shaanxi, People's Republic of China
Chapter 21, "Fetal Echocardiography in China"

Donald C. Watson, Jr., MD
Professor and Director
Division of Pediatric Cardiothoracic Surgery
Department of Surgery and Pediatrics
University of Tennessee, Memphis, College of Medicine
Division of Pediatric Cardiothoracic Surgery
Department of Surgery
LeBonheur Children's Medical Center
Memphis, Tennessee
Chapter 18, "Surgical Interventions and Corrections for
    Congenital Heart Disease"

Foreword

Like it or not, we live in an era of technology and sub-specialization. While many decry this trend in American medicine, we can look with pride to innumerable accomplishments in clinical research and advances in the practice of medicine since the era of Osler. Many of these innovations have been nurtured by strong collaborative research that spanned multiple disciplines, and this book is an example of this rich tradition. Contributions to the field of fetal echocardiography have been made by cardiologists, perinatologists, geneticists, sonographers, pediatricians, physiologists, and biomedical engineers, among others.

Ultrasound has without a doubt been the technology leading to the major perinatal advances of the last decades. It has allowed for accurate and detailed diagnoses of the fetus, as well as for interventional therapy, which are remarkable. Fetal echocardiography has developed as a particular subspecialty for those interested in prenatal diagnosis, whether they be perinatal obstetricians, pediatricians, pediatric cardiologists, sonographers, geneticists, or any of those involved in complex care of fetuses, newborns, and infants with heart disease. If there is a unique role for the maternal-fetal medicine specialist within obstetrics and gynecology, it is in diagnosis and management of specific prenatal conditions using such special techniques as ultrasound, targeted ultrasound and fetal echocardiography, amniocentesis, percutaneous umbilical blood sampling, intrauterine transfusion, and fluorescent in situ hybridization. With advances in diagnostic and therapeutic methodologies, extraordinary precision can now be directed at diagnosis, management, and prognosis of fetuses at risk. In the management of fetuses at risk, fetal echocardiography has become an important service at tertiary and quartenary perinatal centers, which provide such complex prenatal and perinatal management of patients.

Fetal echocardiography is not a technique for use in general practice or the primary care setting, but it is a technique that generalists and all those caring for pregnant women must be aware of, for they must be able to provide comprehensive services for their patients. They must coordinate referrals for appropriate diagnosis and assist in management planning once such diagnosis has been made. They need to be able to provide continuity and resources for these patients, which requires an understanding of the implications and management of the disease processes that are identified. In addition, common fetal prenatal diagnostic techniques, such as routine ultrasound and the acceptance of the four-chamber view as a standard screening technique that can identify conditions associated with congenital heart disease and mandate special fetal cardiographic studies, have increased the importance of fetal echocardiography, as has the widespread application of prenatal genetic testing where chromosomal abnormalities associated with complex congenital heart disease can be identified.

This text, *Fetal Echocardiography*, serves an important role. It will allow those involved in the care of women and children at many levels to obtain the necessary information they need to fulfill their role as either primary care provider or specialist. The risk factors for fetal cardiac disease are broad and need to be understood so that appropriate prereferral counseling can be accomplished. In addition, particular techniques will be used in different clinical situations, and referring physicians would be well served to understand these techniques, such as the role of the four-chamber view in screening for cardiac abnormalities, the role of M-mode echocardiography in the detection and the definition of fetal arrhythmia, and the role of color flow Doppler, all of which are well explored in this book. *Fetal Echocardiography* outlines those conditions that place a pregnancy at risk for fetal cardiac abnormality mandating referral. Many in primary care practice, including nurse practitioners, certified nurse midwives, family physicians, and general obstetricians, as well as perinatologists, will see women with a significant personal history or a previous child with congenital heart disease. Pediatricians and endocrinologists will see women in the reproductive age group who have diabetes and other conditions placing them at risk for fetal cardiac disease. Family physicians and psychiatrists may see women exposed to a broad range of therapeutic drugs that can put their fetus at risk for significant cardiac abnormality.

Just as the generalist must be aware of new and important techniques that can be of use to his or her patients, those specialists who deal with the diagnosis and management of fetal neonatal cardiac disease will be well served by this book. Increasingly, prenatal diagnoses of complex congenital abnormalities, such as hypoplastic left heart and cardiovascular abnormalities associated with diaphragmatic hernia, lead to specialized prenatal referral and management and delivery at specialized centers. Once again a thorough understanding of the diagnostic principles, clinical conditions, and therapeutic and interventional modalities is critical to achieve the best outcome for the patient.

The authors of this text are experienced fetal echocardiographers. L. Wayne Hess, MD, an obstetric perinatologist, has extensive experience in prenatal diagnosis and counseling as well as in management of fetal and perinatal abnormalities. Darla B. Hess, MD, brings the perspective of an echocardiographer and a skilled cardiologist with experience in both adult and child disease and the unique aspects of fetal echocardiography that make diagnosis so difficult. The authors underline the importance of understanding the role that fetal physiology plays in giving special challenges to the fetal echocardiographer.

I have always found that I learn most from clinicians outside my field of expertise, since they have a perspective that is foreign to mine and offer novel and unique insights. *Fetal Echocardiography* offers just such a multidisciplinary approach. It will serve as a key text for the specialist and a useful reference for the generalist. Readers will find much important new information and many new insights in this book. It will improve patient care, it will lead to new knowledge, and I know my copy will be well thumbed.

Timothy R.B. Johnson, MD

Foreword

During the last decade, no field has seen as many advances or made as great an impact on the lives of obstetric patients as antenatal diagnosis. With increasingly sophisticated techniques, both invasive and noninvasive, a much more in-depth assessment of the fetus has been available to clinicians. During this period, fetal cardiology has become an established field in its own right, and in utero echocardiography has been a mainstay of the improvements in this new and exciting area. This progress has led to the expectation on the part of our patients that intrauterine diagnosis, as well as therapy, will solve many of the fetal heart problems that would have been fatal just 10 years ago. This expectation mirrors societal attitudes in general, but specifically it is focused in the area of fetal diagnosis and treatment.

The field of prenatal diagnosis has probably changed more than any single area in medicine. In addition, these alterations have taken place in such a short time. Approximately 40 years ago, invasive fetal diagnosis, using amniocentesis and fetal karyotype, was ushered onto the scene. Beginning approximately 15 years ago, an intricate survey of fetal anatomy with ultrasound revealed much more than we ever thought possible about predicting certain fetal anomalies. During the past decade each 12-month period has proffered tremendous accomplishments. Another phenomenon during the last 20 years that has affected patients and health care providers alike is that the early use of antibiotics has drastically reduced acquired cardiovascular disease complicating pregnancy. This change has brought about an increase in the ratio of acquired versus congenital heart lesions in the adult population. Also, there are now more procedures to ameliorate heart disease in childhood and during adolescence; therefore, even patients with severe cardiac disease are living long enough to reach child-bearing age and able to become pregnant. Furthermore, since more and more of the lesions are congenital, we have begun to

realize the important impact of maternal cardiac disease on inheritance patterns in the offspring. Women with cardiac disease have a drastically increased risk of cardiac problems in their offspring. These clinical imperatives, plus our ability to use new imaging techniques, make fetal echocardiography even more important now than at anytime in its recent development.

All of these advances have not been without controversy or the creation of new and difficult problems. Ethical dilemmas as well as legal issues associated with fetal/neonatal cardiac disease now complicate the lives of health care providers, as well as patients. In the past these thorny issues were usually limited to occurrences after birth, but now they arise with regularity during pregnancy and preconception counseling sessions. Just 10 to 20 years ago, when life-threatening congenital anomalies or fetal demise were present, we rarely knew the etiology until delivery or shortly thereafter when neonatal abnormalities became apparent. Another problem, which stems from the rapid pace of the discovery of the new techniques and the burgeoning amount of information available (and necessary) in this field, centers around the absence of a collective work that assimilates all the knowledge on the subject of fetal echocardiography. Part of this problem, which has prevented the publication of a comprehensive textbook on the subject, is the speed at which advances in the field have made the transition from the research laboratory to the patients' bedside, where they become the standard of care. Another difficulty has been that the subject of fetal echocardiography spans many different and highly technical areas. For example, basic science research physicians, such as embryologists and physiologists, in addition to clinicians in maternal-fetal medicine, pulmonology, neonatology, cardiology, cardiac surgery, and anesthesia, as well as ethicists, lawyers, and consumer advocates are all involved in this ever-expanding area. It is no wonder that a subject that embraces all of these areas and touches so many people's lives would be difficult to bring together in one volume. Nevertheless, this is exactly what Drs. Hess and Hess have accomplished.

In an overview of this important work, it is clear that fetal echocardiography is critical to practitioners of obstetrics, particularly those with an interest in prenatal diagnosis, both in the clinical sphere and from a research standpoint. The reader will finally have all of the basic as well as clinical knowledge for diagnosis and management of fetal cardiac disorders noted during pregnancy and early neonatal life collected in one place. It is necessary that the etiologic basis of congenital fetal heart disease be discussed in detail, as well as the reader understanding the importance of normal fetal/neonatal cardiac physiology, anatomy, and embryology in this field. Cardiac as well as extra-cardiac anomalies associated with fetal heart disease must be included as well as the clinical techniques for diagnosis. In addition to the modalities of cardiac imaging, the operation of an echocardiology laboratory is critiqued. These components include JCAHO requirements, quality assurance, storage or computerization of images, and so forth and address all areas necessary to begin and sustain such an operation. Each specific clinical entity is covered in a way that enables the reader to understand the pathophysiology, the methods of diagnosis, and the techniques of correction. Importantly, sections on patient counseling, legal requirements, and ethical dilemmas are also included.

The unifying approach of using fetal echocardiography to join specialists and subspecialists, basic scientists and clinicians, attorneys and physicians, is not unique, but the specific scope and direction of this volume certainly sets it apart from other, more narrowly focused attempts. This important work is a must-read for clinicians in maternal-fetal medicine, neonatology, and pediatric cardiology who routinely care for fetuses or neonates and counsel their families.

John C. Morrison, MD

Preface

We first began to be regularly involved in ultrasound examinations in 1979. This became a practical reality when ADR[R] provided the first commercially available real-time ultrasound scanner in that year. Shortly thereafter Dr. John Hobbins, Dr. Roger Sanders, Dr. Rudy Sabbagha, and others produced preliminary ultrasound books providing practical advice and education to sharpen the obstetrical sonographers' skills.

Fetal number, viability, presentation, and placental location were obtainable following limited scanning experience in 1979. However, identification of fetal anomalies seldom occurred unless gross defects existed. The possibility of diagnosing fetal cardiac defects was not at that time considered even a "theoretical" possibility by most obstetricians. Maternal-fetal medicine was a recognized specialty with fewer than 75 board certified physicians in the specialty.

In the early to late 1980s, Dr. David Sahn, Dr. Norm Silverman, Dr. Greg DeVore, Dr. Charles Kleinman, and others began to demonstrate that fetal echocardiography was a practical reality. Dr. Greg DeVore, in a series of reviews in the *American Journal of Obstetrics and Gynecology*, introduced the basic concept of fetal echocardiography to obstetricians and gynecologists.

In the early phase of development of fetal echocardiography, Dr. Lindsay Allen published a brief textbook of fetal echocardiography, which was followed by a short monograph on fetal echo by Dr. Kathryn Reed.

In March 1997, the American College of Cardiology and the American Heart Association in their Task Force Guidelines recommended that fetal echo be performed only by trained fetal echocardiographers, with joint involvement of cardiologists and maternal-fetal medicine specialists. This recommendation was probably due to the practical limits of cardiologists and others in recognizing other fetal anomalies that are frequently related to congenital heart defects. It was also related to the practical limits of maternal-fetal medicine specialists in dealing with complex congenital heart defects.

Presently, most fetal echo labs foster a team approach to diagnosis, counseling, and therapy. Our team at the University of Missouri–Columbia Medical Center involves the specialities of Maternal-Fetal Medicine, Adult and Pediatric Cardiology, Pediatric Cardiothoracic Surgery, Human Genetics, Neonatology, Social Services, Pediatric Anesthesia, and the clergy. This team deals with diagnosis and therapy and medical, social and ethical issues related to fetal and neonatal congenital heart disease.

As we developed our fetal echo team, it became obvious that there was a need for a basic introductory textbook on fetal echocardiography to orient new team members to the subject. Numerous articles and books were required to orient new members. Topics such as traditional and contemporary cardiac embryology and physiology, basic fetal echo ultrasound scanning techniques, quantitative and qualitative pulse, continuous wave, and color flow Doppler and power angiography, and basic cardiac surgical repair must be understood to have a quality fetal echo laboratory.

This textbook is an attempt to introduce these basic concepts to newcomers to the area of fetal echocardiography.

Darla B. Hess, MD
L. Wayne Hess, MD

Acknowledgments

L. Wayne Hess would like to express his gratitude to his wife, Darla B. Hess, and children for allowing him the time to work on this book. He would also like to express his gratitude to Dr. Marco Labudovich, his residency program director, for knocking off many of his rough edges and allowing him freedom to develop as a physician; Dr. Robert Cefalo, Dr. Robert Park, Dr. Thomas Kline, Dr. Don Gallup, Dr. Jeff Phelan, Dr. Bill O'Brien, Dr. John Morrison, Dr. Jim Daly, and many others who have served as mentors moving him forward with his career. He would also like to thank his secretary, Mrs. Caprice Forest, and computer analyst, Mr. Joseph Wu, for helping him maintain his sanity during the development of this book.

Darla B. Hess would like to thank her husband, L. Wayne Hess, and her daughter, Ever Marie Hess, for the time spent away from them for the preparation of the book. She would also like to thank Mrs. Kathleen Yates, her secretary, for her endless help with sorting and filing. Darla B. Hess would also like to thank Ever Curtis, MD, for being her foremost role model (the woman who did it all and is still doing it). She would also like to thank Dr. Pravin Shah for inspiring her early interest in echocardiography, Dr. Patrick Lehan for allowing a career in academic medicine to develop, and the many other mentors who taught and inspired a drive for excellence.

Darla B. Hess and L. Wayne Hess would also like to thank Jane Licht, Beth Broadhurst, and others at Appleton & Lange for their patience as this text developed. Their advice and patience was never-ending, as managed care and the changes sweeping medicine eliminated more and more of the contributing authors' time that could be devoted to this text.

Introduction

Darla B. Hess, M.D.
L. Wayne Hess, M.D.

"To study the phenomena of disease without books is to sail an uncharted sea, while to study books without patients is not to go to sea at all."

Sir William Osler

Fetal echocardiography has become the method of choice to diagnose fetal heart disease in the prenatal period. This technique allows cardiologists, perinatologists, geneticists, and other fetal cardiologists the opportunity to evaluate the structure, function, and physiology of the fetal heart in utero. Modern ultrasound technology offers a "window in the womb" to evaluate the fetal heart. Although the fetal heart is developed into the four-chambered heart by approximately 8 weeks' gestation, cardiac function and structure continue to evolve throughout fetal, neonatal, and adolescent life.

This textbook will attempt to provide a "chart" to sail the sea of fetal cardiology. Basic embryology of the fetal heart (both classic and contemporary) will be explored as a separate chapter to allow the reader to appreciate the embryologic basis for most congenital heart disease. The changing physiology of the fetal heart from conception to birth will also receive a devoted chapter. Detailed anatomy of the fetal heart will be covered in depth. These basic concepts will then become the basis to explore diagnosis and treatment in fetal cardiology.

Building from the basic science of the fetal heart, the genetic and nongenetic etiologies of fetal heart disease will be discussed. Sonographic evaluation of the fetal heart—2D, M-mode, color M-mode, pulsed and continuous wave Doppler, color flow mapping, power Doppler (angiography)—will be reviewed in detail. Fe-

tal and neonatal management of fetal heart disease will also receive ample attention. Finally, ethical and legal implications of fetal cardiology and future developments such as 3D ultrasound, harmonic imaging, and Doppler tissue imaging will be covered.

Fetal cardiology has become an exciting field of prenatal diagnosis. It has evolved markedly since its initial inception. However, it is still in its infancy of development. When first performed it was like a small boy with a hammer: everything seen needed to be pounded and the accuracy of the pounding was not established. Slowly the limitations, indications, and accuracy of fetal echo are becoming established. Additionally, what constitutes an adequate fetal echo is becoming well defined. Realism is rapidly supplanting egotism when discussing fetal echocardiographic diagnosis.

INCIDENCE AND DETECTION OF CONGENITAL HEART DISEASE

Improved computer technology and resolution of echocardiographic images have markedly improved the diagnosis of fetal anomalies. Approximately 60–70% of pregnancies undergo an ultrasound examination during pregnancy.[1] Still, most neonates born with congenital heart disease are not diagnosed prenatally. Many of the reasons for a failure of diagnosis include inadequate experience and training of some sonographers, failure to completely evaluate a four-chambered view of the heart, low reliability of the four-chambered heart to screen for congenital heart disease, and failure to refer appropriate patients for a fetal echocardiogram.

The incidence of neonatal congenital heart disease has only recently been evaluated in complete studies. One of the most complete of these studies is the Report of the New England Regional Infant Cardiac Program.[2] Neonates were enrolled in this study if they died of congenital heart disease or required cardiac catheterization or cardiac surgery in the first year of life. This study was performed during the years 1968–1973. The incidence of significant congenital heart disease was 2.3–2.6 cases per 1000 live births. However, these numbers refer only to the prevalence of severe congenital heart disease. Cases of asymptomatic atrial septal or ventricular septal defects, noncritical valvular anomalies, mild coarctation, and so forth are excluded from this study since physical examination alone in the first year of life will miss a significant number of these infants. An estimate of nonlethal neonatal cardiac disease (both mild and severe) from this study is 8 cases per 1000 live births.

Since it is estimated that 30% of fetuses with congenital heart disease die prior to birth, the estimated incidence of fetal congenital heart disease at 20 weeks' gestation is 10 cases per 1000 live births.[3] Estimates of severe, complex fetal cardiac disease at 20 weeks' gestation have varied between 3.0 and 3.6 cases per 1000 live births.[4] It would be reasonable to expect that most severe fetal cardiac diseases would be diagnosed by a complete fetal echocardiogram. However, less severe forms, such as secondary ASD, mild valvular disease, small VSDs, or noncritical coarctation, would quite possibly be missed with a complete fetal echocardiogram.

The initial report by Copel et al[5] in a retrospective review optimistically suggested that 90% of fetal congenital heart disease could be diagnosed by a four-chambered view of the fetal heart alone. However, several retrospective and prospective studies (Table 1) through 1997 have failed to confirm this initial optimism even when a full fetal echocardiogram is performed. There is a wide variation in the sensitivity of these studies to detect fetal congenital heart disease with a range of sensitivity varying from 40–96%. This wide variation may possibly be accounted for by differences in equipment, training, study populations, study design, examination techniques, and case ascertainment methods, which are very important in these studies. Physical examination of the neonate alone following birth will miss 70–80% of ventricular septal defects, or more than 50% of secondary ASDs. A neonatal echocardiogram would be expected to markedly improve case ascertainment. Additionally, because some cases of fetal cardiac disease develop later than 20 weeks' gestation, serial fetal echocardiograms would improve fetal ascertainment. If ascertainment is incomplete, then sensitivity would appear to be improved in these studies.

Buskens et al,[6] in a retrospective study of 3223 "high-risk" fetuses undergoing a complete fetal echo, noted a 43% sensitivity and a 95% specificity. Cooper et al[7] in a similar retrospective study of 915 "high-risk" fetuses noted a 64% sensitivity and 100% specificity to detect fetal cardiac disease. Leslie et al[8] in a retrospective study utilizing a four-chamber view noted only a 38% sensitivity to detect congenital heart disease. Rustico et al[9] in a prospective study of 6623 low-risk fetuses noted a 35% sensitivity overall with a 61% sensitivity for serious congenital heart disease. Ott[10] in a prospective study noted a 14% sensitivity in low-risk fetuses and 82% in high-risk fetuses. Ascertainment in the Rustico study was probably adequate since 9 cases of congenital heart disease per 1000 live births were detected in the study.

These and other studies demonstrate that four-chambered screening alone is inadequate to detect most fetal congenital heart disease with a sensitivity of 4–40%. The four-chambered view could be expected to detect atrioventricular valvular abnormalities or ventricular hypoplasias. However, VSDs, transposition of the great vessels, tetralogy of Fallot, and coarctation of the aorta would be underdetected by a four-chamber view. Since VSD, transposition of the great vessels, tetralogy of Fallot, and coarctation of the aorta are the four most common, severe cardiac diagnoses made in the first year of life, the four-chambered screen alone

TABLE 1. STUDIES EVALUATING PRENATAL CARDIAC DIAGNOSES

Study	Study Population	Study Design	Sensitivity	Specificity
Buskens et al[6]	3223 high-risk patients	Retrospective	43	95
Cooper et al[7]	915 high-risk patients	Retrospective	64	100
Rustico et al[9]	6623 low-risk patients	Prospective	35	100
Ott[10]	1136 low-risk and 68% high-risk patients	Prospective	14 (low-risk) 82 (high-risk)	99
Yagel et al[11]	4961 high-risk and 17,089 low-risk patients	Retrospective	85	95

would not be adequate for detection of most severe fetal and neonatal congenital heart disease.

The study of Yagel et al[11] from Israel in 1997 has been one of the better studies yet published to assess the accuracy and limits of fetal echocardiography. In this study a fetal echocardiogram was performed in the early or late second and third trimesters on 22,050 mixed high- and low-risk fetuses from January 1990 to January 1994. Following delivery, all of these neonates underwent careful evaluation by a pediatrician. Autopsies were performed on fetal or neonatal deaths and pregnancy terminations. Their reported detection rate for congenital heart disease was 7.6 cases per 1000 live births. Therefore, both fetal and neonatal ascertainment should be fairly complete. This group of investigators reported a 85% sensitivity and 95% specificity to detect fetal congenital heart disease. All of these studies demonstrate that four-chamber, outflow tracts, and aortic arch imaging combined with Doppler and color flow mapping markedly improved the sensitivity and specificity of the fetal echocardiogram. "High-risk" fetuses screened in these studies included mothers with a family history of congenital heart disease, maternal insulin-dependent diabetes mellitus, fetal chromosome or other abnormalities, fetal arrhythmias, and fetal teratogen exposure. The sensitivity and specificity for "high-risk" patients was far greater than for low-risk populations.

Presently only those fetuses at high risk for congenital heart disease are screened via fetal echocardiography. Even if fetal echocardiography had a 100% sensitivity and 100% specificity (i.e., a perfect test), most congenital heart disease would not be detected in utero since 75% of neonatal congenital heart disease occurs in the low-risk population. Presently fetal echocardiography for all pregnant women is not recommended. Additionally, fetal echocardiography is not routinely available in all areas. Improvements in the detection of congenital heart disease antepartum would require a complete sonogram and fetal echocardiogram for all pregnant patients. The practicality and cost effectiveness of such an approach has not yet been studied or determined.

REFERENCES

1. Ewigman BG, Crane JP, Frigoletto D, et al.: Effect of prenatal ultrasound on perinatal outcome. *N Engl J Med.* 329:821–7, 1993.
2. Report of the New England Infant Cardiac Program. *Pediatrics.* 85:2, 1980.
3. Allan LD, Crawford DC, Chita SK, et al.: Prenatal screening for congenital heart disease. *Br Med J.* 292:1717–19, 1986.
4. Allan LD, Crawford DC, Henderson RH, et al.: Spectrum of congenital heart disease detected echocardiographically in perinatal life. *Br Heart J.* 54:523–6, 1985.
5. Copel JA, Pilu G, Kleinman CS: Congenital heart disease and extracardiac anomalies: Associations and indications for fetal echocardiography. *Am J Obstet Gynecol.* 154:1121–32, 1986.
6. Buskens E, Stewart P, Hess L, et al.: Efficacy of fetal echocardiography and yield by risk category. *Obstet Gynecol.* 87:423–8, 1996.
7. Cooper MJ, Enderlein MA, Dyson DC, et al.: Fetal echocardiography: Retrospective review of clinical experience and an evaluation of indications. *Obstet Gynecol.* 86:577–82, 1995.
8. Leslie KK, Perautic WH, Draco JA, et al.: Prenatal detection of congenital heart disease by basic ultrasonography at a tertiary care center: What should our expectations be? *J Maternal Fetal Invest.* 6:132–5, 1996.
9. Rustico MA, Bensttoni A, D'Ottavio G, et al.: Fetal heart screening in low risk pregnancies. *Ultrasound Obstet Gynecol.* 6:313–9, 1995.
10. Ott WJ: The accuracy of antenatal fetal echocardiography screening in high and low risk patients. *Am J Obstet Gynecol.* 172:1741–9, 1995.
11. Yagel S, Weissman A, Rotstein Z, et al.: Congenital heart defects—natural course and in utero development. *Circulation.* 96:550–5, 1997.

CHAPTER ONE

Cardiac Embryology

Ronald W. Dudek

Although recent research findings in the area of heart embryology have contributed greatly to our understanding, it is appropriate to begin this chapter with a simple explanation of heart development. Heart formation involves four main events: (1) the formation of a tube with a single lumen; (2) a right-hand folding of the tube, called *dextral looping*; (3) bulging of the tube into vesicles called the *conotruncus, primitive ventricle, primitive atrium,* and *sinus venosus;* and (4) partitioning of the single lumen into four chambers. It is important to realize that the embryonic heart, even though it has undergone dextral looping and growth of vesicles, is still *a tube with a single lumen.* And herein lies the critical issue that the embryo must solve during development: How does a tube with a single lumen partition into four distinct chambers of the adult heart? An optimal solution will result in a "normal" heart, whereas suboptimal solutions will result in a plethora of congenital heart malformations. With this albeit simple explanation of heart development, we can now embellish our description.

PRIMARY HEART TUBE FORMATION

During week 3 of human development, one of the most important events in embryologic development occurs, that is, *gastrulation.* Gastrulation is the process whereby three primary germ layers (ectoderm, mesoderm, and endoderm) are formed. Gastrulation is presaged by the appearance of the primitive streak within the epiblast of the embryo. Epiblast cells located at the rostral part of the primitive streak are already committed to cardiac development by the time they ingress at the primitive streak (Figure 1–1). The exact molecular cues involved in this early commitment process are unknown, but these epiblast cells have been shown to express the antigen JB3, which is related to the protein *fibrillin.*[1,2] These cells (now called *precardiac mesoderm*) reside within the lateral plate mesoderm.

Precardiac mesoderm is bipotential in that it differentiates into two types of cells under the influence of foregut endoderm.[3,4] The first type of cell is the *premyocardial cell,* which forms the adult myocardium and secretes an extracellular matrix called *cardiac jelly.* The second type of cell is the *preendocardial cell,* which forms part of the endocardium.

The embryologic formation of the endocardium is interesting in that the endothelial cells lining the adult endocardium arise from at least two sources.[5–7] The first source is *precardiac mesoderm* that differentiates into preendocardial cells and expresses antigens JB3 and QH1 (i.e., JB3+ and QH1+) under the inductive influence of foregut endoderm. The second source is *noncardiogenic splanchnic mesoderm* or *anterior head mesoderm* that differentiates into preendocardial cells and expresses antigen QH1 but not JB3 (i.e., JB3– and QH1+). Preendocardial cells from both sources form the endothelial lining of the endocardium.

The lateral plate mesoderm eventually splits to form a somatic layer and a splanchnic layer such that the precardiac mesoderm is preferentially concentrated in the splanchnic layer as bilateral *heart-forming regions* (HFRs; see Figure 1–2). The space that forms between the somatic layer of the lateral plate mesoderm and the HFRs via cavitation of lateral mesoderm forms the *pericardial cavity.* In addition, the embryo undergoes two important folding processes (head-and-tail folding and lateral body folding) during the embryonic period, which essentially convert the embryo from a two-dimensional disk to a three-dimensional cylinder. The head-and-tail folding results from the growth of the

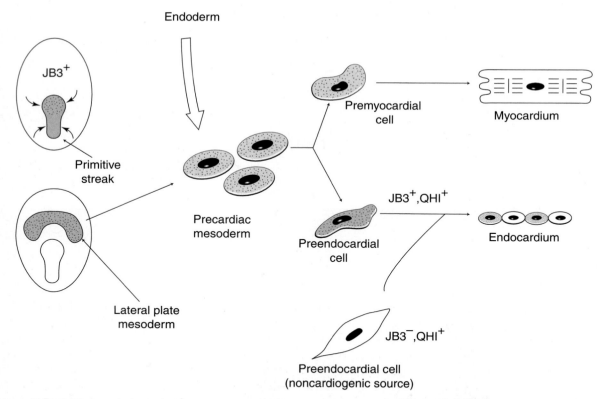

Figure 1–1. Conceptual framework of the events involved in early cardiac morphogenesis. JB3-positive cells at the rostral end of the primitive streak are already committed to cardiac development. Foregut endoderm plays a role in the differentiation of precardiac mesoderm into premyocardial and preendocardial cells. Note that the definitive lining of the endocardium has two embryologic sources: precaridac mesoderm and a noncardiogenic source.

neural tube and is responsible for placing the heart in its adult anatomic location within the middle mediastinum of the thorax. The lateral body folding is due to the growth of the somites and is responsible for fusion of precardiac mesoderm within the HFRs at the midline.

Recent findings[8,9] strongly suggest that the single endocardial tube arises after the fusion of the bilateral HFRs. In light of these recent findings, the endocardial tube may arise by a progressive remodeling of small, discontinous angiogenic vesicles into a single endocardial tube, not by the merging of two separate endocardial tubes as traditionally proposed by Patten and others.[10–12] Consequently, the traditionally held explanation that heart development proceeds via the bilateral formation of two "minihearts" followed by their fusion in the midline into one "complete heart" may not be as robust as once thought. This distinction may be more than academic, because it may point to important clues in the mechanism of endocardial vasculogenesis. Endocardial vasculogenesis occurs beneath the *foregut*

endoderm where the endodermal cells are hypertrophied and markedly different from endodermal cells not associated with HFRs.[13] It may be that foregut endoderm cells are involved in endocardial vasculogenesis by secreting factors that promote vasculogenesis, for example, vascular endothelial growth factor (VEGF).[14] Consequently, foregut endoderm, in addition to its inductive role in lineage separation, i.e., the differentiation of precardiac mesoderm into myocardial cells and preendocaridial cells, may also play a crucial role in endocardial vasculogenesis.

The adult *epicardium* forms as an outgrowth of the coelomic wall near the liver region and is related to coronary artery formation. The outgrowth of the coelomic wall makes initial contact with the heart tube at the sinus venosus and then spreads over the ventricular and atrial surfaces.[15–18] The epicardium thus formed consists of a simple squamous epithelium as the outer lining and a subepicardial layer of connective tissue.

From the above discussion, it should be appreci-

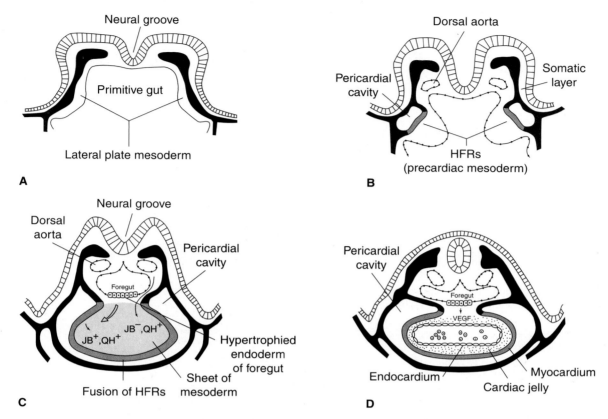

Figure 1–2. Cross sections of an embryo at the level of the developing heart from approximately day 20 to day 22. **A.** The formation of lateral plate mesoderm is shown. **B.** Lateral plate mesoderm splits into a somatic and splanchnic layer, thus forming the pericardial cavity. Precardiac mesoderm is preferentially distributed into the splanchnic layer and patches are now called heart-forming regions (HFRs; dotted area). **C.** Because of lateral folding of the embryo, the HFRs fuse in the midline. Hypertrophied cells of foregut endoderm induce the differentiation of precardiac mesoderm (large curved arrow) within the HFRs to form (JB+, QH+) preendocardial cells. In addition, (JB−, QH+) preendocardial cells from a noncardiogenic source are shown migrating into the cardiogenic region (long arrow). The (JB+, QH+) and (JB−, QH+) preendocardial cells form a continuous sheet of mesoderm (a mesenchymal sheet). **D.** Hypertrophied foregut endoderm secretes vascular endothelial growth factor (VEGF), which induces the mesenchymal sheet of preendocardial cells to form small, discontinuous angiogenic vesicles that eventually get remodeled into a single endocardial tube. This figure depicting early heart tube formation may be at odds with figures found in many textbooks. Here we have tried to incorporate many of the latest research findings into the figure, although they may be somewhat controversial at this time.

ated that we have formed a primary heart tube with its various layers, namely, the *endocardium, cardiac jelly, myocardium,* and *epicardium.* The primary heart tube is initally and very briefly a straight tube that is already specified in a cranial–caudal direction to form the various regions or chambers of the adult heart. Subsequently, the primary heart tube begins rhythmic contractions at day 23 in humans. Soon thereafter, the primary heart tube undergoes dextral looping, which is the first indication of left–right (LR) asymmetry in the embryo.

DEXTRAL LOOPING

The straight primary heart tube is specified in a cranial–caudal direction to form the conotruncus, primitive ventricle, primitive atrium, and sinus venosus, respectively (Figure 1–3). In addition, blood flows into the heart tube at the caudal end (sinus venosus) and out of the heart tube at the cranial end (conotruncus). A closer inspection of the blood flow pattern through the primary heart tube reveals a surprising fact: Blood flows within the heart tube from the sinus venosus →

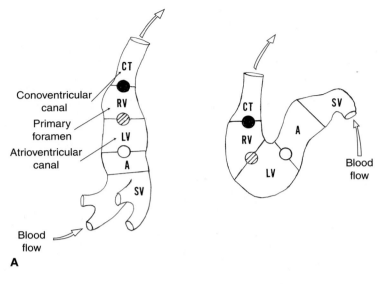

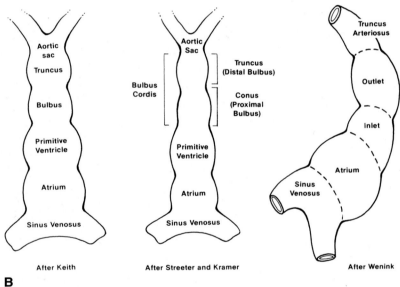

Figure 1–3. The primary heart tube, depicting its specification in the cranial–caudal direction. **A.** The straight primary heart tube can be divided into five distinct areas: conotruncus (CT), right ventricle (RV), left ventricle (LV), primitive atrium (A), and sinus venosus (SV). In addition, there are three orifices or canals that are extremely important to understand since they undergo changes in positioning during dextral looping: the conoventricular canal, the primary foramen, and the atrioventricular canal. **B.** For students of cardiac embryogenesis, the process of heart development is difficult enough to understand without the added hardship of variable nomenclature that exists within the literature. This diagram indicates the different names that have been applied by authors to various areas of the primary heart tube. (*Reprinted with permission from Garson A Jr., Bricker JT, McNamara DG. The Science and Practice of Pediatric Cardiology. Philadelphia: Lea & Febiger; 1990.*)

primitive atrium → atrioventricular canal → presumptive *left* ventricle → primary foramen → presumptive *right* ventricle → conoventricular canal → conotruncus. (Note that venous blood flows through the left ventricle before following through the right ventricle.) It can easily be appreciated that for normal heart development to occur, it is critical that the atrioventricular canal, primary foramen, and conoventricular canal undergo rearrangement. Dextral looping is one of the key events in this rearrangement. When considering the phenomenon of looping, we should distinguish between the *direction* of looping and the *process* of looping.

The direction of looping reflects the overall left–right (LR) asymmetry of the embryo. LR asymmetry has a clear genetic basis since several types of mutations affecting LR asymmetry have been described in mice and humans, which include (1) the *iv/iv* (inversus viscerum) mutation, whereby 50% of the offspring demonstrate a full array of LR reversals and isomerisms;[19] (2) the *inv/inv* (inversion of embryonic turning) mutation, whereby nearly 100% of the offspring demonstrate an LR reversal of heart, viscera, and body–tail orientation;[20] (3) heterotaxia whereby each organ makes an independent decision regarding its LR orientation;[21] (4) the *legless* mutation whereby limb malformations are related to LR orientation of visceral organs;[22] and (5) an autosomal recessive defect for the protein dynein (Kartagener's syndrome) that produces LR reversals.[23]

Since dextral looping occurs in all vertebrate species, a cellular mechanism involving differential gene expression that has been highly conserved throughout evolution may be postulated. In this regard, three genes that are asymmetrically expressed and may participate in dextral looping of the heart have been identified[24]: activin receptor IIa (*cAct-RIIa*), sonic hedgehog (*Shh*), and nodal-related 1 (*cNR-1*).

The process of looping (Figure 1–4) can be divided into three stages, as follows.

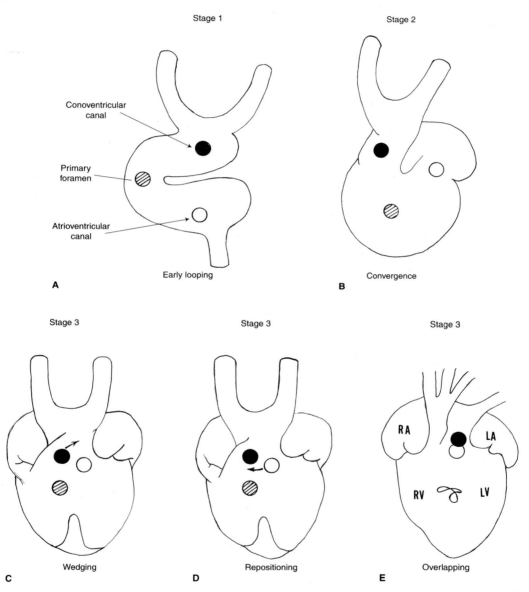

Figure 1–4. The various stages in the process of dextral looping. **A.** Stage 1 of dextral looping shows an early position of the conoventricular canal, primary foramen, and atrioventricular canal. **B.** Stage 2 of dextral looping involves convergence of the conoventricular canal and atrioventricular canal so that both canals are approximately at the same level. **C.** Stage 3 of dextral looping involves wedging, whereby the conoventricular canal moves to the left (arrow) so that it is oriented correctly with the ventricles. **D.** Stage 3 of dextral looping also involves repositioning, whereby the atrioventricular canal moves to the right (arrow) so that it is oriented correctly with the ventricle also. **E.** Stage 3 of dextral looping also involves overlapping (this term has been coined by the present author), whereby the primary foramen undergoes extensive remodeling so that it actually forms three separate openings (see Figure 1–5). RA, right atrium; LA, left atrium; RV, right ventricle; LV, left ventricle.

Stage 1

Stage 1 of looping seems to be inherently programmed within the myocardial cells. Consequently, a number of cellular mechanisms have been implicated in looping; these include differential rates of proliferation of myocardial cells,[25,26] assymetrically located bundles of actin filaments,[27,28] altered cell adhesion[29] and extracellular matrix input.[30]

Stage 2

Stage 2 of looping involves *convergence*[31] of the atrioventricular canal and conoventricular canal, which is imperative if proper alignment of these two canals is to occur.

Stage 3

Stage 3 of looping involves *wedging*,[31] whereby the conoventricular canal is brought into correct orientation with the appropriate ventricles such that the aortic side of the conotruncus is brought to nestle between the mitral and tricuspid valves. Wedging occurs concurrently with the formation of the aortopulmonary septum (AP septum), which divides the conotruncus into the aorta and pulmonary trunk. As long as convergence and wedging occur normally, the AP septum will be in the correct position to fuse with the atrioventricular septum (AV septum) and the interventricular septum (IV septum). If not, a number of congenital heart malformations may occur, namely, double-outlet right ventricle (DORV), persistent truncus arteriosus (PTA) over the right ventricle, or overriding PTA.

Stage 3 of looping also involves a *"repositioning"* of the atrioventricular canal. As the IV septum begins to form, the AV canal is positioned over the presumptive left ventricle so that all the blood from the primitive atrium flows into the presumptive left ventricle. For normal heart development to occur, it is essential that the AV canal become "repositioned" to the right so that the AV canal straddles both the presumptive right and left ventricle. However, the exact mechanism of "repositioning" is still the subject of some controversy in that various mechanisms have been suggested in the literature, for example: (1) a migration of the posterior part of the IV septum to the left,[32] (2) a "shift" of the AV canal to the right,[33] (3) an alignment of the posterior part of the IV septum with the septum primum of the interatrial septum,[34] and (4) formation and expansion of the right AV canal.[35] Whether one or a combination of these particular mechanisms is responsible, "repositioning" must occur for normal heart development.

Stage 3 of looping also involves *"overlapping,"* in which the primary foramen (the opening between the presumptive left ventricle and the presumptive right ventricle) is remodeled (Figures 1–4 and 1–5). This may well be one of the most difficult areas of cardiac embryology to understand fully. Initially, the primary foramen is orientated in a craniocaudal direction. During dextral looping, the primary foramen bends to the right and eventually overlaps itself so that the primary foramen is divided into three separate openings: (1) a sagittal plane opening between the presumptive left and right ventricles, which is completely closed in the adult heart by the IV septum; (2) a frontal plane opening that persists in the adult heart near the orifice of the right atrioventricular canal; and (3) a transverse plane opening that persists in the adult heart near the junction between the left ventricle and the aorta.

SEPTATION

As noted earlier, the critical puzzle the embryo must solve is to partition a tube with a single lumen into the four distinct chambers of the adult heart. This is accomplished by the formation of four septa: (1) the atrioventricular septum, (2) the aortopulmonary septum, (3) the interventricular septum, and (4) the atrial septum.

Atrioventricular Septum

Nomenclature associated with heart development is sometimes more difficult to deal with than is understanding the process of development itself. The atrioventricular (AV) septum, for example, has been given a wide variety of names by various authors, including the atrioventricular cushions, the endocardial cushions, or the inflow septum. Despite the various names, it is necessary to understand that the AV septum plays a key role in partitioning the heart tube (1) because of its central location between the atria and ventricles, thereby separating the common AV canal into the right and left AV canals; and (2) because the other three septa grow toward the AV septum and fuse with it.

Early in heart development, the primitive atrium is separated from the primitive ventricle by localized thickenings (or cushions) of cardiac jelly, which are composed of matrix molecules produced by the myocardium (Figure 1–6). These cushions are oriented in a dorsal–ventral plane and are called the *dorsal endocardial cushion* and the *ventral endocardial cushion*, respectively. Subsequently, the endocardial cushions are invaded by mesenchymal cells that arise from the endocardial endothelial cells. Recent findings have shed light on the mechanism whereby endocardial endothelial cells are transformed into mesenchymal cells of the endocardial cushions.[36] The question of why the endocardial cushions form in an area restricted to the central location between the primi-

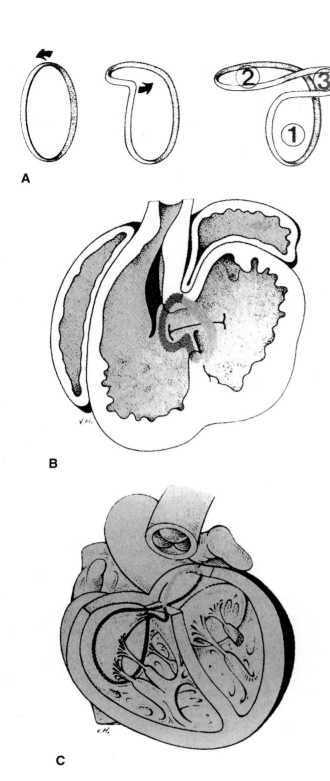

Figure 1–5. A. Changes in shape of the primary foramen (overlapping) that occur during stage 3 of dextral looping and as a result of a remodeling of the myocardium around the primary foramen, called the primary junction. This results in the division of the primary foramen into three orifices: a sagittal plane orifice, called the embryonic interventricular communication; a frontal plane orifice, called the right atrioventricular connection; and a transverse plane orifice found near the presumptive left ventricle and the conotruncus. **B** and **C.** Schematic diagrams show the position of the primary junction located around the primary foramen as identified by the expression of G1N2 (entire gray line in **B**) compared with the position it occupies in the fully developed heart (entire gray line in **C**). In both **B** and **C,** the anterior walls of the right and left ventricles have been removed to allow visualization of the interior of the heart. The light portion of the gray line represents that portion of the primary foramen and primary junction that lies within the part of the heart that has been removed. (*Reprinted with permission from Lamers WH et al. New findings concerning ventricular septation in the human heart.* Circulation: *1992; 86(4):1194–1205.*)

tive atrium and the primitive ventricle seems to be answered by the fact that only myocardial cells in this area express homeobox genes *msx-1*[37] and *mox-1*,[38] TGF-β,[39] and bone morphogenetic protein 4 (BMP-4).[40] In addition, myocardial cells in this area secrete 0.1- to 0.5-μm particles known as *adherons,* which consist of the *ES proteins 28, 46, 93, 130,* and *180kd* and *fibronectin.* Using the collagen gel assay, ES proteins have been shown to play a role in the transformation of endocardial endothelial cells into mesenchymal cells.[41] On binding of ES proteins to cell receptors, endocardial endothelial cells up-regulate

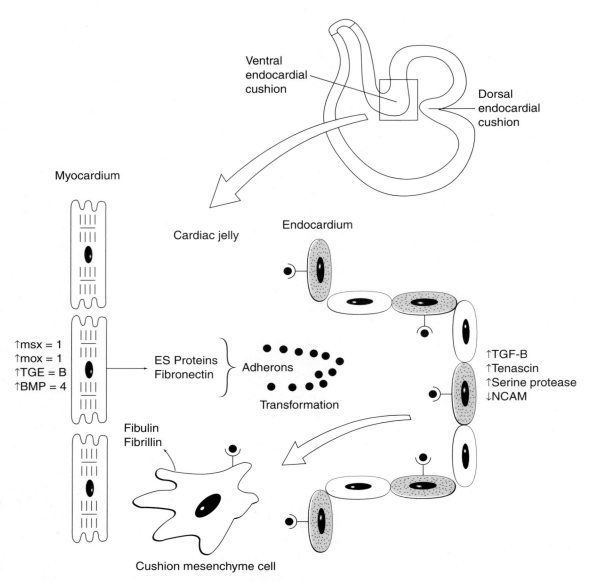

Figure 1–6. Formation of the dorsal and ventral endocardial cushions. The dorsal and ventral endocardial cushions develop as regionalized swellings of cardiac jelly and contain protein complexes of ES proteins and fibronectin. These ES proteins, which are produced by the myocardium, cause the transformation of endocardial cells to cushion mesenchyme cells, which then begin to secrete fibulin and fibrillin.

the expression of *TGF-β*, *msx-1*, tenascin, and serine proteases, but down-regulate *N-CAM*. Once the transformation from endothelial cell to mesechymal cell is complete, cushion mesenchymal cells begin to secrete the extracellular matrix proteins, *fibulin* and *fibrillin*. These complex cell biologic processes direct the fusion of the dorsal and ventral endocardial cushions to form the AV septum.

Aortopulmonary Septum

The aortopulmonary (AP) septum plays a key role in partitioning the conotruncus into the aorta and pulmonary trunk. Proliferation of cells within the walls of the conotruncus forms the *conal cushion* and the *truncal cushion*. The conal and truncal cushions grow in a *spiral* orientation and eventually fuse to form the AP septum. Recent findings have established that *neural crest cells* are responsible for the proliferation of cells within the conal and truncal cushions.[42] In this regard, ablation of premigratory cranial neural crest cells results in a variety of conotruncal anomalies.[43]

Neural crest cells can be subdivided into two major regions: cranial and trunk neural crest. The cranial neural crest region also gives rise to the *cardiac neural crest* region (Figure 1–7). Cardiac neural crest cells, which migrate into the conotruncus, extend from the otic placode to somite 3 along the lateral aspects of the neural tube. En route to the conal and truncal cushions, cardiac neural crest cells migrate into pharyngeal arches 3, 4, and 6, where they form skeletal components of craniofacial anatomy and then continue into the conal and truncal cushions. The largest population of cardiac neural crest cells within the AP septum arrives from pharyngeal arch 4.[44]

The widely held understanding of neural crest cells is that they demonstrate a high degree of plasticity by differentiating into a variety of mature cell types. However, cardiac neural crest cells appear to be a unique population. This is highlighted by experiments

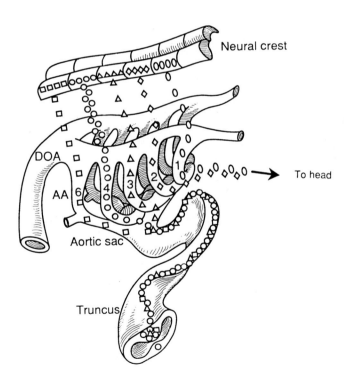

Figure 1–7. Cranial neural crest migratory pathway through the pharyngeal region. Some neural crest cells in pharyngeal arches 3, 4, and 6 continue their migration from the pharyngeal region into the conotruncus of the developing heart, where they participate in the formation of the aortopulmonary septum. AA, aortic arches; DOA, dorsal aorta. (*Reprinted with permission from Kirby ML, Waldo KL. Role of neural crest in congenital heart disease.* Circulation: *1990; 82(2):332.*)

demonstrating that persistent truncus arteriosus (i.e., no formation of the AP septum) results when cardiac neural crest is removed and replaced with cranial or trunk neural crest; this indicates that only cardiac neural crest is capable of AP septum formation.[45]

Ablation of cardiac neural crest has been shown to result in dextroposed aorta, tricuspid atresia, right fourth aortic arch hypoplasia, ventricular septal defects caused by hypoplasia of conal and truncal ridges, and tetralogy of Fallot. These findings have solidified the now well-established role of neural crest cells in heart formation. In addition, the role of neural crest cells serves to explain the connection between craniofacial and heart congenital malformations. The most obvious connection in humans is the *DiGeorge syndrome.*

It is now well appreciated that many heretofore disparate anomalies of the craniofacial and heart regions are related as neurocristopathies. There are two types of neurocristopathies, *dysgenetic (congenital)* and *neoplastic.*[46] The DiGeorge syndrome, which consists of hypoplasia of the thymus and parathyroid glands, craniofacial dysmorphisms, and conotruncal abnormalities of the heart, is a good example of a congenital neurocristopathy. The DiGeorge syndrome has been mapped to chromosome 22q11.2, where deletions and microdeletions have been identified in most cases.[47,48] Other closely related syndromes, such as conotruncal anomaly face syndrome and velocardiofacial syndrome, have also been linked to chromosome 22q11.2,[49] and many authors now term these syndromes associated with chromosome 22 as *CATCH 22* (for *c*ardiac defects, *a*bnormal facies, *t*hymic hypoplasia, *c*left palate, and *h*ypocalemia). A candidate gene (*TUPLE 1*) for the DiGeorge syndrome has been identified.[50] *TUPLE 1* encodes for a protein that contains repeating motifs similar to the WD40 domains of the transducin-like enhancer (TLE) family and other features typical of a transcription control protein.

Interventricular Septum

The interventricular (IV) septum plays a key role in separating the presumptive left and right ventricles. When the IV septum begins to form, it is important to note the configuration of the heart tube (see Figure 1–4D). At this time, the AV canal is positioned over the presumptive left ventricle so that all blood from the primitive atrium flows into the presumptive left ventricle. Consequently, it is essential that the AV canal become "*repositioned*" during the formation of the IV septum so that the right AV canal is oriented over the presumptive right ventricle and the left AV canal is oriented over the presumptive left ventricle. Clearly, dextral looping, as previously discussed, plays a role in "repositioning."

At the junction of the presumptive right and left

ventricles, a *primary IV septum* begins to form at the floor and grow toward the AV septum. It is crucial that the primary IV septum not fuse immediately with the AV septum since this would cut off the left ventricle from the conotruncus. The primary IV septum will eventually form the adult *muscular IV septum*, which demonstrates a trabeculated anterior portion and a smooth posterior portion. On the right side of the muscular IV septum, the junction of the trabeculated and smooth portions is marked by the *septomarginal trabeculae* or *moderator band*.

There has been a long-standing controversy concerning the origin of the muscular IV septum. One school of thought proposes that (1) the primary IV septum gives rise only to the anterior portion of the definitive IV septum and (2) a muscular ridge develops into the inlet septum and forms the posterior portion of the definitive IV septum.[51,52] Others have argued that the primary IV septum gives rise to the entire (both anterior and posterior portions) definitive IV septum.[48,53,54] Recently, using a neural marker called GlN2 in human embryo specimens, Lamers et al.[55] have shown that the primary IV septum gives rise to the entire definitive IV septum. Consequently, although much controversy has existed in the literature concerning the formation of the adult muscular IV septum from two distinct sources, it is now fairly well established that this may not be the case.

The opening between the presumptive left and right ventricles is finally closed off by the formation of the *membranous IV septum* and its fusion with the muscular IV septum. The formation of the membranous IV septum has classically been described as involving

(1) the right conal cushion of the AP septum, (2) the left conal cushion of the AP septum, and (3) the AV septum. It can easily be appreciated that the complex fusion of these various components involved in the formation of the membranous IV septum provides fodder for congenital malformations and, hence, a membranous IV septal defect is a very common congenital heart defect.

Atrial Septum

The primitive atrium is divided into a right atrium and left atrium by the formation of two septa, which undergo modification and subsequently fuse to form the definitive atrial septum found in the adult heart (Figure 1–8). *Septum primum (S1)* appears as an evagination of the dorsocranial wall of the primitive atrium and grows toward the AV septum. As S1 grows toward the AV septum, an opening called the *foramen primum* exists from the free edge of S1 to the AV septum, which is eventually closed. It is well established that before closure of the foramen primum, the free edge of the S1 thickens to form a structure called the *spina vestibuli*. Although the spina vestibuli develop in close vicinity to the AV septum, the spina vestibuli have a distinct origin and histology.[56] The spina vestibuli play a key role in closing the foramen primum, thus separating the sinus venosus/primitive atrium transition zone into right and left parts. Before the foramen primum is closed, perforations appear in the upper part of the S1 that eventually coalesce to form the *foramen secundum*.

Another septum, called the *septum secundum (S2)*, appears as an evagination of the ventrocranial wall of

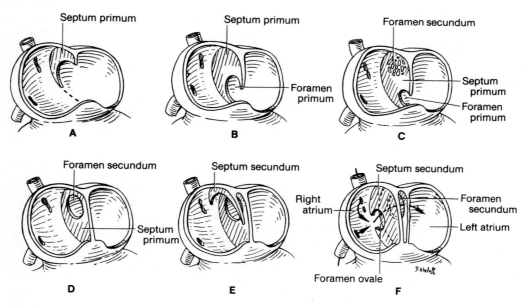

Figure 1–8. The various stages in the formation of the atrial septum. (*Reprinted with permission from Johnson KE. NMS Human Developmental Anatomy. Baltimore: Williams & Wilkins; 1988: p. 149.*)

the primitive atrium immediately to the right of the S1. The S2 grows toward and fuses with the AV septum. However, S2 forms an incomplete partition between the atria, and this opening is called the *foramen ovale*.

The arrangement of S1 and S2 in the fetus allows for an important shunting of blood in the fetal circulation pattern. Before birth, blood returning to the right atrium from the inferior vena cava is shunted to the left atrium via the foramen ovale. After birth, functional closure of the foramen ovale is facilitated by both the decrease in right atrial pressure caused by occlusion of the placental circulation and an increase in left atrial pressure caused by increased pulmonary venous return.

BICUSPID AND TRICUSPID VALVE FORMATION

The formation the bicuspid and tricuspid valves is one of the more complex areas of heart embryogenesis. The difficulty in understanding valve formation is further exacerbated by the conflicting schools of thought that exist in the literature. Questions concerning the relationship between valve formation and heart septation,[57] the contribution of endocardial cushions and the myocardium to the definitive valve,[58,59] and the embryologic origin of the valve leaflets[60–62] remain fertile territory for continued research.

One particular scenario[63,64] of valve development espoused in the literature can be explained as follows (Figure 1–9). At the junction of the primitive atrium and primitive ventricle (atrioventricular junction), mesenchyme (connective tissue) begins to invaginate into the myocardium near the endocardial cushions and forms the *atrioventricular sulcus*. Continued mesenchymal invagination eventually produces a flap that

hangs down into the ventricle and consists of (1) an outer layer of myocardium continuous with the atrium, (2) a middle layer of mesenchymal tissue, (3) an outer layer of myocardium continuous with the ventricle, and (4) an inconspicuous remnant of endocardial tissue at the apex. At the same time that mesenchymal invagination occurs, the inner aspect (closest to the lumen of the ventricle) of the ventricular myocardium is undermined (i.e., degenerates, probably via apoptosis). *Mesenchymal invagination* and *undermining* of the ventricular myocardium result in the formation of an atrioventricular valve consisting of muscular leaflets, muscular cords, and papillary muscles (i.e., a completely muscular valve, albeit for a mesenchymal core and remnant of the endocardial tissue). In the third month of fetal life, the muscular tissue of the leaflets and cords is replaced by connective tissue.

Although valve development can be explained according to the general plan as just described, there are some nuances that can be further addressed. Specifically, the *aortic (anterior) leaflet of the mitral valve* forms (because of its anatomic position) by undermining the myocardium that is associated with the muscular IV septum. This accounts for some interesting facts: (1) No papillary muscles of the mitral valve arise from the definitive IV septum; (2) normal IV septation is a prerequisite for normal formation of the mitral valve; (3) the embryonic relationship of the aortic leaflet of the mitral valve and the primary IV septum may still be recognized by the presence of trabeculations on the ventricular wall between the IV septum and the aortic leaflet (Figure 1–10); and (4) the anterolateral muscle bundle, which is found near the aortic valve leaflet, is probably a remnant of the primary IV septum (see Figure 1–10).

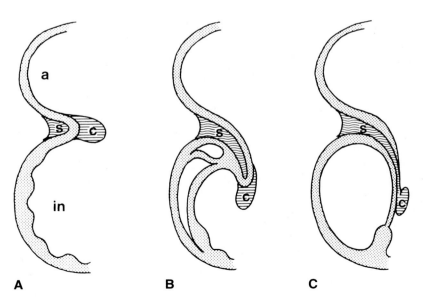

A   **B**   **C**

Figure 1–9. The process of invagination of the atrioventricular junction and the undermining of the myocardium that lead to the formation of the atrioventricular valves. **A.** Before valve formation, endocardial cushion tissue (c) has a valve-like function. **B.** Expansion of the atrium (a) and the ventricles leads to an invagination of sulcus tissue (s). At the same time, the ventricular (inlet) myocardium (in) is undermined to form the tension apparatus of the valve. **C.** After completion of these processes, valve and papillary muscles are present. Further histogenesis leads to a fibrous valve leaflet and tendinous chords. The continuity of atrial and ventricular myocardium has been disrupted by sulcus tissue. (*Reprinted with permission from Wenink ACG et al. Developmental considerations of mitral valve anomalies.* Int J Cardiol: *1986; 11(1):85.*)

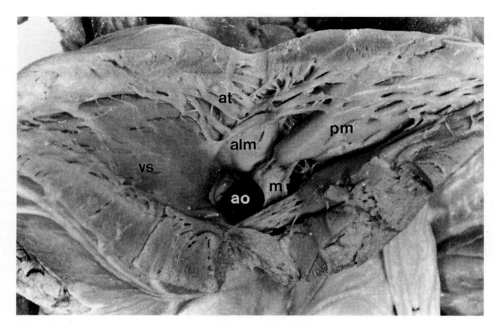

Figure 1–10. Photograph of the left ventricle of a normal heart in which trabeculations on the anterior part of the ventricular septum (vs) and on the anterior ventricular wall (at) form one continuous mass with the anterolateral papillary muscle (pm). An individual anterolateral muscle bundle (alm) may be distinguished as well. ao, arotic orifice; m, mitral valve. (*Reprinted with permission from Wenink ACG, Embryology of the heart. In Anderson RH, Macartney FJ, Shinebourne EA, Tynan M. Pediatric Cardiology. Edinburgh: Churchill Livingstone; 1987: pp 83–107.*)

Recent findings[65] concerning the development of the *tricuspid valve* strongly suggest an alternate scenario for valve formation, in which the following two differences are apparent: (1) Endocardial cushion tissue makes a major contribution and (2) the myocardial contribution comes strictly from the ventricle (no atrial contribution). The development of the tricuspid valve begins when a ridge of myocardium (called the *tricuspid gulley*) forms at the boundary between the AV canal and the primitive right ventricle (Figure 1–11). Eventually, the floor of the tricuspid gulley is undermined, which transforms the anterior rim of the tricuspid gulley into the septomarginal trabeculae of the mature heart. The anterior–lateral portion of the tricuspid gulley is marked by the anterior papillary muscle of the mature heart.

The three leaflets of the tricuspid valve each have a unique origin.

1. The *posterior leaflet* forms by an undermining of the tricuspid gulley and a contribution of endocardial cushion tissue that forms the smooth surface of the valve.
2. The *septal leaflet* forms by an undermining of the muscular IV septum and a contribution of endocardial cushion tissue that forms the smooth surface of the valve.

3. The *anterior leaflet* forms by an undermining of the supraventricular crest and a contribution of endocardial cushion tissue that forms the smooth surface of the valve. In regard to the anterior leaflet, it should be noted that the supraventricular crest forms as the lower portions of the conal cushions of the AP septum fuse at a location interposed between the tricuspid gulley and the future conus arteriosus (smooth part of the right ventricle). Later, the conal cushions of the AP septum become infiltrated by myocardial cells and contribute to the formation of the definitive supraventricular crest. Consequently, the relationship of congenital defects of the anterior leaflet of the tricuspid valve with AP septation can be explained, at least in part, by the embryologic formation.

THE CONDUCTION SYSTEM

The rhythmic beating and sequential contraction of the heart originates in the *sinoatrial node (SA node)*, which lies in the right atrium near the entry of the superior vena cava. The SA node spontaneously depolarizes at about 60 to 100 times per minute. The depolar-

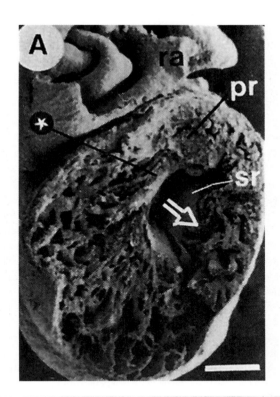

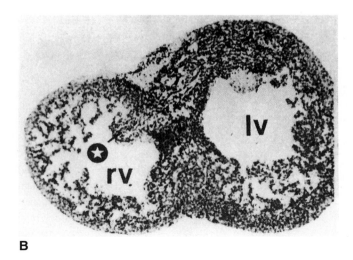

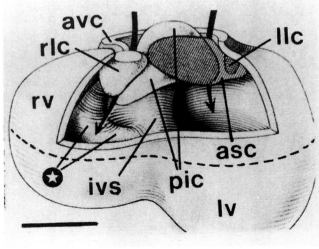

Figure 1–11. A. Scanning electron micrograph of a human heart at stage 16. The lateral wall of the right ventricle is removed to expose the tricuspid orifice. The tricuspid gulley complex (star) is still attached to the ventricular wall via trabeculations. The anterior orifice of the tricuspid valve is indicated by the arrow. Note that the parietal endocardial ridge (pr) is continuous with the tricuspid gulley. The parietal endocardial ridge (pr) and septal endocardial ridge (sr) of the outflow tract (conotruncus) eventually fuse. **B.** Photomicrograph of a human heart at stage 16 stained with toludine blue demonstrating the tricuspid gulley complex (star) with the right ventricle (rv). lv, left ventricle. **C.** A graphic reconstruction of toludine blue–stained sections through a human heart at stage 16, depicting the formation of the tricuspid valve and its close relationship to interventricular septum (ivs) and the right lateral endocardial cushion (rlc). pic, posterior inferior endocardial cushion; asc, anterior superior endocardial cushion; llc, left lateral endocardial cushion; avc, atrioventricular canal. (*Reprinted with permission from Lamers WH. Formation of the tricuspid valve in the human heart.* Circulation: *1995: 91(1):112–21.*)

ization spreads from the SA node through atrial myocardial cells and causes contraction of the atria, which fills the ventricles with blood (diastole). After a slight delay, depolarizations enter the *atrioventricular node (AV node)*. As the atria and ventricles become electrically isolated by the formation of the fibrous skeleton of the heart, the AV node provides the only pathway for depolarizations to flow from the atria to the ventricles. Depolarizations spread from the AV node along the *AV bundle* or *bundle of His*, which runs within the membranous IV septum and splits into the *right AV bundle branch* and *left AV bundle branch* at

the junction of the membranous and muscular IV septum, forming a *"central conduction system."* Finally, depolarizations spread to an *intramural network of Purkinje fibers*, which make up a *"peripheral conduction system."* The main function of the intramural network of Purkinje fibers is to distribute the depolarization rapidly throughout the ventricular myocardial cells and cause ventricular contraction (systole). Consequently, a discussion of the embryologic development of "the conduction system" should include these various components: (1) SA and AV nodal tissue, (2) AV bundle and bundle branches (cental conduction system), and (3) the intramural network of Purkinje fibers (peripheral conduction system).

SA and AV Nodal Tissue

It has been indicated earlier in this review that the primitive heart tube is specified in a cranial–caudal direction to form the conotruncus, primitive ventricle, primitive atrium, and sinus venosus, respectively. In addition, it has long been known that the intrinsic pulsation rate of the primitive heart tube is also specified in a cranial–caudal direction in that slow pulsation rates are found cranially and fast pulsation rates are found caudally.[66] The pulsation rate has been shown to be a constitutive property of individual myocardial cells since isolated myocardial cells from the primitive ventricle pulse more slowly than isolated myocardial cells from the primitive atrium after trypsin disaggregation.[67] Since the intrinsic pulsation rate depends on and is directed by stimulation from "pacemaker" regions, the question arises as to when and where "pacemaker" activity can be identified within the primitive heart tube. In this regard, De Haan[68] cultured cranial fragments, midfragments, and caudal fragments of the chick heart tube at stages 5, 7, and 9 and found that "pacemaker" activity was predominantly restricted to *caudal fragments* as early as stage 5 (Figure 1–12). Recently, the caudal areas of the primitive heart tube have also been found to be associated with the expression of a slow myosin isoform (β-myosin heavy chain), which results in slow contraction velocity,[69] and sarcoplasmic Ca^{2+}-ATPase, which results in a decrease in contraction duration.[70] The expression of both β-myosin heavy chain and Ca^{2+}-ATPase in the caudal area of the primitive heart is in keeping with an area that is going to remain dedicated to "pacemaker" activity versus developing into contractile myocardium.

Recently, the concept of the *primary myocardium* has been put forth to describe the myocardial cells comprising the primitive heart tube.[71] The cells of the primary myocardium share many characteristics, which justifies their classification into a distinct category termed the primary myocardium. The basic feature of the primary myocardium is a *slow* spread of contractile activity.[72,73] The slow conduction rate has been associated with a low density of gap junctions,[74] low expression of connexin 43,[75] and the presence of slow voltage–gated Ca^{2+} ion channels.[76] At day 24 of human development, the primitive atrium and primitive ventricle begin to develop within the primary myocardium and thereby differentiate unique molecular and electrophysiologic properties. The basic feature of the primitive atrium and primitive ventricle is a *fast* spread of contractile activity.[77] The fast spread has been associated with high density of gap junctions,[74] high expression of connexin 43,[78] and the presence of a fast voltage–gated Na^+ ion channel.[77]

As dextral looping of the primitive heart tube occurs, the sinus venosus is incorporated into the right atrium, so a major portion acquires the characteristics of the atrial myocardium, whereas a minor portion retains the characteristics of the primary myocardium that form the SA node (Figure 1–13). The atrioventricular canal is generally assumed to be incorporated into the right atrium, so a major portion acquires the characteristics of the atrial myocardium whereas a minor portion retains the characteristics of the primary myocardium that form the AV node. Consequently, both the SA and AV nodes are embyologic *remnants of the primary myocardium*. In this regard, many textbooks

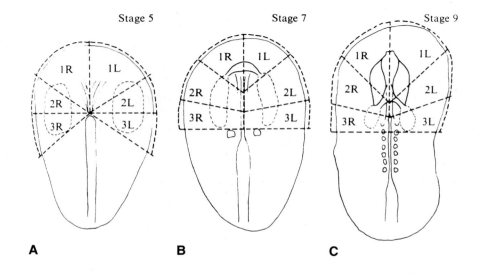

Figure 1–12. Chick embryos at stages 5, 7, and 9. The heavy broken lines represent cuts made to separate the presumptive heart regions into anterior, middle, and posterior fragments. At all stages, fragments 1R and 1L contained presumptive conoventricular mesoderm, 2R and 2L included preventricular cells, and 3R and 3L had sinus venosus and atrium tissue. The fragments included all three primary germ layers. (*Reprinted with permission from DeHaan RL. Regional organization of pre-pacemaker cells in the cardiac primordia of the early chick embryo. J Embryo Exp Morph: 1963; 11(5) 65–76.*)

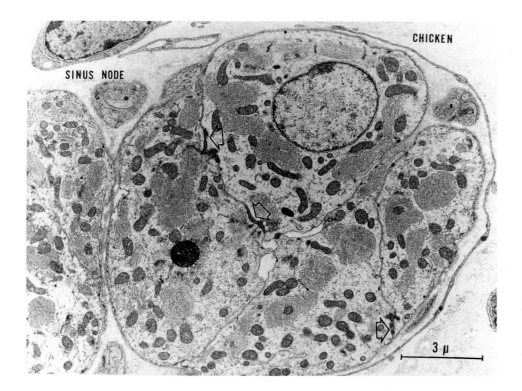

CHICKEN

SINUS NODE

3 μ

Figure 1–13. An electron micrograph of a cell cluster in the chicken sinus node. Myofibrils and several desmosomes (arrows) can be observed. This is the typical ultrastuctural appearance of cells within the primary myocardium. (*Reprinted with permission from Ying Lu et al. Cardiac conduction system in the chicken: Gross anatomy plus light and electron microscopy.* Anat Rec: *1993; 236:493.*)

erroneously describe SA and AV nodal tissue as "specialized" tissue when, in fact (from a embryologic viewpoint), nodal tissue is *not* specialized but is a remnant of the primary myocardium.

AV Bundle and Bundle Branches (Central Conduction System)

With the evolutionary appearance of two ventricles, the AV bundle and bundle branches became essential to ensure the regulated contraction of both ventricles. And herein lies the basis for considering the embryologic development of the AV bundle and bundle branches independently of the development of SA and AV nodes.

In the human heart, a ringlike cluster of cells located at the primary junction and primary foramen near the AV junction (as previously discussed; see Figure 1–5) has been mapped[79] as an initiation site for the development of the central conduction system by immunolabeling with an antibody generated against an extract of the ganglion nodosum of the chicken called G1N2 (Figure 1–14A, B). In addition, cells of the central conduction system can be identified during embryologic development by other markers (which are discussed subsequently) that are generally associated with either neural or muscle tissues. The demonstration of both neural and muscle markers within the myocardium has confounded our understanding of the origin of the central conduction system.

Ikeda et al.[80] found that Leu[7] immunoreactivity coincided with the central conduction system; however, Leu[7] immunoreactivity was also localized within neural components. Using dual immunolabeling technique for both desmin (a muscle marker) and Leu[7], Aoyama et al.[81] specifically identified cells of the central conduction system at the primary junction, the AV bundle, and the right and left bundle branches (Figure 1–14C, D).

Nagakawa et al.[82] found that HNK-1 (a marker for neural crest) immunoreactivity coincided with the developing IV septum and spread to either side of IV septum to form the right and left bundle branches (Figure 1–14E).

Lamers et al.[83] found that acetylcholinesterase immunoreactivity coincided with the developing central conduction system (Figure 1–14F). However, the specificity of acetylcholinesterase as a marker is questionable since intense immunoreactivity was also found in the ventricular myocardial cells and weak immunoreactivity was found in the SA and AV nodes.

In addition to the above-mentioned markers for central conduction system development, *homeotic selector genes* have recently been implicated. The first indication of the existence of homeotic selector genes in general came with the discovery of mutations in *Drosophila* (e.g., *D. antennapedia*) that caused wierd disturbances in the organization of the adult fly (e.g., legs sprout from the head instead of antennae). These muta-

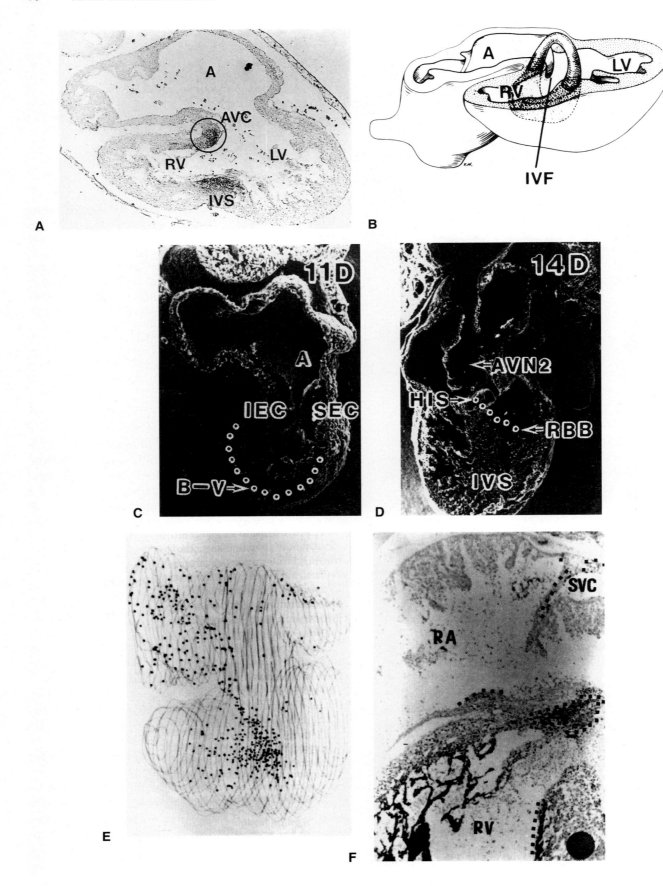

tions, which transform part of the body into structures appropriate to other positions, were termed *homeotic*. The products of homeotic selector genes are gene-regulatory proteins that contain a highly conserved 180-base pair homeobox sequence which codes for a 60-amino acid-long region that has DNA-binding ability (i.e., a DNA binding site). Two recently isolated homeobox genes, *msx-1* and *msx-2* (fomerly called *hox-7* and *hox-8*, respectively) have been identified in a variey of vertebrate species. Chan-Thomas et al.[37] using in situ hybridization, have reported that *msx-2* espression is restricted to a distinct subpopulation of myocardial cells that coincides with the central conduction system in later development (Figure 1–15A, B, C). Specifically, *msx-2* expression was found at the inner curvature of the heart tube, at the primary junction and primary opening, along the crest of the IV septum, and at the right and left bundle branches. However, it is not possible to determine whether myocardial cells expressing *msx-2* at early stages of embryologic development give rise to the entire central conduction system given that Thompson et al.[84] have found a reduced proliferative capacity using BrdU labeling within the area of the heart tube destined to form the central conduction system (Figure 1–15D). Consequently, embryologic formation of the definitive central conduction system may involve recruitment of additional cells rather than proliferation of an early population of *msx-2*-espressing cells.

Intramural Network of Purkinje Fibers (Peripheral Conduction System)

Many investigators have commented on the separate embrylogic genesis of the central conduction system and the intramural network of Purkinje fibers or peripheral conduction system. In this regard, Gourdie et al.,[85] using retroviral labeling, have reported that parental myocardial cells (already contractile when virally labeled) generate intramural Purkinje fibers as well as contractile myocytes within their daughter populations. Consequently, Purkinje cells are modified cardiac muscle cells. In addition, they reported that (1) intramural Purkinje fibers develop in close temporal and spatial association with the coronary arteries, based on the increased number of Purkinje fiber–containing clones; and (2) the central conduction system contributed no parental cells to the development of intramural Purkinje cells.

In that the central conduction system and intramural Purkinje fibers have separate embryologic origins, this raises the question of how the two systems become linked into a sequentially integrated conduction system of the adult heart. This question remains unanswered since the cellular processes that would enable scattered populations of intramural Purkinje fibers, first, to link together and, second, to establish continuity with the central conduction system remain to be characterized.

Figure 1–14. A. Immunohistochemical staining using anti-G1N2 in a human heart at days 31 to 35 of embryonic development. Immunoreactivity is demonstrated in a ringlike cluster of cells in the primary junction surrounding the primary foramen, that is, the opening between the right ventricle (RV) and left ventricle (LV). A, primitive atrium; IVS, interventricular septum. **B.** A diagrammatic reconstruction of various sections of the human heart stained with anti-G1N2 showing G1N2-positive cells in a ringlike fashion surrounding the primary foramen (IVF). G1N2, extract of the ganglion nodosum of the chicken. **C.** Scanning electron micrograph of the rat heart at day 11 (11D). Anti-Leu[7]–positive tracts and nodes are superimposed on the scanning pictures and are indicated by dotted lines and arrrows. This picture shows the bulboventricular ring (BV) located along the edge of the developing interventricular septum. A, primitive atrium. **D.** Scanning electron micrograph of the rat heart at day 14 (14D). Anti-Leu[7]–positive tracts and nodes are superimposed on the scanning pictures and are indicated by dotted lines and arrrows. This picture shows the bundle of His (HIS) extending to the posterior right border of the endocardial cushion. Anterior parts of the BV ring form the right and left bundle branches; only the right bundle branch (RBB) is shown. Note the presence of the AV node (AVN2) at the base of septum secundum. **E.** Computer reconstruction of rat heart stained with HNK-1 antibody. Prominent immunostaining formed a distinct drape across the interventricular septum, clearly associated with the forming left and right bundle branches. Immunostaining in the right atrium was more widely scattered, with a few reactive cells found across the roof of the left atrium. Note the continuity of HNK-1 immunoreactivity across the atrioventricular junction. **F.** A photomicrograph of 16.5-ed rat heart stained with AChE antibody. Prominent immunostaining is found in the trabeculated muscle of the right ventricle (RV), the right bundle branch (dotted line), and the AV node (encircled). Weak immunostaining was observed in the SA node region and the muscle of the right atrium (dotted lines). RA, right atrium; SVC, superior vena cava. (**A-B.** *Reprinted with permission from Wessels A et al. Spatial distribution of "tissue-specific" antigens in the developing human heart and skeletal muscle.* Anat Rec: *1992; 232:97.* **C-F.** *Reprinted with permission from Clark EB, Markwald RR, Takao A.* Developmental Mechanisms of Heart Disease. *Armonk, NY: Futura;1995.*)

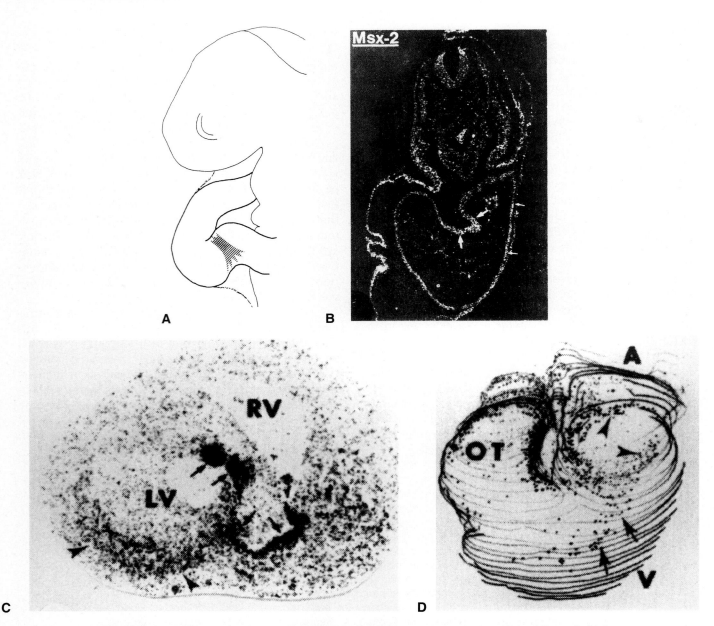

Figure 1–15. A. The approximate distribution of *msx-2* expression in the myocardium of chick heart at HH stage 15+. **B.** Dark-field image of a chick heart at stage 15 hybridized with a probe for *msx-2*. Very weak labeling for *msx-2* was consistently detected over the myocardium in the lesser curvature of the heart (between the large arrows) and along the left margin of the AV junction (between small arrows). **C.** Reverse dark-field image of a chick heart at stage 27 hybridized with a probe for *msx-2*. The expression of *msx-2* can be observed along the crest of the interventricular septum and coursing to the right AV ring (small arrows) with weaker labeling of the left AV canal myocardium (arrowheads). **D.** Chick heart at stage 21 labeled for 24 h with BrdU. Note the nonproliferating zones of the myocardium surrounding the AV canal (arrowheads) and along the earliest ventricular trabeculae (arrows), which seem to correlate with areas destined to form the central conduction system. A, atrium; OT, outflow tract; V, ventricle. (**A-B.** *Reprinted with permission from Chan-Thomas PS et al. Expression of homeobox genes msx-7 (Hox-7) and msx-2 (Hox-2) during cardiac development in the chick.* Dev Dyn: *1993; 197(3):203.* **C-D.** *Reprinted with permission from Clark EB, Markwald RR, Takao A.* Developmental Mechanisms of Heart Disease. *Armonk, NY: Futura; 1995.*)

THE CORONARY ARTERIES

For a long time, it was intuitively, but mistakenly, thought that coronary arteries developed by sprouting from the aortic semilunar sinuses and growing distally into the primitive heart tube. Current research has clearly indicated that this is not the case. Using quail-to-chicken chimeras[86,87] it has been demonstrated that coronary arteries develop as discontinuous endothelial channels, beneath the epicardium (i.e., *in situ vasculogenesis*), that grow proximally toward the conotruncus or the future aorta (Figure 1–16). These endothelial channels eventually form a ring of capillaries around the conotruncus (called the *peritruncal capillary ring*), many of which penetrate the wall of the aorta. Multiple capillaries have been shown to penetrate all three aortic semilunar sinuses (left, right, and posterior). However, the only two capillaries that survive are associated with the right and left aortic semilunar sinuses, and these become the *right and left coronary artery "stems."*

The penetration of peritruncal capillaries into the aortic wall and their selected survival seems to be a highly controlled angiogenic process. At the forefront of controlling factors is a ring of *parasympathetic ganglia and nerves* that encircle the base of the aorta prior to and at the time of penetration of the aorta by peritruncal capillaries. In this regard, it has been shown that parasympathetic ganglia and nerves are associated only with the right and left aortic semilunar sinuses (where the peritruncal capillaries persist and form the right and left coronary artery "stems") and not at the posterior aortic semilunar sinus.[88] In addition, Hood and Rosenquist[89] have suggested that the formation of the aortopulmonary septum via the spiral course of cardiac neural crest migration may influence the placement of the right and left coronary artery "stems."

In looking further into coronary artery development, we can fine tune the discussion to include the embryologic formation of the endothelial cells of the tunica intima, the smooth muscle cells of the tunica media, and the fibroblasts of the tunica adventitia. Indeed, Mikawa and Fischman[90] have demonstrated using retroviral labeling that the endothelial cell, smooth muscle cell, and fibroblast each have their own *separate progenitor cell* that migrates into the heart tube from the liver region.

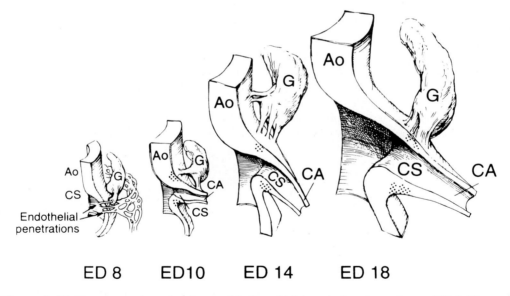

Figure 1–16. Coronary artery development in the chick heart at various stages. ED 8: The peritruncal capillaries penetrate the wall of the nascent coronary sinus (CS). A ganglion (G) embraces one of the penetrating channels. No neural crest cells are in the walls of the aorta (Ao) or the peritruncal capillaries. ED 10: The parasympathetic ganglion has extensions reaching to the wall of the coronary sinus and the coronary artery. Cardiac neural crest cells (dots) are clustered in the tunica media of the aorta at the junction of the coronary artery with the aorta. ED 14: Clusters of neural crest cells (dots) have begun to form in the wall of the coronary sinus at the mouth of the coronary artery. They extend from the tunica media inward toward the lumen. ED 18: The clusters of neural crest cells around the mouth of the coronary artery have moved distally as the coronary sinus expands distally. A rim developing around the ostium of the coronary artery seems related to some of the clusters of neural crest cells. The parasympathetic ganglion has developed well-formed, large connections with the wall of the coronary artery. (*Reprinted with permission from Waldo et al. Association of the cardiac neural crest with development of the coronary arteries in chick embryo. Anat Rec: 1994; 239:315–31.*)

The endothelial cells of the entire coronary artery system (both subepicardial and intramyocardial vessels) develop from endothelium-specific progenitor cells that originate in the *liver* region.[91] These progenitor cells enter the heart tube via the dorsal mesocardium, position themselves beneath the epicardium, later extend into the myocardium, and eventually coalesce into endothelial channels, forming the endothelium of the tunica intima. As the progenitor cells enter the heart tube, they are first observed near the sinus venosus and subsequently spread to the atrioventricular sulcus, to the conotruncus, and finally to the ventricles. The migration of progenitor cells from the liver into the heart tube is presaged by formation of the epicardium, which forms from the coelomic wall near the liver region. In this regard, many studies have clearly shown that coronary artery development is closely associated with epicardium formation.

The smooth muscle cells of the entire coronary artery system develop from smooth muscle–specific progenitor cells that also originate in the liver region. These progenitor cells enter the heart tube via the dorsal mesocardium substantially after the heart tube has begun propulsive contractions. Subsequently, the progenitor cells are attracted toward the endothelial channels by chemotactic mechanisms, differentiate into smooth muscle cells, and encircle the endothelial channels, with spiral colonies forming the tunica media. Restricted to a small area within the tunica media near the ostia and coronary artery "stems," another population of cells has been identified that arises from the migration of cardiac neural crest cells.[88] These cardiac neural crest cells are always associated with the parasympathetic ganglia and nerves also found in this area. Hence, these cardiac neural crest–derived cells may have a sensory or endocrine function (like the carotid body) similar to that described by Hodges.[92]

It is interesting to contrast the embryologic formation of the *tunica media of the coronary arteries* against the *tunica media of the aortic and pulmonary trunks* (i.e., the great vessels). As previously noted, the tunica media of the coronary arteries is derived predominantly from *mesodermal progenitor cells* that migrate into the heart tube from the liver region (with only a small cardiac neural crest component near the ostia and coronary artery "stems" forming parasympathetic ganglia and nerves). However, the tunica media of the aortic and pulmonary trunks is derived predominately from *cardiac neural crest cells*.[93–95]

Although it is clear that fibroblasts of the entire coronary artery system develop from fibroblast-specific progenitor cells that originate in the liver region and migrate into the heart via the dorsal mesocardium, little else is known about the chemotactic mechanisms employed in their organization into the tunica adventitia.

RIGHT ATRIUM AND LEFT ATRIUM FORMATION

The primitive heart begins rhythmic contractions on day 23 in humans and by day 24 blood begins to circulate throughout the embryo. Initially, all venous blood returns to the primitive heart tube via the *common cardinal veins* and enters into a bilaterally symmetrical chamber called the *sinus venosus* (Figure 1–17). Within a few weeks, the entire venous system of the embryo is remodeled such that all systemic venous blood enters the right side of the sinus venosus (*right sinus horn*) via the superior vena cava (SVC) and inferior vena cava (IVC). As the right sinus horn enlarges to keep pace with the growth of the rest of the primitive heart tube, the right sinus horn containing the orifices of the SVC, IVC, and coronary sinus gradually becomes incorporated into the posterior wall of the primitive atrium and eventually forms the *smooth portion of the right atrium* (or the *sinus venarum*) in the adult heart. The primitive atrium forms only the *rough portion of the right atrium*. Because of the remodeling of venous blood return to the right sinus horn, the left side of the sinus venosus (*left sinus horn*) takes on a more diminutive, but still important, role in forming the *coronary sinus* and *left oblique vein* and in sprouting *the pulmonary vein*.

As the definitive right atrium develops as just described, the definitive left atrium forms simultaneously through a somewhat similar process. Although there are conflicting reports as to the origin of the pulmonary vein, it seems fairly well established that the pulmonary vein originates from the left sinus horn.[96,97] At week 4, the left sinus horn sprouts a pulmonary vein that eventually branches a number of times to form four pulmonary veins. These veins grow toward the lungs to make anastomotic connections with veins that are developing in the mesoderm surrounding the lung buds. At week 5, the left sinus horn containing the orifice of the pulmonary vein becomes incorporated into the posterior wall of the primitive atrium. A portion of the sinus venosus near the orifice of the pulmonary vein thickens and evaginates to form the septum primum of the atrial septum. Continued incorporation of the pulmonary vein up to its first two branchings, along with the simultaneous formation of the atrial septum, eventually forms the *smooth portion of the left atrium*. The primitive atrium forms only the *rough portion of the left atrium*. As a result of this incorporation process of the pulmonary veins, the pulmonary venous system initially opens into the primitive atrium via one

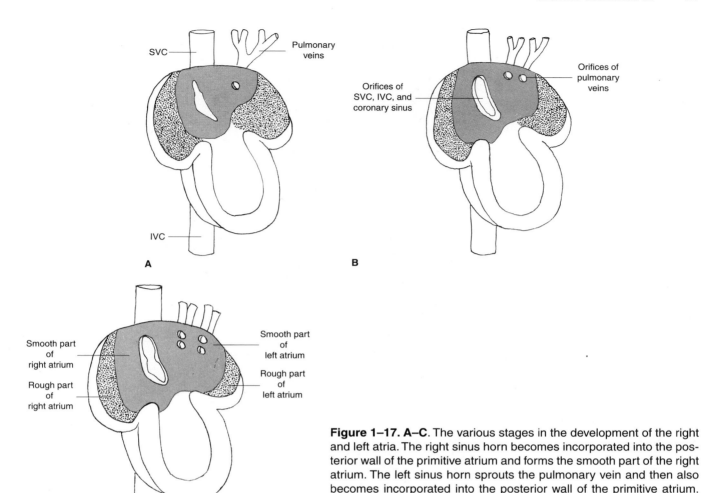

Figure 1–17. A–C. The various stages in the development of the right and left atria. The right sinus horn becomes incorporated into the posterior wall of the primitive atrium and forms the smooth part of the right atrium. The left sinus horn sprouts the pulmonary vein and then also becomes incorporated into the posterior wall of the primitive atrium. Continued incorporation of the pulmonary vein up to its first two branchings will form the smooth part of the left atrium. SVC, superior vena cava; IVC, inferior vena cava.

orifice, transiently via two orifices, and finally via four orifices of the definitive pulmonary veins.

PULMONARY AND AORTIC SEMILUNAR VALVE FORMATION

The pulmonary and aortic semilunar valves form embryologically within the truncus arteriosus *before* the truncus arteriosus is partitioned by the AP septum into the pulmonary trunk and aorta (Figure 1–18). Initially, four endocardial swellings can be observed within the truncus arteriosus, which are named according to their location, i.e., *anterior, posterior, right,* and *left.* These four endocardial swellings are the rudiments of the pulmonary and aortic semilunar valve cusps. As the AP septum divides the truncus arteriosus, it also divides the right and left endocardial swellings, thereby forming the pulmonary trunk and aorta, each with three endocardial swellings. Each endocardial swelling grows and is excavated to form a semilunar valve cusp and its related sinus.

Histologically, the endocardial cells lining the ventricular surface of the semilunar cusps are *simple squamous,* whereas the cells lining the arterial surface (facing the sinus) are *simple cuboidal.* At 23-mm CRL (crown–rump length), the valve cusps are short and thick, but by 30-mm CRL the cusps become thinner and more delicate. At 60-mm CRL, the valve cusps lose their predominantly cellular character and collagen fibers begin forming such that by 150-mm CRL (week 17) a central core of collagen (*lamina fibrosa*) exists that is delicate and thin in each crescent-shaped *lunule* and thick and compact at the central *nodule of Arantius.* At the base of the cusp, the lamina fibrosa is continuous with the fibrous skeleton of the heart. At a 100-mm CRL (week 15), elastic fibers begin to form in the subendocardial layer on the ventricular surface of the semilunar cusp and gradually extend around the cusp tip into the subendocardial layer on the arterial surface such that, at birth, the cusp is completely surrounded by elastic fibers. In the definitive semilunar valve, how-

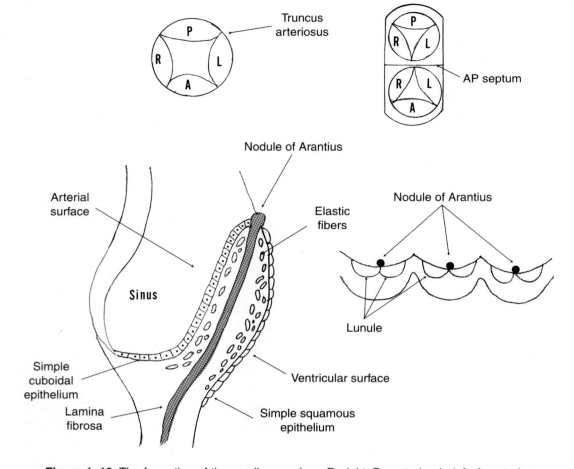

Figure 1–18. The formation of the semilunar valves. R, right; P, posterior; L, left; A, anterior.

ever, elastic fibers are more prominent on the ventricular surface of the cusp, which is exposed to intermittent tension during systole. Collagen fibers, however, are more prominent on the arterial surface of the cusp, which is exposed to the static tension of diastole.

Congenital malformations of the semilunar valves are usually associated with other congenital heart defects. For example, pulmonic stenosis is associated with tetralogy of Fallot and aortic stenosis is associated with coarctation of the aorta. Given these associations, one may ask whether malformations of the semilunar valves occur during or after normal development. After studying 306 human hearts, Moore et al.[98] concluded that malformations of semilunar valves result from congenital heart defects acquired in utero *after* the semilunar valves develop normally. Although the exact mechanism is not clear, it may be that increased or disproportionate blood flow from either the right or the left side of the heart because of various congenital heart defects is the predisposing factor in semilunar valve malformations.

ABNORMAL CARDIAC EMBRYOLOGY

As previously stated, the critical puzzle the embryo must solve is how to partition a tube with a single lumen into four distinct chambers of the adult heart. Clearly, the embryo solves this puzzle by constructing the four septa we have discussed: AV septum, AP septum, IV septum, and atrial septum. An optimal solution, whereby normal construction of the septa occurs, results in a "normal" heart. A suboptimal solution, whereby faulty (or incomplete) construction of the septa occurs, results in an "abnormal" heart or congenital heart defects. Although many congenital heart defects involve more than one septum, congential heart defects are catagorized in this chapter based on the predominant septum that is abnormally constructed.

ATRIOVENTRICULAR SEPTAL DEFECTS

Persistent Common Atrioventricular Canal

Persistent common AV canal (Figure 1–19) is characterized by a crescent-shaped defect in the lowermost

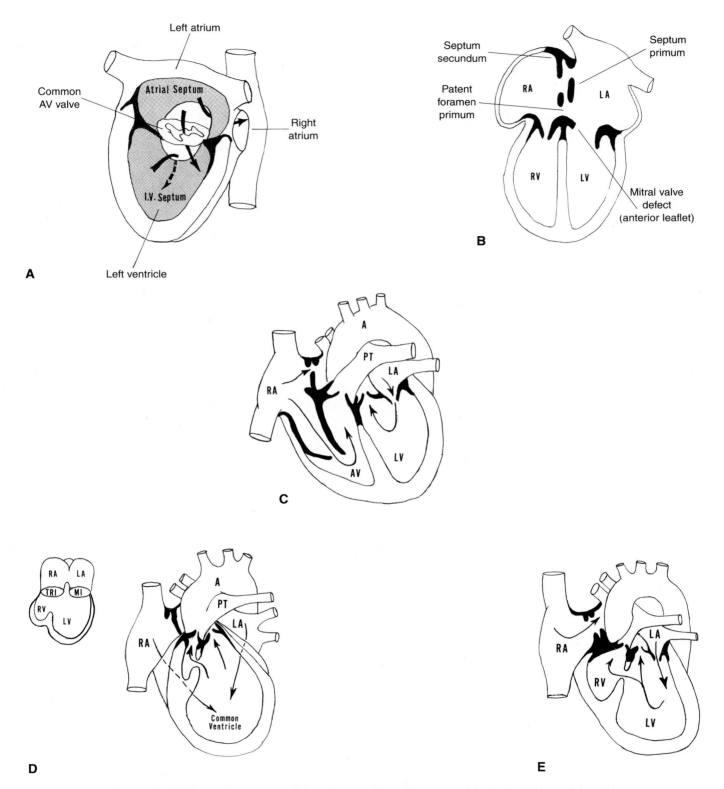

Figure 1–19. The various congenital cardiac malformations associated with defects of the atrio-ventricular (AV) septum. **A.** Persistent common AV canal. **B.** Foramen primum defect. **C.** Ebstein's anomaly. **D.** Univentricular heart. **E.** Tricuspid atresia.

portion of the atrial septum (ASD) and a defect in the upper portion of the IV septum (membranous VSD). In addition, the mitral and tricuspid valves are represented by one valve common to both sides of the heart. There are two common hemodynamic abnormalites found in persistent common AV canal: (1) a L → R shunt of blood from the left atrium to the right atrium that results in an enlarged right atrium and ventricle, and (2) "mitral" regurgitation, which results in an enlarged left atrium and ventricle.

Persistent common AV canal results embryologically when the dorsal and ventral endocardial cushions fail to fuse such that a complete AV septum is never formed. Consequently, the common AV canal is never partitioned into the right and left AV canals so that what results is a large hole in the center of the heart.

Foramen Primum Defect

Foramen primum defect (Figure 1–19B) is a defect in which the AV septum does not fuse with the septum primum such that the foramen primum is never closed. This defect is usually accompanied by a cleft in the anterior leaflet of the mitral valve, whereas the tricuspid valve is normal.

Foramen primum defect probably results embryologically from an insufficient amount of endocardial cushion tissue such that, although the AV septum forms, it is not adequately robust to fuse with septum primum. In addition, an insufficient amount of endocardial cushion tissue also explains the mitral valve defect, since most investigators agree that endocardial tissue makes a major contribution to both the mitral and the tricuspid valves.

Ebstein's Anomaly

Ebstein's anomaly (Figure 1–19C) is a congenital cardiac defect in which the posterior and septal leaflets of the tricuspid valve do not attach normally to the annulus fibrosus but are, instead, displaced inferiorly into the right ventricle. The anterior leaflet of the tricuspid valve is not displaced but is enlarged and abnormally attached. Because the posterior and septal leaflets are displaced into the right ventricle, the right ventricle is divided into a large, upper, "atrialized" portion and a small, lower, functional portion. Because of the small, functional portion of the right ventricle, there is reduced amount of blood available to the pulmonary trunk and a large amount of blood in the right atrium and "atrialized" portion of the right ventricle. An ASD allows a right-to-left shunting of this large amount of blood from the right atrium and "atrialized" portion of the right ventricle into the left atrium.

The posterior and and septal leaflets that are specifically involved in Ebstein's anomaly are formed embryologically from endocardial cushion tissue of the AV septum and the undermining of the myocardium (either the tricuspid gulley or the muscular IV septum, respectively). Although the exact embryologic cause is not known, faulty undermining of the myocardium may be a prime candidate. It is interesting to note that the embryologic formation of the anterior leaflet (which is not specifically involved in Ebstein's anomaly) seems to be more related to the AP septum than to the AV septum.

Univentricular Heart

Univentricular heart (Figure 1–19D) represents a continuum of congenital cardiac defects that are unified by certain similarities but, at the same time, divided by certain differences. This ambiguity is evidenced by the various names that have been applied to this continuum, e.g., single ventricle, common ventricle, cor biatrium triloculare, double-inlet left ventricle, or double-inlet right ventricle. Probably the clearest way to define this continuum of cardiac defects is by the presence of a single ventricular chamber that receives both the tricuspid and the mitral valve or a common atrioventricular valve if present. By this definition, both atria will be found connected to a single ventricular chamber. By far the most commonly observed univentricular heart is one in which the left ventricle is dominant and the right ventricle is extremely reduced. Although the right ventricle is extremely reduced, it still gives rise to the pulmonary trunk, which receives blood from the dominant left ventricle through a VSD.

One specific embryologic process cannot explain all of the defects within this continuum. However, faulty "repositioning" of the AV canal during stage 3 of dextral looping may result in an AV septum extremely skewed to the right, which is then attended by faulty muscular and membranous IV septum formation.

Tricuspid Atresia (Hypoplastic Right Heart)

Tricuspid atresia (Figure 1–19E) is characterized by the complete agenesis of the tricuspid valve such that there is no communication between the right atrium and the right ventricle. Tricuspid atresia is associated with (1) ASD or patent foramen ovale, (2) VSD, (3) underdeveloped (hypoplasia) right ventricle, (4) overdeveloped left ventricle, and (5) pulmonary stenosis. In response to the occlusion of the tricuspid valve, blood circulation is maintained by a right-to-left shunt through the ASD or patent foramen ovale and by a left-to-right shunt through the VSD into the pulmonary trunk, which arises from the hypoplastic right ventricle.

There are three types of tricuspid atresia that are important clinically and are classified based on the position of the great vessels. *Type 1* occurs with normally related great vessels and accounts for 70% of the cases. *Type 2* occurs with a D transposition of the great vessels (complete) and accounts for 23% of the cases. *Type 3* occurs with an L transposition of the great vessels (corrected) and accounts for 7% of the cases.

Tricuspid atresia may result embryologically from an insufficient available amount of endocardial tissue for the formation of the tricuspid valve or from a complete absence of the undermining process. In addition, faulty "repositioning" of the AV canal may play a role since the AV septum is somewhat skewed to the right.

AORTOPULMONARY SEPTAL DEFECTS

The formation of the AP septum involves the migration of cardiac neural crest cells through pharyngeal arches 3, 4, and 6, where they form skeletal components of craniofacial anatomy en route to the conal and truncal cushions of the heart (Figure 1–20). Consequently, congenital heart defects involving the AP septum may be associated with craniofacial malformations (e.g., DiGeorge syndrome). Normally, the AP septum forms in a spiral fashion as the neural crest cells migrate into the conal and truncal cushions. In addition, it must be remembered that AP septum formation is intimately associated with wedging that occurs during stage 3 of dextral looping. Wedging involves the alignment of the conoventricular canal with the appropriate ventricles. All these processes (i.e., neural crest cell migration, spiral AP septal formation, and wedging) are needed to explain adequately the congenital heart defects associated with the AP septum.

PERSISTENT TRUNCUS ARTERIOSUS

Persistent truncus arteriosus (PTA) (Figure 1–20A) results in one large vessel leaving the heart that receives blood from both the right and left ventricles, causing some mixing of arterial and venous blood. This results in early systemic cyanosis and pulmonary hypertension. The semilunar valve found with this one large ves-

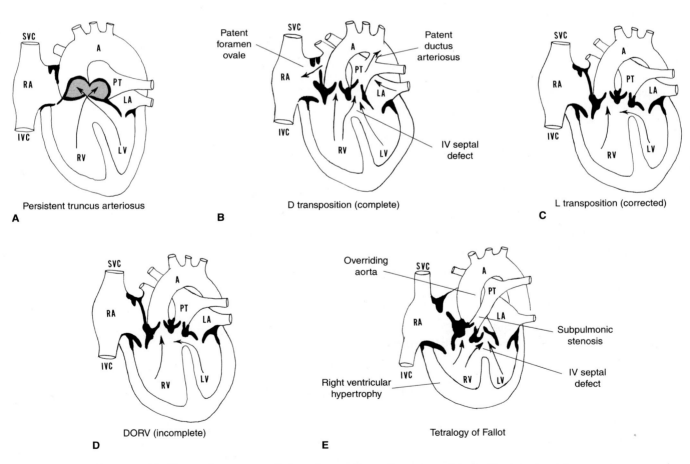

Figure 1–20. The various congenital cardiac malformations associated with defects of the aortopulmonary (AP) septum.

sel may have two, four, or sometimes five cusps. In addition, PTA is associated with membranous VSD.

PTA may arise from a developmental defect involving the abbreviated migration of neural crest cells such that the AP septum does not separate the conotruncus into the aorta and pulmonary trunk along its entire length.

Transposition of the Great Vessels

There are three types of transpositions: D transposition or complete type, L transposition or corrected type, and double-outlet right ventricle or incomplete type.

D Transposition of the Great Vessels (Complete)

D transposition of the great vessils (Figure 1–20B) is a condition wherein the aorta arises from the *right* ventricle and the pulmonary trunk arises from the *left* ventricle. Hence, the systemic and pulmonary circulations are completely separated from each other, which is incompatible with life unless an accompanying shunt exists such as VSD, patent foramen ovale, or patent ductus arteriosus. The VSD may be of varying size and lie entirely in the muscular septum or extend into the membranous septum.

The outlook for a newborn with transposition of the great vessels depends on the degree of blood mixing, magnitude of tissue hypoxia, and ability of the right ventricle to maintain systemic circulation.

Transposition of the great vessels arises from a developmental defect involving the failure of the AP septum to follow its normal spiral course. Instead, the AP septum descends on a straight course toward the endocardial cushions which may depend on the hemodynamic influences within the conotruncus.

L Transpostition of the Great Vessels (Corrected)

A corrected transposition of the great vessels (Figure 1–20C) is an interesting phenomenon in which the aorta and pulmonary trunk are transposed and the ventricles are "inverted" such that the anatomic right ventricle lies on the left side and the anatomic left ventricle lies on the right side. These major deviations in heart anatomy offset one another such that blood flow pattern is normal. Although blood flow pattern is normal, a correct transposition of the great vessels is usually associated with other heart defects such as VSDs, mitral valve insufficiency, subpulmonic stenosis, and complete heart block.

Double-Outlet Right Ventricle (DORV or Incomplete Transposition)

DORV is a continuum of congenital cardiac defects, all of which have the common feature that the aorta and

pulmonary trunk arise primarily from the anatomic right ventricle (Figure 1–20D). In a classic study by Lev.[99] DORV is defined as ". . . an anomaly in which two cusps and part of the third of both semilunar valves arise from the right ventricle." DORV is usually associated with a VSD that is usually cradled between the two limbs of the septomariginal trabeculae. The VSD provides the only outlet for the left ventricle. The aorta and pulmonary trunk can be found arranged in three basic patterns: (1) The aorta is located posterior and to the right of the pulmonary trunk, with a subsequent spiral course of the great vessels; (2) the aorta is located to the right of the pulmonary trunk, with a subsequent parallel course of the great vessels; and (3) the aorta is located anterior and to the left of the pulmonary trunk.

DORV probably results embryologically from faulty wedging during stage 3 of dextral looping whereby the conotruncal canal is abnormally skewed to the right.

Tetralogy of Fallot

Tetralogy of Fallot (Figure 1–20E) involves four cardiac defects: (1) subpulmonic stenosis, (2) overriding aorta or biventricular aortic connection, (3) VSD, and (4) right ventricular hypertrophy. The clinical consequences of tetralogy of Fallot depend primarily on the severity of the subpulmonic stenosis because it determines the direction of blood flow. The subpulmonic stenosis may result not only from the small diameter of the pulmonary trunk but also from pulmonary semilunar valve stenosis. If the subpulmonic stenosis is mild, the tetralogy may present clinically as an isolated IV septal defect with a left-to-right shunting of blood (sometimes called "pink tetralogy"). If the subpulmonic stenosis is severe, the resistance to blood flow out of the right ventricle becomes very high and ultimately causes a right-to-left shunting of blood with subsequent cyanosis.

The VSD may be within the membranous or muscular IV septum. In most cases (80%), a membranous VSD is present whereby there is fibrous continuity between the tricuspid valve and the aortic semilunar valves through the septal defect. In the remaining cases (20%), a muscular VSD is present whereby a muscular strip of tissue along the posterior–inferior rim of the defect separates the tricuspid valve from the aortic semilunar valve. This distinction has surgical importance in that the bundle of His runs along the posterior–inferior rim of the defect and is at risk of damage during surgical correction in the case of a membranous IV septal defect. In the case of a muscular IV septal defect, the muscular strip of tissue provides some protection for the bundle of His during surgery.

Tetralogy of Fallot forms embryologically as a result of the AP septum descending toward the endocardial cushions in a deviated fashion (typically described as an anterior–superior deviation) such that the pulmonary trunk obtains a small diameter while the aorta obtains a large diameter. In addition, faulty wedging during stage 3 of dextral looping results in a situation where the conotruncal canal is skewed to the right.

INTERVENTRICULAR SEPTAL DEFECTS

Interventricular septal defects (VSDs) may involve either the membranous portion or the muscular portion of the IV septum (Figure 1–21). By far the most common defect is one involving the membranous portion of the IV septum. The effect of a VSD on the blood circulation is related more to its size than to its location. A small VSD may be considered a restricted opening such that free flow of blood between the ventricles does not occur. However, a large VSD allows free flow of blood between the ventricles and hence the systolic pressure in both ventricles is equal. A large VSD is initially associated with a left-to-right shunting of blood, increased pulmonary blood flow, and increased pulmonary arterial pressure.

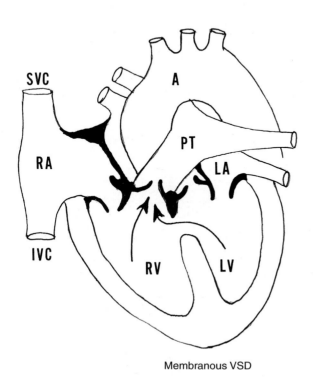

Membranous VSD

Figure 1–21. The most common congenital cardiac malformation associated with a defect of the interventricular (IV) septum: membranous VSD.

One of the secondary effects of a large VSD and its associated pulmonary hypertension is the pathologic alterations in the pulmonary vasculature. Pulmonary muscular arteries and arterioles react to pulmonary hypertension by nonspecfic proliferation of the tunica intima and hypertrophy of the tunica media, which results in narrowing of the lumen. Ultimately, pulmonary vascular resistance resulting from these pathologic changes may result in higher levels than systemic resistance and cause a right-to-left shunting of blood and cyanosis. At this stage, the characteristic of the patient has been termed the *"Eisenmenger complex."*

A VSD usually arises embryologically within the membranous IV septum because of faulty fusion of the right conal cushion, left conal cushion, and the AV septum.

ATRIAL SEPTAL DEFECTS (ASDs)

Foramen Secundum Defect

A foramen secundum defect (Figure 1–22A) is characterized by a large opening between the left and right atria that is generally located near the valve or limbus of the fossa ovalis. A left-to-right shunting of blood occurs largely because pulmonary vascular resistance is considerably lower than systemic vascular resistance and because the compliance of the right ventricle is much greater than that of the left ventricle.

A small foramen secundum defect is usually well tolerated in a newborn and may well remain asymptomatic throughout the life of the individual. A large foramen secundum defect is also well tolerated and may remain asymptomatic in the individual up to 30 years of age.

A foramen secudum defect is caused embryologically by the excessive resorption of septum secundum, septum primum, or both.

Common Atrium (Cor Triloculare Biventriculare)

The most serious of the ASDs is the common atrium defect (Figure 1–22B), which is characterized by the presence of one atrium, as the name suggests. This defect results embryologically from the complete failure of the septum primum and septum secundum to develop. Hence, there is no atrial septum.

OTHER CONGENITAL CARDIAC DEFECTS

Total Anomalous Pulmonary Connection

Total anomalous pulmonary connection (TAPC) is a condition that has several anatomic variations, all of which have the same basic defect in that the pulmonary

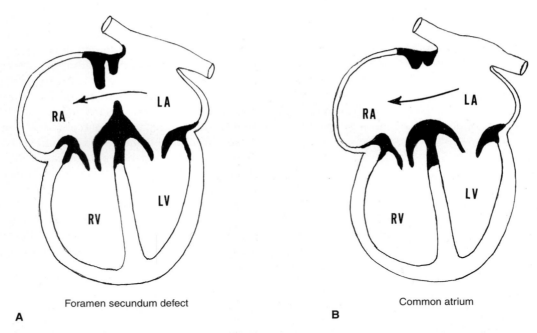

A — Foramen secundum defect

B — Common atrium

Figure 1–22. The various congenital cardiac malformations associated with defects of the atrial septum.

veins do not empty into the left atrium (Figure 1–23A). As a result, pulmonary venous drainage occurs in an anomalous manner. This anomalous pulmonary venous drainage may occur in either a *supradiaphragmatic* or an *infradiaphragmatic* location.

Anomalous pulmonary venous drainage at a supra-diaphragmatic location is usually into veins that are derived embryologically from the *cardinal system of veins* (e.g., *superior vena cava, azygous vein*) but may also drain into the *left brachiocephalic vein* and *coro-*

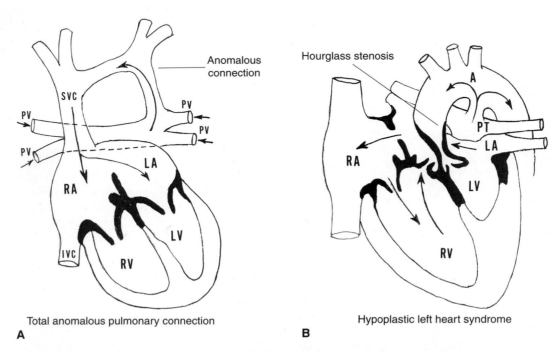

A — Total anomalous pulmonary connection

B — Hypoplastic left heart syndrome

Figure 1–23. Other congenital cardiac malformations not associated with a defect of a specific septum.

nary sinus. Anomalous pulmonary venous drainage at a infradiaphragmatic location is usually into veins that are derived embryologically from the *vitelline system of veins* (e.g., *hepatic veins, portal vein*). Whether the anomalous pulmonary venous drainage is supradiaphragmatic or infradiaphragmatic, all pulmonary venous blood and systemic venous blood will eventually drain into the right atrium, thereby making the right atrium a common mixing chamber. Since TAPC is always associated with a patent foramen ovale or other ASD, mixed blood from the right atrium passes into the left atrium and eventually into the left ventricle for delivery to the arterial systemic circulation.

To understand the etiology of TAPC, it must be recalled that the embryologic origin of the pulmonary vein occurs by sprouting from the left horn of the sinus venosus. The pulmonary vein branches a number of times as it grows toward and makes anastomotic connections with the venous plexus surrounding the lung buds. In TAPC, the pulmonary vein fails to sprout from the sinus venosus so that the venous plexus surrounding the lung buds drains into the systemic venous channels.

Hypoplastic Left Heart Syndrome

Hypoplastic left heart syndrome (HLHS) represents a continuum of congenital cardiac defects, all of which produce a distinctive common feature (i.e., an underdeveloped left ventricle) even though the pathologic lesions associated with it may be varied (Figure 1–23B). An underlying principle of HLHS seems to be the restriction of blood outflow from the left ventricle because of aortic semilunar valve stenosis or atresia.

Severe aortic semilunar valve stenosis or atresia leads to restricted left ventricular outflow with subsequent hypoplasia of the left ventricle and ascending aorta. In these cases, a patent ductus arteriosus, mitral valve stenosis or atresia, an ASD, and a common AV canal can usually be found.

Since the hypoplastic left ventricle is essentially a nonfunctional structure, all the pulmonary venous blood returns to the right atrium by way of an ASD where pulmonary and systemic blood mix. The right ventricle maintains both the pulmonary and the systemic output of the heart, which necessitates a patent ductus arteriosus for systemic circulation to occur. After birth, systemic circulation is maintained as long as the ductus arteriosus remains open. HLHS is nearly always fatal in the first week of life because of the closure of the ductus arteriosus.

Less severe forms of congenital aortic semilunar valve stenosis are usually compatible with long-term survival. The less severe forms can be classified into three categories, as follows.

Valvular Aortic Stenosis

In valvular aortic stenosis, the cusps of the semilunar valves may be either small, thickened, and nodular, or abnormal in number. A bicuspid aortic valve is most common.

Subaortic Stenosis

In subaortic stenosis, a thickened ring (*discrete type*) or collar (*tunnel type*) of dense endocardial fibrous tissue is found beneath the level of the cusps.

Supravalvular Aortic Stenosis

In supravalvular stenosis, the wall of the ascending aorta (tunica media) above the level of the cusps or distal to the coronary arteries is greatly thickened and results in constriction of the aortic lumen. This type of stenosis generally appears in either of three forms. The first form is the most common form and is called the *hourglass type.* The diameter of the ascending aorta is normal except for one area that is abnormally constricted. The second form is the *hypoplastic type,* in which the diameter of the entire ascending aorta is reduced. The third form is the *membranous type,* in which a perforated fibrous membrane encircles the aortic lumen.

Supravalvular aortic stenosis may be related to other developmental disorders [e.g., hypercalcemia of infancy (Williams' syndrome)] and some studies have suggested that mutations in the gene for elastin (elastic fibers) may be involved.

Since there are many pathologic lesions associated with HLHS, there may not be one clear embryologic cause for this defect. In fact, it may well be multifactoral. However, aortic semilunar valve stenosis or atresia plays a leading role. In this regard, it must be remembered that malformations of the semilunar valves are acquired in utero *after* the semilunar valves develop normally, probably as a result of hemodynamic factors. Therefore, the primary embryologic cause of HLHS is most likely not the direct malformation of the aortic semilunar valve.

SUMMARY

This discussion of cardiac embryology began with primary heart tube formation in which some of the more traditionally held views were gently challenged, fully acknowledging the conflicting schools of thought in this area. After primary heart tube formation, dextral looping occurs and results in many important rearrangements that are critical to normal development. Since the primary heart tube is a single-lumen structure, it must be divided by a process called septation so that the normal four-chambered heart is formed. The latest data concerning septation have been reviewed.

Another series of topics has been discussed that usually receive a somewhat cursory treatment, that is, valve formation, conduction system, and coronary arteries. After the discussion of normal cardiac embryology, the reader can readily comprehend abnormal cardiac embryology. Here, various heart malformations have been presented and organized according to the septum that is predominantly involved.

REFERENCES

1. Gallagher BC, Sakai LY, Little CD: Fibrillin delineates the primary axis of the early avian embryo. *Dev Dynamics.* 196:70–8, 1994.

2. Wunsch A, Markwald RR: Cardiac endothelial heterogeneity is demonstrated by the diverse expression of JB3 antigen, a fibrillin-like protein of the endocardial cushion tissue. *Dev Biol.* 165:585–601, 1994.

3. Yukiko S, Lough J: Anterior endoderm is a specific effector of terminal cardiac myocyte differentiation of cells from the embryonic heart forming region. *Dev Dynamics.* 200:155–62, 1994.

4. Schultheiss TM, Xydas S, Lassar AB: Induction of avian cardiac myogenesis by anterior endoderm. *Development.* 121:4203–14, 1995.

5. Bolender DL, Markwald RR: Formation and differentiation of cardiac endocardial endothelium. In Fineberg R, Auerbach R, eds. *Development of the Vascular System,* Vol. 14. New York: Karger; 1990: pp. 109–24.

6. Coffin JD, Poole TJ: Embryonic vascular development: Immuno-histochemical identification of the origin and subsequent morphogenesis of the major vessel primordia in quail embryos. *Development.* 102:735–48, 1988.

7. Noden DM: Origins and patterning of avian outflow tract endocardium. *Development.* 111:857–61, 1991.

8. Sugi Y, Markwald RR: Formation and early morphogenesis of endocardial endothelial precursor cells and the role of endoderm. *Dev Biol.* 175:66–83, 1996.

9. DeRuiter MC, Poelmann RE, Mentink RE, Vaniperen L, Gittenberger-DeGroot AC: Early formation of the vascular system in quail embryos. *Anat Rec.* 235:261–74, 1993.

10. Patten BM: The development of the heart. In Gould SE, ed. *The Pathology of the Heart.* Springfield IL: Charles C Thomas; 1953: pp. 20–88.

11. Manasek FJ: Embryonic development of the heart. 1. A light and electron microscopic study of myocardial development in the early chick embryo. *J Morphol.* 125:329–66, 1968.

12. Virágh SZ, Szabó E, Challice CE: Formation of the primitive myo- and endocardial tubes in the chicken embryo. *J Mol Cell Cardiol.* 21:123–37, 1989.

13. Bolender DL, Markwald RR: Endothelial formation and transformation in early avian heart development: Induction by proteins organized into adherons. In Feinbert RN, Sherer GK, Auerbach R, eds. *The Development of the Vascular System,* Vol. 14 of *Issues in Biomedicine.* Basel: Karger; 1991: pp. 109–24.

14. Drake CJ, Little CD: Exogenous vascular endothelial growth factor induces malformed and hyperfused vessels during embryonic neovascularization. *PNAS.* 92:7657–61, 1995.

15. Kuhn HJ, Liebherr G: The early development of the epicardium in *Tupaia belangeri. Anat Embryol.* 177:225–34, 1988.

16. Shimada Y, Ho E, Toyota N: Epicardial covering over myocardial wall in the chicken embryo as seen with the scanning electron microscope. *Scanning Electron Microsc.* 2:275–80, 1981.

17. Viragh S, Challice CE: The origin of the epicardium and the embryonic myocardial circulation in the mouse. *Anat Rec.* 201:157–68, 1981.

18. Hiruma T, Hirakow R: Epicardial formation in embryonic chick heart: Computer-aided reconstruction, scanning and transmission electron microscopic studies. *Am J Anat.* 184:129–38, 1989.

19. Brueckner M, D'Hoostelaere LA, Calabro A, D'Eustachio P: Linkage mapping of a mouse gene that controls left-right asymmetry of the heart and viscera. *PNAS.* 86:5035, 1989.

20. Yokoyama T, Copeland NG, Jenkins NA, Montgomery CA, Elder FFB, Overbeek PA: Reversal of left-right assymmetry. A situs inversus mutation. *Science.* 260:679–82, 1993.

21. Layton WM, Binder M, Kurnit DM, Hanzlik AJ, Van Keuren M, Biddle FG: Expression of the IV (reversed and/or heterotaxic) phenotype in SWV mice. *Teratology.* 47:595–602, 1993.

22. Schreiner CM, Scott WJ Jr, Supp DM, Potter SS: Correlation of forelimb malformation asymmetries with visceral organ situs in the transgenic mouse insertional mutation, *legless. Dev Biol.* 158:560–2, 1993.

23. Afzelius BA: A human syndrome caused by immotile cilia. *Science.* 193:317–9, 1976.

24. Levin M, Johnson RL, Stern CD, Kuehn M, Tabin C: A molecular pathway determining left-right assymmetry in chick embryogenesis. *Cell.* 82:803–14, 1995.

25. Manasek FJ, Burnside MB, Waterman RE: Myocardial cell shape change as a mechanism of embryonic heart looping. *Dev Biol.* 29:349–71, 1972.

26. Manasek FJ, Kulinlowski RR, Fitzpatrick L: Cytodifferentiation: A causal antecedent of looping? In Rosenquist AW, Bergsma CM, eds. *Morphogenesis and Malformation of the Cardiovascular System,* Vol. 14 of *Birth Defects.* New York: Alan R. Liss; 1978: pp. 161–78.

27. Itasaki N, Nakamura H, Yasuda M: Changes in the arrangement of actin bundles during heart looping in the chick embryo. *Anat Embryol.* 180:413–20, 1989.

28. Itasaki N, Nakamura H, Sumida H, Vasuda M: Actin bundles on the right side of the caudal part of the heart tube play a role in dextral looping in the embryonic chick heart. *Anat Embryol.* 183:29–39, 1991.

29. Baldwin HS, Buck CA: Integrins and other cell adhesion molecules in cardiac development. *Trends Cardio Med.* 1050–738, 1994.

30. Borg TK, Nakagawa M, Carver W, Terracio L: Overview: Extracellular matrix, receptors, and heart development. In Clark EB, Markwald RR, Takao A, eds. *Developmental Mechanisms of Heart Disease:* New York: Futura; 1995: Chapter 17.

31. Kirby ML, Waldo KL: Neural crest and cardiovascular patterning. *Circ Res.* 77:211–5, 1995.

32. Dor X, Corone P: Experimental creation of univentricular heart in the chick embryo. *Herz.* 4: 91–6, 1979.

33. de la Cruz M, Miller B: Double-inlet left ventricle. Two pathological specimens with comments on the embryology and on its relation to single ventricle. *Circulation.* 37:249–60, 1968.

34. Wenink A: Embryology of the heart. In Anderson R, Macartney F, Shinebourne E, Tynan M, eds. *Paedriatric Cardiology.* Edinburgh: Churchill Livingstone; 1987: pp. 57–194.

35. Gittenberger-de Groot A, Bartelings M, Poelmann R: Overview: Cardiac morphogenesis. In Clark EB, Markwald RR, Takao A, eds. *Developmental Mechanisms of Heart Disease.* New York: Futura; 1995: Chapter 15.

36. Eisenberg LM, Markwald RR: Molecular regulation of atrioventricular valvuloseptal morphogenesis. *Circ Res.* 77:1–6, 1995.

37. Chan-Thomas PS, Thompson RP, Yacoub MH, Barton PJR: Expression of homeobox genes *msx-1* (HOX-7) and *msx-2* (HOX-8) during cardiac development of the chick. *Dev Dynamics.* 197:203–16, 1993.

38. Candia AF, Hu J, Crosby J, Lalley PA, Noden D, Nadeau JH, Wright CV: MOX-1 and MOX-2 define a novel homeobox gene subfamily and are differentially expressed during early mesodermal patterning in mouse embryos. *Development.* 116:1123–36, 1992.

39. Nakajima Y, Krug EL, Markwald RR: Myocardial regulation of transforming growth factor-β expression by outflow tract endothelium in the early embryonic chick heart. *Dev Biol.* 165:615–26, 1994.

40. Jones CM, Lyons KM, Hogan BL: Involvement of bone morphogenetic protein-4 (BMP-4) and Vgr-1 in morphogenesis and neurogenesis in the mouse. *Development.* 111:531–42, 1991.

41. Mjaatvedt CH, Markwald RR: Induction of an epithelial-mesenchymal transition by an in vivo adheron-like complex. *Dev Biol.* 136:118–28, 1989.

42. Kirby ML, Waldo KL: Role of neural crest in congenital heart disease. *Circulation.* 82:332–40, 1990.

43. Kirby ML, Gale TF, Stewart DE: Neural crest cells contribute to aorticopulmonary septation. *Science.* 220:1059–61, 1983.

44. Phillips MT, Kirby ML, Forbes G: Analysis of cranial neural crest distribution in the developing heart using quail-chick chimeras. *Circ Res.* 60:27–30, 1987.

45. Kirby ML: Plasticity and predetermination of mesencephalic and trunk neural crest transplanted into the region of the cardiac neural crest. *Dev Biol.* 134:401–12, 1989.

46. Bolande RP: Neurocristopathy: Its growth and development in 20 years. *Pediatr Pathol Lab Med.* 17:1–25, 1997.

47. Driscoll DA, Budarf ML, Emanuel BS: A genetic etiology for DiGeorge syndrome: Consistent deletions and microdeletions of 22q11. *Am J Hum Genet.* 50:924–33, 1992.

48. Demczuk S, Desmaze C, Aikem M, Prieur D, Ledeist F, Sanson M, Rouleau G, Thomas G, Aurias A: Molecular cytogenetic analysis of a series of 23 DiGeorge syndrome patients by fluorescence in situ hybridization. *Ann Genet.* 37:60–5, 1994.

49. Driscoll DA, Spinner NB, Budarf ML, McDonald-McGinn DM, Zackai EH, Goldberg RB, Shpritzen RJ, Saal HM, Zonana J, Jones MC: Deletions and microdeletions of 22q11.2 in velo-cardio-facial syndrome. *Am J Hum Genet.* 44:261–8, 1992.

50. Halford S, Wadey R, Roberts C, Daw SC, Whiting JA, O'Donnell H, Dunham I, Bentley D, Lindsay E, Baldini A: Isolation of a putative transcriptional regulator from the region of 22q11 deleted in DiGeorge syndrome, Shpritzen syndrome and familial congenital heart disease. *Hum Molec Genet.* 2:2099–107, 1993.

51. Anderson R, Becker A, Wilkinson J, Gerlis L: Morphogenesis of univentricular hearts. *Br Heart J.* 38:553–72, 1976.

52. Wenink A, Gittenberger-de Groot A: Left and right trabecular patterns: Consequence of ventricular septation and valve development. *Br Heart J.* 48:462–8, 1982.

53. van Praagh R, Ongley P, Swan H: Anatomic aspects of single or common ventricle in man: Morphologic aspects and geometric aspects of 60 necropsied cases. *Am J Cardiol.* 13:367–86, 1964.

54. Goor D, Edwards J, Lillehei C: The development of the interventricular septum of the human heart: Correlative morphogenetic study. *Chest.* 58:453–67, 1970.

55. Lamers W, Wessels A, Verbeek F, Moorman A, Viragh S, Wenink A, Gittenberger-de Groot A, Anderson R: New findings concerning ventricular septation in the human heart: Implications for maldevelopment. *Circulation.* 86:1194–205, 1992.

56. Igarashi H: Scanning electron microscopic study on the formation of the atrial septum in rat embryos. *Acta Anat Nippon.* 59:28–46, 1984.

57. Wenink A, Gittenberger-de Groot A: Straddling mitral and tricuspid valves: Morphologic differences and developmental backgrounds. *Am J Cardiol.* 49:1959–71, 1982.

58. Ugarte M, de Salamanca E, Quero M: Endocardial cushion defects: an anatomical study of 54 specimens. *Br Heart J.* 38:674–82, 1976.

59. Wenink A, Gittenberger-de Groot A: The role of atrioventricular endocardial cushions in the septation of the heart. *Int J Cardiol.* 8:25–44, 1985.

60. Odgers P: The development of the atrioventricular valves in man. *J Anat.* 73:643–57, 1939.

61. van Mierop L, Alley R, Kause H, Stranahan A: The anatomy and embryology of endocardial cushion defects. *J Thorac Cardiovasc Surg.* 43:71–83, 1962.

62. Victor S, Nayak V: The tricuspid valve is bicuspid. *J Heart Valve Dis.* 3:27–36, 1994.

63. Wenink A, Gittenberger-de Groot A: Embryology of the mitral valve. *Int J Cardiol.* 11:75–84, 1986.

64. Wenink A, Gittenberger-de Groot A, Brom A: Developmental considerations of mitral valve anomalies. *Int J Cardiol.* 11:85–98, 1986.

65. Lamers W, Viragh S, Wessels A, Moorman A, Anderson R: Formation of the tricuspid valve in the human heart. *Circulation.* 91:111–21, 1995.

66. Barry A: Intrinsic pulsation rates of fragments of embryonic chick heart. *J Exp Zool.* 91:119–30, 1942.

67. Cavanaugh M: Pulsation, migration and division in dissociated chick embryo heart cells. *J Exp Zool.* 128:573–89, 1955.

68. DeHaan R: Regional organization of pre-pacemaker cells in the cardiac primordia of the early chick embryo. *J Embryol Exp Morphol.* 11:65–76, 1963.

69. Gonzalez-Sanchez A, Bader D: Characterization of a myosin heavy chain in the conductive system of the adult and developing chicken heart. *J Cell Biol.* 100:270–5, 1985.

70. Oettling G, Schmidt E, Drews U: An embryonic Ca^{++} mobilizing muscarinic system in the chick embryo heart. *J Dev Physiol.* 12:85–94, 1989.

71. Moorman A, Lamers W: Topography of cardiac gene expression in the embryo: From pattern to function. In Clark EB, Markwald RR, Takao A, eds. *Developmental Mechanisms of Heart Disease.* New York: Futura; 1995: Chapter 27.

72. Kamino K: Optical approaches to ontogeny of electrical activity and related functional organization during early heart development. *Physiol Rev.* 71:53–91, 1991.

73. de Jong M, Opthof T, Wilde A: Persisting zones of slow impulse conduction in developing chicken hearts. *Circ Res.* 71:240–50, 1992.

74. Navaratnam V, Kaufman M, Shepper J: Differentiation of the myocardial rudiment of mouse embryos: An ultrastructural study including freeze-fracture replication. *J Anat.* 146: 65–85, 1986.

75. Gourdie R, Severs N, Green C, Rothery S, Germroth P, Thompson R: The spatial distribution and relative abundance of gap junctional connexin-40 and connexin-43 correlate to functional properties of the components of the atrioventricular conduction system. *J Cell Sci.* 105: 985–91, 1993.

76. Galper J, Klein W, Catterall W: Muscarinic acetylcholine receptors in developing chick heart. *J Biol Chem.* 252: 8692–99, 1977.

77. Arguello C, Alanis J, Pantoja O, Valenzuela B: Electrophysiological and ultrastructural study of the atrioventricular canal during the development of the chick embryo. *J Mol Cell Cardiol.* 18:499–510, 1986.

78. van Kempen M, Fromaget C, Gros D: Spatial distribution of connexin-43, the major cardiac gap junction protein, in the developing and adult rat heart. *Circ Res.* 68:1638–51, 1991.

79. Wessels A, Vermeulen J, Verbeek F, Viragh S, Kalman F, Lamers W, Moorman A: Spatial distribution of "tissue-specific" antigens in the developing human heart and skeletal muscle III. An immunohistochemical analysis of the distribution of the neural tissue antigen G1N2 in the embryonic heart; implications for the development of the atrioventricular conduction system. *Anat Rec.* 232:97–111, 1992.

80. Ikeda T, Iwasaki K, Shimokawa I: Leu-7 immunoreactivity in human and rat embryonic heart, with specialized reference to the development of the conduction tissue. *Anat Embryol.* 182:553–62, 1990.

81. Aoyama N, Kikawada R, Yamashina S: Immunohistochemical study on the development of the rat heart conduction system using anti-Leu-7 antibody. *Arch Histol Cytol.* 56:303–15, 1993.

82. Nakagawa M, Thompson RP, Terracio L: Developmental anatomy of HNK-1 immunoreactivity in the embryonic rat heart: Co-distribution with early conduction tissue. *Anat Embryol.* 187:445–60, 1993.

83. Lamers W, Kortshot A, Moorman A: Acetylcholinesterase in prenatal rat heart: a marker for the early development of the cardiac conductive tissue? *Anat Rec.* 217:361–70, 1987.

84. Thompson R, Lindroth J, Wong Y: Regional differences in DNA-synthetic activity in the preseptation myocardium of the chick. In Clark E, Takao A, eds. *Developmental Cardiology: Morphogenesis and Function.* New York: Futura; 1990: pp. 219–34.

85. Gourdie R, Mima T, Thompson R, Mikawa T: Terminal diversification of the myocyte lineage generates Purkinje fibers of the cardiac conduction system. *Development.* 121:1423–31, 1995.

86. Bogers A, Gittenberger-de Groot A, Poelmann R, Peault KB, Huysmans H: Development of the origin of the coronary arteries, a matter of ingrowth or outgrowth? *Anat Embryol.* 180:437–41, 1989.

87. Waldo K, Willner W, Kirby M: Origin of the proximal coronary artery stems and a review of the ventricular vascularization in the chick embryo. *Am J Anat.* 188: 109–20, 1990.

88. Waldo K, Kumiski D, Kirby M: Association of the cardiac neural crest with development of the coronary arteries in the chick embryo. *Anat Rec.* 239:315–31, 1994.

89. Hood L, Rosenquist T: Coronary artery development in the chick: Origin and deployment of smooth muscle cells, and the effects of neural crest ablation. *Anat Rec.* 234:291–300, 1992.

90. Mikawa T, Fischman D: Retroviral analysis of cardiac morphogenesis: Discontinuous formation of coronary vessels. *PNAS.* 89: 9504–8, 1992.

91. Poelmann R, Gittenberger-de Groot A, Mentink M, Bökenkamp R, Hogers B: Development of the cardiac coronary vascular endothelium, studied with antiendothelial antibodies, in chicken-quail chimeras. *Circ Res.* 73:559–68, 1993.

92. Hodges R: *The Histology of the Fowl.* London: Academic Press; 1974.

93. Le Lievre C, Le Douarin N: Mesenchymal derivatives of the neural crest: Analysis of chimeric quail and chick embryos. *J Embryol Exp Morphol.* 34:125–54, 1975.

94. Thompson R, Fitzharris T: Morphogenesis of the truncus arteriosus of the chick embryo heart: The formation and migration of mesenchymal tissue. *Am J Anat.* 154:545–56, 1979.

95. Rosenquist T, McCoy J, Waldo K, Kirby M: Origin and propagation of elastogenesis in the developing cardiovascular system. *Anat Rec.* 221:860–71, 1988.

96. Phillips M, Waldo K, Kirby M: Neural crest ablation does not alter pulmonary vein development in the chick embryo. *Anat Rec.* 223:292–8, 1989.

97. Tasaka H, Krug E, Markwald R: Origin of the orifice of the pulmonary vein in the mouse. In Clark EB, Markwald RR, Takao A, eds. *Developmental Mechanisms of Heart Disease.* New York: Futura; 1995: Chapter 40.

98. Moore G, Hutchins G, Brito J, Kang H: Congenital malformations of the semilunar valves. *Hum Pathol.* 11:367–72, 1980.

99. Lev M: A concept of the double outlet right ventricle. *J Thorac Cardiovasc Surg.* 64:271, 1972.

CHAPTER
TWO

Fetal and Neonatal Cardiac Anatomy

Colin M. Bloor

The foundation for diagnostic and therapeutic considerations in cardiovascular medicine is knowledge of normal cardiovascular anatomy. In pediatric cardiology one also needs to know the evolving structural changes that occur during development since changes occurring during these developmental stages, if not in the usual sequence, result in abnormal development that later presents phenotypically as some form of congenital heart disease. Thus, in this chapter the developmental changes occurring in the cardiovascular system during gestation and the morphologic features of the normal heart at birth, including the normal postnatal developmental changes, are discussed.

DEVELOPMENT OF THE HEART

At all stages of its development, the heart is the sum of the structural and behavioral properties of its cells. During development of the heart its component cells simultaneously and independently participate in growth, differentiation, and morphogenesis. This section briefly describes the fundamentals of cardiac development. The developmental anatomy of the heart is described more completely in other reviews.[1–12]

Formation of the Heart

The cardiac primordia are formed from the splenic mesodermal layer of the primitive pericardial cavity where it lies closely against the developing foregut. Three factors elicit and regulate heart differentiation in the embryo.[13] These are (1) a specific heart inductor in the interior endoderm, which increases the frequency of heart differentiation, (2) a general stimulation in the epidermis, which increases the frequency but not the rate of differentiation, and (3) an inhibitory agent in the

cranial fold in neural tissues, which delays or prevents differentiation. The precardiac portion of the primitive streak is located halfway between the anterior and posterior ends in the embryo.[14] These cardiogenic cells initially migrate into the mesodermal layer laterally and then anteriorly. These cells migrate in an orderly manner from the heart, forming a portion of the primitive streak; that is, the conus portions precede the ventricular portions, which are then followed by the atrial portions. The ventral parts precede the dorsal parts. When cellular transplants are made at different stages in the development of the primitive streak, they migrate to different portions of the heart.[15] This cellular migration follows the cranial–caudal gradient of fibronectin.[16] During development there is a progressive increase in the rate of cell multiplication in the myoepicardial layer.[17] At all stages of development, the rate of cell multiplication in the endocardial layer is greater than that in the myoepicardial layer. Cell multiplication rates differ in various portions of the developing heart. For example, after the early developmental stage the bulbar region has a lower rate of cell multiplication than that observed in the atrial and ventricular portions.

The primordial heart is divided into two layers and into right and left sides. The inner layer is the endocardium, and the outer layer is called the *epimyocardium* since it gives rise to both the muscular layers of the heart wall and its epicardial covering. There is more recent evidence that the epicardium later migrates over the surface of the myocardium.[18,19] There is an asymmetry in the contributions of the right and left precardiac mesoderm to the heart of the early chick embryo.[20] At certain stages significantly more cells are contributed to the epimyocardium from the right side than from the left. This relation persists in the cephalic part of a bulbar ventricular loop at later stages of development. In the caudal part of the loop, the relation is reversed, with an increased number of cells originating from the left side. It is thought that this asymmetry in the number of cells contributed may represent the primary difference between the developmental potencies of right and left heart primordia through which laterality of the heart-loop formation is later determined. The endocardial cells are similarly distributed.

The endocardium first appears as irregular clusters and cords of mesenchymal cells strung between the splanchnic mesoderm and endoderm. Soon after their appearance, the strands acquire a lumen and are then called *endocardial tubes*. These tubes continue beyond the cardiac region to become the primitive ventral aortic route, cranially, and the veins entering the heart, caudally. With closure of the foregut at the level of the heart, the paired endocardial tubes are brought progressively closer together. They finally fuse, forming a single tube lying on the midline. In the same process, the epimyocardial layers are bent medially, completely enveloping the endocardium. At an early stage the embryonic myocardium is metabolically active and shows evidence of enzyme activity,[21] glucose uptake,[22] amino acid transport,[23] and susceptibility to anoxia.[24]

The Cardiac Jelly

The inner endothelial layer of the cardiac tube is bound to the outer epimyocardial layer by the gelantinous cardiac jelly.[25,26] This jelly is an elastic, semisolid gel, composed mainly of sulfated acid mucopolysaccharides, and it is rich in hexosamine and uronic acid.[27] In histologic section, cardiac jelly appears as a delicate mass of coagulated material devoid of cells. Later, cells apparently arrive in the endothelium, invading the cardiac jelly and organizing into a primitive, pliable connective tissue called *endocardial cushion tissue*.

The Histogenesis of Muscle

The layer of the epimyocardium adjacent to the pericardial cavity is mesothelial, and its inner part gives rise to the muscular tissue of the cardiac wall. The inner cells of this primitive myocardium undergo rapid mitosis, differentiating to form loops and strands that interlock with the endocardium and producing the trabecular character of the inner surface of the ventricular chambers.[28] When contractile activity begins, probably at the fourth week of gestation,[29] the nuclei move apart and young myofibrils become conspicuous. They are much larger than the fibrils of mature cardiac muscle, and they display definite dark bands due to local concentration of an isotropic substance. At this time, there are relatively few myofibrils, and these pursue irregular courses, frequently crossing each other. At later stages in the histogenesis of cardiac muscle, strands of myocardium become more regularly arranged as the growing muscle is pulled into spiral bands around the developing chambers of the heart. In the third month, groups of fibers run roughly parallel to each other, crossing other groups of fibers at various angles. The myofibrils become more abundant, and the muscle begins to exhibit its conventional cross-striation. The last of the characteristic histologic features of the cardiac muscle to make their appearance are the intercalated discs.

Primary Divisions of the Heart

Being unattached in its midportion, the primordial heart is free to change both shape and position. Since the heart tube grows longer more rapidly than the pericardial part of the coelom in which it is situated, it soon becomes conspicuously bent. While the cardiac tubes are elongating and bending, their primary regional divisions take shape. They are arranged in the order in which blood flows through them: the sinus venosus, the atrium, the ventricle, and the truncus arteriosus (Figure 2–1). The sinus venosus is a thin-walled chamber formed by the confluence of the great veins entering the heart. From the sinus venosus, the blood passes into the atrium. Guarding this orifice against return blood flow between these two chambers are well-developed flaps known as *valvulae venosae*. The atrial region undergoes extensive transverse enlargement so that it bulges into the pouch-like right and left chambers. From the atrium the blood passes through a constricted region known as the atrioventricular canal to the ventricle, which is formed from the most sharply bent part of the cardiac tube. From the ventricle the blood passes into the truncus arteriosus, and then into the rest of the body via the ventricular aortic roots. During this time the heart is functioning as a simple contractile tube, receiving an undivided blood stream through its sinoatrial end and pumping it out into its ventricular end.

The development of blood flow patterns in the heart of the chick embryo has been described.[30] At the beginning of circulation, separate irregular masses of blood cells are found in the heart. Later, laminar flow appears when the heart rate increases. As flow velocities increase, two blood cell streams form, separated from each other in the heart wall by open, cell-free regions. The hemodynamic force of this blood flow plays an important role in the final molding of the heart.[31] Certain malformations of the ventricular outflow tract have been attributed to aberrant blood flow through the developing conal and truncal regions.[8,34,112] Also, it has been shown experimentally that mechanical interference with blood flow in the developing chick embryo can induce a wide spectrum of congenital cardiac anomalies.[32]

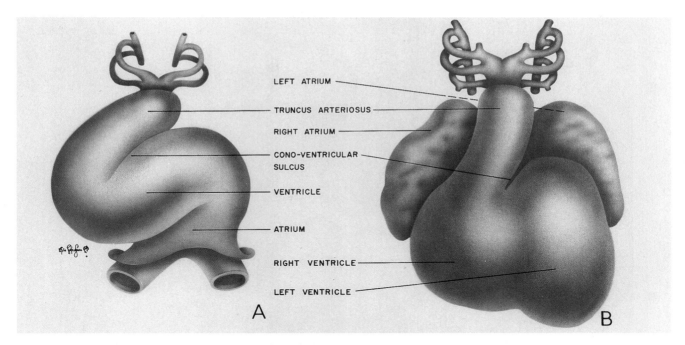

Figure 2–1. Drawing of the primary regional divisions of the embryonic heart. **A.** At first the heart tube elongates and bends on itself to form the primary regional divisions. **B.** Later the atrial and ventricular regions are readily visible. As development continues they divide into right- and left-side chambers. *(Modified, with permission, from Patten BM: The development of the heart. In Gould SE, ed. Pathology of the Heart and Blood Vessels, 3rd ed. Springfield, IL: Charles C. Thomas; 1968.)*

Conversion from the Tubular to the Chambered Heart

The basis of partitioning the heart into right and left sides is established during the second month of development. Since cell multiplication rates are similar on both right and left sides, the hypothesis of cardiac asymmetry is suggested, based upon the assumption that an increase in cellular adhesiveness accompanies differentiation of the heart-forming mesoderm, and upon evidence of an early onset of differentiation on the right side.[20]

The heart tube itself is incurvated. However, the pericardial cavity and the retrocardiac tissue are also necessary factors for normal morphogenesis.[33] Although the difference between the developmental potential of the right and left epicardial primordium causes a normal bending of the heart, the influence upon the cardiac primordium exerted by the neighboring structures and the differences between the morphogenic movements of the two sides of the body are also important factors in bending the cardiac loop to the right. Other factors involved in dextrolooping of the embryonic heart include: (1) features of asymmetry of the embryo, (2) skewness in right dislocation of the plane in which the cardiac primordia are fused, (3) mechanical influence from movements of adjacent tissues, (4) differential elongation of the pericardial cavity in

the heart tube, (5) caudal movement of the whole heart, (6) the mechanism of cell redistribution in the heart mesoderm, (7) disparate patterns of differentiation in the two heart rudiments, (8) the asymmetrical contribution of cells from the two cardiac primordia to the cranial and caudal parts of the conal ventricular loop, and (9) asymmetrical initiation of the heart beat.[34]

During cardiogenesis, the preepimyocardial mesoderm behaves as a coherent sheet. It condenses, stretches, and folds into various forms, but it does not lose its integrity as a sheet, or its continuity with the rest of the layer of splanchnic mesoderm. It does not break up into cells or cell clusters. Endocardial cells do show evidence of dispersing singlets in small groups during formation of the heart tube. Some myocardial cells may die during embryonic development. After losing their intracellular junctions, they spill into the large intercellular spaces, where they are ingested by phagocytes and may eventually be removed from the developing organ.[35]

Atrial Septum

In the separation of the common atrium into right and left chambers, two septa are directly involved (Figure 2–2). Starting as a crescentic ridge on the dorsal cranial part of the atrial wall, the septum primum grows toward

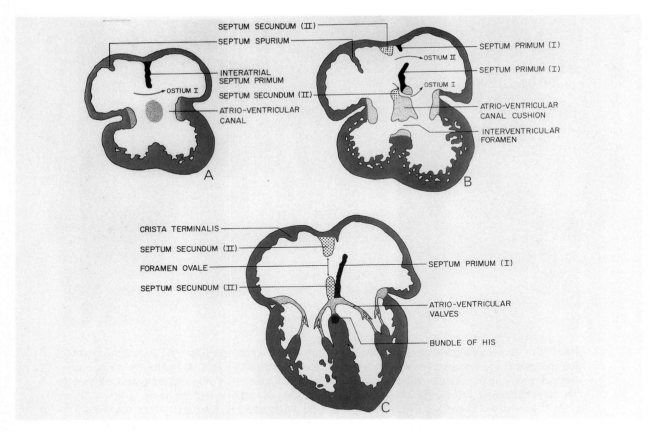

Figure 2–2. Diagram of the development of the cardiac septa. The extent of growth of various cardiac septa at several stages of development is shown. Lightly stippled zones indicate those parts developing from endocardial cushion tissue. Dark stippling indicates the atrial septum secundum. Solid black zones represent the atrial septum primum. *(Modified, with permission, from Patten BM: The development of the heart.* In *Gould SE, ed.* Pathology of the Heart and Blood Vessels, *3rd ed. Springfield, IL: Charles C. Thomas; 1968.)*

the atrioventricular canal. At the same time the septum primum appears, two thickenings, one dorsal and the other ventral, appear in the wall of the atrioventricular canal. These thickenings are the endocardial cushions of the atrioventricular canal, which divide into left and right channels. Each cushion comprises embryonic connective tissue characteristic of tissue that appears at points where septa will fuse, or where elaborate connective tissue structures (such as the cardiac valves) will be molded in the developing heart. During the sixth week of development, these cushions are brought into contact with each other by their own growth, and they fuse to form a common mass dividing the atrioventricular canal.[36] This process leaves an opening between the margin of the septum primum and the growing atrioventricular canal cushion, known as the *ostium primum*. During these developments, the sinus venosus shifts out of the midline so that it opens into the right atrium. When the septum primum is about to fuse with

the endocardial cushion of the atrioventricular canal, closing the interatrial foramen primum, a new opening is established.[37] The cranial part of the septum primum is reabsorbed to form the interatrial foramen secundum. Thus, some of the blood flow into the right atrium still passes into the left atrium. While the ostium secundum is forming in the septum primum, the septum secundum appears. It is crescent-shaped, with its open part directed caudally and dorsally toward the anterior part of the sinus inlet. As its development progresses, the interatrial septum primum and septum secundum consolidate to form that part of the definitive interatrial septum that fuses with the partition dividing the atrioventricular canal. The extension of the septum secundum gradually ceases, leaving a characteristic oval aperture, the foramen ovale. The margin of the septum secundum thus comprises a limbus or annulus fossae ovalis. The ostium secundum is formed so near the cranial wall of the atrium that the unreabsorbed lower part of the septum primum covers the left atrial side of the foramen ovale as a loose flap in the septum secundum.

Ventricular Septum

There are indications that a developing interventricular septum appears at the apex of the ventricular bed when the first interatrial septum appears (Figure 2–2). This leaves the interventricular foramen between the crescentic margin and the bottom of the partition in the atrioventricular canal. In its earliest stages, this appears to be little more than ridged trabeculae carneae.[38] As development progresses, the trabeculae tend to become more compact, and they rearrange to form a relatively solid myocardial mass. The interventricular septum grows towards the atrioventricular canal cushions, reducing the size of the interventricular foramen. The final closure of the interventricular foramen is made by a composite mass of connective tissue. This tissue is de-

rived from the connective tissue margin of the interventricular septum itself, from the base of the endocardial cushions forming the partition in the atrioventricular canal, and from the conal ridges.[39]

Truncus and Valves

Partitioning of the truncus arteriosus starts between the fourth and sixth aortic arches and proceeds through the truncus toward the ventricles. Two ridges composed of young connective tissue, similar to that of the endocardial cushions, grow into the lumen of the truncus and meet to completely partition the truncus into two channels (Figure 2–3). These are the aortic channel, leading into the fourth aortic arch, and the pulmonary channel, leading into the sixth aortic arch.[40–44] Since these truncal ridges pursue a spiral course, the ascending aorta and the main pulmonary trunk twist around each other as they emerge from the ventricles. This twisting brings

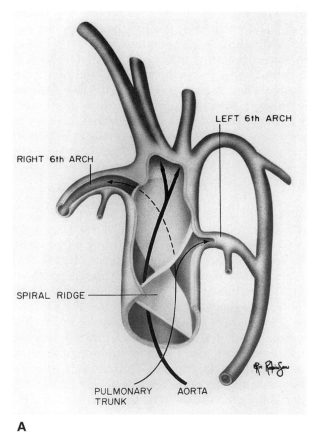

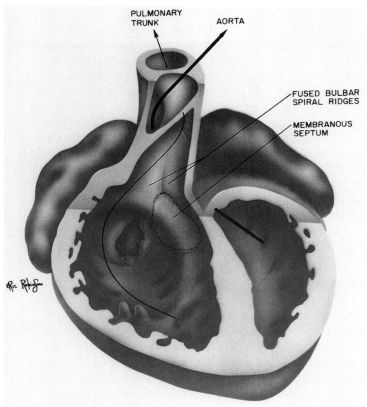

A   **B**

Figure 2–3. Drawings of the partitioning of the truncus arteriosus. **A.** The spiral ridges divide the truncus arteriosus into aortic and pulmonary channels. The latter leads into the sixth aortic arch. The thick line indicates the direction of blood flow through the aortic channel, and the thin line shows directional flow into the pulmonary channels. **B.** The spiral ridges continue into the ventricular outlet and reduce the size of the interventricular foramen. The mass of connective tissue that closes the foramen is the membranous septum.

the aortic channel and the pulmonary channel into apposition with the outflow tracts of the right and left ventricles, respectively. The aortic and pulmonary valves develop at the conus and at the line of demarcation between the truncus arteriosus and the tapering ventricular outlet. Three small pads of endocardial cushion tissue bulge into the lumen from the truncal ridges. The two additional pads of either vessel, which lie adjacent to the point of fusion with the truncal ridges, develop as local enlargements of the ridged tissue. The primordia of the dorsal valve of the aorta and of the ventral valves of the pulmonary trunk are formed by independent local growth centers in the tunica intima opposite the points of fusion of the ridges.[41] Gradually, these masses of endocardial connective tissue become molded into one of the cusps of the semilunar valve of either the aorta or the pulmonary trunk. At later stages of development, the aorta and the pulmonary trunk continue to rotate about each other, with the respective valve cusps rotating with them.

Closing of the Ventricular Foramen

Conal ridges resembling those in the truncus continue on the ventricular side of the aorta and pulmonary valves into the funnel-shaped ventricular outlet. They are a direct continuation of the spiral course of the truncal ridges and are aligned with the crest of the interventricular septum, reducing the size of the interventricular foramen cranially (Figure 2–3). Tubercles on the right margin of the endocardial cushion of the atrioventricular canal enlarge, completing the closure of the interventricular foramen. Although this composite mass of connective tissue is at first bulky and loosely organized, it becomes a thin fibrous sheet as the septal cusps of the tricuspid and mitral valves are formed, and it is known as the membranous part of the interventricular septum.

Atrioventricular Valves and Papillary Muscles

At the point where the right and left atrioventricular canals open into the ventricles, masses of tissue arise from the outer walls of each and project toward the ventricles (Figure 2–2). These masses are a permanent type of connective tissue that resembles that of the endocardial cushion and later differentiates into the flaps of the adult tricuspid and mitral valves. In the early stage, the undivided atrioventricular orifice is encircled by tissue composed almost entirely of developing cardiac muscle. This muscle has a very thin outer epicardial layer and an endothelial layer that has a scanty backing of connective tissue without fiber formation. When the endocardial cushion masses fuse to divide the atrioventricular canal into right and left channels, they serve as foundations for the medial portion of each atrioventricular ring. Simultaneously, the epicardial connective tissue cuts into the myocardium at the atrioventricular groove, and by the eighth week it has met the endocardial tissue, so that ventricular and atrial myocardia are separated by connective tissue. Only slender fascicles of young cardiac myofibers remain, extending from the right atrial floor into the dorsal end and along the crest of the muscular part of the interventricular septum. At this point, the myofibers bifurcate and send fibers into each ventricular wall. This group of myocardial fibers later differentiates into the atrioventricular conduction bundle (bundle of His) and its left and right branches. The connective tissue that separates atrial from ventricular muscle is the primordium of the cardiac skeleton. The connective tissue around each of the atrioventricular orifices differentiates into collagenous fibrous bundles to form the tricuspid and mitral annuli. Similar young connective tissue is molded into flange-like projections that are the primordia of the atrioventricular valve leaflets. As the valve primordia become extended, the trabeculated myocardium is carried out on the ventricular surfaces. Thus, the developing valve comprises loosely organized, young connective tissue, which is continuous with the muscular trabeculae of the heart wall on its ventricular face. In the final molding process, the muscle of the ventricular face retracts and regresses so that the valve flaps become solely connective tissue. As the muscle pulls away from the part of the trabeculae directly adhering to the valves, slender fibrous strands remain, which are forerunners of the chordae tendineae. The basal portions of these same trabeculae become thickened to constitute papillary muscles.

Changes in the Sinus Venosus Region

In early stages of cardiac development, the great veins converge in the sinus venosus, returning blood to the caudal end of the primitive tubular heart (Figure 2–4). In the next phase of development, the opening of the sinus into the atrium shifts from the midline to the right side of the developing interatrial septum. The sinus becomes a lopsided U, bulging out on the dorsal wall of the atrium. With the formation of the left brachiocephalic vein, more blood is shunted through the right side so that the right common cardinal vein enlarges and becomes the superior vena cava. Simultaneously, the left common cardinal vein becomes smaller. The narrow vein crosses the dorsal wall of the left atrium. If it persists in adult life, it is known as the oblique vein of the left atrium (vein of Marshall). The most proximal part of the left common cardinal vein, lying across the dorsal wall of the heart in the atrioventricular groove, acquires new tributaries for the heart itself and becomes the coronary sinus.

While the right common cardinal vein enlarges to

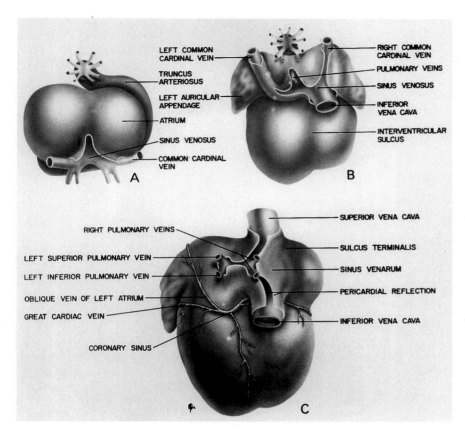

Figure 2–4. Drawings of the heart's development in the region of the sinus venosus. **A.** The sinus venosus returns blood to the caudal end of the tubular heart in a 3- to 4-week-old embryo. **B.** The opening of the sinus venosus shifts from the midline to the right side of the developing interatrial septum in a 5-week-old embryo. **C.** In an 11-week-old embryo the sinus venosus region resembles the stage present at birth. An oblique vein of the left atrium (vein of Marshall) crosses the dorsal wall of the left atrium. *(Modified, with permission, from Patten BM: The development of the heart.* In *Gould SE, ed.* Pathology of the Heart and Blood Vessels, *3rd ed. Springfield, IL: Charles C. Thomas; 1968.)*

form the superior vena cava, the inferior vena cava grows even more strikingly, as systemic, portal, and placental venous returns are redirected to the liver to converge in it. The increase in blood volume returning through the two vena cavae markedly enlarges the original right horn of the sinus venosus to form the sinus venarum. As this horn in the right atrium grows, the external boundaries between them become less distinct. The boundary of the sinus venarum merges medially with the external depression opposite the interatrial septum. On the right side a shallow groove, the sulcus terminalis, marks its boundary. The opening of the sinus venosus into the right atrium is flanked internally by a pair of well-developed valves, the valvae venosae. At the cranial end of the sinus orifice, these valves merge into a flange-like structure that projects into the right atrium from its dorsal cranial wall. This structure, the septum spurium, is eventually reabsorbed, but when this process is completed, vestiges of the right valvae venosae and the septum spurium (Chiari's network) may be found attached along the crista terminalis to the margin of the eustachian and thebesian valves. As the valvae venosae and the septum spurium are reabsorbed and the sinus is partially incorporated into the expanding right atrium, the superior and inferior vena cavae independently open into the right atrium, as does

the coronary sinus. The remains of the right venous valve become the eustachian valve of the inferior vena cava and the thebesian valve of the coronary sinus. Small perforations are frequently present in both of these valves, indicating the resorptive process that they have undergone.

Pericardial Relationship

The pericardial vesicle, which differentiates early, has the potential for developing pericardial as well as myocardial tissue.[45] The tubular form and the S-shaped structure of the heart differentiates only in the presence of the pericardial vesicle, implying that the differentiation of these structures is supported by the pericardial vesicle before their differentiating potency is formally established. The pericardial sac contains the heart and the roots of the great vessels, and it consists of a fibrous and a serous portion (Figure 2–5).[46] The fibrous pericardium attaches to the central tendon of the diaphragm and fuses with the outer coat of the aorta, the pulmonary arteries and veins, and the superior vena cava. The serous pericardium lines the fibrous pericardium as a parietal layer and is reflected onto the heart and great vessels as a visceral layer for the epicardium. A common sheath of the visceral layer in the adult encloses the aorta and pulmonary trunk. Behind

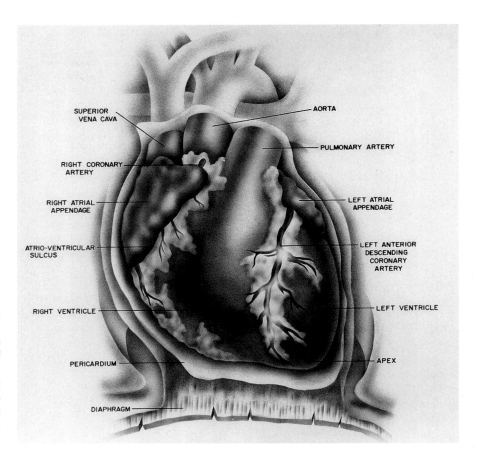

Figure 2–5. Drawing of the relationship of the pericardial sac to adjacent structures. The pericardial sac is opened to show its reflections around the roots of the great vessels. *(Modified, with permission, from Silverman ME, Schlant RC: Anatomy of the cardiovascular system. In Hurst JW, Logue RB, Schlant RC, Wenger NK, eds. The Heart, 3rd ed. New York: McGraw-Hill; 1974.)*

the aorta and pulmonary trunk, and in front of the left atrium and superior vena cava, lies the transverse sinus of the pericardium. The superior and inferior venae cavae and the pulmonary veins are enclosed in a second sheath, which attaches to the parietal layer. The space bounded by irregular attachments is the oblique sinus of the pericardium. When the pericardium is opened on the ventral side, the oblique sinus can be reached from below, where it is open. The fibrous pericardium is attached to the sternum by the sternopericardial ligament. The anterior surface is separated from the sternum by the lungs, except for an area at the sternal ends of the fourth and fifth costal cartilages on the left side of the lower part of the sternum.

Seen microscopically, the pericardium comprises dense fibrous tissue, plus a layer of loose alveolar tissue containing adipose tissue, and a single layer of mesothelium. Initially, the epicardium is a simple epithelium incompletely covering the myocardial surface. As development proceeds, the epicardium covers the heart, and a substantial layer of connective tissue is formed between the epicardial epithelium and the outer myocardial surface.[110] Mesenchymal cells appear within this layer of connective tissue. Collagen bundles are also in the extracellular matrix. Embryonic epicar-

dial cells, in contrast to myocardial cells, do not contain glycogen or myofibrils. When epicardium first appears, the myocardial cells possess myofibrils. The epicardium is not a derivative of the myocardial wall, and therefore the term *epimyocardium* is misleading.

Vessels of the Heart

The development of the coronary arteries has been described in the rat embryo.[12,47] In the rat they appear on the seventeenth fetal day as buds on the aortic wall, joining the intertrabecular and sinusoidal systems of the ventricular myocardium. At the same time, the honeycomb lining of the ventricular cavity disappears, and its trabecular structure forms. By the twentieth day, stems of both coronary arteries, with branches down to the fourth order, are present. In human embryos, the coronary arteries arise from the aorta as buds from the sinus of Valsalva during the seventh week. They enlarge rapidly and pursue their conventional course across the epicardial surface of the heart. Smaller branches of the coronary arteries enter the myocardium and ramify into a rich capillary bed infusing the developing muscle fibers. Most of the blood entering this plexus returns by the way of the coronary veins, but some small vessels connect with endothelium-lined spaces among the trabeculae, which in turn may communicate directly with the atrial or ventricular chambers.

Nerves of the Heart

Our knowledge of the embryologic development of the two categories of nerves supplying the heart is still inadequate, but some basic data are available.[48–50] At the cardiac level, delicate nerve branches follow the developing aortic and pulmonary trunks toward the main mass of the heart. Many migrating neuroblasts are also present in these branches along with the growing nerve fibers. By the seventh week, the main vagal branches of the developing cardiac plexus are clear and recognizable. Before the end of the second month, it is possible to recognize quite clearly both the sympathetic and parasympathetic components of the cardiac plexus in the developing embryo.

Contractile Activity

Electron-microscopic findings contradict the older concept of a cardiac syncytium by showing that discrete cells are present.[51] These discrete cells are in "electrical communication" by "tight" junctions. Not all the cells are capable of spontaneous electrical activity. The early embryonic heart exhibits a coordinated spontaneity, conductivity, and contractility before the definitive appearance of specialized conducting tissues.[52] Underlying the basic function of the conduction system is the extent of coupling between contiguous cells. This is demonstrated in neighboring cells in tissue cultures, which exhibit various degrees of communication related to the proximity and extent of intercellular communications. The potency to develop a heartbeat is established in the heart rudiment of the late gastrula stage.[53] In experiments, heartbeats have appeared before nerves in the embryonic heart,[2] and the heart rate was susceptible to various stimuli, such as temperature[54] and drugs.[55] The development of the electrocardiogram in the embryonic heart also has been described.[56] It is related to the appearance of blood circulation in the embryo and also to the ability of the heart to exhibit atrioventricular block under the influence of digitalis.

Contractile activity develops in the cardiac regions in the same sequence in which those regions are formed. Thus, the initial contractions appear in the conoventricular myocardium before the paired primordia are completely fused in the atrium. The initial rate of contraction in the primitive ventricle is slow. When fusion of the cardiac primordia has extended caudally to form the atrium, this part of the cardiac tube begins to pulsate at a faster rate. The atrium dominates in the control of the contractile rate.[56,57]

It was pointed out when discussing the formation of the fibrous annuli of the atrioventricular valves that a connecting fascicle of muscle fibers persists in the dorsomedial floor of the right atrium, penetrating the fibrous base of the heart and extending along the crest of the muscular interventricular septum. This is the atrioventricular bundle (bundle of His). It retains its capacity for rapidly transmitting contractile impulses. Traced into the ventricular myocardium, this bundle bifurcates into right and left bundle branches that proceed along the septal walls of the two ventricles. These in turn ramify into numerous small strands of atypical cardiac muscle (Purkinje fibers), which lie closely beneath the ventricular endocardium. As these strands develop their characteristic histologic features, the conduction system appears.

The sinoatrial node represents myocardium that is originally associated with the sinus horn. It is the most caudad part of the myocardial primordium. It is also the most rapidly pulsating, and it retains dominance over the contraction rate of the heart as a whole. There is a four-ring theory of development of the cardiac conduction system.[58] Accordingly, specific septations with later invaginations from these rings lead to stepwise formation of the conduction system components.

Before innervation appears, the embryonic heart has cholinergic receptors,[59] and acetylcholine can cause an increase or decrease in heart rate. Sensitivity to contractility increases after innervation appears. Thus, acetylcholine plays a role in regulation of the embryonic cardiac automatism.

ANATOMY OF THE HEART

This section describes the normal gross and microscopic features of the heart and great vessels, including normal postnatal developmental changes. There are other more detailed reviews of the anatomy of the heart.[60,61] With the heart in its normal position, the apex is directed to the left, anteriorly and inferiorly. The atria are located superiorly, posteriorly, and to the right of their respective ventricles. The major surface of the sternocostal aspect of the heart is the right ventricle, and a lesser portion comprises part of the right atrium and right auricular appendage (auricula). A small portion of the left ventricle is also visible (Figure 2–5). A well-marked triangular facet, formed by contact with the diaphragm, disturbs the conical regularity of the ventricular portion of the heart. This area is the diaphragmatic surface, and mainly comprises the left ventricle. Its ventral margin, marked by an abruptly curved edge running to the right from the apex to the atrium, is the acute margin of the heart, and it marks the transition between the diaphragmatic surface and the sternocostal surface. The left surface of the ventricular portion of the heart is called the *obtuse margin*. It forms around the side of the left ventricle and extends from the ventricular apex to the root of the pulmonary trunk. The obtuse margin passes gradually over into the sternocostal surface of the heart. The external demarcation between the atria and the ventricles is the coronary groove or atrioventricular groove. It is well marked along the lateral ventral aspects of the heart, and it contains coronary arteries and veins embedded in a considerable amount of fat. The superior vena cava and right atrium form, when looked at on an anterior–posterior frontal chest x-ray, the right lateral border of the cardiac shadow, whereas the great vessels and left ventricle form the left cardiac border.

External Aspects

The heart lies in the pericardial sac, which normally contains 20 to 50 mL of clear yellow fluid.[62–64] The adult heart, a roughly conical, hollow, muscular organ with a fibrous framework (the cardiac skeleton), has walls comprising three layers: endocardium, myocardium, and epicardium (visceral pericardium). The base of the heart comprises that part in which the great vessels enter or leave and that portion of the heart wall lying between them. The great vessels and the visceral pericardium (epicardium) hold the heart in position within the pericardial cavity, the latter being reflected at the roots of the great vessels to become continuous with the parietal pericardium. The plane of the base is marked by a groove on the epicardial surface, the atrioventricular groove. Two other grooves, the interatrial groove and the interventricular groove, show the positions of the atrial and ventricular septa, respectively. At the base of the heart on the posterior surface these three sulci become confluent to form the "crux cordis." In situ, the apex of the heart points ventrally and caudally to the left, and the base is directed dorsally and to the right. The left ventricle forms the apex, and the left atrium dominates the base.

The interventricular groove, a shallow groove on the surface of the heart, indicates the location of the internal septum separating the two ventricles. In it lie coronary blood vessels, nerves, and various amounts of fat. On the sternocostal surface this groove is the anterior interventricular groove that originates at the left of the root of the pulmonary trunk, runs obliquely over the cranial aspect of the obtuse margin, and courses nearly vertically down the sternocostal surface. As it crosses the acute margin, it forms a slight notch and continues as a posterior interventricular groove on the diaphragmatic surface.

On the ventral surface of the heart, the right and left auricular appendages of the atria protrude to delineate the deep notch in which the ascending aorta and the pulmonary trunk lie. On the dorsal aspect of the right atrium, a slight groove connects the right side of the superior and inferior venae cavae, which is called the sulcus terminalis and represents the lateral boundary of the right horn of the embryonic sinus venosus.

At the level between the second and third costal cartilages, on the left, the pulmonary conus of the right ventricle gives rise to the pulmonary trunk. This vessel curves abruptly, and soon thereafter it bifurcates into right and left pulmonary arteries. The left ventricle gives rise to the ascending aorta, slightly to the left of the midline at the level of the attachment of the third costal cartilage. The aortic orifice lies dorsally, caudally, and slightly to the right of the pulmonary trunk. The aorta has three sections: (1) the ascending aorta, (2) the aortic arch, and (3) the descending aorta. The large arteries supplying the blood to the upper part of the body arise from the aortic arch. A ligament connects the left pulmonary artery to the aortic arch (ligamentum arteriosum), and it represents the fibrous remains of the ductus arteriosus of the fetus.

Internal Aspects

The heart is divided into four chambers: two thin-walled atria, separated by an interatrial septum, and two thick-walled ventricles, separated by an interventricular septum.[65] Different dimensions characterize the size and shape of the ventricles and their valvular orifices, and the relation of these dimensions to age, body, weight, and body length has been described.[66] The atria and ventricles communicate by means of their respective atrioventricular orifices. Blood enters the right atrium from the superior and inferior venae cavae and the coronary sinus. It then passes to the right ventricle, through the right atrioventricular orifice (the tricuspid valve), and is ejected into the pulmonary circulation via the pulmonary orifice (pulmonary valve). Blood returning to the heart from the pulmonary circulation enters the left atrium by four pulmonary veins, and it passes through the left atrioventricular orifice (mitral valve) into the left ventricle, from which it is finally ejected into the systemic circulation via the aortic orifice (aortic valve).

Atrial Septum

The atrial portion of the heart is divided by the interatrial septum into right and left chambers. The septum, a composite structure, is derived from two independent septa of the embryonic atrium, neither of which formed a complete partition in itself (Figure 2–6). Traces of the two originally independent parts of the interatrial septum are clearly recognizable in the adult. The crescentic margin of the old valve of the foramen ovale can be seen adhering to the left side of the septum. The area cranial to this margin was originally the location of the ostium secundum of the interatrial septum primum in the embryo. The main muscular part of

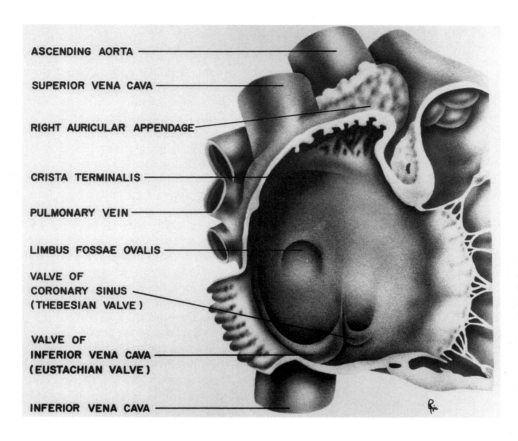

ASCENDING AORTA

SUPERIOR VENA CAVA

RIGHT AURICULAR APPENDAGE

CRISTA TERMINALIS

PULMONARY VEIN

LIMBUS FOSSAE OVALIS

VALVE OF
CORONARY SINUS
(THEBESIAN VALVE)

VALVE OF
INFERIOR VENA CAVA
(EUSTACHIAN VALVE)

INFERIOR VENA CAVA

Figure 2–6. Drawing of the interatrial septum. The interatrial septum is viewed from the right side to show the various structures of the interior of the right atrium. *(Modified, with permission, from Barry A, Patten BM: The structure of the adult heart.* In *Gould SE, ed.* Pathology of the Heart and Blood Vessels, *3rd ed. Springfield, IL: Charles C. Thomas; 1968.)*

the atrial septum is derived from the interatrial septum secundum. It forms somewhat later, immediately to the right of the septum primum. Throughout fetal life, the septum secundum retains an oval opening called the foramen ovale, the margin of which is seen on the right side of the adult interatrial septum in the limbus fossae ovalis. After the valve of the septum primum has fused to the left atrial side of the septum secundum, the foramen ovale becomes a more or less oval depression on the right side of the interatrial septum, called the *fossa ovalis*. In some 20% to 25% of adult hearts, this fusion of the valve of the foramen ovale with the septum secundum is incomplete and remains probe patent.[36] Probe patency, which is not functionally significant, should be sharply distinguished from the total valve defect seen when the valve of the foramen ovale is incompetent to guard the foramen ovale.

Atria

Right atrium

The inferior vena cava enters the caudal side of the right atrium (Figure 2–6). Return flow via this orifice is partially prevented by the valve of the inferior vena cava (eustachian valve) on the ventral aspect. The

opening of the coronary sinus, guarded by the valve of the coronary sinus (thebesian valve), enters the dorsocaudal wall of the right atrium between the atrioventricular orifice and the fossa ovalis. Frequently these valves have a cribiform appearance. The superior vena cava opens into the cranial posterior part of the right atrium. Extending between the right sides of the superior and inferior vena caval orifices is the crista terminalis, the prominent muscular ridge that underlies the sulcus terminalis, a ridge on the external surface of the right atrium. As it extends caudally, it becomes less distinct, and the valve of the inferior vena cava continues its general course. From the crista terminalis, a series of muscular ridges, the pectinate muscles radiate into the anterior wall of the atrium and the right atrial appendage. The smooth-walled portion of the right atrium, which is derived from the right horn of the embryonic sinus venosus, is bounded laterally by the crista terminalis and medially by the interatrial septum. The orifice of the superior vena cava is directed caudally toward the right atrioventricular orifice, and the orifice of the inferior vena cava is directed cranially toward the fossa ovalis. There are numerous small openings into the right atrium, especially on its septal lateral walls, which are the thebesian veins that drain the atrial myocardium.

The anatomic features that specifically characterize the right atrium include the pectinate muscles on its free wall beyond the boundaries of the auricular appendage, the crista terminalis, and the fossa ovalis.

Left atrium

The left atrium, lying dorsal to the root of the aorta, is situated left of and dorsal to the right atrium. Openings into its dorsal wall are the right and left superior and inferior pulmonary veins. The orifices of these four veins have no valves. Also, small thebesian veins enter directly from the left atrial myocardium. The left atrioventricular orifice, guarded by the mitral valve, lies in the ventral side of the atrium facing slightly caudally into the left ventricle. The inner face of the left atrium is relatively smooth, although there are well-marked pectinate muscles on the inner surface of the left auricular appendage. The left side of the atrial septum is derived primarily from the septum primum that is the valve of the foramen ovale during gestation.

The anatomic features that specifically characterize the left atrium include the trabeculations of the pectinate muscles confined to the atrial appendage and the smooth surfaces of the free wall and interatrial septum.

Ventricles

Right ventricle

The right ventricle extends from the right atrium almost to the cardiac apex. On cross-section it appears as a crescentic cavity, with the muscular interventricular septum bulging into its outflow portion. The outer third of its muscular wall is solid, and the inner two thirds of the wall has a distinctly trabeculated pattern. The cranial part of the right ventricle that leads into the pulmonary trunk is called the *pulmonary conus*. It is separated from the rest of the right ventricular cavity by a muscular ridge, the crista supraventricularis (Figure 2–7).[67] Over time there have been controversies over the terminology and grouping of the four muscle bundles comprising the crista supraventricularis. Presently, the prevalent view is that the term *crista supraventricularis* should be reserved for the supraventricular muscle mass of the normal right ventricle.[68] Also, there is consensus that the crista includes the parietal band(s), infundibular septum, and distal (subpulmonary) portion of the septal band. When right ventricular malformations are present, one should describe the individual muscle bundles in anatomic terms for clarity and consistency.[65,68] A large muscular band, the moderator

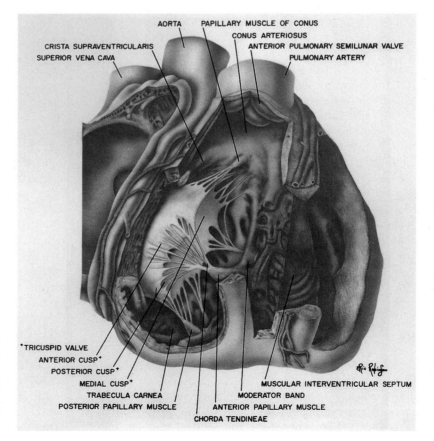

Figure 2–7. Drawing of the right ventricular outflow tract. The wall of the right ventricle is opened to show its internal configuration. A well-developed moderator band is present. *(Modified, with permission, from Barry A, Patten BM: The structure of the adult heart.* In *Gould SE, ed.* Pathology of the Heart and Blood Vessels, *3rd ed. Springfield, IL: Charles C. Thomas; 1968.)*

AORTA PAPILLARY MUSCLE OF CONUS
CONUS ARTERIOSUS
CRISTA SUPRAVENTRICULARIS ANTERIOR PULMONARY SEMILUNAR VALVE
SUPERIOR VENA CAVA PULMONARY ARTERY

*TRICUSPID VALVE
ANTERIOR CUSP*
POSTERIOR CUSP*
MEDIAL CUSP* MUSCULAR INTERVENTRICULAR SEPTUM
TRABECULA CARNEA MODERATOR BAND
POSTERIOR PAPILLARY MUSCLE ANTERIOR PAPILLARY MUSCLE
CHORDA TENDINEAE

band, frequently extends from the septal wall of the right ventricle through the base of the anterior papillary muscle of the right ventricle. When present, it usually contains a portion of the right branch of the atrioventricular bundle.

The anatomic features that specifically characterize the right ventricle include the coarse apical trabeculations, the septal band of the crista supraventricularis, and the muscular separation of the tricuspid (atrioventricular) and pulmonary (semilunar) valves.

Left ventricle

The left ventricle, shaped like a cone, tapers to form the apex of the heart and constitutes the obtuse margin of the heart, approximately half of its diaphragmatic surface, and a small part of the sternocostal aspect. Myocardial ridges of various sizes, the trabeculae carnae, corrugate the greater part of its inner surface. In contrast to the wall of the right ventricle, the outer two thirds of the left ventricular wall is relatively solid muscle. The anatomy of the left ventricular outflow tract, which extends cranially from the apex of the chamber to the aortic valve, has been described.[69] Its cranial part is called the *aortic vestibule*, the anterior wall of which is formed by the juncture of the muscular and membranous parts of the interventricular septum (Figure 2–8). The atrioventricular bundle runs through this junction. The aortic (anterior) leaflet of the mitral valve, which divides the chamber

into its inflow and outflow portions, forms the posterior wall of the vestibule. The vestibule is attached to the cardiac skeleton at its base and at its right and left sides. The interventricular septum is thick and muscular, except for a small area of connective tissue (membranous septum) near the root of the aorta (Figure 2–9). From the left side, the membranous portion of the ventricular septum lies in the angle between the attachments of the right and noncoronary cusps of the aortic valve. Defects of the interventricular septum occur most frequently in the region of the membranous septum. Rarely, they involve the right atrial portion of the membranous septum, in which case they are accompanied by tricuspid valve abnormalities with shunts between the left ventricle and right atrium. The left ventricular free wall and the apical portion of the ventricular septum have extensive muscular trabeculations, the trabeculae carnae. Occasionally, isolated fibromuscular bands may cross the left ventricular cavity near the apex. These may be the source of systolic musical murmurs but have no functional significance.

Two large papillary muscles, the anterolateral and posteromedial, are usually present in the left ventricle. Both of these send chordae tendineae to each of the leaflets, anterior and posterior, of the mitral valve. Each muscle has a major trunk with multiple heads to which the chordae tendineae attach. The anterolateral papillary muscle is slightly larger than the posteromedial

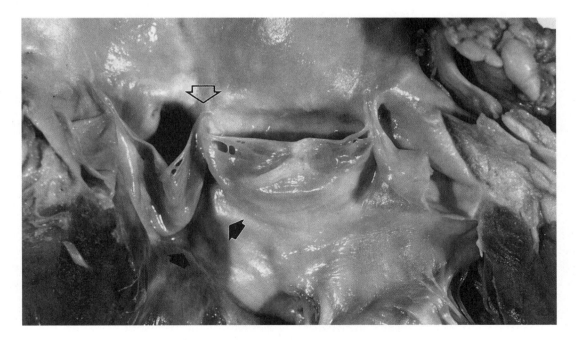

Figure 2–8. Gross specimen showing the left ventricular outflow tract and aortic valve. The membranous portion of the interventricular septum (solid arrows) lies beneath the attachments of the right and noncoronary cusps (open arrows) of the aortic valve.

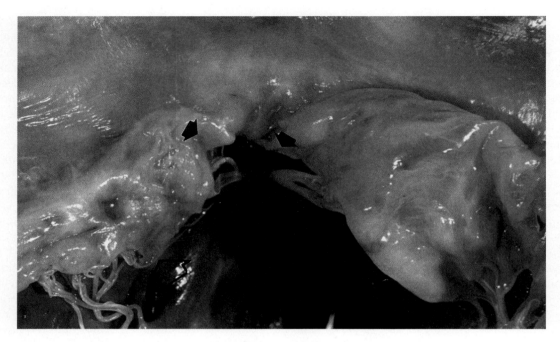

Figure 2–9. Gross specimen showing the membranous portion of the interventricular septum. This view is from the right heart chambers at the level of the tricuspid valve. The membranous portion of the interventricular septum (solid arrows) lies beneath the septal leaflet of the tricuspid valve (open arrow).

one, and the thickness of both muscles is similar to that of the left ventricular free wall.

Atrioventricular and Semilunar Valves

Atrioventricular valves
The atrioventricular valves, the mitral and tricuspid valves, guard the orifices leading from the atria into the ventricles, and the leaflets extend into the cavities of the ventricles. Each valve has a continuous line of attachments, but its free margin is notched, subdividing it into leaflets or cusps.

MITRAL VALVE. The left atrioventricular valve, called the *mitral valve* because of its supposed resemblance to a bishop's miter, is divided into two leaflets (Figure 2–10). The leaflets are joined at the anterolateral and posteromedial commissures. Chordae tendineae hold each valve leaflet to the ventricular papillary muscles. The thinnest chordae are connected to the free edges of the leaflets. Those of intermediate thickness are connected to their ventricular surfaces, a few millimeters from their free margins, and the thickest are connected to the ventricular surfaces near the attached borders of the leaflets. The atrial surfaces of the valve leaflets are smooth and glistening, and the ventricular surfaces are irregular and vesiculated. The two leaflets of the mitral valve are the ventral (anterior) and the dorsal (posterior). Each leaflet receives chordae tendineae from

more than one papillary muscle, and each papillary muscle sends chordae tendineae to more than one valve leaflet. The chordae tendineae of the mitral valve are heavier than the chordae tendineae of the tricuspid valve. They insert into the free margin 6 to 8 mm from the edge or into the basal part of the leaflet.[70,71] The chordae tendineae and papillary muscles act in concert to prevent leaflets of the mitral valve from being forced back into the atria by the pressure buildup in the ventricles during systole.[72] The papillary muscles contract simultaneously with the rest of the ventricular musculature, preventing the loss of tension in the chordae tendineae, which would occur during ventricular systole when the ventricular cavity shrinks. Any alteration in their line of traction can result in incompetence.[73] Contraction of the annulus is also essential, since this reduces the area covered by the mitral leaflets by 20% to 50%.[74]

TRICUSPID VALVE. The right atrioventricular valve is divided into three leaflets that comprise the *tricuspid valve* (Figure 2–11). The atrial surfaces of the valve leaflets are smooth and glistening, and the ventricular surfaces are irregular and vesiculated. The three leaflets of the tricuspid valve are the ventral (anterior), dorsal (posterior), and septal.[75] The junctions between the leaflets are the commissures. In the newborn and neonate occasional tiny blood cysts[76] may be present on the atrial surfaces of the leaflets of the

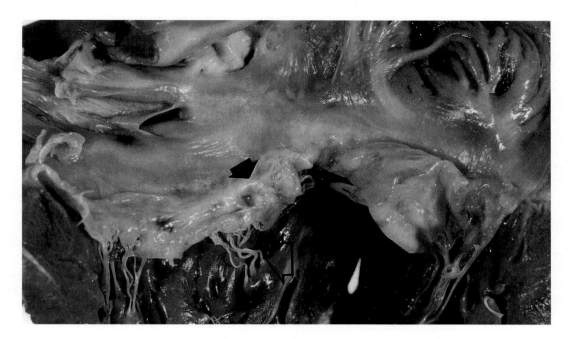

Figure 2–10. Gross specimen of the tricuspid valve. The tricuspid valve has three leaflets: anterior, posterior, and septal (solid arrows). Some chordae tendineae attach to the papillary muscle of the conus (open arrow).

mitral valve. These disappear within the first year. Three papillary muscles, present in the right ventricle, have chordae tendineae attaching to the leaflets of the tricuspid valve. These muscles are the anterior, posterior (inferior), and papillary muscles of the conus. The papillary muscle is frequently indistinct and is named either the muscle of Lancisi or the muscle of Luschka. On its medial aspect the tricuspid valve attaches to the membranous portion of the interventricular septum.

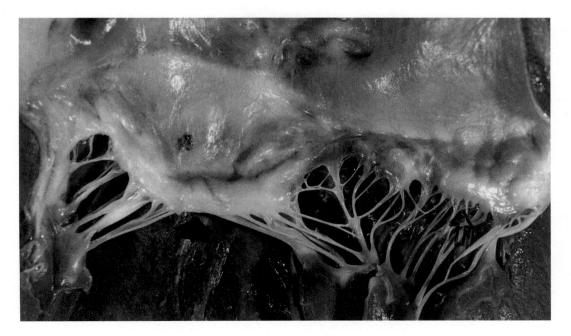

Figure 2–11. Gross specimen of the mitral valve. The mitral valve has two leaflets: anterior (solid arrow) and posterior (open arrow). Chordae tendineae attach to either the anterior or the posterior papillary muscles.

Semilunar valves

The outlet orifices of each ventricle are guarded by the semilunar valves, the aortic and pulmonary valves that have three cusps. Two, four, or five cusps have also been recorded occasionally.[77–80] Each cusp is a pocket-like flap of connective tissue that is covered by endothelium and attached to the annulus fibrosus of the aortic or pulmonary trunk (Figure 2–12). The free margins of these valve cusps are directed away from the ventricle, and in the center of each is a small fibrocartilaginous nodule, the corpus arantii (Figure 2–13).

AORTIC VALVE. The aortic valve cusps are called the right anterior, left anterior, and posterior (noncoronary) cusps. The aortic valve leaflets are thicker and stronger than those of the pulmonary valve because of the higher pressure in the aorta. The spaces between the aortic valve cusps and the aortic wall are called the *aortic sinuses* or the *sinuses of Valsalva* (Figure 2–13). These are the right, left, and posterior (noncoronary) sinuses. The right and left coronary arteries originate from the upper part of the right and left aortic sinuses, respectively. The right aortic sinus is adjacent to the right atrium, right ventricular outflow tract, and right sinus

of the pulmonary valve. The left aortic sinus is adjacent to the left atrium and left sinus of the pulmonary valve. The posterior (noncoronary) sinus of Valsalva is related to the left and right atria and interatrial septum.

PULMONARY VALVE. The pulmonary valve anchored to the infundibulum of the right ventricle and the pulmonary artery trunk has three cusps, the right posterior, left posterior, and anterior. As with the aortic valve, the spaces between the valve cusps and the wall of the pulmonary artery are called the sinuses of Valsalva. Conventionally, the pulmonary valve has three cusps. However, from one to four cusps have been described.[26,48,60] A unicusp valve is stenotic. A bicuspid valve often has no functional significance although patients with congenital pulmonary stenosis frequently have bicuspid valves. The occurrence of a quadricuspid valve is more common in the pulmonary valve than in the aortic valve.

Vasculature of the Heart

The heart's vasculature includes the coronary arteries, the coronary veins, and the cardiac lymphatic vessels.

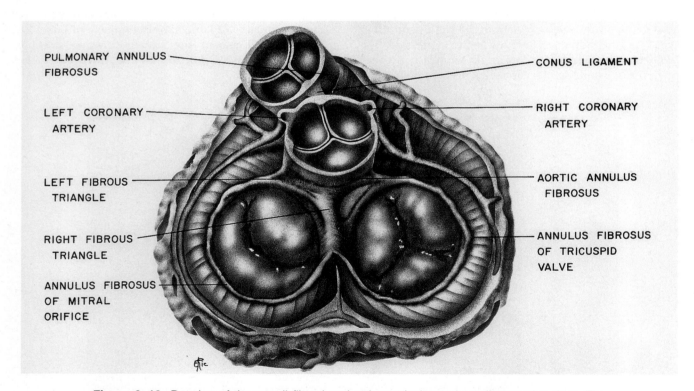

Figure 2–12. Drawing of the annuli fibrosi and atrioventricular and semilunar valve rings. The heart is viewed from above with the atria removed to show the fibrous triangles, the annuli fibrosi, and the attachment of the ventricular muscle bundles to them. *(Modified, with permission, from Barry A, Patten BM: The structure of the adult heart. In Gould SE, ed. Pathology of the Heart and Blood Vessels, 3rd ed. Springfield, IL: Charles C. Thomas; 1968.)*

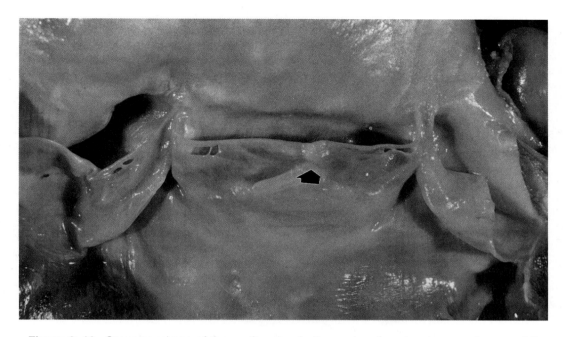

Figure 2–13. Gross specimen of the aortic valve. In the center of each valve cusp is a small fibrocartilaginous nodule, the corpus arantii (arrow).

Coronary Arteries

The heart is supplied by two major coronary arteries, the left and right coronary arteries (Figure 2–14). The left coronary artery ostium is in the left sinus of Valsalva, and the artery runs forward between the root of the pulmonary trunk and the left atrium. The left coronary artery perfuses the entire left ventricle, except for the right half of its posterior wall and the posterior part of the interventricular septum.[81] It soon divides into two major branches, the left anterior descending and the left circumflex branches. The anterior descending branch courses caudally along the anterior inter-

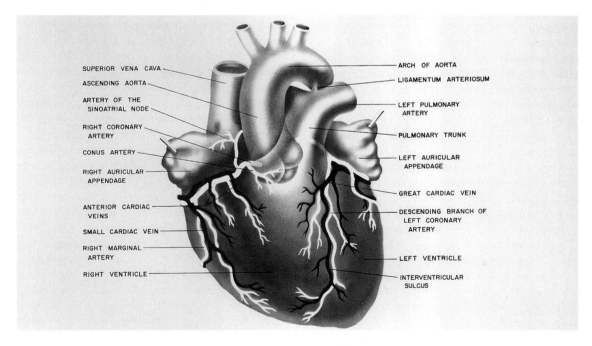

Figure 2–14. Patterns of the coronary arteries and veins. This anterior view of the heart shows the major branches of the coronary arteries and veins.

ventricular groove to the apex of the heart, and then turns upward into the posterior interventricular groove to anastomose with the posterior descending coronary artery. Along its course, the anterior descending branch sends perforating branches into the ventral two thirds of the interventricular septum. Small lateral branches course over the surface of the heart to supply the musculature of the pulmonary conus and the anterior wall of the left ventricle. The left circumflex branch runs in the atrioventricular groove and reaches the diaphragmatic surface of the heart. Along its course, major branches emerge to supply the anterior wall of the left ventricle, the obtuse margin, and the posterior wall of the left ventricle. Other smaller branches supply the left atrium and the root of the aorta.

The ostium of the right coronary artery is in the right sinus of Valsalva. This artery runs laterally in the groove between the pulmonary conus and the right atrium. It then passes around the base of the right atrium to reach the posterior interventricular groove, where it becomes the posterior descending branch, which courses into the groove to anastomose with branches of the left anterior descending branch at the apex of the heart. Smaller branches run from this artery to supply the right and left posterior ventricular walls, and perforating branches supply the dorsal part of the interventricular septum. The conus artery supplies the musculature of the pulmonary conus. It arises as the first ventricular branch of the right coronary artery in 50% of all hearts (Figure 2–14). It has a separate ostium in the right sinus of Valsalva in the other 50%.[82] In all instances, it supplies the musculature of the pulmonary conus.

Several branches of the right coronary artery are of special interest. They are the sinoatrial (SA) node artery, the atrioventricular (AV) node artery, and the right marginal branch. The SA node artery supplies the region of the sinoatrial node. This is the largest atrial artery that passes between the right auricular appendage and the superior vena cava. It courses caudally along the sulcus terminalis to supply the sinoatrial node. The AV node artery arises from a U-shaped bend in the coronary artery at the crux and extends anteriorly along the base of the atrial septum to the AV node. The right marginal branch supplies the acute margins of the heart, and a preventricular branch runs over the ventral wall of the right ventricle. All the branching and straight arteries are similar in both the right and left ventricles.[83]

Although there are many variations in the blood supply of the heart, there are three major patterns[82] that depend on whether the right or left coronary artery supplies the major portion of the ventricular mass. This situation usually equates with the artery that supplies the posterior descending branch that lies in the posterior interventricular groove. The right coronary artery is dominant in 48% of all hearts, the left coronary dom-

inates in 18%, and a balanced distribution between the right and left coronary arteries occurs in 34%. In all instances, the dominant artery supplies nearly all the musculature of the interventricular septum.

Numerous anastomoses (intercoronary collaterals) are present between terminal branches of the left anterior descending and left circumflex coronary arteries, and also between either of these branches and the terminal branches of the right coronary artery. In human hearts these collaterals may occur at all levels of the myocardium, that is, on the epicardial surface, in the midportion of the myocardium, and near the endocardial surface. The subendocardial plexus has been described as a distinctive collateral network.[84] This plexus comprises perforating branches in the proximal portions of the left anterior descending and left circumflex coronary arteries that penetrate the muscular myocardium immediately and then arborize adjacent to the endocardial surface. These collateral communications are of clinical significance when occlusion occurs in a major coronary arterial branch because these channels then serve as alternate routes of blood supply to distal parts of the myocardium.[85] At times loops of atrial or ventricular muscle are present around the coronary arteries. These "myocardial bridges" can produce abnormal configurations of the coronary arterial tree on angiography.[53,86] The incidence of such bridges and loops is related to the pattern of the coronary arterial dominance.[87] They are more frequent in those hearts in which the left coronary artery is dominant.

Coronary Veins

The coronary veins lie in the connective tissue of the epicardium, superficial to the arteries and parallel to the branches of the coronary arteries (Figure 2–14). Most of them drain into the coronary sinus, which opens into the right atrium between the opening of the inferior vena cava and the right atrioventricular orifice (tricuspid valve). The coronary sinus lies in the dorsal part of the coronary groove, parallel to the circumflex branch of the left coronary artery. The major veins draining into the coronary sinus are (1) the great cardiac vein, (2) the middle cardiac vein, (3) the small cardiac vein, (4) the posterior vein of the left ventricle, and (5) the oblique vein (vein of Marshall). The great cardiac vein originates in the epicardium of the anterior interventricular groove near the apex. It parallels the circumflex branch of the left coronary artery, receives branches from the ventricles and left atrium, and terminates in the coronary sinus. The middle cardiac vein runs in the posterior interventricular groove with the posterior descending branch of the right coronary artery, receives blood from the interventricular septum and ventricular walls, and drains into the coronary sinus near its opening into the right atrium. The small cardiac vein runs posteriorly in the coronary groove between the right atrium and ventricle, receives branches from the right atrium and ventricle, and empties into the coronary sinus. The posterior cardiac vein runs over the dorsal aspects of the left ventricle and empties into the distal end of the coronary sinus. The oblique vein of the left atrium, the vein of Marshall,[36] runs down the posterior wall of the left atrium and into the coronary sinus. This vein represents the left common cardinal vein of the embryo. Other anterior cardiac veins lie in the ventral aspect of the right ventricle and empty either into the small cardiac vein or directly into the right atrium.

Thebesian veins were first described in the atria.[88] They open directly into the atrial chamber. Similar vessels, termed *arterioluminal vessels*, also exist in the ventricles.[89,90] These vessels are more numerous in the right atrium. In the ventricles, they are more numerous at the base of the papillary muscles, in the region of the conus, and in the apical musculature of the right ventricle.

Cardiac Lymphatics

Several observers have described these vessels.[68,89,91–93] Two lymphatic plexuses are present in the heart. A deep lymphatic plexus lies under the endocardium and drains through channels in the myocardium into lymphatics of the epicardium. A superficial lymphatic plexus rides adjacent to the endocardium. Left and right branches drain this plexus. The left branch passes upward in the anterior interventricular groove, and, after joining with the large branch of the diaphragmatic surface of the heart, it ascends as a single vessel between the pulmonary artery and the left atrium and ends in the inferior tracheobronchial lymph nodes. The right trunk drains the right atrium and part of the right ventricle and then passes parallel to the right coronary artery in the coronary groove on the ventral side of the aorta, to terminate in one of the innominate lymph nodes.

Fibrous Skeleton of the Heart

In the adult heart, atrial and ventricular myocardia are completely separated, except for the connection between them by the conduction bundle, a fibrous framework (Figure 2–12). This fibrous skeleton also serves as an attachment for the atrial and ventricular musculatures and the atrioventricular and semilunar valve leaflets.[41] This framework (the cardiac skeleton) comprises four rings of dense collagenous fibers and connecting tissue. The rings, annuli fibrosi, surround the two atrioventricular valve orifices (tricuspid and mitral valves) and the semilunar orifices (pulmonary and aortic valves). These annuli also comprise the lines of attachment to the mitral, tricuspid, and semilunar valves. The annuli surrounding the atrioventricular orifices are compact rings of fibrous tissue, whereas the aortic and

pulmonary annuli are short tubes. The pulmonary and aortic annuli are attached to each other by a moderately distinct band of dense fibers, the conus ligament. In the space bounded by the right and left atrioventricular annuli and by the aortic annulus, the fibrous framework is most dense and is called the *right fibrous trigone* (central fibrous body). Through this fibrous triangle passes the atrioventricular conduction bundle (bundle of His). A smaller left fibrous triangle lies in the angle between the aortic and the left atrioventricular annuli. This relatively immobile fibrous skeleton at the base of the heart is the supporting framework for atrial and ventricular contractions and anchors the semilunar valves against the high pressures generated in ventricular systole.

The membranous portion of the interventricular septum extends from the muscular interventricular septum to the bases of the noncoronary and right anterior cusps of the aortic semilunar valves. It is formed of dense collagenous fibers in a manner similar to that of the annuli fibrosi. The line of attachment of the tricuspid valve septal leaflet courses diagonally across the right base of the septum, dividing it into two parts: (1) the interventricular part, which lies below the attachment of the valve and between the right and left ventricular cavities, and (2) the atrioventricular part, which lies above the valve attachment separating the right atrium from the left ventricle. The membranous septum lies in the plane at right angles to the plane of the right and left atrioventricular annuli fibrosi. When viewed from above, it forms the right anterior corner of the right fibrous triangle. Thus, the right fibrous triangle (trigone) actually represents fusion between the right and left atrioventricular annuli fibrosi, the aortic annulus fibrosus, and the membranous septum.

Histologic Features of the Heart

The histologic features of the heart are discussed according to the three major layers of the heart, the endocardium, myocardium, and epicardium. Since the atria, valves, and cardiac lymphatics have some distinctive histologic features, these will also be discussed.

Endocardium

The chambers of the heart are lined with simple, squamous epithelium (endothelium). This single layer of flattened endothelial cells and an underlying layer of fibroelastic connective tissue comprise the endocardium (Figure 2–15). The endocardial connective tissue differentiates into a subendothelial zone of fine collagenous fibers and a deeper layer with many elastic fibers (elastica). The fibers are arranged in wavy lamellae, with collagen fibers in between. Atrial endocardium is thicker than that of the ventricles, especially in the left atrium

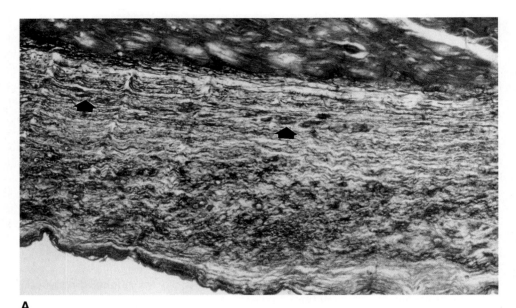

A

Figure 2–15. Photomicrographs of the endocardium. The endocardium comprises a single layer of endothelial cells with an underlying layer of connective tissue. **A.** The endocardium of the atrium is considerably thicker than that of the ventricular endocardium. This section of the left atrial endocardium shows scattered smooth muscle cells (arrows) throughout the connective tissue layer underlying the endothelial cells (hematoxylin and eosin, × 250). **B.** The ventricular endocardium is thinner than the atrial endocardium and has an acellular connective tissue layer beneath the endothelial cells. No smooth muscle cells are present (hematoxylin and eosin, × 250).

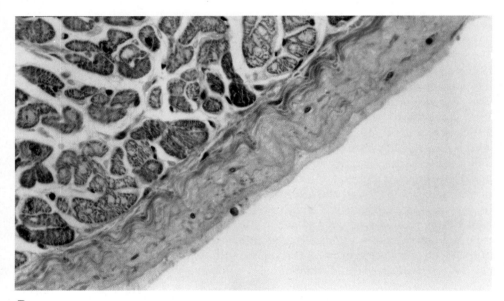

B

where there is an interrupted layer of smooth muscle throughout the endocardial connective tissue. At the base of the heart, the endocardial connective tissue is continuous with the fibrous framework of the heart.

Electron microscopy shows that the endothelium of the atria is similar to other vascular endothelial cells.[94] The subendothelial layer contains thin collagen fibrils with indistinct periodicity, which can be misinterpreted as fibrin. The elastic layer contains collagen and elastic fibers. The endocardium itself is avascular, whereas the subendocardium contains capillaries, metarterioles, and arterioles accompanied by nerve fibers.

Myocardium

The myocardium comprises a branching network of interventricularly and transversely striated muscle and its supporting connective tissue. In the atria, either myocardial fibers are attached to the annuli surrounding the atrioventricular ostia and encircle both atria (superficial fibers), or they are attached to only one annulus and then encircle only one atrium (deeper fibers).

The ventricular myocardium comprises interwoven bundles and bands of muscle fibers that are partially separated from one another by fibroelastic connective tissue (Figure 2–16). The fiber bands adjacent to the en-

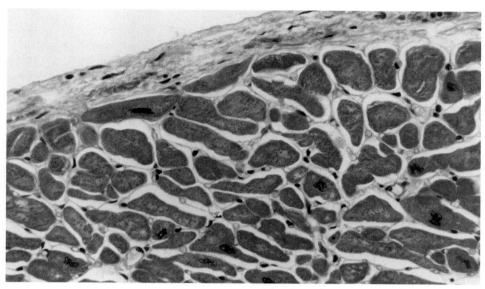

A

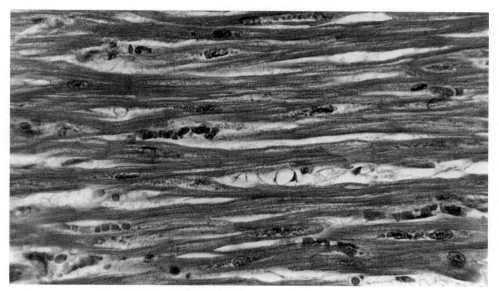

B

Figure 2–16. Photomicrographs of myocardium. **A.** This cross-section of ventricular myocardium shows individual myocyte nuclei to be centrally located (hematoxylin and eosin, × 250). **B.** Longitudinal section of ventricular myocardium shows interwoven bundles of branching muscle fibers. The cross-striations within the fibers are clearly visible (hematoxylin and eosin, × 250).

docardium pursue a course nearly perpendicular to that of the superficial fiber bundles of the same area. The intervening fiber bundles show all degrees of intermediate obliquity. The layer of reticular and collagenous fibers surrounding cardiac muscle fibers is the *endomysium*. Groups of muscle fibers are partly separated from adjacent bundles by denser layers of fibroelastic connective tissue called *perimysium*. The networks of capillaries and lymphatics and the myocardial sinusoids are in these connective tissue networks.

Myocardial nuclei usually are centrally placed, and one or two nuclei may be noted in each individual fiber. There are a variety of nuclear patterns in cardiac mus-

cle fibers. Five types of nuclei are recognized in normal and pathologic conditions.[95] These are (1) double nuclei, (2) "figure-eight" nuclei, (3) rows of nuclei, (4) parallel nuclei, and (5) bifurcated nuclei. Double nuclei and figure-eight nuclei are most frequent, particularly in children and in persons with atrophic hearts. In transverse sections, the highest incidence of nuclear irregularities are observed in cases with hypertrophied hearts and those with aplastic anemia. Patterns of interventricular splitting of nuclei, suggestive of myocardial hyperplasia, are exceedingly rare, and their incidence is not proportional to the heart weight. The high frequency of double nuclei seen in transverse sections of hypertrophied hearts might be related to branching of the nucleus.[95]

The surface layer of myocardial fibers is a thin membrane called the *sarcolemma*, which is in contact with the delicate fibers in the endomysium. The sarcoplasm within the sarcolemma serves as a matrix for the contractile myofibrils that run in the long axis of the fiber and show cross-striation. In light-microscopic sections, the conspicuous striations are alternating A and I bands. These myofibrils are divided into sarcomeres by distinct Z bands. The sarcoplasm around the nucleus contains mitochondria, fat droplets, the Golgi apparatus, and small cytosomes. Mitochondria also frequently are found between the myofibrils. At the poles of the myocardial nuclei, brown pigment granules (lipofuscin) are frequently seen (Figure 2–17). These occur more frequently with age and in certain altered states. The sarcolemma is now known to be a composite structure comprising a cell membrane, basement membrane, and associated fine collagenous reticulum fibers, together with cell processes of interstitial cells. In light-microscopic sections, straight or step-like lines are present in the muscle fibers. These are intercalated discs that run transversely across the fibers and occur in a zone in the middle of the isotropic (I) band. They become more pronounced with age. These discs are cell boundaries, and under electron microscopy they appear very tortuous. They serve as anchoring points for individual myofilaments. They possess both desmosomes and nexus. The latter are specialized to transmit the excitation impulse from cell to cell. Various amounts of glycogen are present in cardiac muscle, but it is not usually seen in autopsy material. Glycogen is unevenly distributed throughout the cell and is present in larger amounts in infant hearts.[96]

Epicardium

The epicardium (visceral pericardium) comprises a simple, squamous epithelial lining (mesothelium) for the layer adjacent to the pericardial cavity and a subjacent layer of fibroelastic connective tissue. There is a considerable amount of fat in the connective tissue of the ventricular epicardium, particularly in the region of the sulci and around the large vessels that lie over the surface of the ventricles (Figure 2–18). The deeper layers of the epicardial connective tissue and the perimysium of the myocardium are contiguous. In regions where there is no mesothelial layer, such as between the reflection of the pericardium and the epicardium, the epicardium connective tissue is continuous with that of the mediastinum. In general, the epicardium of the atria is thinner than that of the ventricles, and it contains relatively few coronary vessels. The atrial epicardium consists of a compact, thin layer of coarse collagenous fibers, with few elastic fibers and sparse amounts of fat. The ventricular epicardium comprises loose connective tissue, with greater amounts of fat and many vessels and nerve bundles running through it.

Atria

Most of the auricular myocardium is arranged in large trabeculae (pectinate muscles), with the myocardium between the trabeculae being extremely thin. In some areas, the myocardium is a loose network of anastomosing bundles of cardiac muscle. The connective tissue of the endocardium and epicardium is continuous through the interstices of this network. The auricular epicardium comprises mesothelium and relatively fine fibroelastic connective tissue containing various amounts of fat. Small coronary arteries and veins in this tissue supply the auricular wall. Characteristic of the auricle,

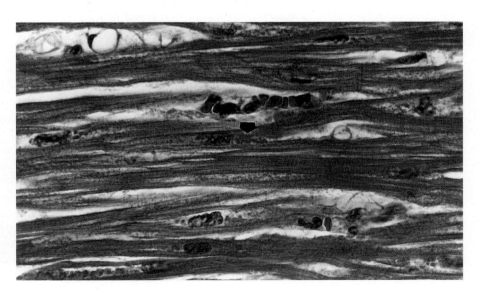

Figure 2–17. Lipofuchsin. The dark-stained pigment granules (lipofuchsin) are located near the poles of the myocyte nuclei (arrow) (hematoxylin and eosin, × 400).

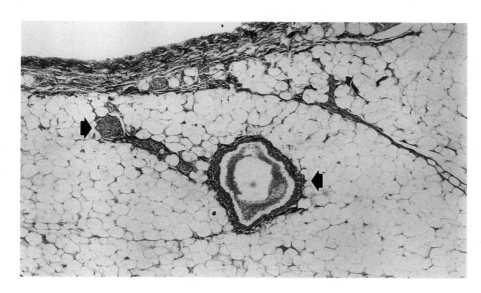

Figure 2–18. Photomicrograph of epicardium. A large number of fat cells are in the epicardium overlying the right ventricle. A layer of mesothelium is at the top. Major vessels and nerve branches run through the epicardium (arrows).

the epicardial vessels communicate directly with the intertrabecular spaces between the pectinate muscles, via the spaces of endothelium-lined channels in the network of myocardial bundles of the wall (arterioluminal channels). In addition, peculiar to the auricular wall is the larger amount of myocardium that comprises the atypical cardiac muscle fibers, those that resemble Purkinje fibers.

Valves

The histology of heart valves has been described in detail.[97] All the valves of the heart have the same basic structure, namely, a fold of collagenous and elastic tissue (fibrosa) lined on the surface by a single layer of flattened endothelial cells (Figure 2–19). The connective tissue layer differentiates into two main layers, one having coarse collagenous bundles for maximum strength and the other having fewer and smaller collagenous fiber bundles and a conspicuous amount of interwoven elastic fibers. The dense collagenous laminar layer is toward the surface of the valve, against which pressure builds when the valve is closed. In the semilunar valve, the central core (fibrosa) consists of dense, collagenous, fine elastic fibers, and it passes into the annulus of the heart, which in turn is contiguous with the media of the aorta and the pulmonary arteries. The fibrosa is covered on both sides with a layer of elastic and collagenous tissue that is continuous with the vessel wall and the ventricular endocardium. Toward the valve tips the fibrosa is looser and often myxomatous in appearance. Immediately beneath the elastic layer derived from the ventricle, the fibrosa appears to be looser and is spongy.

The atrioventricular valves (tricuspid and mitral valves) have a similar structure. The endocardium of the atria and ventricles continues over the fibrosa of the atrioventricular valves to form recognizable layers. In the anterior cusps of the mitral valve, the atrial endocardial smooth muscle layer continues for various distances. In normal hearts there are few, if any, capillaries or small blood vessels in the valve cusp.[98,99] In hearts of elderly people or those with previous pathologic change, rich vascularization of the valve cusp is frequently found.[100–103]

Lymphatics

The histology of the heart lymphatics has been described by several investigators.[104,105] The largest lymphatics accompany the epicardial coronary arteries. Endocardial lymphatics are only visible when dilated. True valves are present in the large lymphatics. Lymph flow goes from the endocardium, through the myocardium, to the epicardial channels. The heart lymphatics change with aging.[106] The superficial and deep layers of the epicardial lymphatics become separated by fat deposits. The decreasing number of capillaries and the appearance of blindly ending capillaries with variously sized networks indicate senility. In the myocardium, the number of capillaries is reduced with age, but there are no signs of involution in the perivascular lymphatics.

Electron-Microscopic Features of the Heart

The electron-microscopic features of the heart have been described by several investigators.[60,107] There are endothelial cells, resembling those of capillaries from other blood vessels, in the endocardium. Immediately beneath the endothelium is a fine fibrillar membrane. The subendothelial layers consist of fine collagenous fibrils with an indistinct periodicity that can readily be

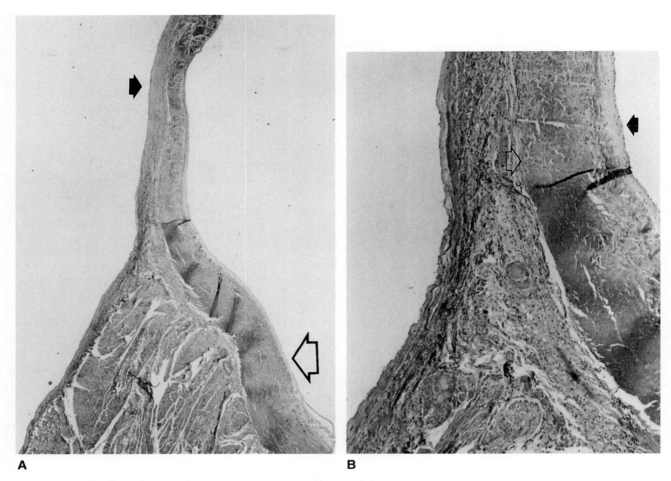

A **B**

Figure 2–19. Photomicrographs of the mitral valve. **A.** At low power, the atrial wall (solid arrow) and the left ventricular wall (open arrow) are seen (hematoxylin and eosin, × 10). **B.** High-power view shows the endothelial covering of the valve leaflet (solid arrow) with the dense fibrous layer beneath it (open arrow) (hematoxylin and eosin, × 40).

mistaken for fibrin. These subperiod bands can be misinterpreted as main bands. The elastica increases in size and complexity toward the subendocardium, and collagen fibers and fibrils increase in thickness. The smooth muscle in the endocardium is similar to that elsewhere. Capillaries and metarterioles can be demonstrated in subendocardium, and they have their characteristic structure. Nonmyelinated nerve fibers are found close to blood vessels in the subendocardium and to smooth muscle in the endocardium. The cells in the endocardium are mainly fibroblasts, undifferentiated cells, and occasionally macrophages.

Heart muscle is composed of individual contractile fibers that are approximately 10 to 20 μm in diameter and 50 to 100 μm in length. At low-level magnification, these cells have centrally located nuclei and a cross-striated appearance. The myofibrils, which contain the contractile elements, are oriented parallel to the long axis of the cells, and they exhibit a repeating band pattern, which accounts for the striations. The sarcolemma, or cell membrane, is approximately 100 Å thick, surrounds the whole cell, and forms the intercalated disc (Figure 2–20). It exhibits the typical trilayered "unit membrane" structure, comprising a bimolecular layer of lipid molecules, with associated protein layers on both surfaces.[108] Numerous membrane-limited vesicles, which appear to form as pinched-off invaginations of the surface membrane, are seen in the periphery of the cells. These vesicles are probably involved in pinocytosis. The cell membrane also participates in the active transport of ions and substrates and in the electrical phenomena associated with myocardial excitation. Intercalated discs form the end-to-end boundaries between adjacent cells of the same muscle column. These discs follow an undulating course, generally at right angles to the long axis of the fibers, and consist of

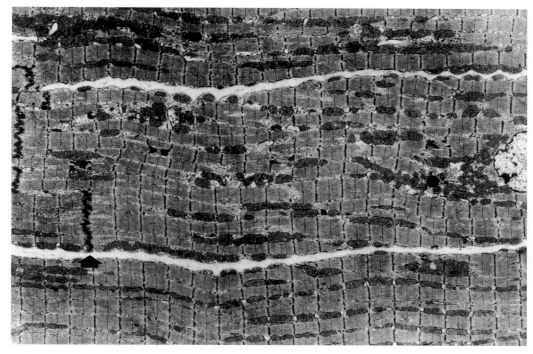

A

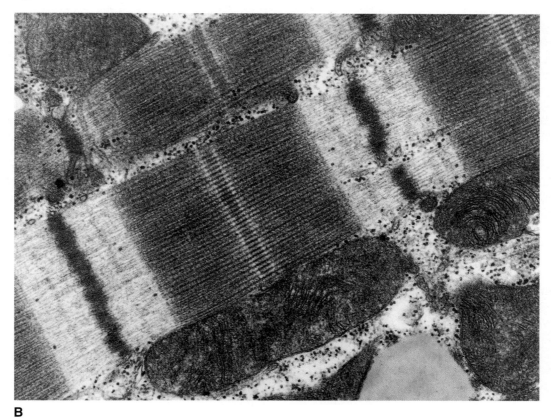

B

Figure 2–20. Electron micrograph of cardiac muscle. **A.** This view show numerous mitochondria, glycogen granules, and myofibrils with banding. At the site of a Z band an intercalated disc (arrow) crosses the fiber (× 4000). **B.** Higher magnification shows a sarcomere with thick and thin filaments (× 39,000).

two apposing, limiting cell membranes with an interposed intercellular space. In rat embryos intercalculated discs and cardiac cells first appear at 10 to 11 days.[109] In early stages of development the discs display limited areas of close apposition to adjacent membranes, with an intercellular gap of 200 to 250 Å. Beneath the plasma membranes, dense osmophilic regions are formed, to which the developing actin myofibrils are anchored. During the later part of the prenatal period, there is a gradual increase in the extent of the intercalated discs. The adult appearance of the intercalated discs is more or less established at birth. The basement membranes of the sarcolemma do not penetrate the intercellular space of the intercalated discs. Three structural modifications of the intercalated discs are evident: (1) simple paired cell membranes separated by an intercellular space that varies in width; (2) limiting cell membranes of greater electron density than those generally seen, which are separated by a narrow intercellular space of uniform width, measuring about 100 Å; and (3) desmosomes, consisting of paired, very dense arcuate cytoplasmic bodies in apposition to the cell membranes (Figure 2–20). The desmosomes aid in maintaining cell-to-cell contacts. The structure of the intercalated discs has been described in detail.[110,111]

The sarcoplasmic reticulum comprises an extensive intercytoplasmic system of membrane-limited channels. It has two components. The first is the transverse or T system, comprising deep invaginations of the sarcolemmal surface membrane of the cell. It is located between myofibrils at the level of the Z line, and it exhibits focal dilatations termed "intermediary vesicles."[111] The second is an interventricular component comprising a system of anastomosing channels that intimately surround the myofibrils. This sleeve of tubules is divided interventricularly into independent units, each limited to one sarcomere. The T system is present only in the myofibers of mammalian cardiac ventricular fibers.[97] Sarcoplasmic reticulum is considered to have two important functional roles: coupling excitation with contraction, and relaxation. Direct continuity of the transverse system of tubules with the sarcolemma has been demonstrated in the muscle of fish.[15]

Mitochondria are extremely abundant in heart muscle, comprising approximately 30% to 50% of the cell volume. They are large, roughly cylindrical bodies distributed between and in close proximity to the interventricularly disposed myofibrils that are the contractile elements (Figure 2–20). Mitochondria are delimited from the sarcoplasm by a double membrane. The inner aspect of this membrane has numerous infoldings that form plate-like projections, or cristae, rather than pairs of membranes, and that transverse the interior of the mitochondria. The cristae are numerous and are closely packed in a relatively ordered arrangement.

Dense granules are also occasionally observed between the cristae. Mitochondria are active in oxidative phosphorylation.[112,113] The closeness of the mitochondrial cristae to the myofibrils facilitates the rapid transfer of high-energy compounds from their source in the mitochondria to their site of utilization in the contracting sarcomere. Other constituents of heart muscle noticed under electron microscopy include glycogen granules, lipid droplets, secretions, droplets of an unknown nature, and lysosomal bodies.

The fundamental unit of contraction in cardiac muscle is the sarcomere, which comprises a carefully ordered interdigitating array of interventricularly disposed contractile protein filaments (Figure 2–20). The sarcomeres themselves are joined end to end to form interventricular intracellular columns known as myofibrils. The myofibrils transverse the length of the muscle fiber, and they are so arranged that the sarcomeres lie in register with respect to the transverse axis of the cell. The characteristic cross-striated appearance of the fiber reflects the banding pattern of the sarcomere. The myofibrils have two parallel filaments: thick, dense filaments of myosin and thin filaments of actin. Special arrangements of these filaments result in the crossbanding. The thick and thin filaments of the myofibers form simultaneously.[114] They are usually accompanied by cross-bridges between them. A and I bands form at the same time; Z lines appear later. Intercalated discs develop from tight functions of primordial cells, and they serve as points of attachment for the developing myofibrils. The myocardium initially has radially oriented cells, with large intercellular spaces that become more tightly packed. The intercellular spaces decrease, and cells assume a circumferential orientation. The myocardial cells remain epithelial throughout the formation of the functional heart tube, and specialized epithelial junctions are modified to form the intercalated discs. Embryonic myocardial cells contain large amounts of free ribosomes, particularly glycogen. This glycogen is often associated with portions of granular reticulum. There is a large amount of granular reticulum in the myocardial cell cytoplasm, and this, along with a hypertrophied Golgi apparatus, suggests that these cells may have a secretory function. These organelles persist during the initial period of fibril formation. Myofibrils apparently form from nonfilamentous precursor material, rather than by alignment of sequentially synthesized components. In electron micrographs the sarcomere is sharply delineated by paired, dense Z lines, which are derived from zonulae or maculae adherents in the embryonic heart.[115] Also evident in the sarcomere are the A band, the I band, the M line, and the L line. The A band is an electron-dense segment in the central part of the sarcomere that is strongly birefringent (anisotropic) and maintains a fixed length of 1.5 μm. The I bands are relatively nonbirefringent (isotropic). They are lighter areas flanking the A bands, and they occupy spaces between the A band and the Z lines. The M–L complex bisects the A band, and it consists of a dark central M line, flanked by the light and rather narrow L line. Thick filaments, measuring 100 Å in diameter and 1.5 μm in length, are confined to the A band to determine its constant length. Peripheral sets of thinner filaments project from the Z line to form the I bands, which then enter the A bands, where they are interposed between thick filaments. The zone of overlap of these two types of filaments is termed "the A band proper." The thin filaments are 1 μm long, and they do not penetrate the M–L complex. Sarcomeres are 2.2 μm or longer. These myofilaments are connected by cross-bridges, and the width of the various bands alters during contraction, as the filaments slide back and forth on each other. Huxley's[116] sliding theory of contraction is still the most satisfactory explanation of contraction of the myocardial fibers. This concept states that the actin (thin) and myosin (thick) filament lengths remain constant. Myocardial contraction results from sliding of the actin filaments relative to the myosin filaments.

Conduction System of the Heart

The three major components of the conduction system are the sinoatrial (SA) node, the atrioventricular (AV) node, and the conduction bundle of His.[117]

Sinoatrial Node

The sinoatrial node (SA node), originally described by Keith and Flack,[118] lies in the sulcus terminalis between the superior vena cava and the right appendage. It is horseshoe-shaped, comprising a main mass with two limbs.[97] One limb extends ventrally and cranially to the entry of the superior vena cava, and the other limb extends caudally in the sulcus terminalis. Histologically, the sinoatrial node is composed of a mass of fusiform muscle cells arranged in a plexiform manner (Figure 2–21). The nodal fibers are more slender than the atrial fibers, and their nuclei are smaller in diameter. These fibers possess a scant number of myofibrils, with cross-striations that are less prominent than those of the atrial musculature. At the edges, the nodal fibers are contiguous with typical myocardial fibers. Although sinoatrial tissue may extend from endocardium to epicardium, it is usually separated from the endocardium by atrial muscle.

Atrioventricular Node

The atrioventricular node (AV node) is located in the floor of the right atrium, between the opening of the coronary sinus and the septal leaflet of the tricuspid valve.[119] Its position is slightly below or adjacent to the central fibrous body, and its fibers are continuous with the musculature of the coronary sinus bed in the right and left atria. It penetrates the central fibrous body to form the bundle of His, which then traverses the lower

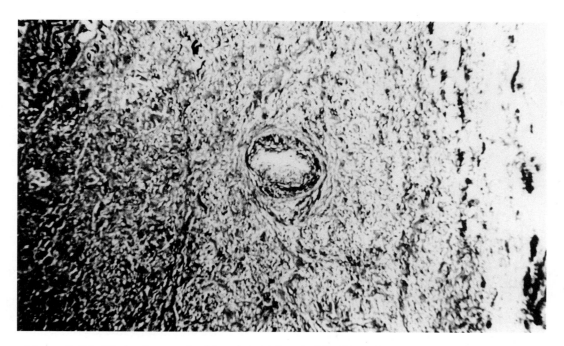

Figure 2–21. Photomicrograph of the sinoatrial node. The SA node contains fine, poorly stained myofibers within a fibrous stroma. These conduction fibers have increased amounts of glycogen. In the center of the nodal tissue lies the central SA node artery (hematoxylin and eosin, × 100).

interatrial septum to the lower part of the membranous portion of the interventricular septum. At its emergence from the central fibrous body, the bundle of His sends forth a thin sheet of fibers that pass down the left side of the interventricular septum immediately beneath the endocardium. This is the left bundle. The right bundle proceeds along the caudal margin of the septal limb of the cristae supraventricularis to the moderator band. If the moderator band is present, the right branch lies within it.

Histologically, the atrioventricular node consists of a network of muscle fibers that are smaller than atrial fibers. The node is richly cellular, containing numerous endothelial-like cells that interlace with the muscle cells. In some places they enclose small spaces (Figure 2–22). The number of elastic fibers in the node is greater than in the atrial or ventricular myocardium, and its reticular network has a more delicate pattern. The atrioventricular bundle also has muscle fibers that are smaller than those of the ventricular myocardium, and they have smaller nuclei as well. They stain more lightly be-

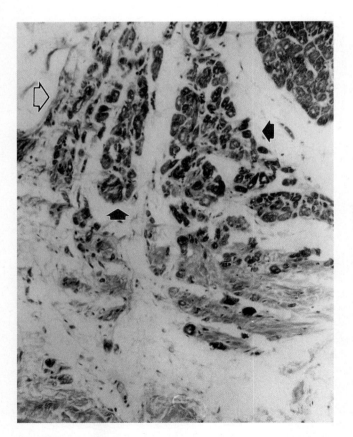

Figure 2–22. Photomicrograph of the atrioventricular node. The central fibrous body lies in the lower third of the field. Atrioventricular nodal tissue (solid arrows) lies above the fibrous body and beneath the right atrial endocardium (open arrow) (hematoxylin and eosin, × 250).

cause of the sparser concentration of striated myofibrils. The number of elastic fibers in the bundle of His and the left and right bundles is greater than in the ventricle. The reticular structure of these bundles also differs from that of the ventricle because the cells are smaller and their arrangement is lobulated. The terminal portions of the right and left bundles resemble Purkinje fibers, and they terminate in the subendocardial network of Purkinje fibers. Purkinje fibers are large with comparatively few myofibrils. They are situated in the periphery of the heart and are pale-staining (Figure 2–23). Their cytoplasm may have a large glycogen content, and they are contiguous with typical ventricular myocardial cells.

Nerve Innervation of the Heart

The nerve supply to the heart has been described in extensive detail.[34,120–122] The heart receives its nerve supply from the sympathetic and parasympathetic divisions of the autonomic nervous system. Cardiac nerves, derived from the superior and middle cervical ganglia, the inferior cervical ganglion, and perhaps the first thoracic ganglion, descend to the region of the ascending aorta and arch of the aorta, around which they anastomose to form the cardiac plexus. Each vagus nerve contributes to this plexus via superior and inferior cervical nerves and thoracic cardiac branches. The thoracic cardiac branches usually arise from the recurrent laryngeal nerve. The cardiac plexus is divided into superficial and deep plexuses. The superficial cardiac plexus spreads over the ventral caudal surface of the arch of the aorta; this plexus is formed by the inferior cervical cardiac branch of the left vagus and the cardiac branch of the superior cervical ganglion of the left sympathetic trunk. Sometimes a small cardiac ganglion is found in this plexus, and it is usually situated below the arch of the aorta and to the right of the ligamentum arteriosum. The deep cardiac plexus lies dorsal to the arch of the aorta between it and the bifurcation of the trachea. The cardiac branches of the vagus, the recurrent laryngeal nerves, the cardiac branches of the cervical and upper thoracic ganglia, and branches from the sympathetic trunks form this plexus with the exception of those branches that supply the superficial cardiac plexus. Extensions of the cardiac plexus are prominent over the atria, particularly in the region of the sinoatrial node. Other ramifications are present in the atrioventricular groove, and they extend along the course of the right and left coronary arteries to form the right and left coronary plexuses. Nerve fibers within the heart run in close proximity to arterioles and capillaries. They are frequently found close to smooth muscle cells in the endocardium. They also form a close association with muscle fibers, but motor end plates have not been

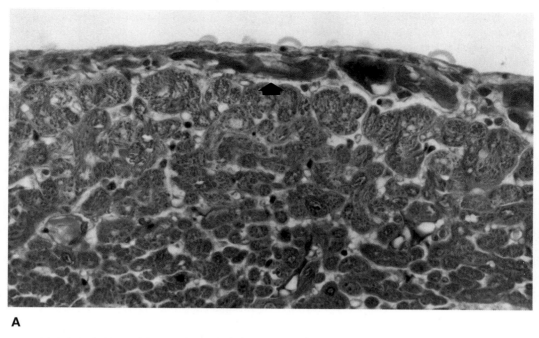

A

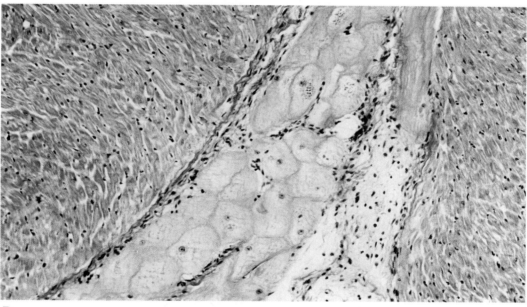

B

Figure 2–23. Photomicrograph of Purkinje fibers. **A.** These fibers are vacuolated (arrow) and lie immediately below the endocardial surface (hematoxylin and eosin, × 250). **B.** The fibers are large with prominent centrally located nuclei. Their cytoplasm is pale because of their increased glycogen content (hematoxylin and eosin, × 100).

demonstrated. Ganglion cells, presumably parasympathetic, are found in the epicardium of the atria. The function of the autonomic nervous system on the heart muscle is regulatory. The sympathetic fibers accelerate the inherent rhythmicity of the heart, whereas the parasympathetic fibers inhibit it.

Morphologic Changes after Birth

The major anatomic changes that occur in the heart after birth include the regression of the ductus arteriosus, the closure of the foramen ovale, and the closure of the interventricular septum. In part these changes represent closure of key shunts present during the uterine life of the embryo. During intrauterine life, with little blood flow going through the pulmonary circulation, the foramen ovale and ductus arteriosus are major right-to-left shunts. With the changes of blood flow through the pulmonary circulation occurring at birth with the expansion of the lungs and metabolic dilation of the pulmonary arterioles, pressure gradients occur between the right and left sides of the heart. Thus, physiologically these shunts close and later the membranous flaps at their orifices actually fuse to the septum for complete closure. In the ductus arteriosus there also is active vasoconstriction of the smooth muscle in its wall induced by the increased oxygen tension.

Atrial Septum
During intrauterine life, blood returning to the right atrium via the inferior vena cava is shunted across the foramen ovale to the left atrium and into the systemic circulation. With the change in pressures between the right and left sides of the heart at birth, there is functional closure of the foramen ovale with the left-side valve of the septum primum closing this opening. During the first few weeks of life, this valve tissue fuses with the interatrial septum for permanent closure, although this channel may remain probe patent in 50% of children through 5 years of age and persist in 25% of adults with no functional significance unless right atrial pressure is greater than left atrial pressure.

Ductus Arteriosus
During uterine life, the ductus arteriosus shunts blood from the pulmonary artery to the aorta, bypassing the pulmonary circulation. At birth the oxygen tension in the ductus arteriosus rises, inducing constriction of the smooth muscle in the wall of the ductus arteriosus and occluding its lumen. Complete closure of the ductus anatomically occurs within the first 6 to 8 weeks of age. If premature closure of the ductus arteriosus occurs during uterine life, there usually is congestive heart failure, right heart dilation, and pulmonary edema caused by right heart overload.

Cardiac Chambers
At birth the cardiac chambers undergo changes. With the closure of the various fetal circulatory shunts, the workload of the heart is redistributed to where the ventricles work in series to supply the otherwise separate pulmonary and systemic circulations. At birth the right and left ventricles appear as symmetrical cone-like structures.[123] This apparent symmetry of the ventricles reflects the relative right ventricular predominance that exists in the newborn. Within 3 to 6 months, the adult ratio of 2.3 : 1 to 3.2 : 1 for left ventricular/right ventricular weights is attained.[123] The mean weight of the heart of a newborn averages 20 to 23 g. By 6 months of

age it is nearly doubled.[60] After this growth spurt during early life the weight of the heart increases in proportion to body weight and averages about 0.5% of body weight.[60,124]

During the first few months of life, physiologic growth of the heart is the result of two processes: hypertrophy and hyperplasia.[124] Hypertrophy is an increase in the size of the myocytes, whereas hyperplasia is an increase in number of myocytes. At birth the myocytes are about 8 μm in diameter, whereas in the adult heart the average diameter of the myocytes is 20 μm in the left ventricle and 16 to 17 μm in the right ventricle.[124] The increase in fiber size is accompanied by an increase in cytoplasmic organelles. Thus, myocardial cell replications play a minor role in the growth of the heart and only during the first 6 months of life.[60,124,125]

Great Arteries
During uterine life and at birth, the walls of the great arteries, the pulmonary artery and aorta, are similar in size, wall thickness, and arrangement of their elastic lamellae.[60] With the change in pressures in the respective circulations after birth, the pressure in the systemic circulation is greater than the pressure in the pulmonary circulation. These pressure differences are reflected in the structures of the walls of the great vessels. By 6 months of age the aortic wall is thicker than the wall of the pulmonary artery. Also, the elastic lamellae are arranged differently in the two great arteries. In the pulmonary arterial wall there is fragmentation of the elastic fibers with a looser arrangement. In the aortic wall the elastic lamellae are widely spaced and short. By 2 years of age the adult structure of the pulmonary artery is present. The average thickness of the aortic wall is nearly 50% greater than that of the pulmonary artery wall. Persistence of the aortic medial pattern of the elastic lamellae in the pulmonary artery wall occurs when pulmonary hypertension is present from birth. This is associated with various congenital heart malformations.

REFERENCES

1. Boyd JD: Development of the heart. In *Handbook of Physiology, Circulation*, Vol. 3. Washington, DC: American Physiological Society; 1959.
2. Cooper MH, O'Rahilly R: The human heart at seven postovulatory weeks. *Acta Anat.* 79:280–99, 1971.
3. DeHaan RL: Embryology of the heart. In Hurst JW, ed. *The Heart.* New York: McGraw-Hill; 1974.
4. Clark EB: Mechanisms in the pathogenesis in congenital cardiac malformations. In Pierpont MEM, Moller J, eds. *The Genetics of Cardiovascular Disease.* Boston: Martinus-Nijhoff; 1986.
5. Clark EB: Cardiac embryology. Its relevance to congenital heart disease. *Am J Dis Child.* 140:41–4, 1986.

6. Ojeda JL, Hurle JM: Establishment of the tubular heart: Role of cell death. In Pexieder T, ed. *Perspectives in Cardiovascular Research*, Vol. 5, *Mechanisms of Cardiac Morphogenesis and Teratogenesis*. New York: Raven Press; 1981.

7. Ruckman RN, Cassling RJ, Clark EB, Rosenquist GC: Cardiac function in the embryonic chick. In Pexieder T, ed. *Perspectives in Cardiovascular Research*, Vol. 5, *Mechanisms of Cardiac Morphogenesis and Teratogenesis*. New York: Raven Press; 1981.

8. Paschoud N, Pexieder T: Patterns of proliferation during the organogenetic phase of heart development. In Pexieder T, ed. *Perspectives in Cardiovascular Research*, Vol. 5, *Mechanisms of Cardiac Morphogenesis and Teratogenesis*. New York: Raven Press; 1981.

9. Arguello C, Servin M: The importance of extracellular matrix components in development of the embryonic chick heart. In Pexieder T, ed. *Perspectives in Cardiovascular Research*, Vol. 5, *Mechanisms of Cardiac Morphogenesis and Teratogenesis*. New York: Raven Press; 1981.

10. Krug EL, Runyan RB, Markwald RR: Protein extracts from early embryonic hearts initiate cardiac endothelial cytodifferentiation. *Dev Biol*. 112:414–26, 1998.

11. Pexieder T: Introduction to section on cell death. In Pexieder T, ed. *Perspectives in Cardiovascular Research*, Vol. 5, *Mechanisms of Cardiac Morphogenesis and Teratogenesis*. New York: Raven Press; 1981.

12. Rychter Z, Rychterova V: Angio- and myoarchitecture of the heart wall under normal and experimentally changed morphogenesis. In Pexieder T, ed. *Perspectives in Cardiovascular Research*, Vol. 5, *Mechanisms of Cardiac Morphogenesis and Teratogenesis*. New York: Raven Press; 1981.

13. Jacobson AG, Duncan JT: Heart induction in salamanders. *J Exp Zool*. 167:104, 1968.

14. Rosenquist GC: Location and movements of cardiogenic cells in the chick embryo: The heart-forming portion of the primitive streak. *Dev Biol*. 22:461–75, 1970.

15. Franzini-Armstrong C, Porter KR: Sarcolemmal invaginations constituting the T system in fish muscle fibers. *J Cell Biol*. 22:675–96, 1964.

16. Linask KK, Lash JW: Precardiac cell migration: Fibronectin localization at mesodermendoderm interface during directional movement. *Dev Biol*. 114:87–101, 1986.

17. Sissman NJ: Cell multiplication rates during development of the primitive cardiac tube in the chick embryo. *Nature*. 210:504–7, 1966.

18. Manasek FJ: Embryonic development of the heart. II. Formation of the epicardium. *J Embryol Exp Morphol*. 22:333–48, 1969.

19. Viragh S, Challice CE: The origin of the epicardium and the embryonic myocardial circulation in the mouse. *Anat Rec*. 201:157–68, 1981.

20. Stalsberg H, DeHaan RL: Regional mitotic activity in the precardiac mesoderm and differentiating heart tube in the chick embryo. *Dev Biol*. 19:128–59, 1969.

21. Gaja G, Loreti L, Ragnotti G, Guidotti G, Foa PP: Adenosine triphosphate-hexose phosphotransferase in devel-

oping chick embryo heart. *Proc Soc Exp Biol Med*. 121:608–11, 1966.

22. Guidotti G, Loreti L, Gaja G, Foa PP: Glucose uptake in the developing chick embryo heart. *Am J Physiol*. 211: 981–7, 1966.

23. Klein RL, Horton CR, Thureson-Klein A: Studies on nuclear amino acid transport and cation content in embryonic myocardium of chick. *Am J Cardiol*. 25:300–10, 1970.

24. Everett NB, Johnson RJ: A physiological and anatomical study of the closure of the ductus arteriosus in the dog. *Anat Rec*. 110:103–11, 1951.

25. Gessner IH, Lorinez AE, Bostrom H: Acid mucopolysaccharide content of the cardiac jelly of the chick embryo. *J Exp Zool*. 160:291–8, 1965.

26. Steding G, Seidl W: Contribution to the development of the heart. Part I: Normal development. *Cardiovasc Surg*. 28:386–409, 1980.

27. Gessner IH, Bostrom H: In vitro studies on 35S-sulfate incorporation into the acid mucopolysaccharide of chick embryo cardiac jelly. *J Exp Zool*. 160:283–90, 1965.

28. Manasek FJ: Embryonic development of the heart. I. A light and electron microscopic study of myocardial development in the early chick embryo. *J Morphol*. 125: 329–66, 1968.

29. DeVries PA, Saunders JBdeCM: Development of the ventricles and spiral outflow tract in the human heart. *Embryol*. 37:87–114, 1962.

30. Jaffee OC: Rheological aspects of the development of blood flow patterns in the chick embryo heart. *Biorheology*. 3:59–62, 1966.

31. Spitzer A: *The Architecture of Normal and Malformed Hearts: A Phylogenetic Theory of Their Development*. Springfield, IL: Charles C. Thomas; 1951.

32. Gessner IH: Spectrum of congenital cardiac anomalies produced in chick embryos by mechanical interference with cardiogenesis. *Circ Res*. 18:625–33, 1966.

33. Llorca FO: Curvature of the heart: Its first appearance and determination. *Acta Anat*. 77:454–68, 1970.

34. Hirsch EF, Borghard-Erdle AM: The innervation of the human heart. II. The papillary muscles. *Arch Path*. 73: 100–17, 1962.

35. Manasek FJ: Myocardial cell death in the embryonic chick ventricle. *J Embryol Exp Morphol*. 21:271–84, 1969.

36. Patten BM: The development of the heart. In Gould SE, ed. *Pathology of the Heart and Blood Vessels*. Springfield, IL: Charles C. Thomas; 1968.

37. Morse DE: Scanning electron microscopy of the developing septa in the chick heart. In Rosenquist GC, Bergsma D, eds. *Morphogenesis and Malformation of the Cardiovascular System*. New York: Alan R. Liss; 1978.

38. Hudson REB: The human conduction system and its examination. *J Clin Pathol*. 16:492–8, 1963.

39. Goor DA, Edwards JE: The development of the interventricular septum of the human heart: Correlative morphogenetic study. *Chest*. 58:453–82, 1970.

40. Frazer JA: Formation of pars membranacea septi. *J Anat Physiol*. 51:19–29, 1917.

41. Kramer TC: The partitioning of the truncus and conus

and the formation of the membranous portion of the interventricular septum in the human heart. *Am J Anat.* 71:343–79, 1942.

42. Odgers PNB: The development of the pars membranacea septi in the human heart. *J Anat.* 72:247–59, 1938.

43. Spitzer A: Uber die Ursachen und den Mechanismus der Aweiteilung des Wirbeltierherzens. Teil II. *Arch Entrv-Mech Organ.* 47:511–70, 1921.

44. Spitzer A: Uber die Ursachen und den Mechanismus der Zweiteilung des Wirbeltierherzens. Teil I. *Arch Entrv-Mech Organ.* 45:686–725, 1919.

45. Ide F, Amano H: Further studies on the differentiation of the amphibian heart rudiment in tissue culture. *Arch Biol.* 80:443–50, 1969.

46. Shabetai R: Function of the pericardium. In Fowler NO, ed. *The Pericardium in Health and Disease.* Mount Kisco, NY: Futura; 1985.

47. Dbaly J, Ostadal B, Rychter Z: Development of the coronary arteries in rat embryos. *Acta Anat.* 71:209–22, 1968.

48. Licata RH: The human embryonic heart in the ninth week. *Am J Anat.* 94:73–125, 1954.

49. Shaner RF: On the development of the nerves to the mammalian heart. *Anat Rec.* 46:23–40, 1930.

50. Streeter GL: Developmental horizons in human embryos. Description of age groups XV, XVI, XVII and XVIII, being the third issue of a survey of the Carnegie collection. *Carnegie Contrib Embryol.* 32:133–204, 1948.

51. DeHaan RL: Cardiac development. A problem in need of synthesis. *Am J Cardiol.* 25:139–40, 1970.

52. Lieberman M: Physiologic development of impulse conduction in embryonic cardiac tissue. *Am J Cardiol.* 25:279–84, 1970.

53. Amano H, Ide F: Differentiation of the amphibian heart rudiment in tissue culture. *Arch Biol.* 80:19–25, 1969.

54. Adolph EF, Ferarri JM: Adaptation to temperature in heart rates of salamander larvae before cardiac innervation. *Am J Physiol.* 215:124–6, 1968.

55. Glanzer ML, Peaslee MH: Inhibition of heart beat development by chloramphenicol in intact and cardiac bifida explanted chick embryos. *Experientia.* 26:370–1, 1970.

56. Paff GH, Boucek RH, Harrall TC: Observations on the development of the electrocardiogram. *Anat Rec.* 160:575–82, 1968.

57. Patten BM, Kramer TC: The initiation of contraction in the embryonic chick heart. *Am J Anat.* 53:349–76, 1933.

58. Wenink ACG: Development of the human cardiac conducting system. *J Anat.* 121:617–38, 1976.

59. Coraboeuf E, Obrecht-Coutris G, LeDouvarin G: Acetylcholine and the embryonic heart. *Am J Cardiol.* 25:285–91, 1970.

60. Titus JL, Kearney DL: Cardiovascular anatomy. In Garson A, Jr, Bricker JT, McNamara DC, eds. *The Science and Practice of Pediatric Cardiology.* Philadelphia: Lea & Febiger; 1990.

61. Silver MM: Gross examination and structure of the heart. In Silver MD, ed. *Cardiovascular Pathology.* New York: Churchill Livingstone; 1983.

62. Holt JP: The normal pericardium. *Am J Cardiol.* 26:455–65, 1970.

63. Edwards WD: Anatomy of the cardiovascular system. In Spitell JA, Jr, ed. *Clinical Medicine.* Philadelphia: Harper & Row; 1984.

64. James TN, Sherf L, Schlant RC, Silverman ME: Anatomy of the heart. In Hurst JW, ed. *The Heart,* 5th ed. New York: McGraw-Hill; 1982.

65. Hagler DJ, Edwards WD, Seward JB, Tajik AJ: Standardized nomenclature of the ventricular septum and ventricular septal defects with application for two-dimensional echocardiography. *Mayo Clin Proc.* 60:741, 1985.

66. Eckner FAO, Brown BW, Davidson DL, Glagov S: Dimensions of normal human hearts. *Arch Path.* 88:497–507, 1969.

67. James TN: Anatomy of the crista supraventricularis: Its importance for understanding right ventricular function, right ventricular infarction and related conditions. *J Am Col Cardio.* 6:1083, 1985.

68. Titus JL, Kim H-S: Blood vessels and lymphatics. In Kissane JM, ed. *Anderson's Pathology,* 8th ed. St. Louis: CV Mosby; 1985.

69. Walmsley R, Watson H: The outflow tract of the left ventricle. *Brit Heart J.* 28:435–47, 1966.

70. Lam JHC, Ranganathan N, Wigle ED, Silver MD: Morphology of the human mitral valve. I. Chordae tendineae; a new classification. *Circulation.* 41:449–58, 1970.

71. Ranganathan N, Lam JHC, Wigle ED, Silver MD: Morphology of the human mitral valve. II. The valve leaflets. *Circulation.* 41:459–67, 1970.

72. Silverman ME, Hurst JW: The mitral complex. Interaction of the anatomy, physiology and pathology of the annulus, mitral valve leaflets, chordae tendineae and papillary muscles. *Am Heart J.* 76:399–418, 1969.

73. Grimm AF, Katele KV, Kubota R, Whitehorn WV: Relation of sarcomere length and muscle length in resting myocardium. *Am J Physiol.* 218:1412–16, 1970.

74. Davis PKB, Kinmouth JB: The movements of the annulus of the mitral valve. *J Cardiovasc Surg.* 4:427–31, 1963.

75. Silver MD, Lam JHC, Ranganathan N, Wigle ED: Morphology of the human tricuspid valve. *Circulation.* 43:333–48, 1971.

76. Zimmerman KG, Paplanus SH, Dong S, Nagle RB: Congenital blood cysts of the heart valves. *Hum Pathol.* 14:699, 1983.

77. Enoch BA: Quadricuspid pulmonary valve. *Brit Heart J.* 30:67–9, 1968.

78. Hurwitz LE, Roberts WC: Quadricuspid semilunar valve. *Am J Cardiol.* 31:623–6, 1973.

79. Peretz DI, Changfoot GH, Gourlay R: Four-cusped aortic valve with significant hemodynamic abnormality. *Am J Cardiol.* 23:291–3, 1969.

80. Roberts WC: The congenitally bicuspid aortic valve. *Am J Cardiol.* 26:72–83, 1970.

81. Gross L: *The Blood Supply to the Heart.* New York: Hoeber; 1921.

82. Schlesinger MJ, Zoll PM, Wessler S: The conus artery: A third coronary artery. *Am Heart J.* 38:823–36, 1949.

83. Farrer-Brown G: Vascular pattern of myocardium of right ventricle of human heart. *Brit Heart J.* 30:679–86, 1968.

84. Estes EH, Entman ML, Dixon H, Hackel DB: Vascular

supply of the left ventricular wall. *Am Heart J*. 71:58–67, 1966.

85. Arluk DJ, Rhodin JA: The ultrastructure of calf heart conducting fibers with special reference to nexuses and their dysfunction. *J Ultrastruct Res*. 49:11–23, 1974.

86. Polacek P: Relation of myocardial bridges and loops on the coronary arteries to coronary occlusions. *Am Heart J*. 61:44–52, 1961.

87. Zechmeister A, Polacek P: The incidence of myocardial bridges and loops relation to the various types of ramifications of the coronary arteries. *Folia Morphol*. 15: 34–44, 1967.

88. Thebesius AC: *Dissertatio Medica de Circulo Sanguinis in Corde. Editio Nova Correctior*. Lugduni Bataborum apud Joh. Arnold; 1716, p. 31.

89. Johnson RA, Blake TM: Lymphatics of the heart. *Circulation*. 33:137–42, 1966.

90. Wearn JT, Mettier SR, Klump TG, Zschiesche LJ: The nature of the vascular communications between the coronary arteries and the chambers of the heart. *Am Heart J*. 9:143–74, 1933.

91. Bradham RR, Parker EF, Barrington BA, Jr, Webb CM, Stallworth JM: The cardiac lymphatics. *Ann Surg*. 171: 899–902, 1970.

92. Johnson RA: The lymphatic system of the heart. *Lymphology*. 2:95–108, 1969.

93. Miller AJ: *Lymphatics of the Heart*. New York: Raven Press; 1982.

94. Lannigan RA, Zaki SA: Ultrastructure of the normal atrial endocardium. *Brit Heart J*. 28:785–95, 1966.

95. Baroldi G, Falzi G, Lampertico P: The nuclear patterns of the cardiac muscle fibers. *Cardiologia*. 51:109–23, 1967.

96. Mowry RW, Bangle R, Jr: Histochemically demonstrable glycogen in the human heart. *Am J Path*. 27:611–26, 1951.

97. Gross L, Kugel MA: Topographic anatomy and histology of the valves in the human heart. *Am J Pathol*. 7:445–74, 1931.

98. Clarke JA: An X-ray microscopic study of the blood supply to the valves of the human heart. *Brit Heart J*. 27: 420–3, 1965.

99. Duran CMG, Gunning AJ: The vascularization of the heart valves: A comparative study. *Cardiovasc Res*. 2: 290–6, 1968.

100. Bayne-Jones S: The blood vessels of the heart valve. *Am J Anat*. 21:449–62, 1917.

101. Koletsky S: Gross vascularity of the mitral valve as a stigma of rheumatic heart disease. *Am J Path*. 22: 351–67, 1946.

102. Kugel MA, Gross L: Gross and microscopical anatomy of the blood vessels in the valves of the human heart. *Am Heart J*. 1:304–14, 1926.

103. Wearn JT, Bromer AW, Zschiesche LJ: The incidence of blood vessels in human heart valves. *Am Heart J*. 11: 22–33, 1936.

104. Goldberg GM, Kozenitzky: The lymphatics of the heart in normal and pathological states. *Path Microbiol*. 30: 738–41, 1967.

105. Kline IK: Lymphatic pathways in the heart. *Arch Path*. 88:638–44, 1969.

106. Fedyai VV: Age changes in the intrinsic lymphatics of the heart. *Fed Proc*. 25:177–80, 1966.

107. Ferrans VJ, Thiedemann K-U: Ultrastructure of the normal heart. In Silver MD, ed. *Cardiovascular Pathology*. New York: Churchill Livingstone; 1983.

108. Spiro D, Spotnitz H, Sonneblick EH: The relation of cardiac fine structure to function. In Gould SE, ed. *Pathology of the Heart and Blood Vessels*. Springfield, IL: Charles C. Thomas; 1968.

109. Melax H, Leeson TS: Fine structure of developing and adult intercalated discs in rat heart. *Cardiovasc Res*. 3: 261–7, 1969.

110. Sjostrand FS, Andersson-Cedergren E, Dewey MM: The ultrastructure of the intercalated discs of frog, mouse and guinea pig cardiac muscle. *J Ultrastruct Res*. 1: 271–87, 1958.

111. Stenger RJ, Spiro D: The ultrastructure of mammalian cardiac muscle. *J Biophysiol Biochem*. 9:325–52, 1961.

112. Green DE, Goldberger RF: Pathways of metabolism in heart muscle. *Am J Med*. 30:666–78, 1961.

113. Lehninger AL: *The Mitochondrion*. New York: Benjamin; 1964.

114. Huang DY: Electron microscopic study of the development of heart muscle of the frog rana pipiens. *J Ultrastruct Res*. 20:211–26, 1967.

115. Hagopian M, Spiro D: Derivation of the Z line in the embryonic chick heart. *J Cell Biol*. 44:683–7, 1970.

116. Huxley HE: The double array of filaments in cross-striated muscle. *J Biophysiol Biochem*. 3:631–47, 1957.

117. Davies MJ, Anderson RH, Becker AE: *The Conduction System of the Heart*. London: Butterworths; 1983.

118. Keith A, Flack MW: The auriculo-ventricular bundle of the human heart. *Lancet*. 2:359–64, 1906.

119. Kistin AD: Observations on the anatomy of the atrioventricular bundle (bundle of His) and the question of other muscular atrioventricular connections in normal human hearts. *Am Heart J*. 37:849–67, 1949.

120. Hirsch EF: Innervation of the human heart. III. The conductive system. *Arch Path*. 74:427–39, 1962.

121. Hirsch EF, Borghard-Erdle AM: The terminal innervation of the heart. I. Quantitative correlations of the myocardial catecholamines with the perimysial plexus in normal cardiac tissues of the rabbit and dog and in the heart of the dog after total extrinsic denervation. *Arch Path*. 76:677–92, 1963.

122. Janes RD, Brandys JC, Hopkins DA, et al.: Anatomy of extrinsic cardiac nerves and ganglia. *Am J Cardiol*. 57:299, 1986.

123. Hort W: The normal heart of the fetus and its metamorphosis in the transition period. In Cassels DE, ed. *The Heart and Circulation in the Newborn and Infant*. New York: Grune & Stratton; 1966.

124. Rakusan K: Cardiac growth, maturation and aging. In Zak R, ed. *Growth of the Heart in Health and Disease*. New York: Raven; 1984.

125. Ferrans VJ: Cardiac hypertrophy: Morphologic aspects. In Zak R, ed. *Growth of the Heart in Health and Disease*. New York: Raven Press; 1984.

CHAPTER THREE

Fetal and Neonatal Cardiac Physiology

Tony L. Creazzo

Approximately 15% of pregnancies are lost because of spontaneous abortions after implantation (see review by Copp[1]). A recent survey of 54 in utero lethal gene knockouts and mutations in mouse suggests that the majority of this loss probably results from defects of the cardiovascular system.[1] This is not surprising considering that other major organ systems, such as the musculoskeletal and central nervous systems, are generally not essential for in utero life. It is well known that even fetuses with the most severe central nervous system defects can come to full term. From numerous studies in experimental animal models, it has become evident that the physiology of the early developing heart is different from later stages and adult. Therefore, it is important to consider both normal development of the basic mechanisms of cardiovascular physiology and what happens when these mechanisms are perturbed either by a genetic defect or some environmental insult.

In organizing this chapter, I have used the three paradigms of analysis of cardiac function suggested by Katz in his excellent book on heart physiology.[2] These are *cell biochemistry* and *biophysics, gene expression,* and *organ physiology.* Over the course of this discussion, it should become apparent to the reader that key cellular systems critical for normal heart function operate quite differently early in development than at later times. This is particularly true of those mechanisms involved in Ca^{2+} handling from beat to beat. Accordingly, it will also become apparent that the pharmacology of drugs commonly used in the treatment of heart disease may affect the fetus and neonate differently from the adult. Moreover, I introduce the concept that the normal development of basic cellular mechanisms of cardiac myocytes can be altered by seemingly unrelated structural defects of the heart.

EXPERIMENTAL MODELS OF HEART DEVELOPMENT

The heart is unique in that it must undergo considerable complex morphologic and functional development while supplying oxygen to the developing embryo. For obvious reasons, much of the biochemistry and biophysics as well as the morphology of heart development have been studied most rigorously in avian species, particularly, the chick embryo. This is especially true of the very early events in heart development. Chick embryos are easily accessed for experimental manipulation; staging of developmental periods is more precise; and they are inexpensive and easily maintained. In the chick, development of various systems in the heart and muscle appears to be somewhat accelerated compared with mammals. This is not surprising considering that the chick must emerge on its own from its shell and must be able to function autonomously very quickly in order to survive. Some neonatal mammalian species have been used in studies of later development, including rat, rabbit, and now the mouse. In these species, the pups are quite helpless at birth and development of mechanisms involved in cardiac contractility is much delayed compared with humans. The rate of development in humans appears to fall somewhere between the chick and these mammalian species. It is important to note that regardless of variations in the rate of development, the fundamental mechanisms of contractility are the same. The specific proteins involved are highly conserved among these species, with a very high degree of amino acid sequence identity.

With the advent of transgenic technology, the mouse has become the most important player with regard to some aspects of heart development. This is especially true of studies of regulatory genes that pertain to very early heart muscle development and genes for myosin and other contractile elements (see Robbins[3]). Most functional studies of transgenic mice have utilized the Langendorf perfused heart attached to a force transducer. Such work is difficult because of the very small size of the hearts (except for lamb) and is feasible only in neonatal animals and older. Because of the very small size of embryonic mouse hearts ($<$ 1 mm) and the scant amount of tissue available, there are almost no published biochemical and biophysical studies of either early embryonic or later fetal heart development. Gene expression studies of proteins other than contractile proteins are also severely lacking. A concept that bears some consideration is that there may be a tendency in adult cardiac heart disease for reexpression of fetal isoforms of proteins important in cardiac contractility. It is generally not known how expression of fetal isoforms differs from adult in terms of cardiac function. There is therefore a need for increased study of cardiac function in relationship to isoform expression during normal development.

It should be apparent from this discussion that work on the timing of functional heart development has been done across a number of species that have different rates of development for the mechanisms involved. Therefore, for the remainder of this chapter, discussion of the relative importance of these mechanisms during development utilizes a generalized timing scheme such as "early" or "late" except where more precise information is available regarding human development.

CARDIAC MYOCYTE PHYSIOLOGY

Cardiac Excitation–Contraction (EC) Coupling

Adult Cardiac EC Coupling

Calcium ion (Ca^{2+}) binding to troponin C is the first step in activation of the contractile apparatus during systole. Thus, there is a transient rise followed by a decline in cytosolic Ca^{2+} with each heart beat, which involves a number of steps that are collectively known as excitation–contraction (EC) coupling. In general, *EC coupling is defined as all the steps between depolarization of the surface membrane and the subsequent release and eventual reuptake of Ca^{2+} by the sarcoplasmic reticulum (SR) and extrusion by Na^+–Ca^+ exchange.* The steps in the EC coupling process of adult cardiac muscle are well described (reviewed by Bers[4]; see Figure 3–1). Briefly, sudden depolarization of the sarcolemma leads to activation of voltage-gated Ca^{2+} channels to produce a Ca^{2+} current (I_{Ca}) that peaks within 2 to 5 ms of depolarization. This current provides net Ca^{2+} entry into the myocyte for approximately 30 ms, after which net Ca^{2+} extrusion occurs via Na^+–Ca^{2+} exchange. Contraction does not occur in

the absence of I_{Ca}, indicating that this current is essential for the EC coupling process. It is thought that I_{Ca} increases the concentration of Ca^{2+} in the vicinity of the terminal cisternae of the SR, which causes release of Ca^{2+} from large stores in the SR. This process is referred to as Ca^{2+}-induced Ca^{2+} release (CICR) and takes place through ryanodine receptor/Ca^{2+} release channels; these appear to be identical to the feet structures that span the space between the sarcolemma and the junctional SR. These channels are in close juxtaposition with the dihydropyridine (DHP)-sensitive L-type Ca^{2+} channels of the sarcolemma. The DHP receptor in adult cardiac muscle appears to function strictly as a Ca^{2+} channel and not as a voltage sensor that directly controls release of Ca^{2+} from the SR, as it does in skeletal muscle. Elevated intracellular Ca^{2+} activates the Ca^{2+}-ATPase of the longitudinal SR, resulting in increased Ca^{2+} uptake, which, along with Na^+–Ca^{2+} exchange, leads to a return of intracellular Ca^{2+} to control levels and relaxation of the heart muscle. Typically, 80% or more of the Ca^{2+} needed for contraction comes from the SR, whereas the rest comes from the extracellular space primarily via Ca^{2+} channels.

Embryonic and Fetal EC Coupling

Present information indicates that the general mechanisms involved in EC coupling for adult myocardium just described are qualitatively similar in developing cardiac muscle. There are some important differences that merit consideration. Embryonic myocytes are small, are mononucleated, lack t-tubules, and have poor myofibrillar organization compared with adult myocytes. This relatively poor cytoplasmic organization is to be expected considering that myocytes have to contract to keep the embryo alive as well as to proliferate. t-Tubule formation, binucleation, and hypertrophy caused by increased myofibrillar organization and growth are probably postnatal events for most mammals. In adult cardiac myocytes, the structural arrangement of the SR and the specialized junctions that form with t-tubules and the surface plasma membrane, although complex, have been well described, and much is known of the functional mechanisms. However, in the embryo, SR development occurs gradually over an extended period of time and the mechanisms that regulate this development are not known. Since t-tubules are not present, SR junctions are first formed on the surface plasma membrane. For a review of the current state of knowledge of this process see Flucher and Franzini-Armstrong.[5] Ca^{2+} channels, in contrast, are present when myocytes first begin to beat in the cardiogenic plate and before heart tube formation.[6,7] *The major difference in cardiac EC coupling between embryo and adult hearts is the primary dependence on extracellular Ca^{2+} for contraction during development.* Adult

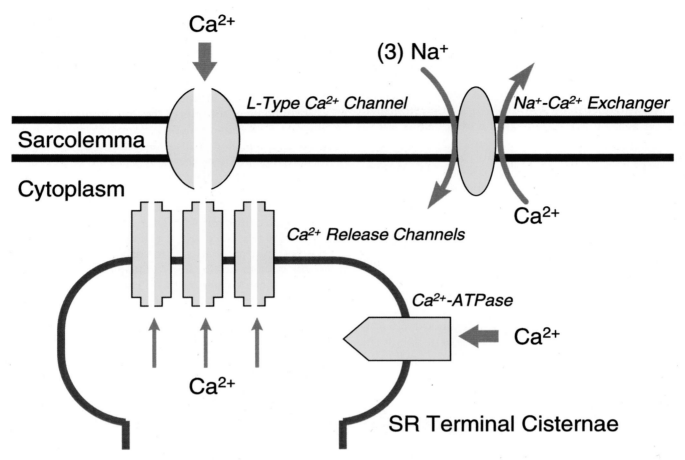

Figure 3–1. Cardiac excitation–contraction coupling. The diagram illustrates the primary mechanism for raising and lowering cytosolic Ca^{2+} during the heart beat. Note that the L-type Ca^{2+} channels in the sarcolemma and the Ca^{2+}-release channels of the terminal cisterna of sarcoplasmic reticulum (SR) are closely opposed. Ca^{2+} entry from T-type Ca^{2+} channels, reversal of the Na^+–Ca^{2+} exchange during peak membrane depolarization in systole, and other Ca^{2+} sources are presumed not to be as effective as the L-type channel in initiating Ca^{2+}-induced Ca^{2+} release from the SR (CICR). Ca^{2+} is removed from the cytosol primarily by the SR Ca^{2+}-ATPase and the Na^+ –Ca^{2+} exchanger, which normally operates in the forward mode, extruding one Ca^{2+} for every three Na^+ coming into the cell. In fetal and newborn hearts, t-tubules are lacking and couplings of the SR with the sarcolemma are at the surface membrane; however, SR is typically sparse in fetal hearts. The obvious implication is that most of the Ca^{2+} entering during systole comes from the extracellular space instead of the SR, as occurs in mature hearts. Further, other sources of extracellular Ca^{2+}, such as from T-type channels and reverse Na^+–Ca^{2+} exchange, may assume greater importance in initiating contraction. Finally, a greater percentage of the systolic Ca^{2+} must be extruded through the Na^+–Ca^{2+} exchanger since SR Ca^{2+}-ATPase is lacking.

myocytes require Ca^{2+} to trigger release from an abundant SR. However, only a small amount of extracellular Ca^{2+} is needed to trigger a much larger cascade from the SR.[4] In embryonic and fetal hearts, most of the Ca^{2+} needed for contraction comes from the extracellular space via sarcolemmal Ca^{2+} channels.[4,5,8] The obvious implication is that embryonic, fetal, and perhaps postnatal hearts are more sensitive to the vast array of drugs in clinical use today that affect Ca^{2+} channel ac-

tivity. Moreover, there is an added consideration associated with early embryonic hearts. This is that the depolarization phase of the cardiac action potential in early heart development is largely Ca^{2+} dependent.[8,9] Na^+ channels are either absent or in an inactive state.[10] However, depolarization is inhibited and can be blocked completely by Ca^{2+} channel blockers.[9]

Following the rise in cytosolic Ca^{2+} contraction during systole, it is necessary to remove the Ca^{2+} in order for the heart muscle to relax for ventricular filling during diastole. There are primarily three mechanisms for removing Ca^{2+} (reviewed in Bers[4]). These are the plasma membrane or sarcolemma Ca^{2+}-ATPase, the SR Ca^{2+}-ATPase, and the Na^+–Ca^{2+} exchanger. Mitochondria can store and release Ca^{2+} but this mechanism is too slow to contribute noticeably to the Ca^{2+} transient during a single beat. Although the sarcolemmal Ca^{2+}-ATPase is sufficient to keep the cytosolic Ca^{2+} low in most cell types, it cannot handle the rapid, large increase associated with a heartbeat. In fact, 80% or more of the Ca^{2+} that is not removed by the SR Ca^{2+}-ATPase is extruded into the extracellular space via the Na^+–Ca^{2+} exchange through the sarcolemma. *Because the SR is sparse or absent in the developing myocardium, a second major difference between embryonic and adult EC coupling is that Ca^{2+} removal during relaxation depends largely on the Na^+–Ca^{2+} exchanger.* Accordingly, there is a decline in the percentage of the systolic Ca^{2+} subject to extrusion by Na^+–Ca^{2+} exchange in parallel with an increasing proportion of Ca^{2+} sequestered by the SR as development proceeds.

Major Proteins in EC Coupling

There are a number of key proteins that play major roles in cardiac EC coupling. These include the Ca^{2+} channels, the SR Ca^{2+}-release channel, the SR Ca^{2+}-ATPase, the Na^+–Ca^{2+} exchanger, and calsequestrin. Except for calsequestrin, these have already been mentioned, at least briefly, in the preceding discussion. These proteins have all been cloned and sequenced in an adult mammalian species and much is known concerning their structure, function, and regulation. There are a number of excellent review articles and books that describe these proteins and their roles in EC coupling in detail.[2,4,11,12] The present discussion is confined to just a few pertinent details relevant to heart development.

L-type Ca²⁺ Channels

The voltage-activated cardiac L-type Ca^{2+} channel is all important in adult heart for providing trigger Ca^{2+} for CICR from the SR. These channels form dense, ordered arrays at junctional sites of the sarcolemma with the SR. It, like other Ca^{2+} channels that have been identified and cloned, mostly in the brain, is a relatively large multimeric protein ($\simeq$ 250,000 daltons). It consist of a cardiac-specific $\alpha 1c$ subunit and β and $\alpha 2$-δ subunits. The $\alpha 1c$ subunit spans the sarcolemma and contains the Ca^{2+} conducting pore. It contains the voltage sensor for membrane depolarization and allosterically coupled binding sites for dihydropyridines, such as nifedipine; phenylalkamines, such as verapamil; and benzodiazapines. The other subunits are essential for normal channel activity because the $\alpha 1c$ subunit functions poorly in their absence. For an excellent and thorough review of Ca^{2+} channel structure and function see McDonald et al.[13] Although there is only a single adult form of $\alpha 1c$, there appears to be one or more fetal isoforms expressed during development.[14] There are likely to be fetal isoforms of the other subunits as well. Whether fetal forms function differently and have different pharmacologies from the adult form remains to be determined. There are several physiologic observations from embryonic chick heart that suggest that there may be relevant differences. These are: (1) The Ca^{2+} current density appears to be larger early in development compared with later development; (2) the probability that the channel will open with depolarization is significantly greater in early development; and (3) the number of dihydropyridine receptors ($\alpha 1c$ subunits) that can be detected with radiolabeled binding is much greater than the number of functional or physiologically detectable channels.[15-18]

T-type Ca²⁺ Channels

Another Ca^{2+} channel, the T-type Ca^{2+} channel, is found in nodal cells, atrial myocytes, and the conducting system, but not in ventricular myocytes. This current appears to be characteristic of myocytes that are capable of generating spontaneous action potentials (i.e., pacemaking myocytes).[13] The gene for this channel has not been cloned in heart and the protein has not been purified. Nothing is known of its structure, nor are there any known specific T-type Ca^{2+} channel agonists or antagonists. It is activated at more hyperpolarized potentials and has faster kinetics than the L-type channel. Its contribution to the total Ca^{2+} current tends to be minor[13,19] and probably does not contribute significantly to CICR because, unlike the L-type channel, it apparently lacks the close association with Ca^{2+} release channels in SR. T-type channels are present in ventricular myocytes, probably throughout most heart development, although expression declines and they are absent at late stages.[20-23] This is consistent with the observation that embryonic ventricular myocytes are capable of pacing, although the exact role of this channel in pacing is not well understood. T-type Ca^{2+} channels may contribute to EC coupling during early development when the SR is sparse or absent, but this has not been studied.

The SR Ca²⁺-Release Channel

The cardiac Ca^{2+}-release channel or the ryanodine receptor, as it is commonly called because of a binding site for this plant alkaloid, is present in the membranes of terminal dilations of the SR, which form junctions with regions of the sarcolemma that contain densely packed arrays of L-type Ca^{2+} channels.[2,4,24] Most importantly, the Ca^{2+}-release channel has a Ca^{2+} binding site and is activated by Ca^{2+} entering via the L-type channel (i.e., CICR). There are only a few nanometers of space separating the release channel from the voltage-activated Ca^{2+} channel; therefore, the release channel "sees" a very high concentration of Ca^{2+} in this restricted space following membrane depolarization. The release channel is also activated by millimolar concentrations of caffeine. The protein is a tetramer with four identical subunits, each weighing 550,000 daltons. This is the largest known ion channel and is readily visible with transmission electron microscopy. An array of these proteins resembles feet walking along the t-tubule, so microscopists have whimsically labeled it the "foot" protein. In development, foot proteins begin to appear in the SR membrane as soon as the SR junction with the sarcolemma forms.[5,25] These slowly accumulate, simultaneously with accumulation of L-type channels in overlying patches in the sarcolemma, until the SR junctional membrane is densely packed with foot proteins and is considered mature. At present, it is not known whether there is expression of fetal isoforms of the ryanodine receptor.

SR Ca^{2+}-ATPase

SR Ca^{2+}-ATPase activity becomes detectable in the developing heart coincident with the time of appearance of the SR junctional complexes.[5] The genes for a number of membrane Ca^{2+}-ATPases have been cloned and the cardiac-specific gene has been labeled *SERCA2*. Study of *SERCA2* has been facilitated by the availability of specific antagonists and much is known of its role in EC coupling.[2,4,5] As expected, the importance of this protein in removing Ca^{2+} from the cytoplasm during relaxation increases as the proportion of the SR contribution to the rise in cytosolic Ca^{2+} during systole increases with development. A second inhibitory protein, phospholamban, exists in close association with the *SERCA2*. Inhibition of the ATPase activity by phospholamban is removed by cyclic andenosine monophosphate (cAMP)-dependent phosphorylation such as that following β-adrenergic receptor stimulation. Phospholamban activity is detectable along with the earliest detection of *SERCA2*.[26-28] The phospholamban gene has been cloned; however, as with *SERCA2*, it is not known whether fetal isoforms exist.

Na^+–Ca^{2+} Exchange

Na^+–Ca^{2+} exchange activity is a potent mechanism for extruding Ca^{2+} in both adult and developing hearts.[5,29] Obviously, its importance in EC coupling in the developing heart, where SR is sparse, is much more significant. Although the gene for this protein has been cloned, study of its physiologic role has been difficult. Specific antagonists for its activity have only recently become available; however, their use is problematic. Study is further complicated by the fact that this protein is always "on." Its activity is highly dependent on the electrochemical gradients for both Na^+ and Ca^{2+}. When there is high cytosolic Ca^{2+} and the membrane is depolarized, such as during peak systole, the Na^+–Ca^{2+} exchange is reversed and it becomes a mechanism for further raising cytosolic Ca^{2+}. This has led to considerable controversy concerning its role in EC coupling. In adult hearts, it seems unlikely that Na^+–Ca^{2+} exchange contributes significantly to CICR since the L-type Ca^{2+} channel appears to have preferential access to the Ca^{2+}-release channel. However, in the embryonic heart, where SR is sparse and the myocytes are relatively small, reverse Na^+–Ca^{2+} exchange could contribute significantly to the Ca^{2+} transient.[27,30] As yet, this hypothesis has not been directly tested.

Calsequestrin

Calsequestrin is a low-affinity Ca^{2+}-binding protein localized to the terminal dilations of junctional SR.[4,5] It is readily detectable by electron microscopy as a follicular density within the SR. Its role is to increase the Ca^{2+} storage capacity of the SR. In heart development, its appearance in the SR is slightly delayed but is detectable shortly after the appearance of foot proteins. The implication is that the early SR cannot store as much Ca^{2+} as more mature SR. This may result in a smaller SR contribution to the Ca^{2+} transient, and the SR can be more easily depleted of its Ca^{2+} store. However, this hypothesis has not been tested.

Action Potentials

Cardiac action potentials in adults have been well described in a number of texts and are not discussed in detail here (see Katz[2] or Fozzard and Arnsdorf[31] for examples and Figure 3–2). For the most part, action potentials in the developing heart are similar to those in the adult. However, the earlier in development one looks, the more the electrical activity of myocytes, including those in the ventricles and certainly earlier in the primitive heart tube, resembles that in myocytes of the adult sinoatrial (SA) node[8] (Figure 3–2). *Indeed, it is fair to say that SA nodal myocytes are in essence embryonic cardiac myocytes.* Like embryonic myocytes, nodal cells are small; they lack t-tubules, their myofibrils are not well organized, and they are spontaneously active. The action potentials of early embryonic myocytes and SA nodal cells have a much slower rate of rise (slow dV/dT, where V is voltage and T is time) and the diastolic potential is more depolarized compared with a mature ventricular myocyte. The dV/dT is slow because voltage-activated Na^+ channels either are absent or are in an inactive state.[10] In the earliest embryonic myocytes, therefore, the rising phase of the ac-

Figure 3–2. Idealized action potentials (APs) from an early embryonic myocyte and an older ventricular myocyte. Embryonic myocytes from the early stages of heart development (e.g., heart tube stage and for a short time after) are capable of spontaneous activity and, therefore, APs resemble those measured in the pacemaking sinoatrial node myocytes of the adult heart. These include a slow diastolic depolarization and a slow upstroke velocity in the first phase of the AP. Also, the peak of the action potential is at a lower potential compared with the mature ventricular AP. See the text for a brief discussion of the ionic basis for these differences. The membrane potential is given in millivolts (mV).

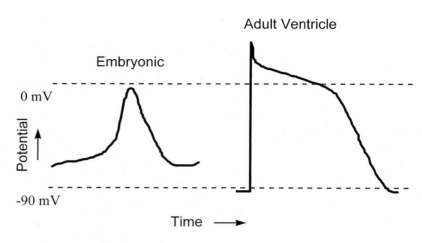

tion potential depends solely on the voltage-dependent activity of L- and T-type Ca^{2+} channels. These action potentials are not affected by Na^+ channel blockers but can be completely inhibited by blocking Ca^{2+} channel activity. The more depolarized diastolic membrane potential is due to poor K^+ permeability resulting from the presence of few background K^+ channels. Thus, the diastolic potential is shifted away from the K^+ equilibrium potential (approximately -95 mV to about -60 to -50 mV).[9,32,33] This brings the membrane potential closer to the activation range for Ca^{2+} channels, especially the T-type channels, which activate at more depolarized potential than the Na^+ channel. In the chick embryo, essentially all of the myocytes in the primitive heart tube and early ventricles beat spontaneously when isolated in cell culture. The percentage of beating myocytes isolated from the ventricles decreases with development such that by midgestation in the chick, spontaneously beating ventricular myocytes are not observed. The ionic basis for the pacemaking diastolic depolarization in spontaneously active cardiac myocytes is controversial and has not been definitively established. Essentially, there is a net inward pacemaking current, probably carried by Na^+ coupled with a slow turning off of a repolarizing K^+ current (I_K). The inward current results either from an as yet unidentified background Na^+ current or from a recently characterized inward current, generally referred to as I_f, which is activated on repolarization of the myocyte. For helpful discussions of the mechanisms of pacemaking, see reviews by Baumgarten & Fozzard[34] and DiFrancesco.[35]

THE CONTRACTILE APPARATUS

During early development of the myocardium, there is a paucity of myofibrils and those that are present are not aligned. Later in development, myofibrils are abundant and aligned.[9,36] In development, there are signifi-

cant changes in the major contractile proteins of the heart which influence the contractile process (see review by Swynghedauw[37]). The study of these changes has been complicated by the fact that differentiation is not synchronous and mitosis can continue while the contractile proteins appear. Myocytes expressing different protein isoforms can be found side by side in the developing myocardium. Nonetheless, much is known and the key points are discussed below.

The contractile apparatus in adult cardiac tissue has been well studied and much is known regarding its structure, biophysics, and molecular biology. The basic contractile mechanisms have been known for many years and are very well described in medical histology and cell biology textbooks. For more detailed consideration, there are a number of excellent books and review articles available, a few of which are recommended here for further reading.[2,12,37] Whereas studies of cardiac function in relationship to the contractile apparatus are lacking, there is good information available on the development of the major contractile proteins. It should be noted that with the advent of transgenic mouse technology, much has been learned recently about the regulation of cardiac gene expression, especially in early development and with respect to the myosin genes. Discussion of gene regulation is beyond the scope of this chapter (see review by Robbins[3]). The present discussion is confined to changes in expression of the major contractile proteins that occur with development and the possible effects of developmental changes on cardiac contractility. It should be noted that expression of myosin and other contractile protein isoforms varies with disease states and that these changes are suggestive of a reactivation of a fetal developmental program of isoform expression.

There are essentially six proteins that are involved in contraction of striated muscle and they are the primary constituents of the sarcomeres, the fundamental units of contraction. The interactions of these proteins require Ca^{2+} and hydrolysis of ATP to generate force. Although there are some exceptions, contractile proteins exhibit more tissue specificity than species specificity.[37] The contractile proteins and their interactions and tissue specificity, along with developmental considerations, are discussed next.

Myosin

Adult Structure and Function

The myosin molecule consist of two heavy chains and two pairs of light chains, with a total molecular weight of about 450,000 daltons. These subunits are members of multigene families.[2,37] The bulk of the protein is made up of the two heavy chain subunits (MHCs), which are the major determinants of contractile AT-Pase activity and the velocity of shortening in living muscle. Each heavy chain consists of a filamentous tail, which lends rigidity to the structure, and a globular head, which pivots or hinges on the tail and contains the site for ATPase activity. There are two heavy chain genes, α and β, and the atria and ventricles each have their own specific set. The α and β heavy chains have fast and slow ATPase activity, respectively. Accordingly, there are three ventricular myosin isoforms: V1 and V2 consist of $\alpha\alpha$ and $\beta\beta$ heavy chains, respectively, and a V3 myosin consists of $\alpha\beta$ heavy chains, which typically exist in smaller amounts than V1 and V2. V1, V2, and V3 have fast, intermediate, and slow ATPase activities, respectively. The ratios of these three isoforms present in ventricles correlates with heart rate (speed of myocyte shortening) in species. Rats and mice, with very fast heart rates, have a high proportion of V1. Intermediate ventricles, such as those in rabbits, have a high proportion of V3. Humans and larger animals have little or no V1. An intermediate $\alpha\beta$ isoform, corresponding to V3, does not exist in atria. A1 and A2 forms in the atria consist of $\alpha\alpha$ and $\beta\beta$ combinations with very fast and slow ATPase activities, respectively. A1 predominates in most mammalian atria.

There are three myosin light chains (MLCs) found in human ventricles, MLC1–MLC3. MLC2 can be phosphorlyated by calcium and calmodulin-dependent protein kinases, and they amply force development during systole. Phosphorylation of MLC2 probably serves to amplify force development during systole when the cytosolic calcium level is high. MLC1 and MLC3 are alternative splice products from the same gene and may contribute to some of the biologic variability among species. Different light chain genes are found in the atria and ventricles. The adult atrium contains mostly MLC2.

Developmental Changes in Myosin

Myosin is probably the earliest of the key contractile proteins to be expressed in the developing heart and can be found in the heart anlagen before formation of the primitive heart tube.[38,39] In the chick embryo, myosin is detected within 6 h of commitment of mesodermal cells to the cardiac myocyte lineage.[39] Interestingly, myocytes begin beating even before sarcomeres and the striated organization of myosin is observed.[38] In rodent ventricle, there is a shift from the V3 to the V1 (slow to fast) form of MHC, which is complete by late fetal life (see Swynghedauw[37] for a review of MHC and MLC expression during development). In larger animals, including humans, V3 is also the predominant isoform expressed in late fetal life; however, V1 is transiently expressed after birth, with V3 becoming the most abundant isoform in adults. The shift to the A1 (fast) isoform in atria probably occurs very early during development in most species, but this has not been well investigated. Rat and fetal human ventricles and atria contain an embryonic MLC isoform that is nonphosphorylatable and appears identical to that observed in fetal skeletal muscle. Phosphorylatable isoforms appear after birth in the ventricles, whereas expression of the fetal isoform is maintained in atria and the conductive Purkinje tissue.

Actin

Actin has a highly conserved structure and is found in all eukaryotic cells. It can exist independently as "globular" G-actin (41,700 daltons) but readily polymerizes in the presence of cations (salts) and ATP to form "fibrous" F-actin. The two most important biologic properties of actin are that it activates myosin ATPase and that it interacts physiochemically with myosin. The F-actin polymer, along with tropomyosin and the troponin complex, constitutes the thin filament component of the sarcomere. In the hearts of small mammals there are two isoforms. The α-skeletal actin is present during fetal life and this is replaced by α-cardiac actin in adult. Human hearts contain mainly α-cardiac actin along with a small amount of skeletal α-actin (reviewed by Katz[2]).

Tropomyosin

The most important function of tropomyosin is its ability, along with troponin, to respond to the calcium signal during systole and to activate the actin–myosin interactions responsible for muscle contraction. It binds stoichiometrically with F-actin and, in this capacity, adds rigidity to the thin filament. The tropomyosin molecule exists as either a homodimer or a heterodimer containing either or both of two isoforms, α and β, each with a molecular weight of 34,000 daltons. Tropomyosin in the hearts of smaller animals is made up mostly of $\alpha2$ dimers, whereas the hearts of larger mammals contain significant amounts of the β subunit. Roughly equal proportions of α and β isoforms exist in adult human atria and ventricles. The proportion of the β isoform is less in the fetus but increases with development. Interestingly, the content of the β isoform in a number of species and developmental stages appears inversely correlated with heart rate (reviewed by Katz[2]).

The Troponin Complex

The troponin complex consist of three proteins, troponin C, I, and T (TN-C, TN-I, and TN-T). It is the binding of calcium to TN-C during the EC coupling process that initiates a conformational change in tropomyosin and exposes the myosin binding sites on actin. Cardiac TN-C differs from the fast skeletal isoform in that it has lost one of the two low-affinity binding sites for calcium. It is the TN-I component that actually regulates the interaction of tropomyosin with actin. TN-T serves to bind the troponin complex to tropomyosin (reviewed by Katz[2]). TN-C is the same in both atrium and ventricle and does not seem to vary with development. Studies in the mammalian heart suggest that a neonatal form of TN-I may play a role in the relative insensitivity of the neonatal contractile apparatus to acidosis.[40-42] Two isoforms of TN-T are expressed in the developing chick heart.[43] One isoform predominates during early development, and this isoform is gradually replaced by an adult form.[43,44] In both mammalian and avian developing heart, it appears that isoform switching to an adult form of TN-T accounts for the developmental decrease in sensitivity of the cardiac contractile apparatus to calcium.[42,45,46]

CONTRACTILITY, HEMODYNAMICS, AND THE FRANK-STARLING RELATIONSHIP

It has been demonstrated in a number of species that muscular strips from fetal myocardium cannot generate the force produced by strips from adult myocardium.[47] This is true at all muscle lengths along the force–tension curve (or pressure–volume relationships; see Figure 3–3). Much of this diminished contractility is probably attributable to a lower density of functioning contractile units. Other factors, such as those already discussed, undoubtedly play a role as well. These could include differences in function of fetal isoforms of contractile and EC coupling proteins, less organized myofibrillar structure, lower SR content, and lack of t-tubules. In contrast, several animal studies have shown an acute increase in myocardial contractility within the first few days after birth to levels above the adult (discussed in Colan et al.[48]). This has been well demonstrated in newborn lamb, a common model for fetal and newborn heart studies because of size similarity with humans (see discussion by Anderson[49]). A recent Doppler and two-dimensional echocardiographic study in normal

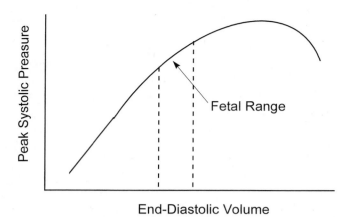

Figure 3–3. An idealized Starling relationship between peak systolic pressure and end-diastolic volume. The heart is able to compensate for increased diastolic filling with an increase in the force of contraction measured as an increase in peak systolic pressure (ascending limb of the curve). If the diastolic volume is too great, then the ability to generate pressure begins to decline (descending limb). The fetal heart appears to operate along a narrow range near the top of the ascending limb of the Starling curve, indicating less of an ability to respond to cardiovascular stress than the adult heart.

human neonates and infants indicates a reduction in contractility and systolic function with growth.[48] This reduced contractility appeared greater than could be accounted for solely by the increased after-load and wall stress that occurs after birth.

Starling's Law

The Frank-Starling relationship, or Starling's law of the heart, is characterized by an increase in systolic pressure with increasing ventricular volume (see Figure 3–3 and descriptions in Katz[2] and Shroff et al.[50]). This is analogous to the increased force (i.e., peak systolic pressure) generated in muscle strips with increased lengthening of sarcomeres (i.e., end-diastolic distention) until the maximum overlap of actin and myosin for cross-bridge interaction is achieved and the A band is at its longest (sarcomere length = 2.2 μm). Obviously, increasing length further will decrease the efficiency of cross-bridge formation and force generation will decrease. This relationship is illustrated by the curve in Figure 3–3, which shows both an ascending and a descending limb with increased volume. The Starling relationship differs from the length–tension curve in that the relationships are between pressure and volume. Second, the high compliance of the myocardium tends to impede high filling levels, which helps protect against overstretching. It is unlikely that the normal ventricle ever dilates to the point that the descending limb of the Starling curve is achieved. Starling's law maintains the balance between the venous return and the cardiac output by increasing stroke volume along the ascending limb when more blood returns to the heart. Thus, the relationship is important in making adjustments to the circulatory system dynamics on a beat-to-beat basis such as occur with changes in body position. More drastic changes in circulatory dynamics, such as with exercise, are mediated by changes in contractility. The result of increased or decreased contractility is the generation of a new Starling curve, with a new maximum higher or lower achievable pressure. As an example, it should be clear from the earlier discussion that interventions that raise or lower cytosolic calcium levels produce corresponding changes in contractility and a new Starling relationship.

Starling's Law in the Developing Heart

The presence of a fetal Frank-Starling relationship has been demonstrated in the developing heart, generally in studies employing the fetal lamb as a model (see excellent reviews by Teital[47] and Anderson[49]). A key observation that has emerged from these studies is that the fetal heart appears to be operating close to the top of the ascending limb of the Starling curve (Figure 3–3). Therefore, there is less reserve in response to circulatory stress. Given the fetal environment (analogous to a "tropical island" according to Teital[47]), a limited Starling response would normally not pose any problems. In agreement with the hemodynamic studies, the isolated fetal myocardium does demonstrate an impaired response to stretch. This diminished response to stretch indicates that some of the impairment of the Starling mechanism is likely to be due to fewer and less mature contractile units. However, there appear to be other contributing and as yet not well-understood factors as well. These include greater myocardial stiffness and differences in the fetal circulation such as a very compliant umbilical–placental unit and an already dilated vascular bed, which limits changes in preload (see discussion by Teital[47]). The marked and immediate increase in left ventricular volume with birth may transiently expend most of the immature heart's Frank-Starling reserve, so that there is even less ability to respond to circulatory stress.[49] The sudden increase in ventricular volume may in some way be related to the rapid increase in contractility seen after birth but this has not been studied.

DEVELOPMENT OF AUTONOMIC REGULATION OF CARDIAC PHYSIOLOGY

The autonomic innervation to the heart exerts profound influence on cardiac physiology. Stimulation by the sympathetic system acts to increase the rate and force of contraction, whereas parasympathetic stimulation serves to antagonize the effects of sympathetic nerves. In the normal heart, there is a balance between these opposing elements. The effects of cholinergic and adrenergic stimulation are achieved primarily by modulation of ion channel activity and SR function in cardiac myocytes. Much is known regarding the cellular mechanisms and these details have been reviewed extensively.[51-55] To facilitate understanding of developmental changes, a brief synopsis of autonomic effects on cardiac myocytes is provided here.

Stimulation of β-adrenergic receptors with norepinephrine (NA) acts on several effector mechanisms via G-protein coupling with adenylate cyclase and subsequent elevation of cytosolic cAMP. The increase in the beat frequency is caused primarily by an increase in the magnitude of the repolarizing K^+ current (I_K; delayed rectifier). This increases the rate of repolarization and thereby shortens the action potential. The pacemaker Na^+ current (I_f) is also increased by NA. This is thought to produce a more rapid pacemaker depolarization. The increase in peak systolic tension is largely due to an increase in the influx of Ca^{2+} during the action potential, caused by increasing the activity of L-type Ca^{2+} channels. Increased influx from sarcolemmal Ca^{2+} channels has an amplifying effect because this Ca^{2+} triggers further release from the SR. In addition, cAMP-dependent phosphorylation of the SR protein phospholamban enhances uptake by the SR Ca^{2+}-ATPase, thereby increasing SR Ca^{2+} stores. This increases the amount of Ca^{2+} available for release and thus further increases cytosolic Ca^{2+} during systole. Muscarinic acetylcholine receptor stimulation from parasympathetic nerves directly antagonizes the effects of sympathetic stimulation by a G-protein–dependent mechanism that inhibits adenylate cyclase. The result is reduced elevation of cytosolic Ca^{2+} from NA stimulation of β-adrenergic receptors and a subsequent decrease in contractility. In addition, cholinergic stimulation, again through a G-protein–dependent mechanism, activates a background K^+ channel, which produces a hyperpolarizing membrane current. The effect is to reduce the beat frequency by slowing the rate of diastolic depolariation. The acetylcholine-activated background K^+ channel does not appear to be present in ventricular myocytes.

In the developing heart, the onset of parasympathetic innervation precedes sympathetic innervation. This has been best characterized in the chick embryo. In the chick, postganglionic parasympathetic neurons and nerve fibers are detected in the heart at about embryonic age day 4 and the system becomes functional at around day 11. This is halfway through the gestation period for the chicken (22 days). Sympathetic fibers are detected at about day 9 and the system is functional by day 16.[56,57] Interestingly, adrenergic and cholinergic receptors and their associated effector mechanisms are present in cardiac myocytes well before autonomic nerve fibers can be found innervating the heart. It is not known why these autonomic receptor–mediated effector mechanisms are present before there is functional innervation. The level of circulating catecholamines in the embryo may be high,[58,59] which could conceivably have a trophic effect on heart growth by interaction with autonomic receptors even in the absence of autonomic innervation. However, this has not been studied. The level of autonomic innervation in the human at birth has been recently documented and has been found to be very similar to the adult pattern and density.[60] Sympathetic fibers are found throughout the atria and ventricular myocardium. Parasympathetic fibers are found throughout the atria but there is a paucity of fibers in the ventricles. This observation is consistent with an absence of muscarinic acetylcholine receptor–activated background K^+ channels in ventricular myocytes that has been seen in other species.[61]

CARDIAC PHYSIOLOGY AND CONGENITAL HEART DISEASE

A number of single-gene mutations of ion channels and contractile proteins have recently been identified in human congenital heart disease. The best characterized of these mutations are associated with long QT disease and familial cardiomyopathy and can have effects on cardiac function ranging from subtle to profound. Other more complex disorders produce structural cardiac defects and may be associated with other, noncardiac defects as well. Probably the best studied of these is the DiGeorge syndrome, which involves abnormalities in the development of neural crest–related structures. The DiGeorge syndrome represents the severest form of a spectrum of defects that has recently been called CATCH 22. CATCH 22 includes *c*ardiac defects, *a*bnormal facies, *t*hymic hypoplasia, *c*left palate, and *h*ypocalcemia, and almost all involve microdeletions of chromosome 22q11.[62,63] Whether abnormal cardiac myocyte physiology is associated with structural cardiac defects is not known. However, it is intriguing that recent studies in animal models of neural crest–related cardiac outflow tract defects indicate that there may be impairment of Ca^{2+}-handling mechanisms in ventricular myocytes from these hearts. Environmental factors undoubtedly can interfere with structural development of the heart but these are poorly understood and are not considered here. The following discussion focuses on the current knowledge of genetic defects with respect to cardiac function.

Inherited Long QT Disease

Inherited long QT disease (LQT) manifests itself in electrocardiogram (ECG) measurements as a prolonga-

tion of the QT interval. LQT can lead to arrhythmias and sudden cardiac death, particularly at a young age. It was generally thought that LQT was the result of an imbalance of the autonomic innervation caused by the overstimulation of the left side of the heart by the sympathetic nervous system. Recently, molecular genetic studies have indicated that the autonomic nervous innervation to the heart is not central to the pathogenesis of autosomal dominant LQT (reviewed by Keating and Sanguinetti[64]). The QT interval reflects the length of the plateau phase of the cardiac action potential and is a useful clinical index of action potential duration. Clearly, ion channel defects that prolong the duration of inward depolarizing membrane currents or decrease outward repolarizing currents increase the action potential duration and are reflected by a prolonged QT interval.

Within the past 2 years three LQT genes have been identified by Keating and others (see review by Keating and Sanguinetti[64]). These are *SCN5A* on chromosome 3, *HERG* on chromosome 7, and *KVLQT1* on chromosome 11. *SCN5A* encodes the α1 or pore-containing subunit of the cardiac Na^+ channel, which produces the fast upstroke and overshoot portion of the cardiac action potential. This protein has been very well characterized in recent years and the gene has been cloned in a number of species.[65] The LQT-associated mutations in *SCN5A* cause a gain of function resulting from destabilization of the inactivation gate of the channel. The result is repetitive channel opening and prolongation of the action potential. The *HERG* gene encodes α subunits that form channels responsible for I_{Kr}, the "rapid" component of the cardiac delayed rectifier or repolarizing potassium current. This current normally contributes to termination of the action potential, but *HERG* mutations result in loss of function in this channel. Despite molecular differences, therefore, the mutations in both *SCN5A* and *HERG* lead to prolongation of the action potential. The physiologic properties of the protein coded by *KVLQT1* are not known; however, sequence analysis suggests that it is a novel type of potassium channel.

LQT can also be acquired. Most commonly, this occurs as a consequence of drug therapy with medications such as certain antiarrhythmics, antihistamines, and antibiotics that can block the *HERG* K^+ channel. These treatments are a mechanism for an induced loss of function of the HERG channel. An understanding of the molecular properties of the HERG and SCN5A can suggest treatments for LQT involving these channels. Individuals with mutations of SCN5A could be treated with sodium channel blockers. Individuals with genetic or acquired LQT involving the HERG channel may be treated with potassium supplementation. Paradoxically, small increases in extracellular K^+ increase the activity of the HERG channel.

Cardiomyopathies

Although most cardiomyopathies are secondary, resulting from hypertension and valvular heart disease, genetic factors are clearly important. Familial hypertrophic cardiomyopathy (FHC), a heterogeneous autosomal dominant disorder, is characterized by thickening of the ventricular walls, impaired relaxation, and reduced ability for the heart to fill.[66,67] Symptoms can range from mild to extreme and there are an estimated 20 to 200 cases per 100,000 people in the United States. Mutations in four genes have been implicated in FHC and all four code for contractile proteins. These are β cardiac myosin heavy chain, a tropomyosin, troponin T, and cardiac binding protein C. It appears that mutations of the myosin gene result in inefficient actin–myosin cross-bridge cycling. The molecular consequences of mutations of the other three contractile genes in FHC are presently unknown.

Dilated cardiomyopathy (DCM) is characterized by enlargement of the cardiac chambers, thinning of the ventricular wall, reduced contractility, heart failure, and death.[67] There are about 37 cases per 100,000 people in the United States, and this disorder is the primary indication for cardiac transplantation. In about 20% to 25% of these cases, genetic factors are key to the pathogenesis. Many of these have been linked to enzymes involved in fatty acid metabolism. Other genetic factors may contribute as well. Discussion of these genetic factors is beyond the scope of this chapter.

Cardiac Myocyte Physiology and Congenital Heart Disease

In adults, pathologic conditions that result in a sustained increase in the hemodynamic burden on the heart lead to cardiac hypertrophy and, eventually, to ventricular dysfunction and heart failure. This process results from the altered expression of normal genes, which is very different from a genetic heart disease, such as LQT and the cardiomyopathies discussed above, involving a deleterious single-gene mutation (see review by Sanguinetti et al.[67]). In the hypertrophied myocyte, a number of changes have been identified that involve almost all subcellular structures. These include altered expression of genes coding for proteins in the contractile apparatus and for proteins involved in EC coupling. In experimental models of pressure overload, isoform switches of both myosin and actin have been characterized. In the rat, pressure overload up-regulates expression of the slow β-MHC, which is the predominate isoform in fetal ventricles. This leads to the theory that reactivation of a fetal program occurs with hemodynamic overloading. However, such data have to be interpreted with caution because in large mammals, such as humans, the β-MHC isoform is predominate both in the fetus and in the adult heart.

And in humans, α-skeletal actin is up-regulated during development and is the predominate isoform of adult normal, hypertrophied, and failing hearts.

In all animal models of heart failure, as well as in human failing myocardium, there is impaired EC coupling. This is frequently manifested by a significant decrease in the systolic Ca^{2+} transient and a slowing of the relaxation rate of the transient. Both of these phenomena can be accounted for by a decrease in the expression of the SR Ca^{2+}-ATPase, which results in slower uptake and less SR storage of Ca^{2+}. Some reports indicate a reduction in the L-type Ca^{2+} current, which could directly contribute to a reduced Ca^{2+} transient as well as to less Ca^{2+} storage by the SR and less Ca^{2+}-induced Ca^{2+} release.[23,68,69] However, other reports indicate no change in L-type Ca^{2+} current.[70,71] The issue of whether L-type Ca^{2+} channel activity is affected in pressure overload models and in failing human heart has yet to be resolved.

Given that hemodynamic overload can alter expression of contractile and Ca^{2+}-handling proteins in mature heart, development of the contractile apparatus and EC coupling mechanisms is likely to be affected by altered hemodynamics. It has been shown that, as anticipated from adult studies, constriction of the outflow tract in the early chick heart produces an enlarged heart.[72] The enlarged heart is due to hyperplasia of myocytes rather than hypertrophy. This has led to speculation that heart size in development is determined to some extent by hemodynamic loading. Studies on the effects of hemodynamic overload later in development are difficult to carry out and have not been performed. However, recent studies on experimental and genetic models of neural crest–related congenital heart defects may shed some light on this question.

In all of the animal models of neural crest–related heart defects, prenatal mortality is too high to be attributed to structural defects of the heart alone. This suggests that there is poor cardiac function because of altered development of the myocardium.[1,62,63] A possible explanation for the morbidity in embryos with outflow tract defects was provided by studies in which persistent truncus arteriosus (PTA), the most severe of the neural crest–related heart defects, was induced experimentally by surgical ablation of the premigratory cardiac neural crest in the chick.[73] In this defect, there is a common outflow from the ventricles caused by a failure to divide into aortic and pulmonary arteries. By midgestation, the embryos with PTA show signs of impending heart failure. The hearts are enlarged with respect to body weight; the embryos are edematous and exhibit reduced contractility. All of the embryos die before hatching. Although the state of the hemodynamic load on these hearts is not known, ventricular myocytes from chick embryos with PTA have reduced L-type Ca^{2+}

current, indicating impaired EC coupling.[20,23] There is less Ca^{2+} available, therefore, for heart muscle contraction. Identical results were obtained in the splotch[2H] mutant mouse embryo, which has PTA[74,75] along with a reduced L-type Ca^{2+} current.[76] At present it is not known whether the neural crest is directly affecting development of the myocardium or whether these changes are due to an indirect effect of the neural crest on hemodynamics.

It is premature to state whether the physiologic studies in the animal models described here are applicable to human fetuses with congenital heart disease. In theory, both animal and human fetuses should be protected from the effects of outflow tract defects because, in the fetal circulatory system, all of the blood is shunted systemically and it should not matter that the outflow is not properly divided. With neural crest defects there are anomalies of the aortic arch arteries and their derivatives that could alter hemodynamics. Resolving the issue of hemodynamics in congenital heart disease awaits further study. However, several clinical studies indicate significant cardiac symptoms in human fetuses in utero with significantly elevated in utero and neonatal mortality compared to fetuses without congenital heart disease (CHD). For example, a 5-year Italian study of women undergoing routine ultrasonographic examinations indicated an incidence of 5.2 fetuses per 1000 with CHD. The in utero fetal death rate in the cases of CHD was 17.9%, and the neonatal mortality rate was 59.4%.[77] In a Czech study of stillborn infants, 2.1% had congenital heart malformations, nearly three times that found in normal populations (0.8%).[78] Other studies demonstrate that in utero CHD significantly alters the normal development of the fetus. An 8-year study conducted in England on nonimmune hydrops found 14 of 31 hydropic babies to have major cardiovascular anomalies, of which 8 were isolated to the heart,[79] in fetuses without known cardiac dysrhythmias. Another study indicates that 20% of babies with intrauterine growth retardation have CHD.[80] There is convincing evidence, therefore, that human fetuses with congenital heart disease have evidence of circulatory insufficiency, which may result in fetal demise in utero and during the neonatal period. However, the mechanisms underlying morbidity and mortality are largely unknown.

It should be clear from the preceding discussion that much remains to be learned regarding the physiology of the fetal and neonatal hearts in congenital heart disease. Within the next few years, recent advances in molecular biology in combination with electrophysiologic approaches and new genetic models should lead to increased understanding of both normal and abnormal heart physiology in development.

SUMMARY

A majority of spontaneous abortions occurring after implantation appear to be the result of defects of the cardiovascular system and may involve impairment of cardiac function. This chapter has considered the normal development of cellular mechanisms of Ca^{2+} handling, contractility, and electrical excitability in heart muscle. Over the course of pre- and postnatal development it is evident that the underlying mechanisms for these processes undergo significant changes that may have relevance in the treatment of heart disease. The chapter has concluded with discussions of specific congenital disorders that involve deleterious perturbations of these mechanisms and have adverse effects on cardiac function.

REFERENCES

1. Copp AJ: Death before birth: Clues from gene knockouts and mutations. *Trends Genet.* 11:87–93, 1995.
2. Katz AM: *Physiology of the Heart.* New York: Raven Press; 1992: p. 687.
3. Robbins J: Regulation of cardiac gene expression during development. *Cardiovasc Res.* 31:E2–E16, 1996.
4. Bers DM: *Excitation-Contraction Coupling and Cardiac Contractile Force.* Boston: Kluwer Academic Publishers; 1991: p. 258.
5. Flucher BE, Franzini-Armstrong C: Formation of junctions involved in excitation - contraction coupling in skeletal and cardiac muscle. *Proc Natl Acad Sci USA.* 93:8101–6, 1996.
6. Van Mierop LHS: Location of pacemaker in chick embryo heart at the time of initiation of the heart beat. *Am J Physiol.* 212:407–15, 1967.
7. Shigenobu K, Scheider JA, Sperelakis N: Blockade of slow Na^+ and Ca^{++} currents in myocardial cells by verapamil. *J Pharmacol Exp Ther.* 190:280–88, 1974.
8. Sperelakis N, Pappano AJ: Physiology and pharmacology of developing heart cells. *Pharmacol Ther.* 22:1–39, 1983.
9. Sperelakis N: Pacemaker mechanisms in myocardial cells during development of embryonic chick heart. In Bouman LN, Jongsna HJ, eds. *Cardiac Rate and Rhythm.* Amsterdam, The Netherlands: Martinus Nijhoff; 1982: pp. 129–165.
10. Fujii S, Ayer RKJ, DeHaan RL: Development of the fast sodium current in early embryonic chick heart cells. *J Membr Biol.* 101:209–23, 1988.
11. Swynghedauw B, Besse S, Assayag P, Carré F, Chevalier B, Charlemagne D, Delcayre C, Hardouin S, Heymes C, Moalic JM: Molecular and cellular biology of the senescent hypertrophied and failing heart. *Am J Cardiol.* 76: 2D–7D, 1995.
12. Fozzard HA, Haber E, Jennings RB, Katz AM, Morgan HE, eds: *The Heart and Cardiovascular System: Scientific Foundations.* New York: Raven Press; 1991: p. 2165.
13. McDonald TF, Pelzer S, Trautwein W, Pelzer DJ: Regulation and modulation of calcium channels in cardiac, skeletal, and smooth muscle cells. *Physiol Rev.* 74:365–507, 1994.

14. Diebold RJ, Koch WJ, Ellinor PT, Wang J-J, Muthuchamy M, Wieczorek DF, Schwartz A: Mutually exclusive exon splicing of the cardiac calcium channel α_1 subunit gene generates developmentally regulated isoforms in the rat heart. *Proc Natl Acad Sci USA.* 89:1497–1501, 1992.

15. Tohse N, Mészáros J, Sperelakis N: Developmental changes in long-opening behavior of L-type Ca^{2+} channels in embryonic chick heart cells. *Circ Res.* 71:376–84, 1992.

16. Aiba S, Creazzo TL: Comparison of the number of dihydropyridine receptors with the number of functional L-type calcium channels in embryonic heart. *Circ Res.* 72:396–402, 1993.

17. Tohse N, Sperelakis N: Long-lasting openings of single slow (L-type) Ca^{2+} channels in chick embryonic heart cells. *Am J Physiol.* 259:H639–H642, 1990.

18. Creazzo TL, Burch J: Calcium current development in the embryonic chick heart. *Biophys J.* 66:A423, 1994 (Abstract).

19. Creazzo TL: Reduced L-type calcium current in the embryonic chick heart with persistent truncus arteriosus. *Circ Res.* 66:1491–98, 1990.

20. Kawano S, DeHaan RL: Analysis of the T-type calcium channel in embryonic chick ventricular myocytes. *J Membr Biol.* 116:9–17, 1990.

21. Wallukat G, Nemecz G, Farkas T, Kuehn H, Wollenberger A: Modulation of the beta-adrenergic response in cultured rat heart cells. I. Beta-adrenergic supersensitivity is induced by lactate via a phospholipase A_2 and 15-lipoxygenase involving pathway. *Mol Cell Biochem.* 102:35–47, 1991.

22. Aiba S, Creazzo TL: Calcium currents in hearts with persistent truncus arteriosus. *Am J Physiol Heart Circ Physiol.* 262:H1182–H1190, 1992.

23. Bean BP: Two kinds of calcium channels in canine atrial cells: Differences in kinetics, selectivity, and pharmacology. *J Gen Physiol.* 86:1–30, 1985.

24. Meissner G: Ryanodine receptor/Ca^{2+} release channels and their regulation by endogenous effectors. *Annu Rev Physiol.* 56:485–508, 1994.

25. Protasi F, Sun XH, Franzini-Armstrong C: Formation and maturation of the calcium release apparatus in developing and adult avian myocardium. *Dev Biol.* 173:265–78, 1996.

26. Will H, Küttner I, Vetter R, Will-Shahab L, Kemsies C: Early presence of phospholamban in developing chick heart. *FEBS Lett.* 155:326-30, 1983.

27. Vetter R, Studer R, Reinecke H, Kolár F, Ostádalová I, Drexler H: Reciprocal changes in the postnatal expression of the sarcolemmal Na^+–Ca^{2+}-exchanger and SERCA2 in rat heart. *J Mol Cell Cardiol.* 27:1689–701, 1995.

28. Vetter R, Will H, Küttner I, Kemsies C, Will-Shahab L: Developmental changes of Ca transport systems in chick heart. *Biomed Biochem.* 45:219–22, 1986.

29. Hilgeman DW, Philipson KD, Vassort G, eds. Sodium–calcium exchange: Proceedings of the third international conference. *Ann NY Acad Sci.* 779:593, 1996.

30. Vetter R, Will H: Sarcolemmal Na-Ca exchange and sarcoplasmic reticulum calcium uptake in developing chick heart. *J Mol Cell Cardiol.* 18:1267–75, 1993.

31. Fozzard HA, Arnsdorf MF: Cardiac electrophysiology. In Fozzard HA, Haber E, Jennings RB, Katz AM, Morgan HE, eds. *The Heart and Cardiovascular System: Scientific Foundations.* New York: Raven Press; 1997: pp. 63–98.

32. Josephson IR, Sperelakis N: Developmental increases in the inwardly-rectifying K^+ current of embryonic chick ventricular myocytes. *Biochim Biophys Acta Mol Cell Res.* 1052:123–7, 1990.

33. Masuda H, Sperelakis N: Inwardly rectifying potassium current in rat fetal and neonatal ventricular cardiomyocytes. *Am J Physiol Heart Circ Physiol.* 265:H1107–H1111, 1993.

34. Baumgarten CM, Fozzard HA: Cardiac resting and pacemaker potentials. In Fozzard HA, Haber E, Jennings RB, Katz AM, Morgan HE, eds. *The Heart and Cardiovascular System: Scientific Foundations.* New York: Raven Press; 1991: pp. 963–1002.

35. DiFrancesco D: Pacemaker mechanisms in cardiac tissue. *Annu Rev Physiol.* 55:455–72, 1993.

36. Manasek FJ: Histogenesis of the embryonic myocardium. *Am J Cardiol.* 25:149–68, 1970.

37. Swynghedauw B: Developmental and functional adaptation of contractile proteins in cardiac and skeletal muscles. *Physiol Rev.* 66:710–71, 1986.

38. Van Der Loop FTL, Schaart G, Langmann W, Ramekers FCS, Viebahn C: Expression and organiation of muscle specific proteins during the early developmental stages of the rabbit heart. *Anat Embryol.* 185:439–50, 1992.

39. Han Y, Dennis JE, Cohen-Gould L, Bader DM, Fischman DA: Expression of sarcomeric myosin in the presumptive myocardium of chicken embryos occurs within six hours of myocyte commitment. *Dev Dynam.* 193:257–65, 1992.

40. Solaro RJ, Lee JA, Kentish JC, Allen DG: Effects of acidosis on ventricular muscle from adult and neonatal rats. *Circ Res.* 63:779–87, 1988.

41. Solaro RJ, El-Saleh SC, Kentish JC, Meyer A, Martin A: Transitions in isoform populations of thick and thin filament proteins and calcium activation of force and ATP hydrolysis by cardiac myofilaments. *Prog Clin Biol Res.* 315:487–502, 1989.

42. Godt RE, Fogaça RTH, Nosek TM: Changes in force and calcium sensitivity in the developing avian heart. *Can J Physiol Pharmacol.* 69:1692–7, 1991.

43. Sabry MA, Dhoot GK: Identification of and changes in the expression of troponin T isoforms in developing avian and mammalian heart. *J Mol Cell Cardiol.* 21:85–91, 1989.

44. Cooper TA, Ordahl CP: A single cardiac troponin T gene generates embryonic and adult isoforms during developmentally regulated alternative splicing. *J Biol Chem.* 260:11140–8, 1985.

45. Reiser PJ, Westfall M, Solaro RJ: Developmental transition in myocardial troponin-T (TnT) isoforms correlates with a change in Ca^{2+} sensitivity. *Biophys J.* 57:549A, 1990 (Abstract).

46. McAuliffe JJ, Gao L, Solaro RJ: Changes in myofibrillar activation and troponin C calcium binding associated with troponin T isoforms switching in developing rabbit heart. *Circ Res.* 66:1204–16, 1990.

47. Teitel DF: Physiologic development of the cardiovascular system in the fetus. In Polin RA, Fox WW, eds. *Fetal and*

Neonatal Physiology. Philadelphia: W.B. Saunders Company; 1992: pp. 609–19.

48. Colan S, Parness IA, Spevak PJ, Sanders SP: Development modulation of myocardial mechanics: Age- and growth-related alterations in afterload and contractility. *JACC.* 19:619–29, 1992.

49. Anderson PAW: Physiology of the fetal, neonatal, and adult heart. In Polin RA, Fox WW, eds. *Fetal and Neonatal Physiology.* Philiadelphia: W.B. Saunders Company; 1992: pp. 722–58.

50. Shroff SG, Janicki JS, Weber KT: Mechanical and energetic behavior of the intact left ventricle. In Fozzard HA, Haber E, Jennings RB, Katz AM, Morgan HE, eds. *The Heart and Cardiovascular System: Scientific Foundations.* New York: Raven Press; 1991: pp. 129–50.

51. Hartzell HC: Regulation of cardiac ion channels by catecholamines, acetylcholine, and second messenger systems. *Prog Biophys Mol Biol.* 52:165–247, 1988.

52. Creazzo TL, Titus L, Hartzell C: Neural regulation of the heart. A model for modulation of voltage-sensitive channels and regulation of cellular metabolism by neurotransmitters. *TINS.* 430–3, 1983.

53. Loffelholz K, Pappano AJ: The parasympathetic neuroeffector junction of the heart. *Pharmacol Rev.* 37:1–24, 1985.

54. Pappano AJ: The development of postsynaptic cardiac autonomic receptors and their regulation of cardiac function during embryonic, fetal, and neonatal life. *Physiol Pathophysiol Heart.* 355–375, 1984.

55. Robinson RB: Autonomic receptor-effector coupling during post-natal development. *Cardiovasc Res.* 31:E68–E76, 1996.

56. Kirby ML, Creazzo TL, Christiansen JL: Chronotropic responses of chick atria to field stimulation after various neural crest ablations. *Circ Res.* 65:1547–54, 1989.

57. Pappano AJ, Higgins D: Initiation of transmitter secretion by adrenergic neurons and its relation to morphological and functional innervation of the embtyonic chick heart. *Cardiac Rate Rhythm.* 631–51, 1982.

58. Stewart D, Kirby ML: Endogenous tyrosine hydroxylase activity in the developing chick heart: A possible source of extraneural catecholamines. *J Mol Cell Cardiol.* 17:389–98, 1985.

59. Kirby ML: Drug modifications of catecholamine synthesis and uptake in early chick embryos. *Brain Res.* 149:443–51, 1978.

60. Tsun-Cheung Chow L, Chow SSM, Anderson RH, Gosling JA: The innervation of the human myocardium at birth. *J Anat.* 187:107–14, 1997.

61. Satoh H, Sperelakis N: Developmental changes and modulation through G-proteins of the hyperpolarization-activated inward current in embryonic chick heart. *Ann NY Acad Sci.* 707:413–6, 1993.

62. Kirby ML, Creazzo TL: Cardiovascular development: Neural crest and new perspectives. *Cardiol Rev.* 3:226–35, 1995.

63. Kirby ML, Waldo KL: Neural crest and cardiovascular patterning. *Circ Res.* 77:211–15, 1995.

64. Keating MT, Sanguinetti MC: Molecular genetic insights into cardiovascular disease. *Science.* 272:681–5, 1996.

65. Fozzard HA, Hanck DA: Structure and function of voltage-dependent sodium channels: Comparison of brain and cardiac isoforms. *Physiol Rev.* 76:887–926, 1996.

66. Edwards JG, Lyons GE, Micales BK, Malhotra A, Factor S, Leinwand LA: Cardiomyopathy in transgenic *myf5* mice. *Circ Res.* 78:379–87, 1996.

67. Sanguinetti MC, Curran ME, Zou AR, Shen JX, Spector PS, Atkinson DL, Keating MT: Coassembly of KvLQT1 and minK(IsK) proteins to form cardiac Iks potassium channel. *Nature.* 384:80–3, 1996.

68. Bouron A, Potreau D, Raymond G: The L-type calcium current in single hypertrophied cardiomycytes isolated from the right ventricle of ferret heart. *Cardiovasc Res.* 26:662–70, 1992.

69. Nuss HB, Houser SR: Voltage dependence of contraction and calcium current in severely hypertrophied feline ventricular myocytes. *J Mol Cell Cardiol.* 23:717–26, 1991.

70. Scamps F, Vassort G: Effect of extracellular ATP on the Na$^+$ current in rat ventricular myocytes. *Circ Res.* 74:710–7, 1994.

71. Cerbai E, Bouchard RA, Li Q, Mugelli A: Ionic basis of action potential prolongation of hypertrophied cardiac myocytes isolated from hypertensive rats of different ages. *Cardiovasc Res.* 28:1180–7, 1994.

72. Clark EB, Hu N, Frommelt P, Vandekieft GK, Dummett JL, Tomanek RJ: Effect of increased pressure on ventricular growth in stage 21 chick embryos. *Am J Physiol.* 257:H55–H61, 1989.

73. Kirby ML, Gale TF, Stewart DE: Neural crest cells contribute to normal aorticopulmonary septation. *Science.* 220:1059–61, 1983.

74. Franz T: Persistent truncus arteriosus in the *Splotch* mutant mouse. *Anat Embryol.* 180:457–64, 1989.

75. Conway SJ, Henderson DJ, Copp AJ: *Pax3* is required for cardiac neural crest migration in the mouse: Evidence from splotch (Sp^{2H}) mutant. *Development.* 124:505–14, 1997.

76. Conway SJ, Godt RE, Greene C, Leatherbury L, Zolotouchnikov VV, Brotto MAP, Henderson DJ, Copp AJ, Kirby ML, Creazzo TL: Neural crest is involved in development of abnormal cardiac function. J *Mol Cellular Cardiol* 29:2675–2685, 1977.

77. Vergani P, Mariani S, Ghidini A, Schiavina R, Cavallone M, Locatelli A, Strobelt N, Cerruti P: Screening for congenital heart disease with the four-chamber view of the fetal heart. *Am J Obstet Gynecol.* 167:1000–3, 1992.

78. Samanek M, Goetzova J, Benesova D: Distribution of congenital heart malformations in autopsied child population. *Int J Cardiol.* 8:235–50, 1985.

79. Gough JD, Keeling JW, Castle B, Lliff PJ: The obstetric management of non-immune hydrops. *Br J Obstet Gynaecol.* 130:828–37, 1986.

80. Paladini D, Calabro R, Palmieri S, D'Andrea T: Prenatal diagnosis of congenital heart disease and fetal karyotyping. *Obstet Gynecol.* 81:679–82, 1993.

CHAPTER Four

Using Doppler Ultrasound to Assess Fetal Circulation

Robert F. Fraser II
and Daniel A. Rightmire

Doppler ultrasound provides a noninvasive technique of direct fetal assessment. Fitzgerald and Drumm[1] were the first to report on the application of Doppler to perinatal medicine. The investigations that followed have not only revealed the potential of Doppler as a management tool in obstetrics but have also contributed to our understanding of fetal physiology and the pathophysiology of abnormal pregnancy. Since its introduction into obstetrics, cumulative experience with this modality has shown a significant association of abnormal Doppler studies and adverse pregnancy outcomes. There is no consensus on the appropriate role of Doppler in obstetrics. However, the utility of Doppler in the management of selected complications of pregnancy is considered convincing based not only on observations but on demonstrated improvements in perinatal outcome.[2–4]

THE DOPPLER PRINCIPLE IN BLOOD FLOW EVALUATION

The Doppler equation expresses the relationship between blood flow velocity and the Doppler frequency shift:

$$f_d = 2(v \cdot \cos \theta)f_0/c \qquad (4\text{--}1)$$

where f_d is the Doppler frequency shift, v is blood flow velocity, θ is the angle between the incident ultrasound beam and blood flow, f_0 is the ultrasound transducer frequency, and c is the speed of sound in tissue. If the transducer frequency is known and the speed of sound in tissue is assumed constant, the equation can be re-

arranged to yield the product of blood flow velocity and the ultrasound incident angle as a function of the observed Doppler frequency shift:

$$v \cdot \cos \theta = c \cdot f_d/(2 \cdot f_0) \qquad (4\text{--}2)$$

In the application of the Doppler principle to assessing blood flow within a vessel, the red blood cells are the elements that reflect the ultrasound waves and produce the Doppler frequency shift. Because blood flow velocities within a vessel are not uniform, the Doppler sample volume contains a large number of blood cells with varying velocities. As a result, the observed Doppler shift signal is a summation of multiple Doppler frequency shifts from the many blood cells within the sample volume. The spectral density of the Doppler signal is determined by the fraction of blood cells within the sample volume moving at the corresponding velocity. The demodulated Doppler signal is typically analyzed by a Fourier transform technique to produce the Doppler shift spectral data, which are quantified and displayed as amplitude in real time. For most transducer frequencies used in practice, the Doppler shift frequency is within the range of human hearing and can be produced audibly.

DOPPLER ULTRASOUND INSTRUMENTATION

The Doppler ultrasound modes utilized in quantitative assessment of the fetal circulation are continuous wave (CW) and pulsed wave (PW). A CW Doppler system utilizes dual transducer elements. One element in the transducer transmits continuously while the adjacent element serves as a receiver. Motion within the region where the fields intersect produces a Doppler frequency shift. CW systems are utilized in umbilical artery velocimetry and electronic fetal heart rate monitoring. These instruments, however, cannot discriminate different Doppler signals within the Doppler sample volume. PW Doppler instruments overcome this limitation by range gating.[5] These instruments transmit signals in short pulses and select a specific depth range within the sample volume based on the arrival time of the reflected Doppler signals. This provides PW Doppler with the ability to target a specific vessel. PW Doppler instruments are limited to a maximum frequency known as the Nyquist limit. Above this limit, which is one-half the Doppler pulse repetition frequency, aliasing occurs and some of the Doppler shifts are interpreted negatively. The potential advantages of a CW Doppler instrument in comparison to a PW instrument include less expense, simplicity of operation, a lower power output, and the ability to measure higher velocities.[4]

The signals received by the Doppler transducer–receiver contain the Doppler frequency shifts produced by blood flow as well as signals from other sources. These signals include low-frequency signals from adjacent tissue structures and high-frequency signals produced by the instrument. These unwanted signals are removed by electronic filters. A low-pass filter removes the unwanted high-frequency noise and a high-pass filter removes low-frequency signals. The high-pass filter is often referred to as a "wall filter," referring to its intended purpose to remove low-frequency signals produced by the vessel structure and the adjacent tissues. A high-pass filter should be used with caution in that a high setting may eliminate Doppler frequency shifts resulting from low-velocity end-diastolic flow. In most obstetrical Doppler applications, a high-pass filter of 50 to 100 Hz suffices.

DOPPLER BLOOD FLOW ANALYSIS

Doppler frequency shifts produced by red blood cells within a blood vessel provide indirect measurements of the blood flow velocity (equation 4–2). Further calculations are required to provide useful quantitative measurements from the Doppler frequency shift data. Calculation of the blood flow velocity using the Doppler equation requires measurement of the ultrasound beam angle of insonation. Furthermore, calculation of volumetric blood flow from blood flow velocity requires multiplication by the vessel cross-sectional area.

DOPPLER VOLUMETRIC BLOOD FLOW

Using the Doppler-derived blood flow velocity, volumetric blood flow can be calculated by three principal

techniques.[6] In the velocity profile technique, the total rate of blood flow is determined by summing the various elements of flow across the vessel:

$$\text{Flow} = \sum_i (v_i \cdot \Delta A_i) \qquad (4\text{–}3)$$

where v_i is the blood flow velocity at element ΔA_i of the cross-sectional area of the vessel. The individual velocity components are determined by a PW Doppler combined with a B-mode real-time ultrasound to measure the vessel dimension.[7] This technique requires a high-resolution PW instrument capable of achieving very small sample sizes.[8] In the uniform insonation method, an intensity-weighted mean Doppler flow velocity profile is determined for the entire cross-sectional area of the vessel and then multiplied by the cross-sectional area to give instantaneous volumetric flow. The volumetric flow rate can be integrated over a time period to provide volume flow per unit time. The assumed velocity profile method assumes that blood flow within the vessel is plug flow, which is characterized by a uniform velocity profile across the vessel.[5] The blood flow velocity is determined as a function of the maximum Doppler frequency shift and then multiplied by the vessel cross-sectional area to provide volumetric flow. Because plug flow is not characteristic of small-diameter vessels, such as the umbilical circulation, although this method is simpler, it is not generally accurate. The assumption of a parabolic flow profile may be more accurate for smaller vessels. Assessment of vessel dimension that utilizes real-time B-mode or M-mode is a significant source of error and a major limitation to all of these techniques. Additionally, vessel diameter varies during a cardiac cycle as a result of the pressure pulsatility. To minimize error, assessment of the vessel diameter and cross-sectional area should optimally occur at the same instant as the Doppler flow velocity determination.[9]

Fetal hemodynamic assessment by volumetric blood flow determination has not been widely utilized in obstetrics. Volumetric flow has been measured in the fetal aorta, umbilical artery, inferior vena cava, and umbilical vein using Doppler techniques.[10–13] The limited use of this methodology in practice is in part due to errors inherent in the above techniques with the present state of ultrasound technology.[14]

DOPPLER WAVEFORM ANALYSIS

Arterial blood flow in the fetal circulation is pulsatile, demonstrating temporal changes over the cardiac cycle. These temporal variations include changes in pressure and flow. The difference in the maximum systolic and minimum diastolic components of blood flow velocity characterizes the pulsatility. The pulsatility depends on several factors, which include the resistance of the vascular bed, the distensibility or compliance of the vessel, and the inertia of the blood column. The maximum Doppler frequency shift waveform represents the peak red blood cell velocity profile within the vessel. The Doppler velocity profile is therefore an indirect assessment of the determinants of pulsatility. Assessment of distal circulatory hemodynamics as a function of the Doppler velocity profile is therefore a rational objective of Doppler blood flow analysis. Because of the error involved in determining the angle of insonation of the ultrasound beam, a method that does not require calculation of the actual blood flow velocity is preferable.

The techniques of quantitative Doppler waveform analysis utilized in obstetrics involve indexes derived from the curve of the maximum Doppler frequency shift throughout the cardiac cycle (Figure 4–1). The pulsatility index (PI) was first described by Goslin and King as a measure of the velocity pulse differential in the peripheral vasculature.[15] It was initially derived in terms of Fourier transform data, but a simpler version was developed as a function of peak-systolic (S), end-diastolic (D), and mean (A) Doppler frequency shifts:

$$PI = \frac{S - D}{A} \qquad (4\text{–}4)$$

The resistance index (RI) described by Pourcelot differs from the PI in that the peak-systolic (S) rather than the mean Doppler frequency shift is used as the denominator[16]:

$$RI = \frac{S - D}{S} \qquad (4\text{–}5)$$

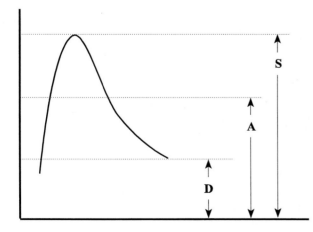

Figure 4–1. Depiction of the Doppler indexes. S = peak systolic, D = end-diastolic, and A = average value of maximun frequency shift waveform over the cardiac cycle. *A/B* ratio = *S/D;* resistance index = (*S* − *D*)/*S;* pulsatility index = (*S* − *D*)/*A;* D/A ratio = D/A.

Stuart et al.[17] described the velocity pulsatility of the umbilical artery in simpler terms. The *A/B* ratio was defined as the ratio of the pulsatile element or highest systolic velocity of blood flow (A) to the continuous element or end-diastolic velocity (B). The *A/B* ratio is also known as the *S/D* ratio:

$$A/B \text{ ratio} = \frac{S}{D} \qquad (4\text{–}6)$$

In most applications of Doppler ultrasound, the characteristics of the diastolic component of the Doppler waveform appear to be the most relevant. Therefore, Maulik et al.[18] have suggested the use of the ratio of diastolic (D) to mean (A) Doppler velocity::

$$\frac{D}{D/A} \qquad (4\text{–}7)$$

Because the Doppler indexes are ratios of Doppler frequency shift data, they are independent of the incident angle of the ultrasound beam, since it is contained in both the numerator and the denominator. Of the Doppler waveform indexes, the PI, the RI, and the *S/D* ratio are most commonly used in obstetric applications. Ultrasound machines designed for Doppler applications typically have software applications incorporated that automatically or semiautomatically analyze the waveform and compute these indexes. Because all of the Doppler indexes are expressions of pulsatility, their diagnostic performances are expected to be similar. In obstetrical applications, however, the diagnostic accuracies of the indexes differ when applied to the prediction of specific perinatal outcomes.[19]

Qualitative assessment of the Doppler waveform when absent or reversed diastolic blood flow is present has diagnostic and prognostic application. Diastolic blood flow is normally present in the umbilical arteries, and its presence is an indicator of the normal low resistance in the placental bed.[20] The absence of diastolic flow indicates abnormal placental development or significant injury with an increase in vascular resistance.[21] Absence of end-diastolic velocity (AEDV) in the fetal umbilical artery is a markedly abnormal situation and is associated with a high risk of perinatal morbidity and mortality.[21,22] Umbilical artery AEDV is an unspecific finding and is associated with a variety of maternal and fetal pathologic entities, including fetal aneuploidy, congenital malformations, intrauterine growth retardation (IUGR), and preeclampsia.[23,24] Reversed umbilical artery blood flow in diastole is an indicator of serious fetal compromise.[25] Doppler investigation of animal and human fetuses with reversed diastolic flow in the umbilical arteries has shown reversed diastolic flow in the central circulation retrograde to the level of the fetal aortic arch.[26,27]

A semiquantitative method of Doppler analysis

**TABLE 4–1. DOPPLER WAVEFORM SEMIQUANTITATIVE
BLOOD FLOW CLASSES (BFC) SCHEME**

Blood Flow Class	Diastolic Flow	Pulsatility Index (PI)
BFC 0	Positive	PI < mean + 2 SD
BFC I	Positive	PI ≥ + 2 SD
BFC II	Absent end-diastolic flow	
BFC III	Absent diastolic flow *or* Reverse flow	

Reprinted, with permission, from Laurin J, Lingman G, Marsal K, Persson PH: Fetal blood flow in pregnancy complicated by intrauterine growth retardation. Obstet Gynecol. *69:895, 1987.*

based on the pulsatility and the diastolic component of the waveform has also been described.[28] This scheme categorizes arterial blood flow into one of four blood flow classes (BFC) based on the Doppler index and the diastolic blood flow (Table 4–1). This technique was applied to aortic blood flow in patients with suspected IUGR and proved to be a more accurate predictor of IUGR and fetal distress than the PI alone.[29] The BFC classification scheme has been applied to fetal umbilical artery waveform analysis as well.[30] A recent implementation of the BFC system uses computer-assisted pattern recognition of the Doppler waveform.[31]

More sophisticated methods of Doppler frequency shift analysis have been proposed.[32–34] These methods are characterized by more detailed assessment of the Doppler waveform. Their capabilities, however, have not been thoroughly investigated.

TECHNIQUES FOR DOPPLER ASSESSMENT OF THE FETAL CIRCULATION

The Umbilical Circulation

The umbilical artery has been the most widely studied of the fetal and uteroplacental circulations. This is in part because of the ease of access of the umbilical circulation with both PW and CW Doppler ultrasound instruments. The CW Doppler technique first involves determination of fetal position with the assumption that the umbilical cord is adjacent to the ventral aspect of the fetus. This can be accomplished by either a clinical exam or with real-time B-mode ultrasound. The transducer is slowly moved over the maternal abdomen in this region until the typical waveform is visualized and an auditory Doppler shift heard. Subtle changes in the angulation of the transducer are used to produce an optimal waveform and the clearest auditory signal. With PW Doppler, real-time B-mode ultrasound is used to localize the umbilical cord, and the Doppler receiver gate is positioned over the cord. A Doppler range gate size should be selected such that it completely encompasses the umbilical cord and therefore achieves maximal insonation of

the umbilical artery's cross-sectional area. Appropriate positioning of the transducer will produce both the umbilical artery waveform and the umbilical venous flow, with opposite polarities. Because of the occasional tortuous path of the artery in the umbilical cord, the umbilical artery waveform and the umbilical venous flow can be produced with the same polarity and be superimposed. The superimposed venous flow can be misinterpreted as umbilical artery diastolic flow, allowing a potentially pathologic finding to go unrecognized. Likewise, both umbilical arteries can be sampled simultaneously, producing mirror image Doppler waveforms of opposite polarity.

The velocity pulsatility of the umbilical artery is gestational age dependent. In normal pregnancy, the values of the *S/D* ratio, PI, and RI decrease with advancing gestational age (Figure 4–2).[20,35–37] The umbilical artery RI is considered to be normally distributed, whereas the *S/D* ratio is not.[36] The decrease in the velocity pulsatility of the umbilical artery indicates a progressive decrease in the resistance of the umbilical–placental vascular bed with advancing gestational age.

Other physiologic factors that affect the blood flow pulsatility and the Doppler waveform are the fetal heart rate (FHR), fetal breathing, and other fetal movements.[38] The predominant effect of FHR on the umbilical artery Doppler waveform is through the influence on the length of diastole. As the FHR decreases, diastole is lengthened, producing a decrease in the end-diastolic blood flow velocity. An increase in FHR shortens diastole and increases the diastolic blood flow velocity. The effect of FHR on the systolic component of the Doppler waveform is minimal in comparison, and the result is an increase in blood flow pulsatility and the calculated Doppler indexes with decreasing FHR.[39,40] This influence is valid for physiologic variations in the FHR. The hemodynamic alterations associated with variable decelerations and umbilical cord compression patterns produce a dissimilar effect on the Doppler waveform.[41] For physiologic variations in the FHR, the relationship between FHR and the umbilical artery Doppler indexes is linear. Correction of the Doppler indexes to a standardized FHR of 140 beats per minute has been recommended.[38] Although normalization of the umbilical artery Doppler indexes to FHR has shown significant reductions in variability, a clinical benefit has not been demonstrated.[40,42] The effect of fetal breathing is theoretically attributed to the fluctuations in intrathoracic pressure, influencing venous return to the fetal heart and therefore cardiac output. The influence of fetal breathing on the umbilical artery RI is reflected in a greater variability of measurements when the Doppler waveform is recorded during episodes of fetal breathing.[43] Fetal breathing also has a similar influence on the fetal aortic blood flow.[44] The fetal behavioral state is

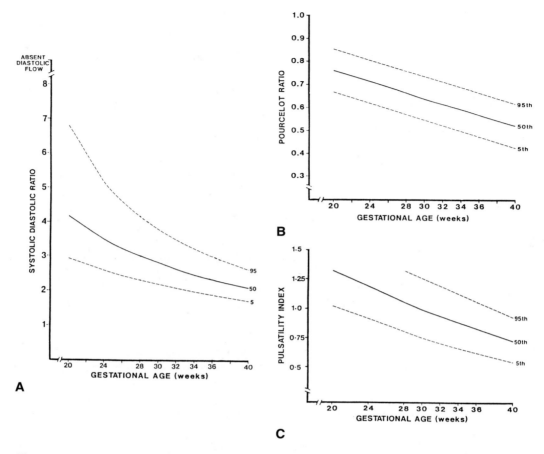

Figure 4–2. Values of the umbilical artery Doppler indexes in normal pregnancy. **A.** Systolic/diastolic ratio or *A/B* ratio. **B.** Pourcelot ratio or resistance index. **C.** Pulsatility index. *(Reprinted, with permission, from Thompson RS, Trudinger BJ, Cook CM, Giles WB: Umbilical artery velocity waveforms: Normal values for A/B ratio and Pourcelot ratio.* Br J Obstet Gynecol. *95:589, 1988.)*

also associated with changes in the umbilical artery Doppler waveform. This, however, appears to be attributable to the influence of fetal movement on the FHR.[38] Doppler assessment of the fetus should optimally be performed in the absence of fetal motion and fetal breathing movements.

The Doppler waveform depends the location of the Doppler sampling site along the umbilical cord. The velocity pulsatility in the umbilical artery is greatest at the fetal insertion and lowest at the placental insertion. Significant differences can be demonstrated in the values obtained for the Doppler indexes depending on the umbilical artery sampling site.[45,46] Likewise, the distribution of normal and elevated values for the RI is altered by the sampling site selection. Maulik et al.[47] compared values of the umbilical artery Doppler indexes obtained at the fetal and placental insertion sites using a PW instrument. The variability component of the Doppler indexes attributable to sampling at the two extremes of the cord was 32% for the RI, 38% for the

S/D ratio, and 46% for the PI. Because the greatest differences in the pulsatility occur at the two extremes of the umbilical cord, the effect of sampling site on the Doppler waveform can be minimized if the two insertion sites are avoided.[48] There is no accepted standard for selection of the umbilical cord Doppler sampling site. Most practitioners prefer a central, free-floating segment of umbilical cord. Variations in the Doppler measurements can be reduced by performing at least two recordings at different sites for comparison.[48] Gudmundsson et al.[49] compared measurements of the umbilical artery PI and *S/D* ratio using both CW and PW instruments. The Doppler indexes obtained by the two methods did not differ significantly. The authors emphasize, however, that operator experience has a significant influence on the reliability of measurements obtained with a CW Doppler instrument.

Two additional aspects of the Doppler technique that affect the measurements are the interobserver and intraobserver variabilities (Table 4–2). Observer vari-

TABLE 4–2. INTEROBSERVER AND INTRAOBSERVER VARIABILITIES OF THE DOPPLER INDEXES DETERMINED WITH A CONTINUOUS WAVE DOPPLER INSTRUMENT

Doppler Index	Interobserver Error Variance (%)	Intraobserver Error Variance (%)
S/D	9.8	4
PI	14.3	5
RI	11.1	8

Reprinted, with permission, from Maulik D, Yarlagadda AP, Youngblood JP, Willoughby L: Components of variability of umbilical arterial Doppler velocimetry—A prospective analysis. Am J Obstet Gynecol. *160:1406, 1989.*

ability introduces a component of measurement error that affects accuracy and decreases the clinical utility of the Doppler technique.[47] The proportion of variability these contribute to Doppler measurements is not expected to be consistent for all techniques or all Doppler laboratories.[49] Periodic determination of the interobserver and intraobserver variabilities is appropriate for an ultrasound laboratory that reports Doppler measurements.

Fetal Aortic Circulation

Doppler assessment of the fetal aortic blood flow was initially described by Eik-Nes et al.[10] The technique requires real-time B-mode ultrasound for vessel localization combined with a PW Doppler instrument. Although not required, color flow Doppler may assist in identification of the aorta. Quantitative Doppler studies of the aorta are typically limited to the descending aorta distal to the ductus arteriosus. Doppler studies

proximal to the ductus are hindered by interference from the proximity of the great vessels within the fetal mediastinum.[51] The Doppler waveform of the fetal descending aorta is influenced by the resistance in its distal branches, which supply the fetal kidneys, abdominal viscera, umbilical–placental circulation, and lower extremities. Physiologic variation in renal and visceral blood flow may therefore introduce variability into serial Doppler examinations.[52] In a sagittal section, the fetal diaphragm serves as a reference for the Doppler sampling location of the fetal descending aorta. The Doppler sampling site should be at or just above the diaphragm for the thoracic aorta and below the renal arteries, 1 to 2 cm above the aortic bifurcation, for the abdominal aorta.[51] A Doppler ultrasound incident angle of 45° is technically obtainable in most clinical situations. A standardized angle of insonation and a well-defined sampling site are recommended for reproducibility. A 100-Hz high-pass filter is suitable for eliminating noise from wall motion in Doppler assessment of fetal aortic blood flow.[44]

The Doppler shift spectrum of the fetal descending aorta is characterized by a narrow distribution of high velocities during systole and a wider distribution of lower velocities throughout diastole (Figure 4–3). The Doppler waveforms obtained from the thoracic and abdominal regions of the fetal aorta differ in that systolic velocities are greater and diastolic velocities less in the thoracic aorta as compared to the abdominal aorta.[6] Likewise, the Doppler PI of the fetal aorta in the abdominal region is lower than in the thoracic region. As opposed to the fetal umbilical artery, the PI of the fetal descending aorta does not change appreciably in the third trimester of pregnancy.[53,54]

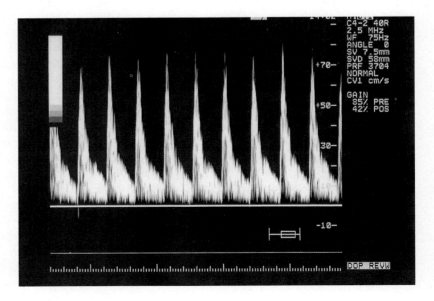

Figure 4–3. Doppler waveform of the abdominal fetal descending aorta at 30 weeks gestation.

Carotid and Cerebral Circulation

The Doppler waveforms of the fetal head and neck circulation have been measured in the common carotid,[55] the internal carotid,[56] and the fetal cerebral arteries.[57] Doppler examination of these vessels requires a combination of B-mode real-time ultrasound and Doppler ultrasound. The common carotid is visualized in a sagittal view of the fetal head and neck. The ability to identify and perform Doppler assessment of the fetal common carotid depends on the fetal position as well as the degree of flexion of the head. Doppler interrogation of the internal carotid artery is performed at its bifurcation into the middle and anterior cerebral vessels. This is best achieved in a transverse view of the fetal cerebrum at the level of the orbits, where the internal carotid is located anterolateral to the cerebral peduncles. The middle cerebral artery is best visualized more cephalad in the standard biparietal diameter plane, where its pulsations can be seen coursing anterolateral in the sylvian sulcus. Landmarks at this level include the thalami and the cavum septum pellucidum. Although not required, color flow Doppler may be used to facilitate identification of the appropriate vessel (Figure 4–4).[58]

The diastolic component of blood flow in the main cerebral arteries is proportionately low before the third trimester of pregnancy (Figure 4–5).[59] During this time, it can be masked by a 100-Hz high-pass filter. The diastolic component of blood flow in the cerebral vessels gradually increases during the third trimester of pregnancy and is accompanied by a decrease in the velocity pulsatility and the Doppler waveform indexes.[57,60,61] The increase in diastolic flow and the decrease in velocity pulsatility is less pronounced in the fetal internal carotid artery as compared to its distal branch, the middle cerebral artery.[59,62,63] This has been interpreted as a mechanism of physiologic distribution to accommodate fetal brain development. The fetal middle cerebral artery is considered the best suited of the cerebral vessels for Doppler assessment.[64] This is in part because of its accessibility to Doppler ultrasound. The middle cerebral artery is sensitive to fetal hypoxia, which produces a significant reduction in the Doppler PI.[65]

In pregnancies complicated by IUGR and uteropla-

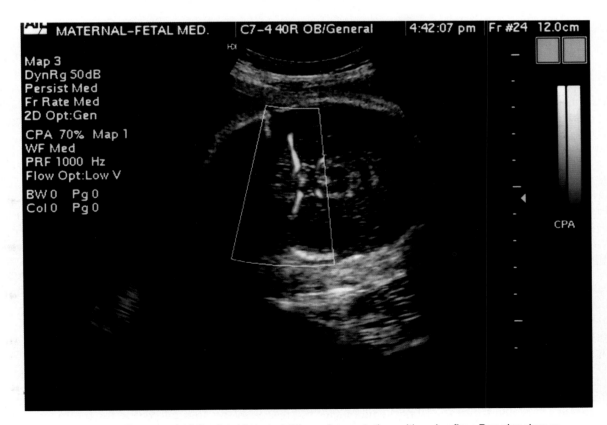

Figure 4–4. Ultrasound of the fetal head at 32 weeks gestation with color flow Doppler demonstrating the middle cerebral artery in the sylvian fissure.

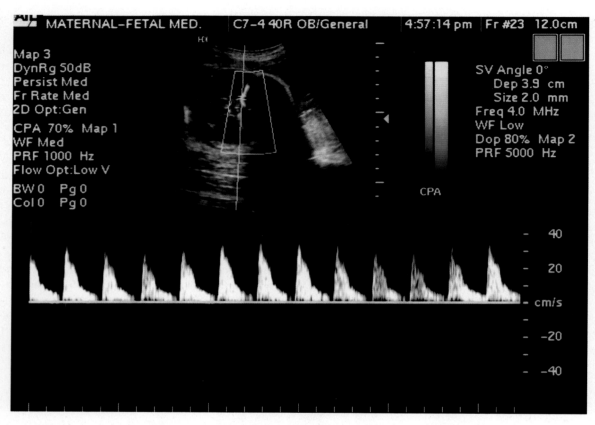

Figure 4–5. Doppler waveform of the fetal middle cerebral artery at 32 weeks gestation recorded with a pulsed wave Doppler instrument.

cental insufficiency, the umbilical artery velocity pulsatility increases while the pulsatility in the cerebral vessels decreases.[61–63] This decrease in the pulsatility of cerebral blood flow and the calculated Doppler indexes indicates a lowering of the vascular impedance and an increase in diastolic blood flow. This mechanism is interpreted as a "brain sparing" effect that redirects blood flow to the fetal brain in a state of relative fetal hypoxia.[66] The existence of such a mechanism was supported by animal studies in which induced fetal hypoxia produced relative redistribution of blood flow to the fetal brain.[67,68] Fetal blood sampling has also shown a relationship between fetal hypoxia and a reduction in the middle cerebral artery pulsatility.[69] The relationship did demonstrate physiologic limitations, however, and an increase in pulsatility in severely hypoxic fetuses was attributed to cerebral edema. The Doppler cerebroplacental ratio described by Arbeille et al.[57] is a quantitative measure of the redistribution effect. The ratio was calculated as the RI of the fetal anterior cerebral artery divided by the RI of the umbilical artery. It was noted that minor elevations in the umbilical artery RI were associated with clearly abnormal

values of the ratio. The cerebroplacental ratio is greater than 1 in normal pregnancy and values less than 1 are considered abnormal.

CLINICAL APPLICATIONS

A principal goal of antenatal fetal assessment is to identify pregnancies at risk for perinatal morbidity and mortality. A number of investigations have demonstrated associations between Doppler studies of the fetal circulation and abnormal pregnancy at risk for adverse outcome. The majority of this research has focused on the ability of Doppler to identify pregnancies complicated by uteroplacental insufficiency, IUGR, and/or intrauterine hypoxia.

Intrauterine Growth Retardation

IUGR is second only to premature birth as a major contributor to perinatal morbidity and mortality.[70,71] The most commonly used definition of IUGR is fetal weight less than the 10th percentile for the pregnancy gestational age.[72,73] Typically, fetal weight is estimated from formulas that incorporate one or more fetal measurements and is then categorized according to gestational age–dependent standards.[74–78] It is recognized that a fetus identified as small for gestational age (SGA) may be constitutionally small because of biologic variability or growth-restricted as a result of an underlying pathologic process.[79] The goal of Doppler in management of pregnancy at risk for IUGR is to aid in making this distinction and in identifying the growth-restricted fetus at risk of becoming hypoxemic. A second role of Doppler is to assist in the management of the pregnancy complicated by IUGR, which largely consists of antenatal assessment of the fetal condition and determination of the timing of delivery.[80]

The application of umbilical artery Doppler to predicting IUGR and the associated perinatal morbidity and mortality has been the focus of several observational studies.[81–85] In the earliest of these, Trudinger et al.[85] used a continuous wave instrument to perform umbilical artery Doppler studies on 172 high-risk pregnancies within 10 days of delivery. Of the fetuses in the study, 53 had a birthweight at or below the 10th percentile, and 34 of those had a Doppler S/D ratio greater than the 95th percentile. Those pregnancies with an abnormal S/D ratio required delivery earlier than those with a normal ratio (average 34 versus 37 weeks) and had a fourfold higher incidence of neonatal intensive care unit admission. Of the six neonatal deaths in the low-birthweight group, all were in the subgroup with an abnormal S/D ratio. The correlation of IUGR and abnormal umbilical artery Doppler demonstrated by this investigation is further emphasized by its unbiased design. Because the umbilical artery Doppler measurements were not available to the investigators for clinical decision making, the outcome was not biased by the normal or abnormal results. Fleischer et al.[81] used a CW Doppler instrument to measure the umbilical artery S/D ratio in 189 women. Approximately one half of the patients in the group had risk factors for IUGR. With two or more examinations at 31 to 39 weeks gestation, and using an S/D ratio of ≥ 3 as abnormal, Doppler demonstrated a sensitivity of 78%, with a specificity of 85%, to identify fetuses with birthweight < 10th percentile. The positive and negative predictive values of Doppler with an overall 16% prevalence of birthweight < 10th percentile in this study were 49% and 95%, respectively.

Various modifications of the Doppler cerebroplacental ratio have been applied to the detection of IUGR pregnancies. Wladimiroff et al.[62] used the ratio of the PI in the umbilical artery to the PI of the fetal internal carotid artery as a test to identify IUGR pregnancies. A decrease in the carotid PI with an increase in the umbilical PI in cases of IUGR suggested the brain sparing effect. The sensitivity of the umbilical PI alone to detect IUGR was 60% and the sensitivity of the umbilical/internal carotid ratio was 78%. Arduini et al.,[86] also

using the ratio of the umbilical artery PI and the internal carotid artery PI to identify IUGR pregnancies, reported a sensitivity of 70%, with a specificity of 92% and a positive predictive value of 81%. Gramellini et al.[87] determined the cerebroplacental ratio of the PIs from the fetal middle cerebral and umbilical arteries in 45 IUGR and 45 appropriately grown fetuses. The diagnostic accuracy of the ratio was 70%, as compared to 65% for the umbilical artery PI alone. An additional finding was a 90% diagnostic accuracy of the ratio to predict adverse perinatal outcome. Although not conclusive, the findings of these investigations suggest improved accuracy of the cerebral/placental ratio over the individual vessel studies.

Management of High-Risk Pregnancy

Trudinger et al.[88] first applied Doppler to antenatal surveillance in high-risk pregnancy. In a group of 170 high-risk pregnancies undergoing antenatal surveillance by fetal heart rate monitoring, the umbilical artery Doppler S/D ratio was measured approximately weekly. The sensitivity of Doppler to detect fetal compromise was 60%, with a specificity of 85%, compared to 17% and 69%, respectively, for fetal heart rate monitoring. Farmakides et al.[89] evaluated the umbilical artery Doppler S/D ratio compared to conventional nonstress testing (NST) in 140 pregnancies with one or more risk factors. Overall, pregnancies with a normal NST but an abnormal Doppler study had worse outcomes than those with an abnormal NST and a normal Doppler study. The group with both tests abnormal had the greatest perinatal morbidity. An abnormal NST was associated with a 32% need for cesarean section delivery. When both tests were abnormal, the need for cesarean section was 75%, with a 63% neonatal intensive care unit admission rate. Two thirds of the pregnancies with an abnormal Doppler S/D ratio were complicated by IUGR, indicating a chronic disease process. The authors conclude that the two tests assess different fetal functions. The NST reflects the status of fetal oxygenation and central nervous system function, whereas the umbilical artery Doppler identifies impaired fetal placental circulation. Devoe et al.[90] evaluated the NST, amniotic fluid measurements, and the umbilical artery Doppler S/D ratio as surveillance tools in 1000 high-risk pregnancies complicated by either postdates, suspected IUGR, hypertension, or diabetes mellitus. The clinical outcomes assessed included perinatal mortality, intrapartum fetal distress, and indirect measures of perinatal morbidity. The overall sensitivity of the Doppler S/D ratio as an individual test was 21% compared to 69% for the NST. The highest sensitivities of Doppler were in the hypertension and IUGR subgroups but were below 50%. The authors concluded that Doppler velocimetry alone was not adequate as a primary antepartum screening test but might be a useful adjunct. This study illustrates that Doppler ultrasound is not a replacement for the established methods of fetal assessment but is complementary in the appropriate clinical scenarios.

The efficacy of fetal Doppler assessment as a surveillance tool has been the focus of randomized clinical trials. In the first of these, Trudinger et al.[91] randomized 300 patients to umbilical artery Doppler velocimetry or conventional surveillance. The timing of delivery was similar for both groups, but the clinical decision making in the Doppler-managed group demonstrated a reduction in fetal distress in labor. As a result, the need for emergent cesarean section was 23% in the control group and 13% in the Doppler group. Almstrom et al.[92] randomized 426 high-risk pregnancies from four participating centers to umbilical artery Doppler or surveillance with cardiotocography. In the Doppler group, the umbilical artery PI and the semiquantitative BFC determined the intensity of fetal surveillance. Fetuses with absent or reversed diastolic flow were delivered by cesarean section immediately. Although the number of cesarean sections in the Doppler and cardiotocography groups did not differ, there were significantly more cesarean sections and operative deliveries for fetal distress in the cardiotocography group (14% versus 23%). Omtzigt et al.[93] evaluated the impact of Doppler availability on obstetrical management and pregnancy outcome in 1598 pregnancies of low to high risk. In the Doppler group, umbilical artery Doppler was performed if indicated by events or findings associated with perinatal morbidity. There was a greater than 50% reduction in perinatal mortality in the Doppler group compared to the controls. The analysis, however, did not reveal any appreciable difference in obstetrical management between the two groups. Pattinson et al.[94] randomized 212 hypertensive and/or SGA pregnancies to management with or without the availability of the umbilical artery Doppler RI results. The study was halted prematurely after six perinatal deaths had occurred in the control group, all in fetuses with umbilical artery AEDV. In addition to a reduction in perinatal mortality, management with the Doppler result available produced a decrease in fetal distress (0% versus 9%) and neonatal morbidity (0% versus 9%) in fetuses with IUGR and AEDV. As these studies have demonstrated, an additional benefit of Doppler surveillance is the ability to identify those pregnancies at risk for intrapartum fetal distress requiring emergent intervention.

Alfirevic and Neilson recently performed a systematic review and meta-analysis of the randomized trials of Doppler ultrasound in high-risk pregnancy.[95] The analysis includes studies based solely on Doppler assessment of the fetal circulation as well as those complemented by Doppler assessment of the uteroplacental circulation. The review collected data on 24 prespeci-

fied perinatal outcomes, and the analysis was based on intention to treat. The analysis revealed a perinatal death rate of 1.6% in Doppler-managed pregnancies and 2.5% in controls. The odds ratio for perinatal death was 0.62 with Doppler management of high-risk pregnancy, and the effect was consistent across the reviewed trials. There were also reductions in hospital admissions, labor inductions, and cesarean sections for fetal distress in the Doppler groups. The authors conclude that the evidence supporting the use of Doppler ultrasound in high-risk pregnancy is compelling.

Multifetal Gestation

In abnormal multifetal pregnancy, placentation is a predominant problem.[96] Abnormalities of the placental circulation are responsible for IUGR, discordant fetal growth, and twin–twin transfusion syndrome. Because Doppler ultrasonography identifies placental dysfunction, it is expected to be useful in these complications. Histologic evidence of microvascular disease has been demonstrated in the placentas of fetuses of twin pregnancies with abnormal umbilical artery Doppler studies.[97] The umbilical artery S/D ratios throughout gestation of normal twin pregnancies are similar to those of singleton pregnancies.[98,99]

Giles, Trudinger, and Cook[98] were the first to describe a relationship between Doppler ultrasound measurements and IUGR in twin pregnancies. In 33 of the 76 twin pregnancies they studied, at least one fetus was SGA. Of the SGA pregnancies, 78% had an abnormal S/D ratio. In a study of 207 twin pregnancies that followed, the potential of Doppler ultrasonography in management of twin gestation was demonstrated.[100] All of the pregnancies had umbilical artery Doppler examinations, but the results were not made available to the clinician in the first group of 95 patients. The availability of the Doppler results in the second group of 112 pregnancies was associated with a decrease in the corrected perinatal mortality from 42.1 per 1000 to 8.9 per 1000. This was achieved without any difference in the gestational age at delivery or mode of delivery. Farmakides et al.[101] studied the relationship of the umbilical artery Doppler S/D ratio and neonatal weight difference in 43 twin pregnancies. An average difference in the S/D ratios of 0.4 or more was predictive of a weight difference of ≥ 350 g, with a sensitivity of 73% and specificity of 82%. Gerson et al.[102] evaluated 56 multifetal pregnancies for evidence of discordant growth using traditional ultrasound methods as well as umbilical artery Doppler S/D ratios and umbilical venous blood flow measurements. The Doppler studies were normal in 44 of the 45 pregnancies with concordant fetal growth and were abnormal in 9 of 11 pregnancies with discordant fetuses. The sensitivity and specificity of the Doppler studies to detect discordant growth were 81% and 97%, respectively. In the majority of cases, the Doppler studies were noted to be abnormal several weeks before the detection of discordance by the traditional ultrasound methods. Hastie et al.,[103] in a study of 89 twin pregnancies, found the umbilical artery *S/D* ratio to have a sensitivity of 29% and a positive predictive value of only 34% in detecting SGA infants. The study did, however, show an association of persistent AEDV and poor perinatal outcome.

The relationship of Doppler studies and fetal growth in the twin–twin transfusion syndrome appears to be complex.[104] Intertwin comparisons of Doppler measurements have produced variable results. Giles et al.[105] found the umbilical artery *S/D* ratios of the two fetuses to be concordant in the twin–twin transfusion syndrome. Others have reported quantitative differences in the umbilical artery Doppler indexes in association with this condition.[101,104,106–108] An intertwin difference in the umbilical artery *S/D* ratios of 0.4 or more may be useful in the antenatal diagnosis of the twin–twin transfusion syndrome.[109]

Screening in Low-Risk Pregnancy

Because investigations of Doppler in complicated pregnancy have had encouraging results, its utility as a screening tool in patients without clinically identifiable disease or risk factors has also been examined. Beatie and Dornan[110] evaluated CW Doppler ultrasonography as a screening tool for IUGR and adverse perinatal outcome in 2097 unselected pregnancies. The three common umbilical artery Doppler waveform indexes—the PI, the *S/D* ratio, and the RI—were evaluated. Using any Doppler index above the 90th percentile as abnormal, 17% of pregnancies were identified to be at risk for IUGR. The sensitivity of Doppler to predict birthweight below the fifth percentile was only 43%. The authors concluded that this was unacceptably low for a condition that affected only 5% of the population. Umbilical artery Doppler indexes correlated poorly with Apgar scores, cord artery pH, and the development of fetal distress requiring emergent operative delivery. There was an apparent association of unexplained stillbirth and abnormal umbilical artery Doppler indexes, but the predictive value was again low. The authors cautioned against the indiscriminate use of Doppler as a screening tool until its proper role had been defined. In a multicenter study of 916 low-risk pregnancies, Todros et al.[111] evaluated umbilical artery Doppler as a screening tool for pregnancy-induced hypertension, low birthweight, and associated complications. The prevalences of pregnancy-induced hypertension and low birthweight in this low-risk group were 3.4% and 4.6%, respectively. An umbilical artery Doppler *S/D* ratio > 3.5 in the early third trimester demonstrated a sensitivity of 43%, with a specificity of 80%, to identify fetuses with low birthweight. The positive predictive value of the test, however, was only 7%. For all of the outcomes evaluated, the positive predictive value of umbilical artery Doppler was under 8%. The authors concluded that the positive predictive value of the test was too low to be of use as a screening tool in a low-risk population. Other investigators have evaluated the performance of Doppler ultrasound in low-risk pregnancies with similar results.[112,113]

SUMMARY

Doppler ultrasound provides a noninvasive means for assessment of the fetal circulation. Various components of the fetal circulation are accessible to Doppler study. Evaluation of the fetal umbilical circulation has received the greatest attention. Doppler ultrasound can be applied to assessment of volume blood flow or, more commonly, vessel resistance across the cardiac cycle. Doppler indexes derived from the blood flow velocity waveform provide an indirect measure of the impedance to flow in the vessel of interest. Because the commonly used Doppler indexes are ratios, they are independent of the ultrasound angle of insonation.

Management of high-risk pregnancy using Doppler ultrasound of the fetal umbilical artery improves perinatal outcome. Doppler ultrasound is clinically useful in diagnosing IUGR pregnancy and in identifying those pregnancies at greatest risk for intrapartum distress and the requirement for operative delivery. Combined Doppler assessment of the cerebral and umbilical circulation may provide additional predictive value in identifying those pregnancies at greatest risk for intrapartum distress. The clinical utility of the information derived from Doppler assessment of the fetal aortic circulation is comparable to that of the umbilical circulation. Use of Doppler ultrasound in unselected and low-risk pregnancies is not of benefit.

REFERENCES

1. Fitzgerald DE, Drumm JE: Noninvasive measurement of the fetal circulation using ultrasound: A new method. *Br Med J.* 2:1450, 1977.
2. Marsal K: Rational use of Doppler ultrasound in perinatal medicine. *J Perinat Med.* 22:463, 1994.
3. Maulik D: Doppler for clinical management: What is its place? *Obstet Gynecol Clin N Am.* 18:853, 1991.
4. Farmakides G, Weiner Z, Mammapoulos M, Nikolaides P: Doppler velocimetry. Where does it belong in evaluation of fetal status? *Clin Perinatol.* 21:849, 1994.
5. Kremkau FW: *Doppler Ultrasound: Principles and Instruments.* Philadelphia: W. B. Saunders; 1995.
6. Gill RW: Measurement of blood flow by ultrasound: Ac-

curacy and sources of error. *Ultrasound Med Biol.* 11:625, 1985.

7. Eik-Nes SH, Brubakk AO, Ulstein MK: Measurement of human fetal blood flow. *Br Med J.* 280:283, 1980.

8. Eik-Nes SH, Marsal K, Kristoffersen K: Methodology and basic problems related to blood flow studies in the human fetus. *Ultrasound Med Biol.* 10:329, 1984.

9. Sindberg Eriksen P, Gennser G, Lindstrom K: Physiological characteristics of diameter pulses in the fetal descending aorta. *Acta Obstet Gynecol Scand.* 63:355, 1984.

10. Eik-Nes SH, Marsal K, Brubakk AO, Kristofferson K, Ulstein M: Ultrasonic measurement of human fetal blood flow. *J Biomed Eng.* 4:28, 1982.

11. Lingman G, Marsal K: Fetal central blood circulation in the third trimester of normal pregnancy—A longitudinal study. I. Aortic and umbilical blood flow. *Early Hum Dev.* 13:137, 1986.

12. Gill RW: Pulsed Doppler with B-mode imaging for quantitative blood flow measurements. *Ultrasound Med Biol.* 5:223, 1979.

13. Indik JH, Chen V, Reed KL: Association of umbilical venous with inferior vena cava blood flow velocities. *Obstet Gynecol.* 77:551, 1991.

14. Trudinger B: Doppler ultrasound assessment of blood flow. In Creasy RK, Resnik R, eds. *Maternal-Fetal Medicine: Principles and Practice.* Philadelphia, W. B. Saunders; 1994: pp. 194–224.

15. Gosling RG, King DH: Ultrasound angiology. In Harcus AW, Adamson L, Clarke CA, eds. *Arteries and Veins.* Edinburgh: Churchill-Livingston; 1975: pp. 72–98.

16. Pourcelot L: Applications clinique de l'examen Doppler transcutane. In Pourcelot L, ed. *Velocimetric Ultrasonore Doppler.* Paris: INSERM; 1974: pp. 169–193.

17. Stuart B, Drumm J, Fitzgerald DE, et al. Fetal blood velocity waveforms in normal pregnancy. *Br J Obstet Gynaecol.* 87:780, 1980.

18. Maulik D, Nanda NC, Saini VD: Fetal Doppler echocardiography: Methods and characterization of normal and abnormal hemodynamics. *Am J Cardiol.* 53:572, 1984.

19. Maulik D, Yarlagadda P, Youngblood JP, Ciston P: Comparative efficacy of umbilical arterial Doppler indices for predicting adverse perinatal outcome. *Am J Obstet Gynecol.* 164:1434, 1991.

20. Schulman H, Fleischer A, Stern W, et al.: Umbilical velocity wave ratios in human pregnancy. *Am J Obstet Gynecol.* 148:985, 1984.

21. Rochelson B, Schulman H, Farmakides G: The significance of absent end-diastolic velocity in umbilical artery velocity waveforms. *Am J Obstet Gynecol.* 156:1213, 1987.

22. Woo JSK, Liang ST, Lo RLS: Significance of an absent or reversed end diastolic flow in Doppler umbilical artery waveforms. *J Ultrasound Med.* 6:291, 1987.

23. Arduini D, Rizzo G, Romanini C: The development of abnormal heart rate patterns after absent end-diastolic velocity in umbilical artery: Analysis of risk factors. *Am J Obstet Gynecol.* 168:43, 1993.

24. Wenstrom K, Weiner C, Williamson R: Diverse maternal and fetal pathology associated with absent diastolic flow in the umbilical artery of high-risk fetuses. *Obstet Gynecol.* 77:374, 1991.

25. Malcom G, Ellwood D, Devonald K, et al.: Absent or re-versed end diastolic flow velocity in the umbilical artery and necrotizing enterocolitis. *Arch Dis Child.* 66:805, 1991.

26. Fouron JC, Teyssier G, Maroto E, et al.: Diastolic circulatory dynamics in the presence of elevated placental resistance and retrograde diastolic flow in the umbilical artery. An experimental Doppler echographic study. *Am J Obstet Gynecol.* 164:195, 1991.

27. Fouron JC, Teyssier G, Shalaby L, et al.: Fetal central blood flow alterations in human fetuses with umbilical artery reverse diastolic flow. *Am J Perinatol.* 10:197, 1993.

28. Laurin J, Lingman G, Marsal K, Persson PH: Fetal blood flow in pregnancy complicated by intrauterine growth retardation. *Obstet Gynecol.* 69:895, 1987.

29. Laurin J, Marsal K, Persson P, Lingman G: Ultrasound measurement of fetal blood flow in predicting fetal outcome. *Br J Obstet Gynaecol.* 94:940, 1987.

30. Gudmundsson S, Marsal K: Umbilical and uteroplacental blood flow velocity waveforms in pregnancies with fetal growth retardation. *Eur J Obstet Gynecol Reprod Biol.* 27:187, 1988.

31. Malcus P, Andersson J, Marsal K, Olofsson P: Waveform pattern recognition—A new semiquantitative method for analysis of fetal aortic and umbilical artery blood flow velocity recorded by Doppler ultrasound. *Ultrasound Med Biol.* 17:453, 1991.

32. Maulik D, Saini VD, Nanda NC, Rosenzweig MS: Doppler evaluation of fetal hemodynamics. *Ultrasound Med Biol.* 8:705, 1982.

33. Campbell S, Diaz-Recasens J, Griffin DR, et al.: New Doppler technique for assessing uteroplacental blood flow. *Lancet.* 1 (8326 Pt 1):675, 1983.

34. Thompson RS, Trudinger BJ, Cook CM: Doppler ultrasound waveforms in the fetal umbilical artery: Quantitative analysis technique. *Ultrasound Med Biol.* 11:707, 1985.

35. Erskine RL, Ritchie JW: Umbilical artery blood flow characteristics in normal and growth-retarded fetuses. *Br J Obstet Gynaecol.* 92:605, 1985.

36. Thompson RS, Trudinger BJ, Cook CM, Giles WB: Umbilical artery velocity waveforms: Normal reference values for A/B ratio and Pourcelot ratio. *Br J Obstet Gynaecol.* 95:589, 1988.

37. Arstrom K, Eliasson A, Hareide JH, Marsal K: Fetal blood velocity waveforms in normal pregnancy. *Acta Obstet Gynecol Scand.* 68:171, 1989.

38. Mulders LG, Muijsers GJ, Jongsma HW, et al.: The umbilical artery blood flow velocity waveform in relation to fetal breathing movements, fetal heart rate and fetal behavioural states in normal pregnancy at 37 to 39 weeks. *Early Hum Dev.* 14:283, 1986.

39. Mires G, Dempster J, Patel NB, et al.: The effect of fetal heart rate on umbilical artery flow velocity waveform. *Br J Obstet Gynaecol.* 94:665, 1987.

40. Yarlagadda P, Willoughby L, Maulik D: Effect of fetal heart rate on umbilical arterial Doppler indices. *J Ultrasound Med.* 8:215, 1989.

41. Weiss E, Hitschold T, Berle P: Umbilical artery blood flow velocity waveforms during variable decelerations of the fetal heart rate. *Am J Obstet Gynecol.* 164:534, 1991.

42. Hoskins PR, Johnstone FD, Chambers SE, et al.: Heart-rate variation of umbilical artery Doppler waveforms. *Ultrasound Med Biol.* 15:101, 1989.

43. Mulders LGM, Muijsers JJM, Jongsma HW, et al.: The umbilical artery blood flow velocity waveform in relation to fetal breathing movement, fetal heart rate, and fetal behavioural states in normal pregnancy at 37 to 39 weeks. *Early Hum Dev.* 14:283, 1986.

44. Marsal K, Eik-Nes SH, Lindblad A, Lingman G: Blood flow in the fetal descending aorta. Intrinsic factors affecting fetal blood flow, i.e., fetal breathing movements and cardiac arrhythmia. *Ultrasound Med Biol.* 10:339, 1984.

45. Mehalek KE, Rosenberg J, Berkowitz GS, et al.: Umbilical and uterine artery flow velocity waveforms. Effect of the sampling site on Doppler ratios. *J Ultrasound Med.* 8:171, 1989.

46. Kay HH, Carroll BA, Bowie JD, et al.: Nonuniformity of fetal umbilical systolic/diastolic ratios as determined with duplex Doppler sonography. *J Ultrasound Med.* 8:417, 1989.

47. Maulik D, Yarlagadda AP, Youngblood JP, Willoughby L: Components of variability of umbilical arterial Doppler velocimetry—A prospective analysis. *Am J Obstet Gynecol.* 160:1406, 1989.

48. Trudinger BJ: Obstetric Doppler applications. In Fleischer AC, Romero R, Manning FA, et al., eds. *The Principles and Practice of Ultrasonography in Obstetrics & Gynecology.* East Norwalk, CT: Appleton and Lange; 1991: pp. 101–198.

49. Gudmundsson S, Fairlie F, Lingman G, Marsal K: Recording of blood flow velocity waveforms in the utero-placental and umbilical circulation: Reproducibility study and comparison of pulsed and continuous wave Doppler ultrasonography. *J Clin Ultrasound.* 18:97, 1990.

50. Sauders JB, Wright N, Lewis KO: Measurement of human fetal blood flow. *Br Med J.* 280:283, 1980.

51. Marsal K, Laurin J, Lindblad A, Lingman G: Blood flow in the fetal descending aorta. *Semin Perinatol.* 11:322, 1987.

52. de Koekkoek-Doll PK, Stijnen T, Wladimiroff JW: Behavioural state dependency of renal artery and descending aorta velocimetry and micturition in the normal term fetus. *Br J Obstet Gynaecol.* 101:975, 1994.

53. Lingman G, Marsal K: Fetal central blood circulation in the third trimester of normal pregnancy—a longitudinal study. II. Aortic blood velocity waveform. *Early Hum Dev.* 13:151, 1986.

54. Campbell S, Vyrias S, Nicolaides KH: Doppler investigation of the fetal circulation. *J Perinat Med.* 19:21, 1991.

55. Arabin B, Berkman P, Saling E: Simultaneous assessment of blood flow velocity waveforms in utero-placental vessels, the umbilical artery, the fetal aorta and the fetal common carotid artery. *Fetal Ther.* 2:17, 1987.

56. Wladimiroff JW, Tonge HM, Stewart PA: Doppler ultrasound assessment of cerebral blood flow in the human fetus. *Br J Obstet Gynaecol.* 93:471, 1986.

57. Arbeille P, Roncin A, Berson M, Patal F, Pourcelot L: Exploration of the fetal cerebral blood flow by duplex Doppler-linear array system in normal and pathological pregnancies. *Ultrasound Med Biol.* 13:329, 1987.

58. Locci M, Nazzaro G, De Placido G, Montemagno U: Fetal cerebral hemodynamic adaptation: a progressive mechanism? Pulsed and color Doppler evaluation. *J Perinat Med.* 20:337, 1992.

59. Arstrom K, Eliasson A, Hareide JH, Marsal K: Fetal blood velocity waveforms in normal pregnancies. A longitudinal study. *Acta Obstet Gynecol Scand.* 68:171, 1989.

60. Woo JS, Liang ST, Lo RL, Chan FY: Middle cerebral artery Doppler flow velocity waveforms. *Obstet Gynecol.* 70: 613, 1987.

61. Kirkinen P, Muller R, Huch R, Huch A: Blood flow velocity waveforms in human fetal intracranial arteries. *Obstet Gynecol.* 70:617, 1987.

62. Wladimiroff JW, Wijngaard JA, Degani S, et al.: Cerebral and umbilical arterial blood flow velocity waveforms in normal and growth-retarded pregnancies. *Obstet Gynecol.* 69:705, 1987.

63. Wladimiroff JW, Tonge HM, Stewart PA: Doppler ultrasound assessment of cerebral blood flow in the human fetus. *Br J Obstet Gynaecol.* 93:471, 1986.

64. Mari G, Moise KJ, Deter RL, et al.: Doppler assessment of the pulsatility index in the cerebral circulation of the human fetus. *Am J Obstet Gynecol.* 160:698, 1989.

65. Chandran R, Serra-Serra V, Sellers SM, Redman CWG: Fetal cerebral Doppler in the recognition of fetal compromise. *Br J Obstet Gynaecol.* 100:139, 1993.

66. Scherjon SA, Smolders-DeHaas H, Kok JH, Zondervan HA: The brain-sparing effect: Antenatal cerebral Doppler findings in relation to neurologic outcome in very preterm infants. *Am J Obstet Gynecol.* 169:169, 1993.

67. Kjellmer I, Karlsson K, Olsson T, Rosen KG: Cerebral reactions during intrauterine asphyxia in the sheep. I. Circulation and oxygen consumption in the fetal brain. *Pediatr Res.* 8:50, 1974.

68. Sheldon RE, Peeters LLH, Jones DM, et al.: Redistribution of cardiac output and oxygen delivery in the hypoxemic fetal lamb. *Am J Obstet Gynecol.* 135:1071, 1979.

69. Vyas S, Nicolaides KH, Bower S, Campbell S: Middle cerebral artery flow velocity waveforms in fetal hypoxaemia. *Br J Obstet Gynaecol.* 97:797, 1990.

70. Kramer MS: Determinants of low birth weight: Methodological assessment and meta-analysis. *Bull WHO.* 65: 663, 1987.

71. Witter FR: Perinatal mortality and intrauterine growth retardation. *Curr Opinion Obstet Gynecol.* 5:56, 1993.

72. Ott WJ: The diagnosis of altered fetal growth. *Obstet Gynecol Clin N Am.* 15:237, 1988.

73. Read MS, et al. Intrauterine growth retardation—Identification of research needs and goals. *Semin Perinatol.* 8:2, 1984.

74. Campbell S, Wilkin D: Ultrasound measurements of fetal abdominal circumference in the estimation of fetal weight. *Br J Obstet Gynaecol.* 82:689, 1975.

75. Shephard MJ, et al. An evaluation of two equations for predicting fetal weight by ultrasound. *Am J Obstet Gynecol.* 142:47, 1982.

76. Hadlock FP, et al.: Sonographic estimation of fetal weight. *Radiology.* 150:535, 1984.

77. Lubchenco LO, Hansman C, Boyd E: Intrauterine growth in length and head circumference as estimated from live

births at gestational ages from 26 to 42 weeks. *Pediatrics.* 37:403, 1966.

78. Brenner WE, Edelman DA, Hendrics CH: A standard of fetal growth for the United States of America. *Am J Obstet Gynecol.* 126:555, 1976.

79. Wilcox AJ: Intrauterine growth retardation: Beyond birthweight criteria. *Early Hum Dev.* 8:189, 1983.

80. Visser GHA, Stigter RH, Bruinse HW: Management of the growth-retarded fetus. *Eur J Obst Gynecol Reprod Biol.* 42:S73, 1991.

81. Fleischer A, et al. Umbilical artery velocity waveforms and intrauterine growth retardation. *Am J Obstet Gynecol.* 151:502, 1985.

82. Erskine RL, Ritchie JW: Umbilical artery blood flow characteristics in normal and growth-retarded fetuses. *Br J Obstet Gynaecol.* 92:605, 1985.

83. Reuwer PJ, Bruinse HW, Stoutenbeek P, Haspels AA: Doppler assessment of the fetoplacental circulation in normal and growth-retarded fetuses. *Eur J Obstet Gynecol Reprod Biol.* 18:199, 1984.

84. Gudmundsson S, Marsal K: Blood velocity waveforms in the fetal aorta and umbilical artery as predictors of fetal outcome: A comparison. *Am J Perinatol.* 8:1, 1991.

85. Trudinger BJ, Giles WB, Cook CM: Flow velocity waveforms in the maternal uteroplacental and fetal umbilical placental circulation. *Am J Obstet Gynecol.* 152:155, 1985.

86. Arduini D, Rizzo G, Romanini C, Mancuso S: Fetal blood flow waveforms as predictors of growth retardation. *Obstet Gynecol.* 70:7, 1987.

87. Gramellini D, Folli MC, Raboni S, et al.: Cerebral-umbilical Doppler ratio as a predictor of adverse perinatal outcome. *Obstet Gynecol.* 79:416, 1992.

88. Trudinger BJ, Cook CM, Jones L, Giles WB: A comparison of fetal heart rate monitoring and umbilical artery waveforms in the recognition of fetal compromise. *Br J Obstet Gynaecol.* 93:171, 1986.

89. Farmakides G, Schulman H, Winter D, Ducey J, et al.: Prenatal surveillance using nonstress testing and Doppler velocimetry. *Obstet Gynecol.* 71:184, 1988.

90. Devoe LD, Gardner P, Dear C, Castillo RA: The diagnostic values of concurrent nonstress testing, amniotic fluid measurement, and Doppler velocimetry in screening a general high-risk population. *Am J Obstet Gynecol.* 163:1040, 1990.

91. Trudinger BJ, Cook CM, Giles WB, et al.: Umbilical artery flow velocity waveforms in high-risk pregnancy: Randomized controlled trial. *Lancet.* i:188, 1987.

92. Almstrom H, Axelsson O, Cnattingius S, et al.: Comparison of umbilical-artery velocimetry and cardiotocography for surveillance of small-for-gestational-age fetuses. *Lancet.* 340:936, 1992.

93. Omtzigt AMWJ, Reuwer PJHM, Bruinse HW: A randomized controlled trial on the clinical value of umbilical Doppler velocimetry in antenatal care. *Am J Obstet Gynecol.* 170:625, 1994.

94. Pattinson RC, Norman K, Odendaal HJ: The role of Doppler velocimetry in the management of high-risk pregnancies. *Br J Obstet Gynaecol.* 101:114, 1994.

95. Alfirevic Z, Neilson JP: Doppler ultrasonography in high-risk pregnancies: Systematic review with meta-analysis. *Am J Obstet Gynecol.* 172:1379, 1995.

96. Farmakides G, Schulman H, Schneider E, et al.: Umbilical artery velocimetry in multiple pregnancy. *Clin Obstet Gynecol.* 32:687, 1989.

97. Giles W, Trudinger B, Cook C, Connelly A: Placental microvascular changes in twin pregnancies with abnormal umbilical artery waveforms. *Obstet Gynecol.* 81:556, 1993.

98. Giles WB, Trudinger BJ, Cook CM: Fetal umbilical artery flow velocity-time waveforms in twin pregnancies. *Br J Obstet Gynaecol.* 92:490, 1985.

99. Shah YG, Gragg LA, Moodley S, Williams GW: Doppler velocimetry in concordant and discordant twin gestations. *Obstet Gynecol.* 80:272, 1992.

100. Giles WB, Trudinger BJ, Cook CM: Umbilical artery flow velocity waveforms and twin pregnancy outcome. *Obstet Gynecol.* 72:894, 1988.

101. Farmakides G, Schulman H, Saldana LR, et al.: Surveillance of twin pregnancy with umbilical arterial velocimetry. *Obstet Gynecol.* 153:789, 1985.

102. Gerson AG, Wallace DM, Bridgens NK, et al.: Duplex Doppler ultrasound in the evaluation of growth in twin pregnancies. *Obstet Gynecol.* 70:419, 1987.

103. Hastie SJ, Danskin F, Neilson JP, Whittle MJ: Prediction of the small for gestational age twin fetus by Doppler umbilical artery waveform analysis. *Obstet Gynecol.* 74:730, 1989.

104. Pretorius DH, Manchester D, Barkin S, et al.: Doppler ultrasound of twin transfusion syndrome. *J Ultrasound Med.* 7:117, 1988.

105. Giles WB, Trudinger BJ, Cook CM, Connelly AJ: Doppler umbilical artery studies in the twin-twin transfusion syndrome. *Obstet Gynecol.* 76:1097, 1990.

106. Hecher K, Ville Y, Snijders R, Nicolaides K: Doppler studies of the fetal circulation in twin-twin transfusion syndrome. *Ultrasound Obstet Gynecol.* 5:318, 1995.

107. Ohno Y, Ando H, Tanamura A, et al.: The value of Doppler ultrasound in the diagnosis and management of twin-to-twin transfusion syndrome. *Arch Gynecol Obstet.* 255:37, 1994.

108. Ishimatsu J, Yoshimura O, Manage A, et al.: Ultrasonography and Doppler studies in twin-to-twin transfusion syndrome. *Asia-Oceania J Obstet Gynecol.* 18:325, 1992.

109. Blickstein I: The twin-twin transfusion syndrome. *Obstet Gynecol.* 76:714, 1990.

110. Beattie RB, Dornan JC: Antenatal screening for intrauterine growth retardation with umbilical artery Doppler ultrasonography. *Br Med J.* 298:631, 1989.

111. Todros T, et al.: Performance of Doppler ultrasonography as a screening test in low risk pregnancies: Results of a multicentric study. *J Ultrasound Med.* 14:343, 1995.

112. Newnham JP, Patterson LL, Ian JR, et al.: An evaluation of the efficacy of Doppler flow velocity waveform analysis as a screening test in pregnancy. *Am J Obstet Gynecol.* 162:403, 1990.

113. Davies JA, Gallivan S, Spencer JAD: Randomised controlled trial of Doppler ultrasound screening of placental perfusion during pregnancy. *Lancet.* 340:1299, 1992.

CHAPTER FIVE

Cardiac Function in the Late-Gestation Fetus

Mark D. Reller and Kent L. Thornburg

It is well recognized that the fetal circulation differs significantly from that seen postnatally. One of the important differences is that both the right and left ventricles function together, each contributing to the fetal systemic cardiac output with "in parallel" circuits. In addition, quite unlike the postnatal circulation, the two ventricles have similar filling (atrial) and systolic ventricular pressures. Because both fetal ventricles contribute to the systemic output, many investigators refer to the fetal cardiac output as the "combined ventricular output,"[1,2] and this output is high when compared to adult cardiac output indexed per unit body weight. It is important to emphasize, however, that although both fetal ventricles contribute to the cardiac output and function in similar hemodynamic environments, the two ventricles have important differences in both their morphology and their function. The purpose of this chapter is to review what is known about fetal cardiac physiology in the late-gestation fetus, emphasizing information that has been learned from investigations obtained primarily from the fetal lamb model. In this chapter we review: (1) normal cardiac hemodynamics as they relate to fetal ventricular function (preload, afterload, etc.); (2) the distribution of fetal cardiac output; (3) changes that take place in the transitional circulation at birth; (4) the effects of hypoxemia on fetal ventricular function; and (5) important new findings regarding the regulation of coronary flow in the fetus.

CONCEPTS OF PRELOAD RESERVE AND RIGHT VENTRICULAR DOMINANCE

Numerous studies have documented that the fetal right ventricle ejects a larger stroke volume than does the left ventricle and contributes a greater proportion of the combined fetal ventricular output.[1-5] Using ventricular function curves that relate fetal cardiac stroke volume to an index of filling pressure (mean atrial pressure), Gilbert demonstrated that fetal biventricular output is normally nearly maximal and increases little on raising filling pressure above baseline control levels.[6] These data were the first, using ventricular function curves, to emphasize the concept of limited preload reserve in the fetus. To assess the relative contributions of the two ventricles, fetal right and left ventricular stroke volumes have been separately measured both at baseline and during changes in filling pressure produced by hemorrhage and saline infusion (i.e., by generating ventricular funciton curves).[3-5] These studies have consistently shown that the right ventricular function curve relating stroke volume to atrial pressure has a shape similar to the left ventricular function curve but differs importantly in that it is positioned "above" the left ventricular curve (Figure 5–1). Both curves were composed of a steep *ascending limb*, where ventricular stroke volume increased rapidly as mean atrial presure increased, and a *plateau limb*, where stroke volumes were only minimally affected by further increases in atrial filling pressure. The mean atrial pressure seen at the *breakpoint* of these two limbs has been invariably shown to be quite similar to that seen in the fetus in its baseline resting state. The left and right ventricular function curves data clearly demonstrate that, for any given filling pressure, right ventricular stroke volume exceeds left ventricular stroke volume (Figure 5–1), indicating right ventricular dominance at physiologic filling pressures. Data from human fetuses are obviously more difficult to obtain, but noninvasive studies

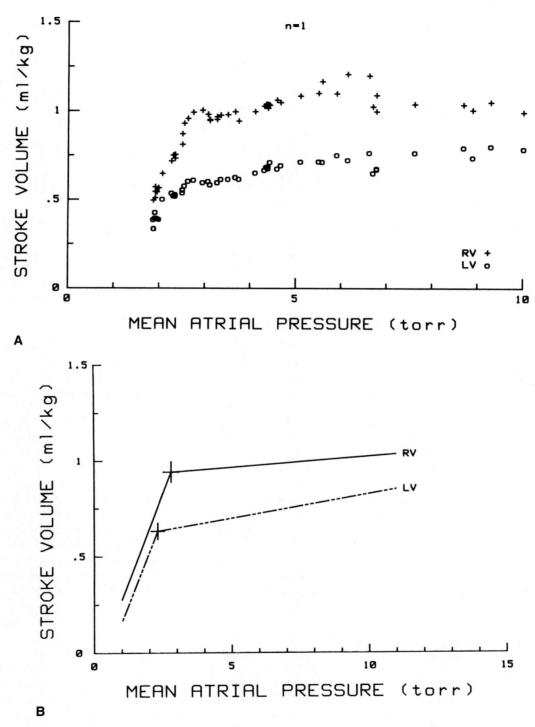

Figure 5–1. A. Simultaneous stroke volumes are shown for the right ventricle (+) and the left ventricle (□) of a fetus during alterations of mean right and left atrial pressures produced by rapid hemorrhage and reinfusion. Each data point represents a 5-s average. Each function curve consists of a steep ascending limb at low atrial pressures and a plateau limb at elevated atrial pressures. **B.** The average simultaneous function curves for 12 fetuses were determined by forcing the average regression coefficients for the ascending and plateau limbs of the right and left ventricular function curves through their rspective average breakpoint stroke volume-mean atrial pressure coordinates. The left ventricular stroke volume intercept is significantly lower than the right ventricular stroke volume at all common filling pressures ($p < .001$).

using Doppler and two-dimensional echocardiographic data to assess ventricular outputs have similarly demonstrated right ventricular dominance in our own species.[7,8]

In an attempt to assess whether anatomic features explain these in vivo studies showing right ventricular dominance, careful volumetric and morphometric analysis of the mature fetal lamb heart has been performed.[9] In these investigations, the fetal right ventricle has been shown to have a greater radius of curvature and a greater chamber volume than the left ventricle at all common transmural filling pressures. These data therefore indicate that although the fetal right ventricle has a similar wall thickness (and a similar wall mass) as the fetal left ventricle, it is a more compliant chamber. These findings are graphically demonstrated by showing the pressure–volume curves, wherein the right ventricle is seen to be shifted to the right (Figure 5–2). From these data, it can be deduced that if the right and left ventricles have similar ejection fractions, the fetal right ventricle will have a larger stroke volume than the left.

In summary, all of the hemodynamic data currently available indicate that the right ventricular output exceeds the left ventricular output in the late-gestation fetus. Using both ventricular function curve data and data derived using radiolabeled microspheres, it can be seen that the right ventricular output comprises from 55% to 67% of the combined fetal cardiac output in the fetal lamb,[1–5,10,11] and the ratio is probably similar in the human.[7,8]

DISTRIBUTION OF FETAL CARDIAC OUTPUT

Although the fetal ventricles both contribute to the systemic cardiac output, important differences exist in the proportion of cardiac output from each chamber that is distributed to the various organ systems within the fetal circulation. Because of preferential streaming of the more highly oxygenated umbilical blood across the foramen ovale (directed by the eustachian valve), left ventricular output carries a somewhat higher oxygen content than does blood ejected from the right ventricle[2,11] (Figure 5–3). Importantly, the fetal left ventricle delivers the majority of its output to the heart, the brain, and the upper body, with only a small proportion (<10%) crossing the aortic isthmus to the descending aorta.[1,2,11] Conversely, the fetal right ventricle receives essentially all of the more poorly saturated blood flow from the superior vena cava and coronary sinus and a greater percentage of the inferior caval flow from the lower body. Because of the high pulmonary vascular resistance (under 10% of the combined ventricular output is directed to the pulmonary circulation in late gestation), the fetal right ventricle delivers the majority of its output across the ductus arteriosus, down the descending aorta, and to the umbilical–placental circulation. To a certain extent, therefore, the fetal ventricles perform similar functions to those seen postnatally. That is, the majority of the more poorly oxygenated right ventricular output is delivered to the placenta for oxygen uptake, whereas the fetal left ventricle delivers

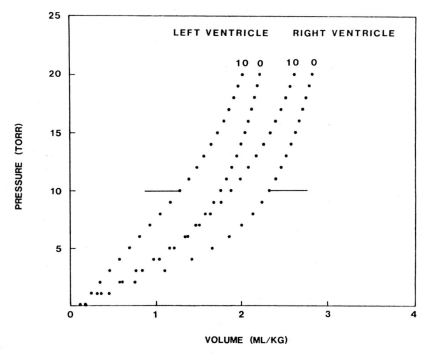

Figure 5–2. Pressure–volume relationship seen in K$^+$-arrested fetal hearts in vitro. Curves were made by rapidly infusing isotonic saline into left ventricular and right ventricular chambers through a plug in the valve annulus while simultaneous pressure measurements were made. Measurements are also shown with the contralateral ventricle at 10 mm Hg transmural pressure and the pericardium in place. Increased pressure in the contralateral ventricle shifts the pressure–volume curve to the left. Note that for any filling pressure, the right ventricular curve is shifted to the right (greater volume).

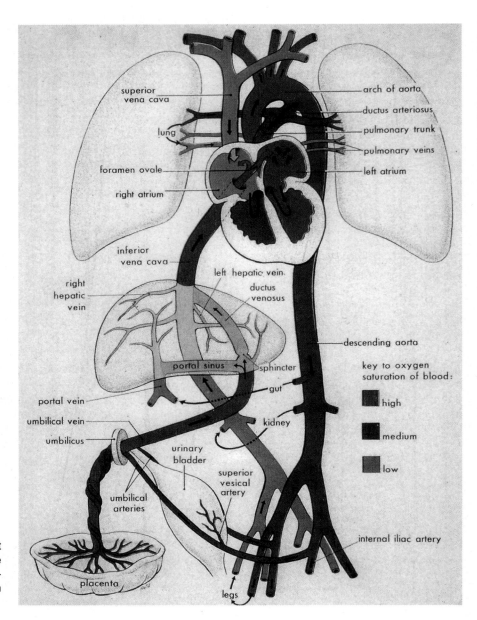

Figure 5–3. Fetal circulation. Note that mixing of the circulation occurs at the level of the ductus venosus (intrahepatic), at the atrial septum (foramen ovale), and at the ductus arteriosus.

the majority of its output to the body (especially the heart and cerebral circulation).

VENTRICULAR SENSITIVITY TO CHANGES IN ARTERIAL PRESSURE

It has been recognized for years that fetal ventricular output and changes in arterial blood pressure are inversely related.[12] More recent information has indicated that when the individual ventricular output responses to changes in arterial pressure are assessed, the two ventricles differ significantly.[3–5] Using electromagnetic flow probes to evaluate ventricular outputs, we were able to measure the changes in stroke volume directly during

increases in arterial pressure produced by occlusion of the descending aorta. During increases in arterial pressure above baseline, both ventricular stroke volumes are decreased. However, the decrement in ventricular output per unit increase in arterial pressure was almost fivefold greater for the fetal right ventricle than for the left (Figure 5–4). It is now apparent, therefore, that the inverse relationship between ventricular stroke volume and arterial pressure resides largely with the right ventricle. The best explanation for this differential sensitivity to arterial pressure may be in the differing morphology of the fetal ventricles previously alluded to.[9] Not only is the fetal right ventricular chamber larger than the left ventricle, but the circumferential radius of curvature to

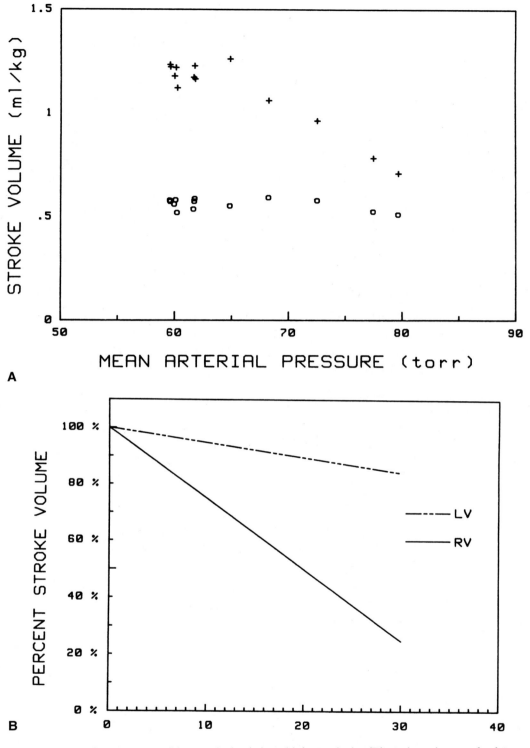

Figure 5–4. A. Simultaneous right ventricular (+) and left ventricular (□) stroke volumes of a fetus are shown during stepwise increases in arterial pressure produced by inflation of an occluder on the descending aorta. Each data point represents a 5-s average. Although right ventricular stroke volume is greater than left ventricular stroke volume under control conditions, right ventricular stroke volume is much more sensitive to increased arterial pressure than left ventricular stroke volume. **B.** The simultaneous average responses of the right and left ventricles to increased arterial pressure are shown for nine fetuses. Stroke volume is expressed as a percentage of control value and arterial pressure as the increment above control. The linear regression coefficient for each ventricle was calculated, the average slope forced through 100% on the *y* axis, and the lines extended through the pressure range studied. The right ventricular pressure sensitivity ($-2.5 \pm 1.4\%$ stroke volume·torr^{-1}) was more than five times the left ventricular pressure sensitivity ($-.5 \pm .7\%$ stroke volume·torr^{-1}) ($p < .001$).

wall thickness ratio is nearly twice as great in the right than in the left ventricle.[9] This ratio, an important determinant of wall stress and, therefore, of after-load, indicates that the fetal right ventricle likely has a much higher after-load at any given arterial pressure than does the left ventricle. This puts the right ventricle at a severe mechanical disadvantage compared to the left.

In more recent investigations, the hypothesis that limitation of coronary blood flow could contribute to the fetal right ventricle's increased sensitivity to changes in arterial pressure (wall stress) was evaluated. Although limited data are currently available in the fetus, numerous studies in the adult indicate that myocardial blood flow is tightly linked to changes in myocardial oxygen consumption. Therefore, changes in wall stress would be expected to result in metabolically mediated coronary vasodilatation. Because previous studies have shown that resting myocardial blood flow to the right ventricle exceeds that of the left,[13] it is possible that the right ventricle may be more vulnerable to ischemia during acute hemodynamic stress. Recent studies, however, have clearly demonstrated that acute increases in maximally tolerated right ventricular pressure are associated with a doubling of myocardial blood flow from baseline values, and that this blood flow response is well below the maximal vasodilatory *flow reserve*.[14] There is therefore no evidence that any limitation of myocardial blood flow delivery contributes to the right ventricle's enhanced sensitivity to increases in arterial pressure.

CIRCULATORY ADJUSTMENTS AT THE TIME OF BIRTH

The successful adaptation of the fetus from its in utero environment to extrauterine life involves dramatic changes in all aspects of the cardiopulmonary, hemodynamic, metabolic, and neurohormonal milieu. To better understand these important cardiovascular changes, several investigators have used the fetal lamb model of in utero ventilation to assess the changes that occur.[5,11,15] From these studies, it is known that in utero ventilation results in a significant decrease in placental flow; that foramenal flow from right atrium to left atrium is nearly abolished; that pulmonary blood flow is dramatically increased; and that ductal flow is reversed. Thus, in many ways, in utero ventilation simulates birth; yet, by circumventing the birth process itself, it is easier to study the precise hemodynamic events sequentially. In utero ventilation results in a doubling of the fetal arterial oxygen content to postnatal levels.[5] In addition, it is known that in utero ventilation results in doubling of left ventricular output[5,11] and is associated with a dramatic shift upward in the left ventricular function curve (Figure 5–5). Using noninvasive Doppler echocardiographic studies, similar findings of increased left ventricular stroke volume are known to be present in the human as well.[16] The precise mechanisms for the dramatic increase in left ventricular output are uncertain, but fundamental to the changes that occur at birth are the dramatic increase in pulmonary blood flow that re-

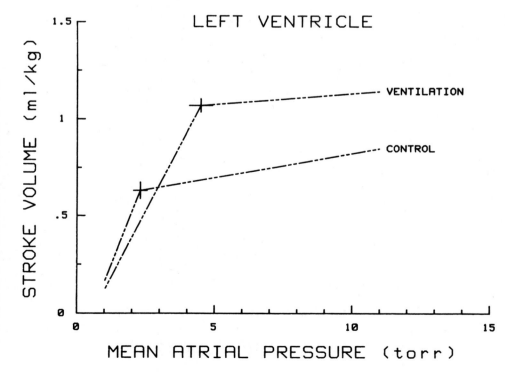

Figure 5–5. Average function curves (*n* = 8) for the left ventricle before and during in utero ventilation were constructed as described in Figure 5–1. The left ventricular function curve was shifted upward during in utero ventilation (analysis of covariance, *p* < .001). The breakpoint stroke volume increased from .63 ± .15 to 1.07 ± .09 mL·kg^{-1}, while atrial pressure increased from 2.3 ± .8 to 4.5 ± 1.1 torr (*p* < .001) during ventilation. The ascending limb slopes, .36 ± .26 and .27 ± .10 mL·kg^{-1}·torr^{-1}, and plateau limb slopes, .03 ± .02 and .01 ± .02 mL·kg^{-1}·torr^{-1}, were not different between control and ventilation, respectively.

sults in a doubling of left atrial pressure and the increase in left ventricular end-diastolic volume.[5,15,16] The fact that a stroke volume increase of this magnitude cannot be brought about by increased left atrial pressure alone before birth[4,5] suggests that the left ventricular pressure–volume relationship is dramatically altered at birth and with in utero ventilation. We have hypothesized that this shift in the left ventricular pressure–volume relationship could be explained by the concept of ventricular interaction through the establishment of a left to right atrial pressure gradient.[5] Recent elegant work by Lewinsky and colleagues assessing left ventricular pressure–volume data obtained using a conductance catheter has demonstrated that the major determinants of the increased left ventricular stroke volume at birth are due to an increase in end-diastolic volume (which results from increased pulmonary blood flow) as well as a possible reduction in the effective after-load.[17] Further, these authors concluded that this increase in left ventricular stroke volume occurred in the absence of any apparent change in ventricular contractility.

Following functional closure of the ductus arteriosus in the first several days of life and removal of the atrial shunt, the circulation is dramatically altered from that seen in the fetal circulation to two separate pulmonary and systemic circulations that function in series. In the absence of any anatomic cardiac shunts, the outputs of the two circulations are equal and are recognized clinically as the cardiac output.

THE EFFECT OF HYPOXEMIA ON FETAL VENTRICULAR FUNCTION

Several studies in the fetal lamb have characterized the hemodynamic response to acute hypoxemia as including: (1) a reduction in cardiac output and heart rate, (2) an increase in arterial pressure, and (3) major redistribution of regional blood flow.[18–21] Further, the fetus strongly regulates its myocardial blood flow in an inverse relationship to changes in arterial oxygen content.[22] Fisher and colleagues have previously demonstrated that the coronary flow reserve in the fetus is sufficient to maintain adequate aerobic myocardial metabolism, even with 50% reductions in fetal arterial oxygen content.[23,24] Based on these data, the mechanism for reduced cardiac output with hypoxemia appears to result from some factor other than myocardial hypoxia. Previous work has suggested that the predominant mechanism for reduced cardiac stroke volume with acute hypoxemia is increases in arterial pressure and after-load that are often associated with acute hypoxemia.[25] Further, it has been shown that the decrease in fetal cardiac output with hypoxemia is almost exclusively caused by a decrease in right ventricular output, and that this decrease is due to the fetal right ventricular sensitivity to arterial pressure. In an earlier investigation of chronic hypoxemia, where arterial pressure was not found to be increased, right ventricular output was not altered from normal values in spite of comparable decreases in arterial oxygen content.[26] In summary, therefore, these data indicate that changes in fetal cardiac output with hypoxemia are secondary to acute increases in ventricular after-load and not a result of any limitation in coronary blood flow.

REGULATION OF FETAL CORONARY BLOOD FLOW AND THE RESPONSE TO ACUTE HYPOXEMIA AND CHRONIC HYPOXEMIA

In the adult circulation, it is well established that left ventricular coronary blood flow and left ventricular myocardial oxygen consumption are tightly linked. Futhermore, it is generally recognized that the major determinants of myocardial oxygen consumption are myocardial contractility, wall stress, and heart rate.[27] Although much less is known about the regulation of the fetal coronary vascular bed, Fisher and colleagues have shown that myocardial oxygen consumption per unit myocardium is similar in fetuses and adults in their resting states.[28] The finding that fetal myocardial oxygen consumption is similar to that seen in the adult heart is remarkable given the reduced level of arterial oxygen content in the fetus. However, resting myocardial blood flow per gram tissue is approximately twice that of the adult, so myocardial oxygen delivery as well as oxygen consumption are comparable despite the low fetal arterial oxygen content.[13,28]

Maximal coronary vasodilator flow reserve has been used in the adult circulation to give useful information as to the potential flow response obtainable during maximal stress at a given arterial pressure.[29] Recent investigations have indicated that the fetal coronary vasodilator flow reserve (using the vasodilatory cardiac nucleoside, adenosine) exceeds baseline flows by at least threefold.[14] In addition, right ventricular myocardial blood flow exceeds the left by approximately 30%, both at baseline and during the adenosine infusion. Therefore, the adenosine-mediated myocardial blood flow reserve appears to be similar for the two fetal ventricles.

The role of the nitric oxide synthase (NOS) pathway for the regulation of the fetal coronary vascular bed both under basal conditions and during the response to acute hypoxemia was recently investigated.[30] During an infusion of N-nitro-L-arginine (L-NNA), a competitive inhibitor of NOS, we found that the myocardial flow to the fetal left ventricle decreased to approximately 70% of basal flow. We concluded from these data that nitric oxide (presumably endothelial in origin) exerts a basal coronary vasodilatory effect in the fetus. In addition, although the double product index of myocardial work was comparable, infusion of L-NNA was associated with a significant reduction in myocardial oxygen consumption from that seen in the resting state. These data therefore further suggest that nitric oxide plays a potential role as a modulator of myocardial oxygen consumption in the fetus.[30]

In assessing the myocardial blood flow response to extreme levels of acute hypoxemia (reducing arterial oxygen content to levels approximately 20% of basal levels), we were able to demonstrate that the NOS pathway may also be involved in mediating an important vasodilatory reserve that exceeds the maximal flow obtainable with adenosine.[30] If confirmed, this NOS-mediated coronary flow reserve appears to be unique to the fetal heart and may be an important adaptive response to acute hypoxemic stress. Last, the influence of chronic hypoxemia on the coronary vascular bed is largely unexplored. Recent preliminary data suggest that chronic hypoxemia is associated with an increase in the adenosine-mediated myocardial blood flow reserve, which is significantly greater than that seen in normoxemic fetuses (Figure 5–6).[31] Although the exact mechanism behind this finding remains unclear, the data suggest that an important alteration in the coronary vascular bed can occur in response to hypoxemia. This finding indicates the potential for plasticity of the coronary vascular bed in utero.

In summarizing these myocardial flow data in the fetus, it should be emphasized that the maximal flows exceed maximal adult myocardial flow values by at least twofold.[32] Remarkably, these fetal myocardial flows occur at an arterial perfusion pressure less than half that seen in the adult circulation. These data therefore unequivocally indicate that the conductance of the coronary vascular bed is significantly greater than that seen in the adult. As such, the fetal heart has a substantially greater maximal capacity for myocardial perfusion than does the adult, as well as the possibility of making important adaptive changes in response to stress.

SUMMARY

The purpose of this review has been to focus on several areas of fetal cardiac function as well as the important new findings regarding the regulation of coronary flow in the fetus. The primary areas covered include the evaluation of fetal ventricular function, distribution of cardiac output, cardiac adaptations that take place at birth, and the effects of hypoxemia both on ventricular function and on the coronary flow response to this acute stress. Future research is anticipated to be directed toward the understanding of the mechanisms by

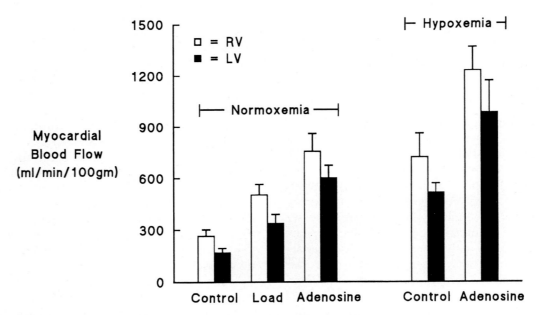

Figure 5–6. Right ventricular (RV) and left ventricular (LV) myocardial blood flow using the radiolabeled microsphere technique. Myocardial flows were measured in normoxemic fetuses ($n = 7$) at baseline (Control), during acute right ventricular pressure loading (Load), and their maximal myocardial flow was assessed (Adenosine). Myocardial blood flow was also measured in a group of hypoxemic fetuses ($n = 4$) at baseline (Control), and their maximal myocardial flow was assessed (Adenosine). Maximal myocardial flow with adenosine in the hypoxemic fetuses was significantly greater than any other measured flow. Baseline (Control) hypoxemic myocardial blood flow was not different from maximal myocardial blood flow seen in normoxemic fetuses.

which the fetal heart (and its coronary vasculature) adapts or remodels to perturbations (i.e., hypoxemia, congenital heart disease) in the fetal circulatory environment. These studies will not only improve our basic understanding of the developing myocardium but will also enhance our knowledge of adaptive mechanisms potentially available to the adult.

REFERENCES

1. Rudolph AM: Distribution of blood flow in the fetal and neonatal lamb. *Circ Res.* 57:811–21, 1985.
2. Heymann MA, Creasy RK, Rudolph AM: Quantitation of blood flow pattern in the foetal lamb in utero. In Comline KS, Dawes GS, Nathanielsz PW, eds. *Foetal and Neonatal Physiology.* Cambridge, England: Cambridge University Press; 1973: pp. 129–35.
3. Thornburg KL, Morton MJ: Filling and arterial pressures as determinants of RV stroke volume in the sheep fetus. *Am J Physiol.* 244:H656–H663, 1983.
4. Thornburg KL, Morton MJ: Filling and arterial pressures as determinants of left ventricular stroke volume in fetal lambs. *Am J Physiol.* 251:H961–H968, 1986.
5. Reller MD, Morton MJ, Reid DL, Thornburg KL: Fetal lamb ventricles respond differently to filling and arterial pressures and to in utero ventilation. *Pediatr Res.* 22:621–6, 1987.
6. Gilbert RD. Control of fetal cardiac output during changes in blood volume. *Am J Physiol.* 238, 1980; *Heart Circ Physiol.* 7:H80–H86.
7. Kenny JF, Plappert T, Doubilet P, Saltzman DH, Cartier M, Zollars L, Leatherman GF, St John-Sutton MG: Changes in intracardiac blood flow velocities and right and left ventricular stroke volumes with gestational age in the normal human fetus: A prospective Doppler echocardiographic study. *Circulation.* 74:1208–16, 1986.
8. Reed KL, Meijboom EJ, Sahn DJ, Seagnelli SA, Valdes-Cruz LM, Shenker L: Cardiac Doppler flow velocities in human fetuses. *Circulation.* 73:41–6, 1986.
9. Pinson CW, Morton MJ, Thornburg KL: An anatomic basis for fetal right ventricular dominance and arterial pressure sensitivity. *J Dev Physiol.* 9:253–71, 1987.
10. Anderson DF, Bissonnette JM, Faber JJ, Thornburg KL: Central shunt flows and pressures in the mature fetal lamb. *Am J Physiol.* 241:H60–H66, 1981.
11. Teitel DF: Circulatory adjustments to postnatal life. *Semin Perinatol.* 12(2):96–103, 1982.
12. Gilbert RD: Effects of afterload and baroreceptors on cardiac function in fetal lambs. *J Dev Physiol.* 4:299–310, 1982.
13. Fisher DJ, Heymann MA, Rudolph AM: Regional myocardial blood flow and oxygen delivery in fetal, newborn, and adult sheep. *Am J Physiol.* 243:H729–H731, 1982.
14. Reller MD, Morton MJ, Giraud GD, Wu DE, Thornburg KL: Severe right ventricular pressure loading in fetal sheep augments global myocardial blood flow to submaximal levels. *Circulation.* 86:581–8, 1992.
15. Teitel DF, Iwamoto HS, Rudolph AM: Changes in the pulmonary circulation during birth-related events. *Pediatr Res.* 27:372–8, 1990.
16. Agata Y, Hiraishi S, Oguchi K, Misawa H, Horiguchi Y, Fujino N, Yashiro K, Shimada N: Changes in left ventricular output from fetal to early neonatal life. *J Pediatr.* 119:441–5, 1991.
17. Lewinsky RM, Szwarc RS, Benson LN, Ritchie JW: Determinants of increased left ventricular output during in utero ventilation in fetal sheep. *Pediatr Res.* 36:373–9, 1994.
18. Cohn HE, Sacks EJ, Heymann MA, Rudolph AM: Cardiovascular responses to hypoxemia and acidemia in fetal lambs. *Am J Obstet Gynecol.* 120:817–24, 1974.
19. Cohen WR, Piasecki GJ, Jackson BT: Plasma catecholamines during hypoxemia in fetal lambs. *Am J Physiol.* 243:R520–R525, 1982.
20. Itskovitz J, Goetzman BW, Rudolph AM: The mechanism of late deceleration of the heart rate and its relationship to oxygenation in normoxemic and chronically hypoxemic fetal lambs. *Am J Obstet Gynecol.* 142:66–73, 1982.
21. Itskovitz J, La Gamma EF, Rudolph AM: Baroreflex control of the circulation in chronically-instrumented fetal lambs. *Circ Res.* 52:589–96, 1983.
22. Peeters LLH, Sheldon RE, Jones, Jr, MD, Makowski EL, Meschia G: Blood flow to fetal organs as a function of arterial oxygen content. *Am J Obstet Gynecol.* 135:637–46, 1979.
23. Fisher DJ, Heymann MA, Rudolph AM: Fetal myocardial oxygen and carbohydrate consumption during acutely induced hypoxemia. *Am J Physiol.* 242:H657–H661, 1982.
24. Fisher DJ, Heymann MA, Rudolph AM: Fetal and myocardial oxygen and carbohydrate metabolism in sustained hypoxemia in utero. *Am J Physiol.* 243:H959–H963, 1982.
25. Reller MD, Morton MJ, Giraud GD, Reid DL, Thornburg KL: The effect of acute hypoxaemia on ventricular function during beta-adrenergic and cholinergic blockade in the fetal sheep. *J Dev Physiol.* 11:263–9, 1989.
26. Reller MD, Morton MJ, Thornburg KL: Right ventricular function in the hypoxemic fetal sheep. *J Dev Physiol.* 8:159–66, 1986.
27. Braunwald E: Control of myocardial oxygen consumption: Physiologic and clinical considerations. *Am J Cardiol.* 27:416–32, 1971.
28. Fisher DJ, Heymann MA, Rudolph AM: Myocardial oxygen and carbohydrate consumption in fetal lambs and in adult sheep. *Am J Physiol.* 238, 1980; *Heart Circ Physiol.* 7:H399–H405.
29. Hoffman JIE: Maximal coronary flow and the concept of coronary vascular reserve. *Circulation.* 70:153–9, 1984.
30. Reller MD, Burson MA, Lohr JL, Morton MJ, Thornburg KL: Nitric oxide is an important determinant of coronary flow at rest and during hypoxemic stress in fetal lambs. *Am J Physiol.* 269, 1995; *Heart Circ Physiol.* 38:H2074–H2081.
31. Reller MD, Morton MJ, Giraud GD, Wu DE, Thornburg KL: Maximal myocardial blood flow is enhanced by chronic hypoxemia in late gestation fetal sheep. *Am J Physiol.* 263, 1992; *Heart Circ Physiol.* 32:H1327–H1329.
32. Barnard RJ, Duncan HW, Livesay JJ, Buckberg GD: Coronary vasodilator reserve and flow distribution during near maximal exercise in dogs. *J Appl Physiol.* 43:988–92, 1977.

CHAPTER SIX

The Etiology of Congenital Heart Disease

Randall C. Floyd

Congenital heart disease (CHD) is one of the most frequent major birth defects in infants in the United States. The current incidence is approximately 0.8%, varying from 0.5% to 1% depending on the study reviewed [1-4] and accounting for 10% to 25% of all congenital anomalies.[5] This is second only to club foot and is therefore the most common life-threatening birth defect.[6] Half of infants with CHD will die before 1 year of age unless their defect is recognized and adequately treated.[7] Identifying the causes of CHD has been the pursuit of many distinguished physicians over the years; however, the etiology remains unclear. This chapter reviews the etiology of some of the particular types of CHD and discusses areas in which research is currently making progress in the definition of further causation.

Congenital anomalies have aroused our curiosity for many centuries. Explanations of their etiology and pathogenesis have been based on supernatural forces, fatalism, and mysticism, as well as on both proper and improper scientific reasoning. The explanation for cardiac anomalies has been one of the more sought after, perhaps because of their profound impact on the individual. At present the emphases for investigation of the etiology of congenital heart disease lie in genetics and teratogenics. Numerous types of studies, from epidemiologic to laboratory research, utilizing animal embryos, continue to be performed in an effort to discover the specific causes and formulate preventive measures to decrease the incidence of CHD in children.

This review discusses structural congenital heart diseases from an embryologic perspective, with an attempt to correlate these defects with possible genetic, metabolic, or teratogenic influences. These influences are then analyzed with specific attention to current knowledge and to areas in which research is currently ongoing. This is by no means intended to be an exhaustive review of the various agents involved in the areas discussed; for this the reader is referred to the various targeted reviews of these respective areas.[8]

The etiology of congenital heart disease can be broken down to its simplest explanation of inherent defect or external influence. This complex topic requires much more discussion than these two very straightforward areas initially imply. The area of inherent defect is becoming much more complex daily. This field now includes traditional inheritance patterns, with which the majority of the readership is familiar, and the newer inheritance mechanisms termed *nontraditional inheritance*.

Teratogenic influences have always been complex and difficult to evaluate. This difficulty results from our inability to isolate influences on human development. Unlike the methods in animal studies, we cannot isolate pregnant humans and evaluate effects of exposure to various agents. Even if this were possible, it would not take into account the effects of the complex interactions of the numerous food additives, industrial chemicals, and over-the-counter and prescription medications to which we are daily exposed. There appear to be many pathogenic mechanisms for any specific cardiac malformation. This strongly suggests that cardiac defects are the outcomes of various influences on heart development at susceptible stages of cardiogenesis. These vulnerable periods of time are noted in Table 6–1. This review will discuss these various influences as they relate to our current knowledge of congenital heart disease.

TABLE 6–1. VULNERABLE PERIODS FOR TERATOGENIC INFLUENCE

Abnormality	Embryonic Event Completed (Days)	Most Sensitive Vulnerable Period (Days)	Limits of Vulnerable Period (Days)
Conotruncal	34	18–29	14–34
Endocardial cushion	38	18–33	14–38
Ventricular septum	38–44	18–39	14–?
Atrial septum (secundum)	55	18–50	14–?
Semilunar valves	55	18–50	14–?
Ductus arteriosus		18–60	14–?
Coarctation of aorta		18–60	14–?

The area of multifactorial inheritance, felt by some to represent an overlap of an inherent disorder (tendency toward abnormality) with teratogenesis (extrinsic influence)[9–11] is discussed along with traditional inheritance. Other possible explanations for this type of inheritance pattern are reviewed in the discussion of nontraditional inheritance. The discussion of teratogenesis includes chemical agents, including drugs and agricultural and industrial chemicals. Possible infectious etiologies, as well as environmental influences such as heat and various forms of radiation, are also discussed as teratogens.

EMBRYOLOGY OF CONGENITAL HEART DISEASE

An understanding of the etiology of congenital heart disease must be founded on an understanding of the embryology of the heart or cardiogenesis.[12] Development of the heart begins with the straight tube heart, which is composed of the prospective segments of right and left atria, primitive ventricle, bulbus cordis, conus, and truncus. The straight tube heart is formed by mesenchymal cells migrating from the bilateral neural crest areas in the dorsal and cephalic regions of the embryo. Thus, the cardiac structures, except for those structures originating from the caudal extremes of the primitive heart, are formed from a fusion of cells of these two primordia. These two cardiogenic areas are imbued with differential growth characteristics and determinants of sidedness. Experiments with chick embryos in which these areas have been disturbed or rearranged have shown that developmental errors at this stage may lead to anomalies such as situs inversus and situs ambiguous (dexter or sinister), as well as conotruncal abnormalities.[13–16]

Cardiac looping, the acquired morphologic asymmetry that leads to development of the ventricles, occurs under the influence of continuous cell migration and multiplication. The bulboventricular segments normally loop or fold in a clockwise direction (D loop). This leads to a folding that forms the two ventricles. A counterclockwise, or L looping, of these segments leads to a transposition of the ventricles, with the pulmonary outflow tract on the positionally left ventricle and the aorta on the right. More complex looping sequences can lead to arterioventricular dissociation, with the great vessels in the D configuration and transposed ventricles in the L configuration.

At this point in development the heart is a folded tube with the potential future ventricles side-by-side. The left ventricular outflow tract and the right ventricular inflow tract now begin to form. The primitive ventricle becomes the left ventricle with development of the muscular septum. The atrioventricular canal widens to the right, extending into the bulbus cordis or future right ventricle, forming the primitive right ventricular inflow tract. The bulboventricular flange resorbs and the conus shifts leftward, forming a common outflow tract at this point. Persistence of this stage without the leftward shift can lead to double-outlet right ventricle. Other consequences of developmental abnormalities at this stage include a double-inlet left ventricle and abnormalities of the mitral and tricuspid valve formation.

The complex process of atrial septation, which involves ingrowths of tissue from various regions as well as duplication, fusion, and resorption, now begins. Appearance of a membrane structure on the posterosuperior aspect of the common primitive atrium is the first occurrence. This is the septum primum, which grows caudally and anteriorly until it meets the medial atrioventricular (AV) cushion. Fusion of the septum primum with the anterior and posterior medial AV cushions closes the ostium primum. The septum secundum, a new membrane, appears just to the right of the septum primum before closure of the ostium primum is complete. This septum grows to cover the septum primum with a central round defect, called the fossa ovalis. Through this defect and an acquired defect (the ostium secundum) in the septum primum, blood flows from the right atrium to the left atrium before birth. After birth, the septum primum and septum secundum coalesce, closing the foramen ovale.

Defects in the formation of the atrial septum can lead to a number of abnormalities. Typical defects occur at certain sites in variable sizes and include:

- *Ostium primum atrial septal defect* (ASD). This is a defect in the caudal portions of both the septum primum and the septum secundum, usually caused by failure of fusion with the two medial AV cushions. This is usually associated with some form of AV canal defect or cleft in the mitral and tricuspid septal leaflets.
- *Fossa ovalis (secundum)* ASD. This is formed from resorption of the portion of the septum primum, which usually forms the floor of the fossa ovale.
- *Sinus venosus* ASD. This defect is formed when the portion of the septum secundum, which usually covers the ostium secundum, is resorbed or does not form.
- *Coronary sinus* ASD. A defect in the caudal posterior aspect atrium above where the coronary sinus normally drains. In these cases the coronary veins drain directly into the right and left atria.
- *Single atria* ASD. This defect is due to complete failure of formation of the atrial septum. This is usually associated with abnormal mitral and tricuspid valves or complete AV canal.

At the time the atrial septum is developing, the ventricular septum and the mitral and tricuspid valves are also forming. Closure of the ventricular septum is usually complete by the 45th day of development in the human embryo. Appropriate development and fusion of the primitive ventricular septum, as well as the posterior and anterior AV cushions and the dextrodorsal and sinistroventral conal ridges, must occur in order for complete closure of the ventricular septum to occur. Development of these latter four structures occurs with duplication of the AV canal and conus as they form the outflow tracts of both ventricles.

The fibrous or membranous ventricular septum is the last portion to close and failure of this closure leads to *type-II (membranous or perimembranous) ventricular septal defect* (VSD). This defect is located in the left ventricular outflow tract just below the noncoronary and right coronary cusps of the aorta. Occasionally, this defect can manifest as a left ventricle to right atrium communication just above the anteromedial commissure of the tricuspid valve.

Other typical ventricular septal defects include:

- *The supracristal or conal septal defect, (type-I VSD).* The type-I VSD is located in the right ventricular outflow tract just below the pulmonary valve. In the left ventricle the defect is located just below the right coronary cusp of the aortic valve leading to prolapse of this cusp in the defect and functional closure in diastole and aortic regurgitation. This defect is located in the midline of the conal septum and represents a failure of the contribution of this structure to closure of the ventricle.
- *Type-III VSD or AV canal.* Type-III VSD is caused by a failure of the development of the uppermost component of the ventricular septum. This is likely secondary to a failure of adequate development of the medial AV cushions. This defect involves variable defects in the AV valves that can range from a common AV valve to clefting of the septal leaflets.
- *Muscular septal defect (VSD type IV).* Type-IV VSD is a result of one or more defects in the primitive ventricular septum. They are usually small and variably located. Common ventricle is a defect in which there is minimal, if any, residual of the muscular septum. This defect is most likely due to absence of the primitive ventricular septum and AV cushion components.

The final area of embryologic development is the formation of the aortic and pulmonary trunks. These structures originate as the conus and truncus of the primitive straight tube heart. Their division into two channels occurs simultaneously, beginning at different levels in each. The caudal ends of the truncal ridges form the cushions that are involved in the development of the aortic and pulmonary valves. At the same time, the conus duplicates its inner lumen with the formation of the dextrodorsal and sinistroventral conal ridges. These eventually fuse in the midline, forming part of the ventricular septum and separating the pulmonary and aortic outflow tracts.

Damage to the neural crest early appears to lead to conotruncal abnormalities such as common truncus or transposition of the great vessels, as previously mentioned. The conotruncal septum normally demonstrates a 180° rotation. Variations in this rotation can lead to transposition of the great vessels in which the aorta and pulmonary artery are parallel and the conotruncal septum is straight (0° rotation). Double-outlet right ventricle is most commonly seen with intermediate rotation (90°) of the conotruncal septum and a side-by-side positioning of the aorta and pulmonary artery.

Other malformations of the great vessels can occur as abnormalities not of the rotation of the conotruncal septum but as failure or uneven development of the septum. These can lead to such abnormalities as truncus arteriosus or hypoplasia or stenosis or atresia of either of the great vessels. Tetralogy of Fallot and type I-VSD (conus only) and aortopulmonary window (truncus only) are examples of this type of developmental failure.

TRADITIONAL INHERITANCE

Chromosomal abnormalities are found in 6% to 10% of all newborns with CHD.[10, 17-19] These chromosomal abnormalities include trisomies, such as Down syndrome, and other types of aneuploidy. The incidence of CHD associated with aneuploidy varies from 40% in Down syndrome to near 100% in trisomies 13 and 18.[20] These defects range from endocardial cushion defect (50% in Down syndrome) to VSD and patent ductus arteriosus (PDA). Some of the more commonly known chromosomal abnormalities and their associated defects are noted in Table 6–2. The developmental mechanisms of the inheritance of these defects remain unclear.

A new area of exploration in this category includes the study of microdeletions, which have recently been implicated in causation of syndromes that involve CHD. The microdeletion 22q11.2, found in some cases of DiGeorge and Shprintzen syndromes, is an illustration.[21-25] This defect has also been described in patients with no accompanying noncardiac anomalies. The development of fluorescent in situ hybridization (FISH) techniques has made this area of research much easier.

Single mutant genes in nuclear DNA are associated with 3% to 4% of congenital heart disease.[19, 26] The defects produced by a single mutant gene usually are part of a syndrome such as Ullrich-Noonan, Apert, and Holt-Oram. These are just a few of these types of syndromes, which all have CHD as a major abnormality noted within the disease process. Table 6–3 lists some of the more common sequences, syndromes, and associations that have CHDs as one of their prominent manifestations. The inheritance patterns in these syndromes include autosomal-dominant, autosomal-recessive, and several types of X-linked syndromes, including focal dermal hypoplasia and incontinentia pigmentosa. The caution here is to beware of the simulation of Mendelism that can be seen in multifactorial inheritance.

Multifactorial inheritance is a concept that has long been accepted as an etiology for a large percentage of isolated CHD. This mode of inheritance is believed to best explain the majority of familial cases of CHD and involves the concepts of genetic–environmental interaction and threshold exposure levels.[27] Multifactorial inheritance may be conceived of as an outcome produced by the interaction of a number of genes and/or a single gene interacting with environmental triggers. The environmental agents that lead to

TABLE 6–2. CARDIAC ABNORMALITIES ASSOCIATED WITH CHROMOSOMAL ABNORMALITIES

Cardiac Abnormality	Chromosomal Abnormality
Trisomy 8 (mosaic)	Ventricular septal defect, patent ductus arteriosus
Trisomy 9 (mosaic)	Ventricular septal defect, coarctation, double-outlet right ventricle
Trisomy 13	Ventricular septal defect, patent ductus arteriosus, atrial septal defect, double-outlet right ventricle
Trisomy 18	Ventricular septal defect, patent ductus arteriosus, pulmonary stenosis
Trisomy 21	Endocardial cushion defect, ventricular septal defect, atrial septal defect, patent ductus arteriosus
Trisomy 22	Atrial septal defect, ventricular septal defect, patent ductus arteriosus
Partial trisomy 22 (cat-eye)	Complex forms of cyanotic heart defects, total anomalous pulmonary venous return
Del(4p−) (Wolf-Hirschorn)	Atrial septal defect, patent ductus arteriosus
Del(5−) (cri-du-chat)	Ventricular septal defect, patent ductus arteriosus
Del(22q11) (DiGeorge, velocardial-facial)	Conotruncal anomalies, right-sided aortic arch, interrupted aorta, patent ductus arteriosus
45,X0 (Turner)	Aortic stenosis, pulmonary stenosis, coarctation, atrial septal defect
Del(4q)	Ventricular septal defect, patent ductus arteriosus, peripheral pulmonic stenosis, aortic stenosis, tricuspid artresia, atrial septal defect, aortic coarctation, tetralogy of Fallot
Del(9p)	Ventricular septal defects, patent ductus arteriosus
Del(11q)	Multiple cardiac defects
Del(13q)	Multiple cardiac defects
Del(18q)	Multiple cardiac defects
Duplication (3q)	Multiple cardiac defects
Duplication (10q)	Multiple cardiac defects
Duplication (15q)	Multiple cardiac defects
Trisomy 9 mosaic	Multiple cardiac defects
XXXXX syndrome (Penta X)	Patent ductus arteriosus, ventricular septal defect

TABLE 6–3. COMMON SYNDROMES AND SEQUENCES ASSOCIATED WITH CARDIAC DEFECTS

Syndrome or Sequence	Cardiac Defect
Apert syndrome	Pulmonic stenosis, overriding aorta, ventricular septal defect, endocardial fibroelastosis
CHARGE association	Tetralogy of Fallot, patent ductus arteriosus, double-outlet right ventricle, ventricular septal defect, atrial septal defect, right-sided aorta
Ellis-van Crevald syndrome	Atrial septal defect (single atrium)
Holt-Oram syndrome	Ostium secundum atrial septal defect, ventricular septal defect
Kabuki syndrome	Coarctation of aorta, bicuspid aortic valve, mitral valve prolapse, membranous ventricular septal defect, tetralogy of Fallot, double-outlet right ventricle, valvular stenosis
Kartagener syndrome	Situs inversus, septal defects
Laterality sequences	Asplenia (bilateral left sidedness), polysplenia (bilateral right sidedness), multiple complex cardiac abnormalities, more serious anomalies associated with polysplenia
Noonan syndrome	Pulmonary valve stenosis, left ventricular hypertrophy, septal defects, patent ductus arteriosus
Radial aplasia–trhombocytopenia syndrome	Tetralogy of Fallot, atrial septal defect
Rubenstein-Taybi syndrome	Patent ductus arteriosus, ventricular septal defect, atrial septal defect
VATER association	Ventricular septal defect
Williams syndrome	Supravavlular aortic stenosis, peripheral pulmonary artery stenosis, pulmonary valve stenosis, ventricular and atrial septal defects

development of the anomaly may be external sources or internal sources, such as epigenesis (development directed by genes) or epistasis. This development pattern of CHD depends on exposure to the environmental triggers at a vulnerable period of embryogenesis in a susceptible individual. The fact that these same environmental influences do not lead to the development of abnormalities in all fetuses exposed gives credence to one of the basic tenets of multifactorial inheritance, i.e., that there is a genetic predisposition to the development of the defect based on the inheritance of the organism.

Research into the biochemical nature of predisposition has implicated the inability of embryologic cells to transform and detoxify chemicals to which they are exposed.[28] The mechanism of clearance for many drugs and chemicals involves cytosolic receptors or phase-I oxidative enzymes, reactive intermediates, and phase II-conjugating enzymes. The cytochrome P450[29,30] enzyme system is the prototype phase-I system, and although primarily located in the liver, is present to some degree in all tissues. The embryo has an inducible cytochrome P450 system but is deficient in phase-II enzymes.[31] Therefore, the chemical to which the embryo is exposed may be metabolized to a reactive intermediate with an inability to complete the detoxification.[32–35] This reactive intermediate may react with a critical macromolecule in the same cell or in a distant cell, leading to the production of a major abnormality in the organ system affected.

The control of these enzyme systems appears to be transmitted to offspring genetically. This may form at least a part of the genetic component of the genetic–environmental interaction of multifactorial inheritance. The fetus who has inherited the paternal allele for response to chemical stimuli, carried by a mother who does not possess the allele, would appear to be at much greater risk for development of congenital anomalies secondary to teratogenic exposure.

NONTRADITIONAL INHERITANCE

Newer areas of exploration into the etiology of CHD include what has been termed the area of nontraditional inheritance. The three categories included in this area are mitochondrial inheritance, germ line mosaicism, and imprinting, including a discussion of uniparental disomy. These inheritance patterns have been recently delineated and are currently being explored as possible explanations for a number of different, apparently inherited abnormalities not readily explained by Mendelian inheritance patterns. This includes a large number of diseases that have been termed multifactorial in the past. Mitochondrial inheritance is a relatively straightforward inheritance pattern and appears to show promise as an explanation for some familial ASDs.[36, 37] The other mechanisms include germ line mosaicism, imprinting, and uniparental disomy and are less easily evaluated and diagnosed; but they may play at least a small role in the inheritance of CHD.

Mitochondrial inheritance is based upon the transmission via the maternal cell line of cytoplasmic DNA. This DNA is contained in the mitochondria and consists of a genome or chromosome consisting of 16,569 base pairs in a circular structure in two strands, one heavy and one light. Both of these strands are transcribed and translated, in contrast to the strands in nuclear DNA. Each mitochondrion contains 2 to 10 copies of the circular chromosomes and each cell contains about 100,000 mitochondria. The mitochrondial genome is transcribed as a single messenger RNA, which is cleaved into various components participating in a number of functions.

The most important function of mitochondrial DNA is the control and production of polypeptides required for oxidative phosphorylation. The mutation rate of mitochondrial DNA is felt to be three to five times that of nuclear DNA. When cells divide, their mitochondria independently replicate and then distribute randomly into daughter cells. This leads to variable phenotypes and a wide range of bioenergetic capabilities. Normal and mutant mitochondrial DNA (mtDNA) coexist within cells and tissues. The effect a mutation in mtDNA has on a cell's function depends on the number of mutant organelles in a cell compared to the number of normal, or wild type, present. This coexistence, termed *heteroplasmy*, may be seen as a protective mechanism necessary to prevent the threat to survival possible should mitochondrial mutants take control.[38] Different persons in the same pedigree may have differing clinical manifestations based on the quantities of normal and mutant mitochondrial DNA in their tissues.

Development of CHD is secondary to a malfunction of the embryologic development of the heart; this depends on numerous complex interactions, including cell migration and multiplication, programmed cell death (apoptosis), and cell differentiation. The effect of these variable bioenergetic capabilities on the complex processes involved in development of the heart may explain some cases of inheritable CHD.[39] One of the examples of CHD that may be explained with mitochondrial inheritance is ASD. There are families in which transmission of this defect appears to be matrilineal.[36,40] In review of the development of the atrial septum it is not difficult to comprehend how such variations in bioenergetic capabilities can influence this complicated process.

Germ line mosaicism and uniparental disomy are the two other areas of nontraditional inheritance that may affect the inheritance of CHD. Germ line mosaicism is unlikely to have a large impact on the incidence of heart disease; however, it may explain some situations in which a condition most often considered to be autosomally dominant may be inherited from two parents with no evidence of disease.[41] These cases have been explained as new mutations in the past. Genetic counseling of these parents would require modification if germ line mosaicism is found to be of significant incidence because the recurrence risk of a dominant disorder would be much higher in these situations.

Uniparental disomy is a condition in which both homologs of the same chromosome are inherited from the same parent.[42] This may occur from loss of one homolog, with duplication of the other, at an early stage in development or from loss of a homolog after a trisomic fertilization of a gamete with two homologs with subsequent loss of one of the trisomic chromosomes. The chromosomes may be copies of the same chromosome (*isodisomy*), different (*heterodisomy*) or a combination of the two maternally or paternally derived chromosomes.

Expression of a recessive disorder may be seen in a situation in which only the one parent is a carrier; in X-linked recessive disorders, transmitted from father to son; or in homozygous form if transmission is to a daughter of an affected father and noncarrier mother. This type of inheritance has been demonstrated in a case of cystic fibrosis in which the child received two copies of the same chromosome from the carrier mother and none from the noncarrier father.[42] This mode of inheritance may be more precisely ascertained by use of DNA markers or alpha satellite probes to determine the origin of the chromosome.

Uniparental disomy also becomes important with consideration of the impact of genomic imprinting. Genomic imprinting is a differential expression of genetic material at either a chromosomal or an allelic level, depending on whether the genetic material has come from the male or the female parent. This goes against Mendelian principles, which hold that the sex of the parent providing an autosomal gene to an offspring should not influence the expression of this gene. This process involves modification of nuclear DNA, causing a difference in phenotype. The modification is *imprinting* and the action is to suppress the allele of interest, whether normal or abnormal. Imprinting of DNA appears to occur during gametogenesis and is reversible.[43, 44] Traditionally, in the study of inheritance, it is taught that the transmission of a normal or abnormal gene leads to a normal or abnormal phenotype. Imprinting, however, reverses this expectation; it is the transmission of the suppression of an allele.

Evidence for this process occurs in the inheritance of Prader-Willi and Angelman syndromes. Both of these syndromes are felt to be manifestations of a microdeletion of the short arm regions q11–q13 of chromosome 15.[43] In patients manifesting these syndromes without deletions of these regions, it was noted that both chromosomes 15 were inherited from a single parent. Patients manifesting Prader-Willi syndrome derive both chromosomes 15 from the mother. This appears to indicate that the area corresponding to the microdeletion in those patients with Prader-Willi, the short arm region q11–q13 of chromosome 15, is suppressed in maternal chromosomes. Patients with Angelman syndrome, who have no evidence of deletion, have subsequently been shown to derive both chromosomes from paternal origin.[44]

These findings demonstrate that imprinting produces suppression and not expression of a trait. There are a number of human disorders in which the severity of the disease appears to depend on the sex of the parent transmitting the disease. These diseases, including neurofibromatosis type II, spinal–cerebellar ataxia, and Beckwith-Wiedemann syndrome, are suspect for being influenced by imprinting based on these findings. Imprinting appears to depend on a methylation modification of DNA ,which may determine whether a particular allele is inactivated or not.[45] The fact that expression of CHD, ventricular septal defect, for example, is much higher in the offspring of an affected mother than in that of an affected father raises the possibility of imprinting as an influence on this disease process.

METABOLIC DISORDERS

The effects of metabolic disorders in the mother or the patient are responsible for 1% to 2% of cardiac abnormalities.[27] Two metabolic diseases, diabetes mellitus and phenylketonuria, have been implicated in abnormal cardiovascular development. The most common metabolic disorder contributing to the incidence of congenital heart disease is diabetes mellitus. The incidence of CHD in the infants of mothers with type-I diabetes mellitus is approximately 4% (2.3% to 6.3%),[46–48] with the most common abnormalities being conotruncal, including double-outlet right ventricle, truncus arteriosus, and transposition of the great vessels as well as VSD and coarctation.[49] These abnormalities are similar to those associated with disturbance of the cardiac neural crest in chick embryos. Maternal hyperglycemia appears to be the most important pathogenic factor.[50, 51] Elevated glucose concentration leads to glycosolation of protein. This glycosolation may lead to disruption of the complex processes that must occur with critical timing during cardiogenesis. Increased efforts directed at strict control of blood sugars before conception should lead to a decrease in these cardiac anomalies.

Other metabolic abnormalities associated with CHD include patients with phenylalanine metabolism abnormalities and patients with metabolic storage disorders. Patients with phenylketonuria have been shown to have a risk of CHD in their offspring that is dose dependent, with an incidence of 10.3%.[52] Control of circulating phenylalanine levels does appear to decrease this risk significantly. An increased risk of CHD

has also been found in infants with phenylketonuria as well as in the children of heterozygous carriers.

Children with inherited disorders of metabolism, including abnormal carbohydrate metabolism (glycogen storage diseases, polysaccharide storage diseases, and mucopolysaccharidoses) and abnormal protein metabolism, amino acid metabolism, lipid metabolism, purine metabolism, and pigment metabolism, have been noted to have associated cardiac abnormalities.[53] These abnormalities are associated with the effects of the metabolic abnormalities on the structure and function of the heart. The classic example of this type of effect is Pompe's disease.[53] The disease is transmitted as an autosomal-recessive trait in which glycogen deposits are found principally in skeletal and cardiac muscle tissue. These glycogen deposits replace myofibrils, decreasing contractility and increasing cardiac mass. These changes lead to cardiomegaly and congestive heart failure.

TERATOGENIC ETIOLOGIES

Infectious etiologies, specifically viral infections, have been suspected as the pathophysiologic mechanisms for CHD since confirmation of the teratogenesis of rubella.[54] Viruses are suspect as likely causative agents because of their ubiquitousness and their predisposition to attack rapidly dividing immature cells. Viral infections, including cytomegalovirus, Coxsackie B virus, mumps, echoviruses, and poliovirus, have been evaluated as potential etiologic agents of CHD.[55] To date, rubella virus is the only documented viral agent that can be identified as a cardiac teratogen in fetuses, causing under 1% of congenital heart disease.[19, 26, 56]

Rubella was first described as a teratogen by Gregg in 1941.[54] The incidence of CHD in children exposed to rubella in utero varies from 20% to 50% depending on the timing of exposure.[57–59] This is consistent with the principles of teratology, which state that exposure must occur during a susceptible time in the development of the affected organ. The most commonly associated defects include patent ductus, pulmonary artery stenosis, and pulmonary valve stenosis. Ventricular septal defect and ASD are less frequent. Vaccination is the appropriate and effective preventive measure for this teratogenic influence. The incidence of CHD associated with inadvertent administration of the vaccine near conception and during the first 3 months of gestation appears to be 1.7%.[60]

The cardiovascular anomalies that were caused by thalidomide in the 1960s were a sobering reminder of the need for a thorough evaluation of medications before their utilization in pregnant women. Luckily, only a few therapeutic drugs have been proved to be human teratogens.[61] These include folic acid antagonists,

TABLE 6–4. COMMON TERATOGENS AND ASSOCIATED CARDIOVASCULAR DEFECTS

Teratogen	Cardiovascular Defect
Alcohol	Ventricular septal defects, atrial septal defects, tetralogy of Fallot
Anticonvulsants	Ventricular septal defects, atrial septal defects, tetralogy of Fallot
Thalidomide	Ventricular septal defects, tetralogy of Fallot, truncus arteriosus
Isotretinoin	Conotruncal and aortic arch defects
Maternal rubella	Patent ductus arteriosus, pulmonary stenosis, pulmonary valve stenosis
Maternal diabetes, type 1	Ventricular septal defect, coarctation, transposition of great arteries
Maternal hyperphenylalaninemia, phenylketonuria	Patent ductus arteriosus, ventricular septal defect, tetralogy of Fallot

isotretinoin, and other vitamin A congeners. There are also a number of drugs that are suspected cardiac teratogens, including lithium, dicumarol (warfarin), anticonvulsants, and amphetamines.[62] Of the drugs that are proven teratogens, only the vitamin A congeners appear to be direct cardiac teratogens. Table 6–4 lists those substances that are thought of as known and potential cardiac teratogens. The prudent course of action remains the utilization of medications only when the benefits of use clearly outweigh the potential risks.

Nontherapeutic agents that may act as teratogens are numerous. These include drugs of abuse, such as alcohol, cocaine[63] and methamphetamine,[62] as well as chemicals utilized in agriculture and manufacturing. There are also case control studies from Finland[64–66] that describe maternal hyperthermia during pregnancy as a risk for the increased incidence for congenital cardiovascular abnormalities. These studies also evaluated the risks of exposure to radiation from computer monitors and microwave ovens and found no increase in risk.[67, 68] There have been several studies that have evaluated the risk of smoking and exposure to secondhand smoke; these have found no increased risk. Maternal consumption of caffeine in pregnant women also does not appear to increase the risk for cardiac abnormalities in their children.[66] The difficulty in evaluating these various exposures as potential etiologic agents for congenital heart disease is the numerous confounding factors that are associated, particularly in patients with exposure to drugs of abuse or alcohol. These confounding factors include poor nutrition, socioeconomic status, multiple drug exposures, and tobacco use. Ideally, exposure to all agents such as these and to agricultural and manufacturing chemicals should be limited during the early part of pregnancy.

The developmental etiologies of congenital heart disease have obviously been relatively well delineated, although research into these areas continues. The current focus of a large proportion of congenital heart disease research is concerned with linkage of genetic, metabolic, or teratogenic influences to these specific

abnormalities. The ultimate goal of this research is not only elucidation of these mechanisms but prevention of congenital heart disease. The area of what is currently termed *multifactorial inheritance* is a very promising field of research. Research into the biochemical nature of genetic predisposition is ongoing and promises new understanding and potential interventions. The area of nontraditional inheritance continues to be investigated and, likewise, promises new understanding of the etiology not only of congenital heart disease but of many other as yet poorly explained inherited abnormalities. Continued research into metabolic disorders promises potentially curative genetic therapies not only for the diseases increasing the risk of CHD but for a number of chronic diseases that plague humankind.

REFERENCES

1. Higgins JTT: The epidemiology of congenital heart disease. *J Chronic Dis.* 18:699, 1965.
2. Carter CO: Genetics of common single malformations. *Br. Med Bull.* 32:21–6, 1976.
3. Leck I, Record RG, McKeown T, Edwards JH: The incidence of malformations in Birmingham, England 1950–59. *Teratology.* 1:263–80, 1968.
4. Ferencz C, Rubin JD, McCarter RJ, Brenner JL, Neill CA, Perry LW, Hepner SL, Downing JW: Congenital heart disease. Prevalence at livebirth. *Am J Epidemiol.* 121:31–6, 1985.
5. Campbell M: Causes of malformations of the heart. *Brit Med J.* 2:895–902, 1965.
6. Leck I, Record RG, McKeown T, Edwards JH: The Incidence of malformations in Birmingham, England 1950–59. *Teratology.* 1:263–80, 1968.
7. Nora JJ, Nora AH: Genetics and environmental factors in the etiology of congenital heart disease. *Southern Med J.* 69(7):919–26, 1976.
8. Bruyere HJ Jr, Kargas SA, Levy JM: The causes and underlying developmental mechanisms of congenital cardiovascular malformations: A critical review. *Am J Med Gen Suppl.* 3:411–31, 1987.
9. Rose V, Gold RJM, Lindsay G, Allen M: A possible in-

crease in the incidence of congenital heart defects among the offspring of affected patients. *J Am Coll Cardiol.* 6:376–82, 1985.

10. Angelina P: Embryology and congential heart diseases: The genetic–environmental interaction. *Circulation.* 38: 604–17, 1968.

11. Nora JJ, Nora AH: The genetic epidemiology of congenital heart diseases. *Prog Med Genet.* 5:91–137, 1983.

12. Angelini P: Embryology and congenital heart diseases. *Texas Heart Inst J.* 22(1):1–12, 1995.

13. Broekhuizen MLA, Wladimiroff JW, Tibboel D, Peoelmann RE, Wenink ACC, Gittenberger-de Groot, AC: Induction of cardiac anomalies with all-trans retinoic acid in the chick embryo. *Cardiol Young.* 2:311–7, 1992.

14. Kirby ML, Gale TF, Stewart DE: Neural crest cells contribute to normal aorticopulmonary septation. *Science.* 220:1059–61, 1983.

15. Manner J, Seidl W, Steding G: Experimental study on the significance of abnormal cardiac looping for the development of cardiovascular anomalies in neural crest-ablated chick embryos. *Anat Embryol.* 194:289–300, 1996.

16. Kirby ML: Cellular and molecular contribution of the cardiac neural crest to cardiovascular development. *Trends Cardiovasc Med.* 3:18–23, 1993.

17. Schinzel AA: Cardiovascular defects associated with chromosomal aberrations and malformation syndromes. *Prog Med Gen.* 5:303–79, 1983.

18. Hoffman JIE, Christianson CH: Congenital heart disease in a cohort of 19,502 births, the long term follow-up. *Am J Cardiol.* 42:641–7, 1978.

19. Pexieder T: Genetic aspects of congenital heart disease. In Pexieder T, ed. *Perspectives in Cardiovascular Research,* vol. 5. 1981:383–7.

20. Hamerton JL, Canning N, Smith S: A cytogenetic survey of 14,069 newborn infants. Incidence of chromosome abnormalities. *Clin Genet.* 8:223–43, 1975.

21. Wilson DI, Goodship JA, Burn J, Cross IE, Schrambler PJ: Deletions within chromosome 22q11 in familial congenital heart disease. *Lancet.* 340:573–5, 1992.

22. Wilson DI, Burn J, Schrambler P, et al: DiGeorge syndrome: Part of CATCH 22. *J Med Genet.* 30:852–6, 1993.

23. Kelley RI, Zachai EH, Emauel BS: The association of DiGeorge anomalad with partial monosomy of chromosome 22. *J Pediatr.* 101:197, 1982.

24. Driscoll DA, Salvin J, Sellinger B, et al: Prevalence of syndromes: Implications for genetic counseling and prenatal diagnosis. *J Med Genet.* 30:813–7, 1993.

25. Goldmuntz E, Driscoll D, Budarf ML, et al.: Microdeletions of chromosomal region 22q11 in patients with congenital conotruncal cardiac defects. *J Med Genet.* 30:807–12, 1993.

26. Nora JJ, Nora AH: The evolution of specific genetic and environmental counseling in congenital heart diseases. *Circulation.* 57:205–13, 1978.

27. Nora JJ, Nora AH: The evolution of specific genetic and environmental counseling in congenital heart diseases (review). *Circulation.* 57(2):205–13, 1978.

28. Nebert DW, Biegelow SW: Genetic control of drug metabolism. Relationship to birth defects. *Semin Perinatol.* 6:105–15, 1982.

29. Pelkonen O, Jouppila P, Karki NT: Effect of maternal cigarette smoking on 3,4-benzpyrene and *N*-methylaniline metabolism in human fetal liver and placenta. *Toxicol Appl Pharmacol.* 23:399–407, 1972.

30. Galloway SM, Perry PE, Menesis J, Nebert DW, Pedersen RA: Cultural mouse embryos metabolize benzo [a] pyrene during early gestation: Genetic differences detectable by sister chromatid exchange. *Proc Natl Acad Sci USA.* 77(6):3524–8, 1980 (June).

31. Dutton GJ: Developmental aspects of drug conjugation, with special reference to glucuronidation. *Ann Rev Pharmacol Toxicol.* 18:17–36, 1978.

32. Gordon GB, Speilberg SP, Benke DA, Balasubramanian V: Thalidomide teratogenesis. Evidence for a toxic arene oxide metabolite. *Proc Natl Acad Sci USA.* 78:2545–8, 1978.

33. Martz F, Fallinger C, Blake DA: Phenytoin teratogenesis. Correlation between embryopathic effect and covalent binding of putative arene oxide metabolite in gestational tissue. *J Pharmacol Exp Ther.* 203:231–9, 1977.

34. Nebert DW, Biegelow SW: Genetic control of drug metabolism. Relationship to birth defects. *Sem Perinatol.* 6: 105–15, 1982.

35. Shum S, Jensen NM, Nebert DW: The AH locus. In utero toxicity and teratogenesis associated with genetic differences in benzo [a] pyrene metabolism. *Teratology.* 20:365–76, 1979.

36. Nora JJ, Nora AH: Maternal transmission of congenital heart diseases: New recurrence risk figures and the questions of cytoplasmic inheritance and vulnerability to teratogens. *Am J Cardiol.* 59:459–63, 1987.

37. Nora JJ: Causes of congenital heart diseases: Old and new modes, mechanisms, and models. *Am Heart J.* 125(5):1409–19, 1993.

38. Wallace D: Diseases of mitochondrial DNA. *Ann Rev Biochem.* 61:1175–1212, 1992.

39. Shoffner JMM, Wallace DC: Heart disease and mitochondrial mutations. *Heart Dis Stroke.* 1:235–41, 1992.

40. Johns DR: Mitochondrial DNA and disease. *N Engl J Med.* 333:638–44, 1995.

41. Edwards JH: Familiarity, recessivity and germline mosaicism. *Ann Hum Genet.* 53:33–43, 1989.

42. Spence JE, Perciaccante RG, Greig GM, Willard HF, Ledbetter DH, Hejtmancik JF, Pollack MS, Obrien WE, Beaudet AL: Uniparental disomy as a mechanism for human disease. *Am J Hum Genet.* 42:217–26, 1988.

43. Nicholls RD, Knoll JHM, Butler MG, Karam S, LaLande M: Genetic imprinting suggested by maternal heterodisomy in nondeletion Prader–Willi syndrome. *Nature.* 342:281–5, 1989.

44. Hall JG: Genomic imprinting and its clinical implications. *N Engl J Med.* 326:827–9, 1992.

45. Nicholls RD, Pai GS, Gottlieb W, Cantu ES: Paternal uniparental disomy of chromosome 15 in a child with Angelman syndrome. *Ann Neurol.* 32(4):512–8, 1992 (Oct).

46. Comess LJ, Bennett PH, Burch TA, Miller M: Congenital anomalies and diabetes in the Pima indians of Arizona. *Diabetes.* 18:471–477, 1969.

47. Mitchell SC, Sellman EH, Westphal MC: Etiologic correlates in study of congenital heart disease in 56,190 births. *Am J Cardiol.* 28:653–7, 1971.

48. Soler NG, Walsh CH, Malins JM: Congenital malformations in infants of diabetic mothers. *Q J Med.* 45:303–13, 1976.

49. Rowland TW, Hubbel JP, Nadas AS: Congenital heart disease in infants of diabetic mothers. *J Pediatr.* 83:815–20, 1973.

50. Brownlee M, Vlassara H, Cerami A: Measurement of glycosylated amino acids and peptides from urine of diabetic patients using affinity chromatography. *Diabetes.* 29:1044–7, 1980.

51. Cohen MP, Urdanivia E, Surma M, Wu VY: Increased glycosylation of glomerular basement membrane collagen in diabetes. *Biochem Biophys Res Commun.* 95:765–9, 1980.

52. Lenke RR, Levy HL: Maternal phenylketonuria and hyperphenylalanemia. *N Engl J Med.* 393:1202–8, 1980.

53. Blieden LC, Moller JH: Cardiac involvement in inherited disorders of metabolism. *Prog Cardiovasr Dis.* 16(6): 615–31, 1974.

54. Gregg NM: Congenital cataract following german measles in the mother. *Trans Ophthalmol Soc (Australia).* 3:35, 1941.

55. Sever JL: Viruses and the fetus. *Int J Gynecol Obstet.* 8: 763–9, 1970.

56. Wagner HR: Cardiac disease in congenital infections. *Clin Perinatol.* 8:481–97, 1981.

57. Cooper LZ, Ziring PR, Ockerse AB, et al.: Rubella: Clinical manifestations and management. *Am J Dis Child.* 118:18, 1969.

58. Dudgeon JA: Maternal rubella and its effect on the fetus. *Arch Dis Child.* 42:110, 1967.

59. Forrest JM, Menser MA: Congenital rubella in school children and adolescents. *Arch Dis Child.* 45:63, 1979.

60. Stray-Pedersen B: New aspects of perinatal infections. *Ann Med.* 25:295–300, 1993.

61. Ferencz C, Boughman JA: Congenital heart disease in adolescents and adults. Teratology, genetics, and recurrence risks. *Cardiol Clin.* 11(4):557–67, 1993 (Nov).

62. Nora JJ, Nora AH, Wexler P: Hereditary and environmental aspects as they affect the fetus and newborn. *Clin Obstet Gynecol.* 24(3):851–61, 1981.

63. Shepard TH, Fantel AG, Kapur RP: Fetal coronary thrombosis as a cause of single ventricular heart. *Teratology.* 43:113–7, 1991.

64. Tikkanen J, Heinonen OP: Maternal hyperthermia during pregnancy and cardiovascular malformations in the offspring. *Eur J Epidemiol.* 7(6):628–35, 1991.

65. Tikkanen J, Heinonen OP: Maternal exposure to chemical and physical factors during pregnancy and cardiovascular malformations in the offspring. *Teratology.* 43:591–600, 1991.

66. Tikkanen J, Heinonen OP: Risk factors for atrial septal defect. *Eur J Epidemiol.* 8(4):509–15, 1992 (July).

67. Yerushalmy J: Congenital heart disease and maternal smoking habits. *Nature.* 242(5395):262–3, 1973.

68. Fedrick J, Alberman ED, Goldstein H: Possible teratogenic effect of cigarette smoking. *Nature.* 231:529–30, 1971.

CHAPTER SEVEN

Recurrence Risks for Cardiac Malformations

Noam Lazebnik

Congenital heart defect (CHD) is the most common form of birth defect, affecting about 8 in 1000 newborns.[1] Rapid advances in cardiovascular science have expanded our knowledge of the mechanisms of heart development. Epidemiologists have defined the prevalence of congenital cardiovascular malformations, developmental biologists have delineated cascades of cell lineage, and molecular geneticists have identified mutations and locuses associated with familial heart and vascular defects. The availability of pre- and postnatal diagnosis of CHDs, coupled with improved surgical advances, has resulted in better prognosis and enabled affected patients to reproduce. Hence, it has become clear that more awareness on the part of pediatricians, obstetricians, and geneticists to make early diagnoses and to comment on recurrence risk is mandatory.

When faced with the reality of a family member with CHD, patients usually ask the following questions: Why did it happen? Will it happen again? A genetic cause has been clearly established for some forms of cardiovascular disease, and new understandings in the molecular genetics of CHD have provided further insight. Progress has been quite impressive for some cardiovascular abnormalities, whereas in other areas the findings are more preliminary. For example, the molecular genetic cause of supravalvular aortic stenosis and the heart disease associated with Marfan's syndrome has been clearly established.[2] Impressive progress has been made in conotruncal defects, Holt-Oram syndrome, Alagille syndrome, and total anomalous pulmonary venous connection.[2] In other areas, such as patent ductus arteriosus and atrioventricular septal defect, the findings are more preliminary. Nevertheless, despite years of intense research, researchers are yet unable to explain the mechanism(s) behind the majority of CHDs, even when the molecular and biochemical defects are clear.

Significant progress has been made in providing recurrence risk for the majority of CHDs. By using traditional genetic tools such as family pedigree to look for possible Mendelian patterns of inheritance and exposure to a known teratogen and population-based studies to infer the empiric risk, recurrence risk figures can be provided for family members of the affected individual. Ideally, aside from providing recurrence risks, clinicians would like to offer their patients a definite test that would look for the molecular abnormality behind the CHD.

For risk assessment, information on the affected individual is critical. Patients are frequently requested to bring any documentation of medical evaluations that have been done, such as chromosome analysis, laboratory test results, photographs, x-ray reports, or autopsy. If the affected individual is living, an evaluation by a pediatric geneticist or adult medical geneticist may be indicated to see whether the diagnosis or etiology of the abnormality can be found. Once a correct diagnosis is made the CHD may fall into one of the following categories:

- Isolated CHD
- Chromosome abnormality
- Syndromes involving cardiac defects
- Metabolic disorder affecting the heart
- Environmental cause
- Maternal medical condition known to increase the risk of CHD

About 2% of CHDs are thought to be due to environmental factors, including rubella, maternal insulin-dependent diabetes, maternal lupus, and exposure to medications. However, it is very possible that even these cases may have genetic components that affect sensitivity to exogenous factors. Approximately 5% to 6% are due to recognized chromosomal abnormalities, and about 3% to 5% to a single-gene disorder, for example, phenylketonuria. The remaining 85% to 90% of CHDs have no identifiable cause and are generally considered to be of multifactorial origin.

As with all birth defects, chromosomal aneuploidy should be suspected in any newborn with congenital heart disease. The association of CHD with a specific dysmorphic pattern may suggest a syndrome. Meticulous maternal history may identify an exposure to a known teratogen as the possible cause of the malformation. Clinical examination may identify cases liable to be associated with a chromosomal deletion not apparent on routine karyotype analysis. A family history of multiple individuals with complex congenital malformations, mental retardation, and recurrent pregnancy loss may suggest chromosomal rearrangement such as translocation, inversion, insertion, duplication, and deletion, mandating karyotype study in similar cases.

The phenomenon of repetition of an adverse reproductive outcome is well known and may have different explanations. The first and obvious one is that the adverse outcome is inherited by a recessive or dominant gene(s). These cases are characteristic of a syndrome that includes multiple abnormalities. The degree of expression of the various abnormal features, as well as the severity of any given congenital anomaly within the specific syndrome, can vary between individuals. Hence, the recurrence risk figure addresses the likelihood of the syndrome's reoccurrence in another family member, rather than that the same CHD of identical severity will reoccur. In such cases the recurrence risk is 25% and 50%, for the recessive and dominant disorder, respectively.

Isolated CHDs not known to be part of a syndrome, whether single-gene disorder or environmentally caused, are counseled as being multifactorial unless the family history indicates a specific pattern of transmission. Assessing the risk for such cases is based on empiric data developed from vast population studies. A starting point for analysis of empiric data on heart defects in siblings and offspring has been the polygenic threshold model. A number of expectations of a polygenic trait allows observational data to be tested against this model:

1. Risk to a first-degree relative equates the square root of the population incidence.
2. Risk to siblings and offspring should be equal.
3. Risk for more distant relatives declines rapidly.
4. Risk increases when there are multiple affected family members.
5. Risk increases with the severity of the disorder.
6. Risk is greater among relatives of the more rarely affected sex.

Recurrence risk for CHDs based on empiric data is given in Table 7–1. The recurrence risk figure addresses the likelihood of any CHD's reoccurrence in another family member rather than recurrence of the same CHD of identical severity. It is widely accepted that the risk for siblings of children with CHDs falls in the range of 2% to 5%.[3] The recurrence risk for a sibling of an individual with a specific CHD is given in Table 7–2. Of interest is the fact that the risk is higher among offspring of affected parents.[4] The incidence of CHD was studied in children of 219 probands with one of the following selected defects: atrial septal defect, coarctation of the aorta, aortic valve stenosis, or complex dextrocardia. Of the offspring, 8.8% had substantial congenital cardiac defects. This incidence was much higher than that reported in most comparable studies and was statistically significant. A later study by Nora and Nora[5] reviewed a total of eight studies involving 3996 offspring of parents who have congenital heart disease. The data showed that the risk for all defects was substantially higher if the affected parent was the mother rather than the father. The risk ratio ranged from a high of 6.39 for aortic stenosis to a low of 1.48 for patent ductus arteriosus (Table 7–3). The risk was severalfold higher for aortic stenosis, atrioventricular canal, and ventricular septal defects. The possible reasons for the preponderance of affected offspring of mothers with a congenital heart disease were studied in the context of various modes of inheritance and maternal physiology. The authors concluded that although many familial cases of CHD are compatible with multifactorial inheritance and vulnerability to teratogens, an important subset of cases, particularly in some high-risk families, may be better explained by mitochondrial inheritance, maternal vulnerability to teratogens, or genomic imprinting, rather than by multifactorial or Mendelian modes.

TABLE 7–1. EMPIRIC RECURRENCE RISK FOR ISOLATED CONGENITAL HEART DEFECT

Affective Relative	Recurrence Risk for Affected Offspring (%)
One affected child	2–5
Affected parent (father)	1.5–3
Affected parent (mother)	2.5–18
Two affected children	5–10
More than two affected first-degree relatives	50
Second- or third-degree relative	Risk is mildly increased over the general population

TABLE 7–2. RISK THAT A SIBLING OF AN INDIVIDUAL WITH A CONGENITAL HEART DEFECT WILL HAVE A HEART DEFECT

Congenital Heart Defect	Risk (%)
Ventricular septal defect	3
Pulmonary stenosis	2
Patent ductus arteriosus	3
Atrial septal defect	3
Coarctation of aorta	2
Aortic stenosis	3
Tetralogy of Fallot	2
Atrioventricular canal	2
Transposition of the great vessels	2

Adapted with permission, from Ardinger RH: Genetic counseling in congenital heart disease. Pediatr Ann. 26:99,1997.

Environmental causes of human malformations include therapeutic medications, maternal chemical dependence, occupational exposures to chemicals and irradiation, and fetal infections. As a group they account for approximately 10% of all malformations. Under 1% of all human malformations are related to prescription drugs, chemicals, or irradiation exposure. For the most part, malformations caused by drugs and therapeutic agents are important because these exposures are preventable. Embryonic stage at exposure, dose, and magnitude of exposure are believed to affect the odds for the newborn to be affected by a teratogen. An example of such association was recently published.[6] Exposure to twice the recommended dose (5000 IU) of vitamin A per day of supplemental vitamin A resulted in a significant risk for fetal malformations: 1 infant in 57. The increased frequency of defects was concentrated among the babies born to women who had consumed high levels of vitamin A, more than 10,000 IU, per day in the form of supplements, before the seventh week of gestation.[6] Occasionally, exposure to a given medication may result in a unique type of CHD. A well-known example is the CHD associated with lithium exposure, Ebstein's anomaly, and tricuspid atresia, which are generally rare CHDs.

The recurrence risk for CHD in future pregnancy is presumably very low. Avoiding future exposure minimizes the risk to that of the general population. For more details regarding risk estimate and type of potential anomalies associated with a given teratogen or medication researchers should consult with a computerized database such as Reprotox.[7] The database provides information regarding the impact of the physical and chemical environment on human reproduction and development. Data presented cover all aspects of reproduction, including fertility; male exposures; lactation; reproductive influence of industrial and environmental chemicals; prescription, over-the-counter, and recreational drugs; and nutritional agents.

A unique situation of congenital malformations resulting from environmental cause arises from maternal characteristics that do not vary between pregnancies, such as maternal medical complications. Although the severity of the medical condition may vary between pregnancies, a woman with insulin-dependent diabetes mellitus (IDDM) or epilepsy during the first pregnancy will most likely have the disease during the following pregnancies and so will have an increased risk of giving birth to an affected offspring.

In general, it is agreed that an increased incidence of cardiac anomalies occurs among offspring of women with IDDM.[8-10] The type of malformation varies with different studies. The most frequent cardiac anomalies are ventricular septal defects (VSDs), transposition of the great vessels, coarctation of the aorta, single ventricle, hypoplastic left ventricle, and pulmonic atresia.[10] A direct relationship between the overall rate and/or the duration of the disease and the level of glycemic control within 3 months before conception and through the first trimester has been reported.[11] The overall risk for CHDs has been reported to be about 4%.[9] The relationship between the level of hemoglobin A1 (Hb A1) in the first trimester and major malformations was examined by Green et al. in 303 insulin-requiring diabetic gravidas.[11] The risk for major malformation, including CHDs, was 3.0% with Hb A1c, less than or equal to 9.3%, and 40% with Hb A1 greater than 14.4% (risk ratio 13.2; 95% confidence interval 4.3 to 40.4). Although the risk for congenital malformations was markedly elevated following a first trimester in very poor metabolic control, there was a broad range of control over which the risk was not substantially elevated.

TABLE 7–3. SUGGESTED OFFSPRING RECURRENCE RISK FOR EIGHT CONGENITAL HEART DEFECTS GIVEN ONE AFFECTED PARENT

Defect	Father Affected (%)	Mother Affected (%)
Aortic stenosis	3	13–18
Atrial septal defect	1.5	4–4.5
Atrioventricular canal	1	14
Coarctation of aorta	2	4
Patent ductus arteriosus	2.5	3.5–4
Pulmonary stenosis	2	4–6.5
Tetralogy of Fallot	1.5	2.5
Ventricular septal defect	2	6–10

Adapted, with permission, from Nora JJ, Nora AH: Maternal transmission of congenital heart diseases: New recurrence risk figures and the questions of cytoplasmic inheritance and vulnerability to teratogens. Am J Cardiol. 59:1369, 1987.

The authors concluded that to keep malformations to a minimum among diabetic women does not require "excellent" control; there seems to be a fairly broad range of "acceptable" control. Hence, an attempt to achieve a Hb A1C level of ≤9% before conception may result in a recurrence risk of <3%.

It is widely acknowledged that there is an increased risk of malformation in children born to epileptic women, whether they are on antiepileptic medications or not.[12,13] Patients who have high seizure frequency and require large doses of antiepileptic drugs have a higher malformation rate in their offspring.[14] The most common major malformations are facial clefts and CHDs. The risk for any malformation is about 7%, and that for a major malformation is about 2% to 3%.

When the patient is pregnant, recurrence risk estimate should be provided in accordance with the above guidelines. Nevertheless, whenever applicable the option of prenatal diagnosis should be suggested through chorionic villus sampling or amniocentesis. A qualified physician can perform either procedure with a miscarriage rate of no higher than 1 in 200. Prenatal diagnosis to detect an inherited disease can be done by applying various types of studies. The most commonly used are chromosome studies, biochemical assays, and various molecular studies.

Standard metaphase preparations will identify fetal aneuploidy and the majority of chromosome rearrangements such as translocation, inversion, duplication, deletions, isochromosomes, and ring chromosomes. High-resolution banding, also called prophase or prometaphase banding (550 to 800 bands), can identify more subtle structural abnormalities of chromosome rearrangement.

When the underlying biochemical defect is known and is expressed in obtainable specimens of fetal tissue (chorionic villi) or cells (trophoblast, amniotic fluid cells, fetal erythrocytes, and leukocytes), prenatal diagnosis is ultimately based on analysis of the enzyme or other protein primarily involved. In other cases, the test is based on measurement of secondary biochemical events such as elevation or absence of particular metabolite(s) or protein(s) in cell-free amniotic fluid or in fetal plasma or serum.

Recently, two very powerful molecular techniques have emerged and revolutionized the field of genetics. These are the polymerase chain reaction (PCR) and fluorescent in situ hybridization (FISH). PCR is able to amplify in vitro a specific piece of DNA from a complex background, a millionfold or more, enabling the researcher to perform mutation screening whenever the gene for the disorder has already been cloned. FISH is beginning to play a larger role in prenatal diagnosis. It has proved to be extremely useful for the identification of subtle structural abnormalities of chromosome re-arrangement, as well as a rapid method for evaluating a large number of cells in order to determine the level of mosaicism in a wide variety of tissues.

When the disease gene in question is unknown or has not yet been cloned and DNA sequence information is unavailable, linkage analysis has been used as an aid to molecular disease diagnosis. In suitable families, the inheritance of a particular disease gene in utero can be detected genetically by following the transmission of other, closely linked locuses called *marker locuses*. Depending on the physical distance between the disease gene and the marker locus, a prediction for or against inheriting the disease gene can be made with an accuracy of ≥95%.

CHROMOSOMAL DEFECTS AND CONGENITAL HEART DEFECTS

Aneuploidy Syndromes

As a general rule, chromosome analysis should be performed in any infant presenting with isolated CHD or a heart defect associated with other malformations. In most cases of aneuploidy there is no specific type of heart defect, and counseling is based on the underlying karyotype.

Cytogeneticists use the term *aneuploidy* to apply to any chromosome number that is not an exact multiple of the haploid number (46) of chromosomes: monosomies, trisomies, and tetrasomies. The most common aneuploidy syndromes that are associated with CHD are trisomies 21, 18, and 13, monosomy 45,X- or Turner's syndrome, and to a much lesser extent, tetrasomies (cat-eye and Pallister-Killian syndromes).

Trisomy 21 (Down Syndrome)

Trisomy 21 is the most important association between a major chromosome defect and CHD. About 30% of newborns with Down syndrome have a heart defect; almost half of these cases are diagnosed with the otherwise rare atrioventricular canal defect.[15] The critical region for the Down phenotype was localized to a small segment of chromosome 21 to the telomeric segment beyond 21q22.12.[16]

If the newborn has standard trisomy 21 or is a 47,+21/46 mosaic, it is unnecessary to study the parent's chromosomes because it can be assumed that they will be 46,XX and 46,XY. For a mother under 30 years old at the birth of the Down syndrome child, the risk for recurrence of Down syndrome in a liveborn child is about 0.7% (1 in 150) and for any chromosomal abnormality at the time of amniocentesis is about 1%. A woman in her 30s or 40s runs the same risk as any other woman of her age.

Down syndrome can result from chromosomal rearrangement as well. The most common example is Robertsonian translocation, resulting from the fusion of two acrocentric chromosomes (chromosomes 13, 14, 15, 21, 22). The history of a child with Robertsonian translocation Down syndrome should result in chromosomal study of the parents. For the de novo translocation (both parents are normal), a recurrence risk figure of <1% is applicable. In familial Robertsonian translocation Down syndrome, the risk can be up to 10% for a newborn with Down syndrome and up to 15% at the time of amniocentesis.

In the rare instance that translocation Down syndrome is associated with a familial reciprocal translocation it becomes necessary to consult with a geneticist because the precise risk estimate needs to be based on the actual cytogenetic imbalance.

Trisomy 18 (Edwards' Syndrome) and Trisomy 13 (Patau's Syndrome)

Trisomy 18 is the second most common autosomal aneuploidy after Down syndrome, with an incidence of 1 in 8000 newborns.[17] It is associated with multiple malformations, severe mental retardation, and short life expectancy.[17] CHDs are a recognized association and are usually the reason for early demise. Of fetuses in a recent study, 87% showed CHD.[17] There is no particular heart defect associated with the syndrome. However, ventricular septal defect, atrioventricular canal, and hypoplastic left heart are common.[17]

Trisomy 13 has an incidence of 1 in 13,000 newborns.[18] This syndrome is also associated with multiple malformations, severe mental retardation, and short survival. There is a high incidence of cardiac defects, in particular atrioventricular or ventricular septal defects, valvular abnormalities, and either narrowing of the isthmus or truncus arteriosus.[18] Abnormality of cardiac position, including dextrocardia, is also common.[18]

Like trisomy 21, trisomies 18 and 13 show a maternal age effect. Recurrences of trisomies 18 and 13 are extremely rare. Therefore, a decision regarding prenatal diagnosis in future pregnancy should be based on maternal age. Nevertheless, offering prenatal diagnosis may be elected for reassurance. If any aneuploidy should be identified, a 45,X or trisomy 21 may be more likely than trisomy 18 or 13. The recurrence risk for partial trisomy 18 or 13 resulting from either parent's having a balanced chromosome rearrangement mandates genetic counseling for a precise risk estimate based on the actual cytogenetic imbalance.

45,X Turner's Syndrome

Absence of the second sex chromosome results in short stature, gonadal dysgenesis, and variable dysmorphic features. The incidence of female newborns

with 45,X or one of its many variants is 1 in 1800. The most common CHD associated with Turner's syndrome is coarctation of the aorta, followed by bicuspid aortic valve and mitral valve prolapse.[18] There is an association between some dysmorphic features such as neck webbing and CHD. Studies of parental origin of the missing sex chromosome suggest evidence for imprinting.[19] Patients who retained the paternal sex chromosome showed a lower incidence of CHD and neck webbing. These findings suggest paternal expression of gene(s) on the sex chromosome in the normal development of the aorta and its surrounding structures.

The syndrome is not known to show association with maternal age. The recurrence risk for parents with a child with Turner syndrome is that of the general population.

Tetrasomy 22p (Cat-Eye Syndrome)

This syndrome results from the presence of a marker chromosome, the inv (inversion) dup (duplication) (22)(ptr-q11.2).[20] As a result of the extra genetic material stored in the marker chromosome individuals with the syndrome have four copies of the critical region. Therefore, they are tetrasomic for this region. The syndrome is characterized by ear tags, imperforated anus, and iris colobomata. There is a very strong association between this syndrome and total anomalous pulmonary venous drainage of the lungs, which leads to pulmonary hypertension.[21]

Most cases arise de novo, but familial transmission is recorded, including familial mosaicism for the marker chromosome. For de novo cases the recurrence risk is very low and equals the risk in the general population. The risk is significantly higher if either parent is hetrozygotic or shows mosaics for the marker chromosome. In such cases prenatal diagnosis should be offered.

Tetrasomy 12p (Pallister-Killian Syndrome)

Pallister-Killian is a rare syndrome characterized by the presence of an isochromosome for the short arm of chromosome 12, I(12p). About 25% of newborns with tetrasomy 12p have CHDs, VSD being the most common one.[22] Other defects such as coarctation of the aorta, aortic stenosis and atrial septal defect are also reported. Another abnormal feature of the syndrome is diaphragmatic hernia, which may be present in up to 50% of patients. Analysis of skin fibroblasts or bone marrow aspirate is required to confirm the diagnosis, because the isochromosome is usually not detected in cultured peripheral blood leukocytes. In utero, the diagnosis can be made through amniocentesis or CVS (chorionic villus sampling). Fluorescent in situ hybridization has proved to be useful in the diagnosis of the isochromosome.[23] Isochromosomes arise somatically, at least most of the time, so the mosaic state is usual. No correlation was found between the degree of the mosaicism in the tissue studied and the severity of the syndrome.[23] In the Pallister-Killian syndrome, the 12p isochromosome can vary from being in the majority of cells sampled to none at all. Because isochromosomes arise somatically most of the time, the recurrence risk for future pregnancy is very low.

CHROMOSOME DELETION SYNDROMES

Chromosome deletion syndromes result from the loss of genetic material from one or more chromosomes. Deletions that are amenable to traditional cytogenetic techniques for diagnosis are known as *deletion syndromes*. Those that are detected through molecular analysis such as FISH are termed *microdeletion syndromes*, because the deleted DNA segment is too small to be detected by conventional cytogenetic techniques. The deletion produces a monosomy for the region of the chromosome that has been removed, and locuses in this segment are therefore underexpressed.

Wolf-Hirschhorn Syndrome (del 4p)

The Wolf-Hirschhorn deletion syndrome results from a deletion of a segment of the short arm of chromosome 4. The deleted chromosome segment is often of paternal origin. Subtle as well as unsubtle deletions occur, and sometimes FISH may be necessary for definitive identification of the former. The extent of the deletion and the specific segment deleted can be correlated with components of the phenotype.[24] The CHDs are frequent but not specific to the syndrome and include aortic and pulmonary stenosis, ASD, and VSD.

The majority of Wolf-Hirschhorn syndrome cases occur de novo, and therefore carry low recurrence risk but not zero, because the rare situation cannot be excluded of parental occult mosaicism not detected by routine blood chromosome study. The abnormal line may be gonadal (confined to gametic tissue) or somatic but does not include blood. The observation of rarity of recurrence allows the counselor to propose a risk of under 0.5%. The few cases recorded were parental balanced translocation and resulted in unbalanced offspring with the syndrome.[25] Hence, parental chromosome and FISH studies should be considered. In these cases a substantial recurrence risk is probable, and appropriate consultation should be sought.

Williams Syndrome

Williams syndrome is a complex genetic syndrome caused by a submicroscopic deletion in chromosome 7q13.[26] Its main clinical findings include a characteristic facial appearance, cardiovascular anomalies, mental re-

tardation or developmental delay, and neurobehavioral abnormalities. It is relatively common, with an overall incidence of approximately 1 in 20,000 newborns.[26]

A major component of Williams syndrome is the cardiovascular defects. The most characteristic anomaly is supravalvular aortic stenosis, but also very common is peripheral pulmonic stenosis or narrowing of other major muscular arteries such as the renal, carotid, and cerebral arteries. In addition, CHDs such as ASD and VSD are common.[26]

The Williams syndrome locus was mapped to 7q11.23.[27] Deletions and mutations in the elastin gene were reported. More than 90% of patients were found to be hemizygous at the elastin locus.[27] The syndrome is an autosomal-dominant disorder, but all but a few cases represent new mutations. Demonstration of the deletion by FISH should be done to confirm the diagnosis. The deletion may equally be of paternal or maternal origin. The degree of the clinical severity is related to the number of locuses deleted. Deletion of the elastin locus alone produces the characteristic cardiac defect in isolation. There is no record of recurrence in siblings of undoubted Williams syndrome to normal parents. However, rare instances of parent to child transmission were recorded.[28] In the rare situation that either parent tests positive for the deletion the recurrence risk is 50%.

Alagille Syndrome

The characteristic features of Alagille syndrome are stenosis of the peripheral pulmonary arteries and insufficient development of bile ducts within the liver, along with eye and skeletal defects and a distinctive facies.[29] An autosomal-dominant mode of genetic transmission with variable penetrance seems likely. In about 10% of cases a deletion involving 20p11.2–20p12 is found.

Velocardiofacial and DiGeorge Syndromes (del 22q11)

Velocardiofacial syndrome and DiGeorge syndrome result from a microdeletion on the long arm of chromosome 22. The 22q11 deletion results in a spectrum of clinical disorders, which include the velocardiofacial syndrome and DiGeorge syndrome. Cleft palate or velopharyngeal insufficiency, conotruncal heart defects, and characteristic facies characterize the velocardiofacial syndrome. DiGeorge syndrome is characterized by conotruncal heart defect, hypocalcemia, and thymic hypoplasia.

The CHD is seen in about 35% of patients with the deletion. The type of CHD is fairly specific and includes those lesions classified as conotruncal heart defects: truncus arteriosus, interrupted aortic arch, tetralogy of Fallot, left-sided aortic arch, vascular rings, and some types of VSDs.

The two syndromes are caused by deletion in 22q11. In most cases these are submicroscopic, requiring FISH technology to detect the missing segment. About 90% of cases are de novo, and thus carry low recurrence risk.[30] Familial cases in more than one generation pointed to a possible Mendelian inheritance pattern.[31] Presumed parental gonadal mosaicism has been described as well, and prenatal diagnosis using FISH may be considered in a subsequent pregnancy to cover these possibilities.[32]

OTHER MAJOR CARDIAC SYNDROMES

More than 270 syndromes have been described with CHD so far.[33] These syndromes show a Mendelian pattern of inheritance: autosomal dominant, autosomal recessive, X-linked recessive, and X-linked dominant, as well as sporadic cases. Some of these syndromes are discussed in this section.

Noonan Syndrome

The Noonan syndrome phenotype is quite variable and shares some abnormal features with Turner's syndrome, such as webbing of the neck, widely spaced nipples, short stature, and mild learning difficulties. However, unlike the case in Turner's syndrome, the karyotype is normal.[34]

About two thirds of children with Noonan syndrome are diagnosed with CHD.[35] Valvular pulmonary stenosis is a very common finding among affected individuals (50%). Other common CHDs among these cases are ASD, asymmetric septal hypertrophy, and persistent ductus arteriosus. VSD occurs in about 5%.[35] The inheritance pattern is autosomal dominant.

Holt-Oram Syndrome

This syndrome is characterized by CHD and limb abnormalities. The limb defects can vary from phocomelia to minor anomalies of the joint, radial defects, absent thumb, or triphalangeal thumb. The most common CHD is a secundum ASD.[36] Occasional cases of VSD, as well as atrioventricular canal, have been reported. The inheritance pattern is autosomal dominant.

Ellis-van Creveld Syndrome

Ellis-van Creveld syndrome is a rare syndrome characterized by intrauterine growth retardation, short limbs, postaxial polydactyly, club foot, small chest, renal cysts, and CHD.[37] About 60% of cases show CHD. The most common reported cardiac anomaly is ASD.[37] Abnormalities of the AV valves are also commonly present. Rarely, atrioventricular canal anomalies have been reported. The inheritance pattern is believed to be autosomal recessive.

CONGENITAL HEART DEFECTS AND METABOLIC DISORDERS

For many years it was known that metabolic disorders affected the heart. However, it was generally accepted that the effect on the heart resulted from accumulation within the cells of an abnormal metabolite. A typical example of such mechanism is the mucopolysaccharidoses, wherein deposition of abnormal metabolite results in dysfunction of the cardiac valves and abnormalities within the muscle, as in Pompe's disease. We are now aware of a different type of cardiac anomalies, which are part of the syndrome and are not secondary to abnormal storage of any metabolite. This section presents two of these disorders.

Zellweger Syndrome

The pathology of this condition is characterized by an absence of normal peroxisomes, and the result is failure to form multiprotein complexes.[38] Severely affected infants present with dysmorphic features, including abnormal facies, profound neurologic impairment, and renal, hepatic, and cardiac abnormalities. Death usually occurs within the first few months of life. At least five genes have been shown to be affected in patients with Zellweger syndrome. The CHD associated with this syndrome is outflow tract malformation.[38] The inheritance pattern is autosomal recessive.

Smith-Lemli-Opitz Syndrome

Smith-Lemli-Opitz (SLO) syndrome is characterized by severe learning disability, cleft palate, hypospadias in males, and syndactyly. The discovery of the deficiency of 7-dehydrocholesterol reductase as a causative factor of the SLO syndrome[39] made this syndrome the first true metabolic syndrome of multiple congenital malformations. The CHDs reported with this syndrome are tetralogy of Fallot, VSD, ASD, atrioventricular canal, and anomalous pulmonary venous drainage.[40] The inheritance pattern is autosomal recessive.

RISK REDUCTION METHODS

Aside from providing recurrence risk figures the clinician should address the issue of risk reduction in future pregnancies. Gene therapy and preimplantation testing are very attractive methods for risk reduction. However, they are as yet far from being clinically relevant options. Presently, there are several methods of risk reduction that have proved to be efficacious. In the case of a clear Mendelian inheritance of a disorder, and profound phenotypic abnormality, artificial insemination or egg donation may be suggested depending on the mode of inheritance and whether the dominant disorder is maternally or paternally derived. If the congenital abnormality has resulted from exposure to a known teratogen, avoiding future exposure will minimize the risk. For multifactorial congenital defects periconceptional use of folic acid should be considered. The preventive efficacy of the periconceptional use of folic acid is well established for neural tube defects, but much less so for other birth defects.[41] Maternal use of folic acid before conception and through the first trimester has been shown to reduce the risk for neural tube defects substantially. In addition, other birth defects may be prevented by the periconceptional use of folic acid. Homocysteine–methionine metabolism appears to be altered in women with pregnancies affected by neural tube defects; however, the specific mechanisms of causation are not yet known.[41]

In a recent study by Botto et al.,[42] the authors conducted a population-based, case–control study to assess the effects of multivitamin use on the risk for conotruncal defects, a group of severe heart defects that includes transposition of the great arteries, tetralogy of Fallot, and truncus arteriosus. They have identified 158 cases of infants with conotruncal defects and 3026 unaffected, randomly chosen control infants. Periconceptional multivitamin use was defined as reported regular use from 3 months before conception through the third month of pregnancy. Pregnant women who reported periconceptional multivitamin use had a 43% lower risk of having infants with conotruncal defects (odds ratio, 0.57; 95% confidence interval, CI = 0.33 to 1.00) than did pregnant women who reported no use. The estimated relative risk was lowest for isolated conotruncal defects (odds ratio, 0.41; 95% CI = 0.20 to 0.84) compared with those associated with noncardiac defects (odds ratio, 0.91; 95% CI = 0.33 to 2.52) or a recognized syndrome (odds ratio, 1.82; 95% CI = 0.31 to 10.67). Among anatomic subgroups of defects, transposition of the great arteries showed the greatest reduction in risk (odds ratio, 0.36; 95% CI = 0.15 to 0.89). These findings could have major implications for the prevention of these and other birth defects in the future.

SUMMARY

Establishing a definite diagnosis for a CHD is a prerequisite before any estimation of recurrence risks can be provided. A meticulous family pedigree and review of pertinent medical records, combined with state of the art cytogenetic and molecular studies of the affected individual(s), can help to ascertain mode of inheritance and diagnosis. Only then can recurrence risk figures be provided. Whenever a molecular test is available to ascertain the presence of a genetic disorder such tests should be offered to provide a more definite risk figure.

Risk reduction methods should be discussed and patients should be encouraged to take advantage of the benefit provided through periconceptional folic acid therapy.

REFERENCES

1. Hsieh CC, Kuo DM, Chiu TH, Hsieh TT: Prenatal diagnosis of major congenital cardiovascular malformations. *Gynecol Obstet Invest*. 42:84, 1996.
2. Benson DW, Basson CT, MacRae CA: New understandings in the genetics of congenital heart disease. *Curr Opin Pediatr*. 8:505, 1996.
3. Ardinger RH: Genetic counseling in congenital heart disease. *Pediatr Ann*. 26:99, 1997.
4. Rose V, Morley RJ, Lindsay GG, et al.: Possible increase in the incidence of congenital heart defects among the offspring of affected parents. *J Am Coll Cardiol*. 6:376, 1985.
5. Nora JJ, Nora AH: Maternal transmission of congenital heart diseases: New recurrence risk figures and the questions of cytoplasmic inheritance and vulnerability to teratogens. *Am J Cardiol*. 59:459, 1987.
6. Rothman KJ, Moore LL, Singer MR, et al.: Teratogenicity of high vitamin A intake. *N Engl J Med*. 333:1369, 1995.
7. Reprotox: Reproductive hazard information, environmental impact of human reproduction and development.
8. Kucera J: Rate and type of congenital anomalies among offspring of diabetic women. *J Reprod Med*. 7:61, 1971.
9. Rowland TW, Hubble JP, Nadas AS: Congenital heart disease in infants of diabetic mothers. *J Pediatr*. 83:815, 1973.
10. Meyer-Wittkopf M, Simpson JM, Sharland GK: Incidence of congenital heart defects in fetuses of diabetic mothers: A retrospective study of 326 cases. *Ultrasound Obstet Gynecol*. 8:8, 1996.
11. Greene MF, Hare JW, Cloherty JP, et al.: First-trimester hemoglobin A1 and risk for major malformation and spontaneous abortion in diabetic pregnancy. *Teratology*. 39:225, 1989.
12. Committee on Educational Bulletins of the American College of Obstetricians and Gynecologists: *Seizure disorders in pregnancy*. ACOG Educational Bulletin No. 231, December 1996.
13. Nulman I, Scolnik D, Chitayat D, et al.: Findings in children exposed in utero to phenytoin and carbamazepine monotherapy: Independent effects of epilepsy and medications. *Am J Med Genet*. 68:18, 1997.
14. Dravet C, Julian C, Legras C: Epilepsy, antiepileptic drugs and malformations in children of women with epilepsy: A French prospective study. *Neurology*. Suppl. 42:75, 1992.
15. Kallen B, Mastroiacovo P, Robert E: Major congenital malformations in Down syndrome. *Am J Med Genet*. 65:160, 1996.
16. Reish O, Berry SA, Dewald G, et al.: Duplication of 7p: Further delineation of the phenotype and restriction of the critical region to the distal part of the short arm. *Am J Med Genet*. 61:21, 1996.

17. Embleton ND, Wyllie JP, Wright MJ, et al.: Natural history of trisomy 18. *Arch Dis Child Fetal Neonatal Ed.* 75:38, 1996.

18. Hyett J, Moscoso G, Nicolaides K: Abnormalities of the heart and great arteries in first trimester chromosomally abnormal fetuses. *Am J Med Genet.* 69:207, 1997.

19. Chu CE, Donaldson MD, Kelnar CJ, et al.: Possible role of imprinting in the Turner phenotype. *J Med Genet.* 31:840, 1994.

20. Wenger SL, Surti U, Nwokoro NA, et al.: Cytogenetic characterization of cat eye syndrome marker chromosome. *Ann Genet.* 37:33, 1994.

21. Paul T, Reimer A, Wilken M, et al.: Complex cyanotic heart defect in a newborn infant with cat eye syndrome. *Monatsschr Kinderheilkd.* 139:228, 1991.

22. Smulian J, Guzman E, Mohan C, et al.: Genetics casebook. Pallister-Killian syndrome. *J Perinatol.* 5:406, 1996.

23. Mowery-Rusthon PA, Stadler MP, Kochmar SJ, et al.: The use of interfase FISH for prenatal diagnosis of Pallister-Killian syndrome. *Prenat Diag.* 17:255, 1997.

24. Estabrooks LL, Lamb AN, Aylsworth AS, et al.: Molecular characterization of chromosome 4p deletions resulting in Wolf-Hirschhorn syndrome. *J Med Genet.* 3:103, 1994.

25. Reid E, Morrison N, Barron L, et al.: Familial Wolf-Hirschhorn syndrome resulting from a cryptic translocation: A clinical and molecular study. *J Med Genet.* 33:197, 1996.

26. Hirota H, Matsuoka R, Kimura M, et al.: Molecular cytogenetic diagnosis of Williams syndrome. *Am J Med Genet.* 64:473, 1996.

27. Lowery MC, Morris CA, Ewart A, et al.: Strong correlation of elastin deletions, detected by FISH with Williams syndrome: Evaluation of 235 patients. *Am J Hum Genet.* 57:49, 1995.

28. Morris CA, Thomas IT, Greenberg F: Williams syndrome: Autosomal dominant inheritance. *Am J Med Genet.* 47:478, 1993.

29. Alagille D: Alagille syndrome today. *Clin Invest Med.* 19:325, 1996.

30. Demczuk S, Aledo R, Zucman J, et al.: Cloning of a balanced translocation breakpoint in the DiGeorge syndrome critical region and isolation of a novel potential adhesion receptor gene in the vicinity. *Hum Molec Genet.* 4:551, 1995.

31. Greenberg F, Crowder WE, Paschall V, et al.: Familial DiGeorge syndrome and associated partial monosomy of chromosome 22. *Hum Genet.* 65:317, 1995.

32. Driscoll DA, Slavin J, Sellinger B, et al.: Prevalence of 22q11 microdeletions in DiGeorge and velocardiofacial syndromes: Implications for genetic counseling and prenatal diagnosis. *J Med Genet.* 30:813, 1993.

33. Burn J, Goodship J: In Rimoin DL, Connor JM, Pyeritz RE, eds. *Emery and Rimoin's Principles and Practice of Medical Genetics.* New York: Churchill Livingstone; 1996: pp. 804–28.

34. Noonan JA: Hypertelorism with Turner phenotype. A new syndrome with associated congenital heart disease. *Am J Dis Child.* 116:373, 1986.

35. Zubeldia Sanchez J, Cabrera Duro A, Sanchez Obregon M, et al.: Cardiopathy in Noonan syndrome. Review of 29 cases. *Ann Esp Pediatr.* 30:104, 1989.

36. Newbury-Ecob RA, Leanage R, Raeburn JA, et al.: Holt-Oram syndrome: A clinical genetic study. *J Med Genet.* 33:300, 1996.

37. Blackburn MG, Belliveau RE: Ellis-van Creveld syndrome: A report of previously undescribed anomalies in two siblings. *Am J Dis Child.* 122:267, 1971.

38. Goldfischer S, Moore CL, Johnson AB, et al.: Peroxisomal and mitochondrial defects in the cerebro-hepato-renal syndrome. *Science.* 182:62, 1973.

39. Tint GS, Irons M, Elias ER, et al.: Defective cholesterol biosynthesis associated with the Smith-Lemli-Opitz syndrome. *New Engl J Med.* 330:107, 1994.

40. Seller MJ, Flinter FA, Docherty Z, et al.: Phenotypic diversity in the Smith-Lemli-Opitz syndrome. *Clin Dysmorphol.* 6:69, 1997.

41. Allen WP: Folic acid in the prevention of birth defects. *Curr Opin Pediatr.* 8:630, 1996.

42. Botto LD, Khoury MJ, Mulinare J, et al.: Periconceptional multivitamin use and the occurrence of conotruncal heart defects: Results from a population-based, case-control study. *Pediatrics.* 98:911, 1996.

CHAPTER EIGHT

Cardiac Defects and Extracardiac Anomalies

Kenneth G. Perry, Jr.
William E. Roberts

Cross-sectional diagnosis of structural congenital heart malformations with two-dimensional (2D) imaging became established in the 1970s.[64,99] Shortly thereafter, investigators utilizing these same techniques began to perform fetal echocardiography.[1,2,117] Their initial efforts to document the anatomic correlates and the assessment of cardiac function in the fetus were soon followed by an ability to diagnose and characterize a variety of congenital heart defects antenatally in the fetus.[26,30] Continued improvements in the resolution capability of ultrasound, coupled with further expansion of our knowledge in this field, have allowed transition of fetal echocardiography from a research tool into a valuable clinical diagnostic test. This development is of paramount importance since congenital heart disease (CHD) is not only the most common structural abnormality seen in liveborn infants but is also associated with over 50% of deaths from lethal malformations in childhood.[51,63]

Cardiac defects occur with a frequency of 8 per 1000 live births but are seen four to five times more often in stillbirths.[50] CHD is over six times more common than other chromosomal abnormalities and is seen with a frequency of over four times that of neural tube defects.[67] However, the exact etiology of most CHD is still unknown. Approximately 90% of CHD cases are felt to be multifactorial in origin. Accordingly, the majority of infants with CHD are born to women without previously known risk factors. As a result, a systematic prenatal screening protocol of the heart as part of a routine ultrasound examination is advocated by both the American College of Obstetricians and Gynecologists[4] and the American Institute of Ultrasound in Medicine.[3]

At a time of intense scrutiny of medical costs, such a recommendation must pass muster in evidence-based medicine. It is no longer possible to justify performing a certain procedure simply because the technology exists. Instead, the procedure must be safe and make a difference in outcome. This chapter provides evidence that the antenatal diagnosis of CHD does meet the criteria of safety and efficacy. In addition, this chapter provides a logical approach to maximizing screening efforts to ensure the best one is provided for the most patients at a reasonable cost.

SCREENING APPROACH

The antenatal diagnosis of CHD has value since it can have a substantial impact on the management and outcome of an affected pregnancy.[26,70,103] The antenatal diagnosis of a CHD can be beneficial to parents and other family members by providing them with time to prepare for the medical, emotional, and socioeconomic consequences of a child with CHD. Finally, by the timely detection of a fetus with CHD, obstetric health care providers often have sufficient time to categorize the disorder fully. This permits more accurate counseling of parents regarding prognosis and management options such as pregnancy termination or referral to a tertiary health care facility for specialized maternal and newborn care.

To maximize health-related resources and utilize

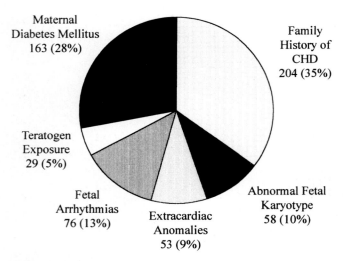

Figure 8–1. Fetal echocardiography experience at the University of Mississippi Medical Center, July 1, 1993–June 30, 1996. N = 583.

TABLE 8–1. RISK FOR CONGENITAL HEART DISEASE

Screening Parameter	Risk for CHD (%)	Reference
Positive family history		
Sibling affected	1–3	16
Mother affected	2.5	17
Father affected	1 – 3	17
Maternal diabetes	2 – 4	15
Fetal arrhythmia	1 – 2	18
Teratogen exposure	2	18
Extracardiac anomaly		19
CNS	2.5 – 25	
Tracheo-esophageal fistula	15 – 40	
Gastrointestinal	5 – 22	
Omphalocele	20 – 32	
Diaphragmatic hernia	10 – 23	
Genitourinary	2 – 43	
Chromosomal anomaly	25	19

diagnostic capabilities efficiently, a determination must be made regarding which pregnancies are at risk for CHD. Any person whose risk of having a fetus with CHD that exceeds that of the general obstetric population ideally should undergo fetal echocardiography. These include patients with a positive family history of CHD, those exposed to teratogens such as lithium, women with overt diabetes mellitus before pregnancy, and those with a fetal arrhythmia.

Figure 8–1 depicts the recent experience with fetal echocardiography at The University of Mississippi Medical Center. Over a 3-year period from July 1993 through June 1996, 583 maternity patients underwent fetal echocardiography. The majority of these (81%) had one or more of the previously mentioned indications of CHD, with the most common indication a family history of CHD. However, these common indications for fetal echocardiography led to the detection of only a minority of cases. The reason for this apparent paradox is shown in Table 8–1. These high-risk conditions are associated with a < 5% incidence of CHD. On the other hand, the fraction of patients (19%) who underwent fetal echocardiography for chromosomal and/or extracardiac anomalies was much more likely to be associated with CHD. This latter group of pregnancies forms the basis for this chapter.

CHROMOSOMAL ABERRATIONS

Publications of fetal echocardiographic patient series indicate that a number of chromosomal defects are characteristically associated with CHD. Any attempt at

the development of a thorough list of associations must necessarily be incomplete since many autosomal abnormalities result in first-trimester abortions. Rarely in such losses is an accurate evaluation of cardiac structure performed. Even so, one can construct relevant information on the association of liveborn chromosomal aberrations and CHD. Of special note is that other somatic malformations are also associated with these chromosomal abnormalities but a complete cataloging is beyond the scope of this chapter.

Trisomy 21

Trisomy 21 (Down syndrome) is the most common autosomal chromosomal abnormality, affecting 1 in 660 liveborn infants (Table 8–2). Although there is a definite association of Down syndrome with advanced maternal age, 80% of Down syndrome infants are born to women younger than age 35. Measuring maternal serum α-fetoprotein (MSAFP) and adjusting for the mother's age improves the detection rate of Down syndrome among low-risk patients from 0% to 30%. The addition of human chorionic gonadotropin (hCG) with or without a plasma estriol measurement (uE$_3$) further improves the detection rate in low-risk patients to 40%.[11]

Because of poor sensitivity, ultrasound is not used as a primary screen for Down syndrome. However, Down syndrome is associated with two pathologic processes with obvious sonographic features that should prompt the ultrasonographer to perform a complete examination and offer genetic amniocentesis. These two pathologic processes are an atrioventricular

TABLE 8–2. CONGENITAL HEART DISEASE IN SELECTED CHROMOSOMAL ABERRATIONS

Conditions	Prevalence	Incidence of CHD (%)	Observed Loss Rate 16 Weeks–Term (%)	CHD in Decreasing Frequency[a]
Trisomy 21	1 in 660	50	30	AVSD, VSD
Trisomy 18	1 in 6,250	95	68	VSD, PDA, PS
Trisomy 13	1 in 12,000	90	43	DORV, VSD, HLHS
Turner's syndrome	1 in 4,200	35	75	COA, AS, ASD

[a]AVSD, atrioventricular septal defect; VSD, ventricular septal defect; PDA, patent ductus arteriosus; PS, pulmonary stenosis; DORV, double-outlet right ventricle; HLHS, hypoplastic left heart syndrome; COA, coarctation of aorta; AS, aortic stenosis; ASD, atrial septal defect.

septal defect (AVSD) and duodenal atresia. Visualization of a "double-bubble" sign is suggestive of duodenal atresia and is associated with a 20% to 30% risk of trisomy 21.

About 50% of Down syndrome infants have a cardiac anomaly, of which 50% are AVSDs. These defects are also known as endocardial cushion defects or atrioventricular canal defects. During fetal life, the endocardial cushion grows and contributes to the closure of the lower part of the atrial septum and the upper portion of the ventricular septum (Figure 8–2). The failure of the endocardial cushion to form and grow results in a complete AVSD in which the center of the heart is missing. This produces a septum primum atrial septal defect (ASD) and/or a ventricular septal defect (VSD). Also, because the endocardial cushion participates in the development of the atrioventricular valve, AVSDs usually are associated with abnormalities of the mitral and tricuspid valves (Figure 8–3).

The diagnosis of a complete AVSD is made in the absence of the atrial septum in conjunction with a single atrioventricular valve and a shortened interventricular septum. Although incomplete forms of AVSDs exist, they are difficult to differentiate from an atrial primum septal defect. Because AVSDs involve the interatrial septum, fetal bradycardia caused by complete atrioventricular block is not uncommon. The prognosis of complete AVSD is poor, with only a 14% survival rate in one recent series.[68] In this series of cases, 50% of AVSDs were associated with aneuploidy, 60% of which were trisomy 21 and 25% trisomy 18.

Although AVSD is the most common cardiac lesion seen in conjunction with Down syndrome, VSDs also occur frequently and are seen in 20% of such infants. The VSD is usually perimembranous in location and, depending on the size, can be difficult to visualize by ultrasound. However, recently a group of investigators has correlated the size of the VSD with the presence of

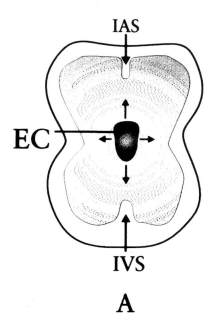

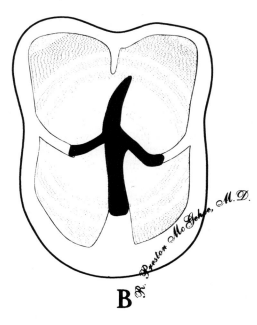

Figure 8–2. The endocardial cushion (EC) grows to meet the interatrial septum (IAS) and the interventricular septum (IVS) (**A**). This embryonic process divides the primitive atrioventricular canal (**B**). (*Courtesy of R. Preston McGehee, MD.*)

LV   RV

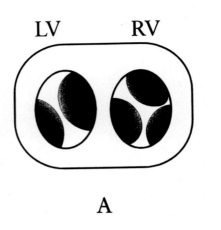

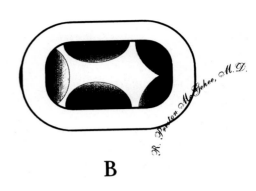

Figure 8–3. The contribution to the atrioventricular valves by the atrioventricular cushion (shown in dark). **A.** As seen in a normal heart from above. **B.** As seen from above in a heart with an atrioventricular septal defect. (*Courtesy of R. Preston McGehee, MD.*)

A   B

nuchal translucency.[59] If the nuchal translucency is 4 mm or more, 75% of fetuses with Down syndrome have a VSD, whereas only 10% of such fetuses have a VSD if the nuchal translucency is 3 mm or less. The proposed mechanism for this association of VSD and nuchal translucency purportedly is increased blood flow through the aortic arch with increasing size of the VSD. This could result in increased perfusion of the fetal head and neck with the development of nuchal edema, which can serve as a valuable marker for the presence of a VSD in the Down syndrome fetus. Isolated VSDs in Down syndrome infants have a clinical course similar to VSDs in other infants, with a spontaneous closure rate of 45% within 1 year.[75]

Trisomy 18

Trisomy 18, or Edwards' syndrome, is the second most frequent trisomy at birth, with a prevalence of 1 in 6250 live births (Table 8–2).[55] The hallmark of trisomy 18 is hydramnios with intrauterine growth restriction and fetal congenital abnormalities. As in Down syndrome, the incidence of trisomy 18 at the time of genetic amniocentesis is different from that observed at birth. In trisomy 21 the intrauterine lethality is 30%, whereas the rate is more than doubled (68%) with trisomy 18.[54] Unlike Down syndrome, trisomy 18 is a lethal condition. Therefore, aggressive obstetric management and/or intervention is not warranted. Furthermore, postnatal studies and interventions are inappropriate and no results of various treatment modalities are available for review.

In the early 1990s, several groups reported an association of choriod plexus cysts (CPCs) and trisomy 18.[9,86] Because 50% of trisomy 18 fetuses in the mid-trimester of pregnancy have sonographically detectable CPCs, some have advocated a genetic amniocentesis whenever this finding has been encountered. On the other hand, because CPCs occur in 1% of chromoso-

mally normal fetuses, others have been concerned that a genetic amniocentesis in the presence of an isolated CPC would result in more procedure-related losses than could be justified through the detection of trisomy 18 fetuses. Recently, Snijders and colleagues[104] provided helpful information for this dilemma; their investigation revealed that 97% of trisomy 18 fetuses have additional anomalies identified on ultrasound.

Presently, there is consensus that the presence of a CPC should stimulate the sonographer to perform a targeted examination with special emphasis on other features associated with trisomy 18. These include ventriculomegaly, absent corpus callosum, enlarged cisterna magna, facial cleft, micrognathia, nuchal translucency, cardiac defect, diaphragmatic hernia, renal defects, esophageal atresia, rocker-bottom feet, hydramnios, and fetal growth restriction. If the CPC is isolated, the risk for trisomy 18 is minimally increased and maternal age should be the primary factor for performance of an amniocentesis.

Congenital heart disease, primarily VSDs, occurs in more than 95% of trisomy 18 infants. In a recent report where thorough pathologic examination was conducted after pregnancy termination, all 19 fetuses with trisomy 18 had cardiac defects, 84% of which were VSDs.[58] Most VSDs were perimembranous and the size of the lesion appeared to be the limiting factor in demonstrating the VSD with ultrasound. Because this series of trisomy 18 fetuses has been identified with chorionic villous sampling after visualization of increased fetal nuchal translucency on sonography, this latter finding appears to be a valuable marker for the concomitant presence of a VSD in trisomy 21 and 18 fetuses.

Trisomy 13

Trisomy 13, also referred to as Patau's syndrome, is the third most frequent trisomy noted at birth, with a prevalence of 1 in 12,000 live births (Table 8–2).[53] As in trisomy

18 fetuses, the number of trisomy 13 fetuses observed at 16 weeks of gestation is markedly different from the number seen at term. In trisomy 13, the spontaneous, intrauterine death rate is approximately 43%.[54] Also, like trisomy 18, trisomy 13 is a lethal condition with a mean survival of 130 days.

Intracranial abnormalities occur more commonly in fetuses with trisomy 13 than in the other trisomies. A characteristic ultrasound finding, seen in two thirds of fetuses with trisomy 13, is holoprosencephaly.[102] In affected fetuses, there is absence of the third ventricle, fusion of the thalamus, and a single horseshoe-shaped ventricle replacing the two lateral ventricles. All three forms of holoprosencephaly are associated with severe mental retardation. Trisomy 13 is present in half of the cases where holoprosencephaly is found.[20]

Congenital heart disease occurs in 90% of infants with trisomy 13.[82] The most often seen lesions are double-outlet right ventricle, hypoplastic left ventricle, VSD, AVSD, and dextrocardia. Because many of these lesions result in either an increased blood flow through the proximal aorta or a hindrance of blood return through the superior vena cava, increased nuchal translucency is also noted in trisomy 13 fetuses. As with trisomy 18, the degree of nuchal transparency appears critical. One group of researchers reported that all trisomy 13 fetuses had a nuchal translucency thickness of 3 mm or more.[90]

Turner's Syndrome

Turner's syndrome (monosomy X) is common, affecting 1 in 70 conceptions. However, the intrauterine wastage is impressive since the prevalence of Turner's syndrome is only 1 in 4200 live births (Table 8–2).[56] Although most abort in the first trimester, the intrauterine lethality continues into the second trimester, with an observed loss rate of 75% from 16 weeks to term.[54]

A characteristic ultrasound finding in Turner's syndrome is nuchal cystic hygroma, a condition considered to result from a failure of the development of a communication between the jugular lymphatic sac and the jugular vein. Thus, lymphatic stasis develops and fluid accumulates in the contiguous tissue. The prenatal diagnosis of nuchal cystic hygroma requires demonstration of a bilateral, separated, cystic structure located in the occipitocervical region. This condition should be differentiated from nuchal edema or translucency in which the separating nuchal ligament is not visualized. Nuchal edema is associated with trisomies but not with Turner's syndrome.

Antenatally diagnosed cystic hygromas are associated with hydrops fetalis (40% to 100%), congenital heart defects (0% to 92%), and chromosomal defects (46% to 90%). The most common associated chromosomal abnormality is Turner's syndrome (70%). Congenital heart defects occur in approximately 20% of infants with Turner's syndrome. When these occur, left-sided lesions predominate, with coarctation of the aorta being the most common anomaly (70%).[6] Other heart defects include aortic stenosis and hypoplastic left heart.

EXTRACARDIAC MALFORMATIONS

The incidence of extracardiac anomalies in children with CHD varies from 25% to 44%[36,43,114] (Table 8–3). Even when cases are excluded in which the noncardiac lesion is part of a syndrome or inheritable disorder, the incidence can be as high as 37%.[32] This wide range depends in part on how each cardiac defect has been detected. For example, cardiac anomalies in cases complicated by extracardiac malformations severe enough to cause stillbirth or neonatal death may not have been apparent clinically and only discovered at autopsy, if detected at all. The incidence of extracardiac malformations in children with CHD would therefore be lower in those diagnosed clinically. In addition, the frequency

TABLE 8–3. INCIDENCE OF ASSOCIATED SYSTEMIC MALFORMATIONS WITH CONGENITAL HEART DISEASE

System	Greenwood et al.[43] $n = 1566$		Gallo et al.[36] $n = 1354$		Wallgren et al.[114] $n = 100$	
	Number	*Percentage*	*Number*	*Percentage*	*Number*	*Percentage*
Central nervous	107	6.9	44	3.2	60	6.0
Respiratory	58	3.8	109	8.0	52	5.2
Gastrointestinal	65	4.2	*a*	—	155	15.5
Genitourinary	83	5.3	*a*	—	131	13.1
Musculoskeletal	137	8.8	62	4.5	161	16.1
TOTAL	395	25.2	446	32.9	439	43.9

*a*Original report contained overlap between subgroups.
Adapted, with permission, from Copel JA, Pilu G, Kleinman CS. Congenital heart disease and extracardiac anomalies: Associations and indications for fetal echocardiography. Am J Obstet Gynecol: 1986;154:1121.

of extracardiac anomalies may be related to the specific cardiac malformation present. Based on large studies determining the incidence of extracardiac malformations associated with specific congenital heart lesions, defects involving the septum are the most common[43,76] (Table 8–4). The remainder of this chapter focuses on the anomalies of various organ systems in which there is an increased risk of coexisting CHD.

Central Nervous System

Lesions of the central nervous system (CNS) are one of the most common congenital anomalies diagnosed prenatally or during the neonatal period. CNS malformations have been associated with cardiac malformations and the overall frequency ranges from 3.2% to 6.9%.[36,43] One study examining CNS anomalies discovered in 1000 children with either clinical CHD or CHD noted at the time of autopsy found 60 children affected with CNS lesions.[114] Of these 60 cases, 22 had unspecified brain abnormalities, 17 had hydrocephalus, 12 had meningomyelocele, and 17 had anomalies of the eyes or ears. Most investigators have failed to find a relationship between the type of CNS anomaly and the CHD, whereas others have noted a propensity toward ventricular septal defects in patients with CNS malformations.[36]

Hydrocephalus is one of the most common CNS malformations and is characterized by an abnormal accumulation of cerebrospinal fluid (CSF), resulting in an enlargement of the cerebroventricular system. In the majority of cases, this accumulation of CSF is the consequence of obstruction to the normal flow of CSF. Hydrocephalus often exists with other congenital anomalies, the most common of which is neural tube defects.[52] Less frequently, hydrocephalus is associated with cardiac malformations. Burton identified 9 cases of cardiac anomalies among a series of 205 patients with isolated congenital hydrocephalus.[13]

Congenital hydrocephalus is diagnosed prenatally with ultrasound by comparing the width of the body of the lateral ventricle to the width of the fetal head or by measuring the diameter of the lateral ventricle. In contrast to postnatally diagnosed hydrocephalus associated with CHD, as many as 15% of the cases of hydrocephalus diagnosed prenatally also have a cardiac malformation. Chervenak [19] found that four of 27 cases of prenatally diagnosed hydrocephalies were also complicated by cardiac anomalies. Of the four infants with cardiac malformations, two had ventricular septal defects, one had tricuspid hypoplasia, and one had tetralogy of Fallot. In another series of 31 cases of prenatally diagnosed hydrocephalus, there were three cardiac malformations identified.[93] Two of the cases had atrio-ventricular septal defects and one case was complicated by pulmonary atresia.

Borderline lateral cerebral ventricular enlargement has also been associated with congenital heart abnormalities. In a series of 55 cases of mild lateral ventriculomegaly (defined as an atrial diameter of 10 to 15 mm), three cardiac anomalies were found.[37] In another series, 4 of 44 cases of mild lateral ventriculomegaly had coexisting CHD.[12] Cardiac lesions reported with bor-

TABLE 8–4. EXTRACARDIAC MALFORMATIONS ASSOCIATED WITH SPECIFIC CARDIAC LESIONS

	Greenwood[43]		Moller[76] New England		Moller[76] Great Plains	
Cardiac Malformation	Number of Infants	Percentage with ECM[a]	Number of Infants	Percentage with ECM[a]	Number of Infants	Percentage with ECM[a]
Congenital atrioventricular septal defect	75	51	119	63	349	74
Atrioventricular septal defect	36	36	70	43	96	40
Ventricular septal defect	233	29	374	33	537	43
Tetralogy of Fallot	104	30	212	31	262	28
Coarctation	111	24	179	26	273	19
Truncus arteriosus	37	14	33	48	72	21
Heterotaxia	—	—	95	32	28	43
Hypoplastic left heart	122	12	177	12	150	14
Patent ductus arteriosus	116	36	146	40	519	65
TOTAL	1566	25	2251	28	4110	33

[a]ECM, extracardiac congenital malformations.
Adapted, with permission, from Copel Semin Perinatol: *1993;17:89–105.*

derline lateral ventricular enlargement were mainly atrial and ventricular septal defects.

Dandy-Walker malformation, another CNS anomaly, is characterized by varying degrees of hydrocephalus, a cyst in the posterior fossa, and a defect in the cerebellar vermis. Dandy-Walker malformation is frequently associated with other congenital anomalies and the incidence of cardiovascular abnormalities ranges from 2.5% to 47%.[49,98,100] Ventricular septal defects appear to be the most common CHD found in conjunction with Dandy-Walker malformation.[88,98]

The corpus callosum is a collection of white matter that connects the cerebral hemispheres. Absence or partial absence of this structure, known as agenesis of the corpus callosum, has been associated with other structural anomalies, including CHD.[45] The diagnosis of agenesis of the corpus callosum is confirmed by demonstrating an increased separation of the lateral ventricles, an enlargement of the lateral ventricles at the level of the atrium, and the upper displacement of the third ventricle. Cardiac defects were reported in seven cases of a 47-patient series diagnosed with agenesis of the corpus callosum.[91] In a study of 35 prenatally diagnosed cases of agenesis of the corpus callosum, 14% had cardiac anomalies.[94] The cardiac defects were predominantly ventriculoarterial lesions and included three fetuses with double-outlet ventricle and one fetus with tetralogy of Fallot.

As previously stated, cardiac abnormalities have also been described in association with holoprosencephaly.[102] Such a relationship exists because holoprosencephaly is commonly observed in fetuses with trisomy 13 and cardiac anomalies are found in as many as 90% of trisomy 13 fetuses.[20,82] Nonetheless, CHD has also been described in cases of holoprosencephaly without coexisting trisomy 13.

In general, isolated anencephaly, spina bifida, porencephaly, and hydranencephaly are not associated with an increased incidence of cardiac malformations above that of the general population. However, cephalocele, a specific type of neural tube defect, has been noted in cases also complicated by congenital cardiac defects. Cephalocele is characterized by herniation of intercranial contents through a defect in the calvarium. Cardiac malformations associated with cephalocele are primarily limited to cases of Meckel-Gruber syndrome, which involves a cephalocele in conjunction with polycystic kidneys and polydactyly. The incidence of CHD in cases of Meckel-Gruber syndrome has been reported to be as high as 14%.[89] Cardiac abnormalities described in cases of Meckel-Gruber syndrome include atrial or ventricular septal defects, aortic hypoplasia or coarctation, aortic valvular stenosis, and rotational anomalies.[87]

Mediastinum and/or Chest

Esophageal atresia is the most common anomaly of the mediastinum, with an incidence that varies between 1 in 800 to 1 in 5000 live births. In the majority of cases, this malformation coexists with a tracheoesophageal fistula. The most common tracheoesophageal abnormality involves esophageal atresia with a fistula between the distal portion of the esophagus and the trachea.

The prenatal diagnosis of isolated esophageal atresia is suspected when there is failure to visualize the stomach on serial ultrasound examinations, especially when hydramnios is present.[97] Because of the coexisting tracheoesophageal fistulae, only in 10% of fetuses with esophageal atresia can the diagnosis be confirmed prenatally because the fistulae allow pulmonary secretions to enter into the stomach.

There is a well-established association between tracheoesophageal malformations and cardiac as well as noncardiac anomalies. Easily recognizable acronyms have been given to the more common syndromes involving tracheoesophageal anomalies and include VATER (vertebral, anal, tracheoesophageal, radial, and/or renal), VACTEL (vertebral, anal, cardiac, tracheoesophageal, limb), and VACTERL (a combination of VATER and VACTEL).

The overall incidence of esophageal atresia with or without tracheoesophageal fistulae in patients with CHD varies. In a study of 1000 cases of postnatally diagnosed CHD, there were 47 cases of esophageal atresia.[114] Other investigators have been unable to demonstrate as high an incidence of esophageal atresia and/or tracheoesophageal fistulae in their series. Gallo et al.[36] noted only 14 cases of esophageal atresia in over 1300 patients with congenital heart defects. Greenwood identified 8 cases of tracheoesophageal fistulae or esophageal atresia in 1566 cases of CHD.[43] Five of the eight cases had additional extracardiac malformations.

Table 8–5 outlines the frequency of cardiac defects among cases of tracheoesophageal fistulae with and without esophageal atresia. In a series of 28 patients diagnosed with esophageal atresia and/or tracheoesophageal fistulae, Landing[65] noted that 39% had coexisting CHD. The majority of these (10 of 11) involved atrial and/or ventricular septal defects, one of which had tetralogy of Fallot. In a series of 183 patients with esophageal atresia and/or tracheoesophageal fistulae, Mellins and Blumenthal[74] described 48 cases of cardiac malformations. Although the majority of these cases involved either atrial or ventricular septal defects, there were five patients with coarctation of the aorta and three patients with tetralogy of Fallot. In a series of 39 autopsies with tracheoesophageal fistulae, Mehrizi et al.[73] reported 13 cases of CHD. Greenwood and Rosenthal[38] described a 15% incidence of congenital cardiac anomalies in a study of 326 patients with tracheoesophageal

TABLE 8–5. CARDIAC DEFECTS ASSOCIATED WITH TRACHEOESOPHAGEAL FISTULA WITH AND WITHOUT ESOPHAGEAL ATRESIA

	Septal Defects			Other Defects	Total CHD	
Series	Atrial	Ventricular[a]	Both		Incidence	Percentage
Mellins[74]	20	15	2	11	48 in 184	26
Mehrizi[73]	2	55	2	4	13 in 39	33
Landing[65]	2	5	3	1	11 in 28	39
Greenwood[38]	5	23	—	20	48 in 326	15

[a]Includes patients with tetralogy of Fallot.
[b]Tracheoesophageal fistula only.

Adapted, with permission, from Copel JA, Kleinman CS. Congenital heart disease and extracardiac anomalies: Associations and indications for fetal echocardiography. Am J Obstet Gynecol:1986;154:1121–32.

fistulae and/or esophageal atresia. The overall incidence of CHD, however, was related to the presence of other coexisting extracardiac defects. For example, only 8.3% of patients with isolated tracheoesophageal fistulae and/or esophageal atresia had cardiac malformations. In contrast, the incidence of CHD was 22% if additional extracardiac malformations were demonstrated.

Diaphragmatic hernia is a malformation characterized by protrusion of abdominal organs into the thoracic cavity through a defect in the diaphragm. It is associated with cardiac as well as extracardiac defects. The overall incidence of diaphragmatic hernia varies but has been reported to be as high as 5 per 10,000. Diaphragmatic hernias are generally classified according to their location. The defects are predominantly located either posterolateral (Bochdaleck's hernia) or parasternal (Morgagni's hernia), shifting the position of the heart within the chest as abdominal organs herniate into the thoracic cavity.

In a series of 1566 infants born with congenital heart disease, 5 were identified as having diaphragmatic hernia.[43] In a series of 48 cases of postnatally diagnosed diaphragmatic hernia, Greenwood et al.[42] reported 11 patients with congenital heart disease. Of these 11 cases, one was also complicated by omphalocele, another had coexisting pentalogy of Cantrell, whereas two had Down syndrome. There was a 13% incidence of cardiac abnormalities in a series of 45 neonates diagnosed with diaphragmatic hernia.[17]

The prenatal diagnosis of congenital diaphragmatic hernia relies on the presence of intraabdominal organs in the chest cavity, which is often apparent during ultrasound examination. Several studies have reported the relationship between cardiac anomalies and prenatally diagnosed diaphragmatic hernia (Table 8–6). Thorpe-Beeston et al.[109] described a 14% incidence of congenital heart malformations in a group of 36 prenatally diagnosed diaphragmatic hernias. Of the 36 fetuses,

11 of the cases were complicated by chromosome abnormalities, 3 of which also had congenital heart defects. In a similar investigation of 19 cases of prenatally diagnosed congenital diaphragmatic hernia, Crawford et al.[27] noted three cases of coexisting congenital heart anomalies. One of the three fetuses also had trisomy 18. Fogel et al.[34] reported an 18% incidence of CHD in 11 fetuses with diaphragmatic hernia. They observed a 36% overall incidence of aneuploidy among these cases. Clinically, in a series of 51 cases of prenatally diagnosed diaphragmatic hernia, Cannon et al.[17] reported 8 cases complicated by cardiac anomalies.

Gastrointestinal System

The pathologic defects of the gastrointestinal system predominantly manifest as bowel obstructions. Duodenal atresia is the most common form of congenital small bowel obstruction and is mainly a result of failure of recanalization of the primitive bowel by the 11th week of gestation. In contrast, bowel atresias of the jejunum, ileum, or colon are less frequent and result primarily from vascular accidents, volvulus, or intus-

TABLE 8–6. PRENATAL DIAGNOSIS OF DIAPHRAGMATIC HERNIA AND THE ASSOCIATION OF CARDIAC MALFORMATIONS AND ANEUPLOIDY

Series	n	Cardiac Defect	Aneuploidy
Thorpe-Beeston et al.[109]	36	5 (14%)	11 (31%)[a]
Crawford et al.[27]	19	3 (16%)	1 (5%)
Fogel et al.[34]	11	2 (18%)	4 (36%)[b]
Cannon et al.[17]	51	8 (15%)	23 (20%)
TOTAL	117	18 (15%)	23 (20%)

[a] 3 of 11 had cardiac defects.
[b] 2 of 4 had cardiac defects.

susception. In addition, intestinal obstruction can be the result of meconium ileus, with or without bowel perforation.

Although the incidence of gastrointestinal abnormalities varies among reports, the presence of a congenital cardiac anomaly increases the risk. In a series of over 1500 cases of congenital heart disease, the incidence of gastrointestinal abnormalities in general was 4.2%.[43] In a similar study involving 1354 patients with congenital heart anomalies, Gallo et al.[36] noted a 7% incidence of intestinal malformations, although the exact anomalies were not categorized. Intestinal obstruction was observed in 2.2% of the cases in another series of infants with CHD.[114] These cases were grouped and no attempt was made to divide the results according to the location of the obstruction. By comparison, 32% of neonates in a 166-patient series diagnosed with congenital gastrointestinal anomalies had coexisting cardiac defects.[112]

There is a definite association between congenital bowel obstruction and CHD. Duodenal atresia, the most common form of small bowel obstruction, is often seen in conjunction with other anomalies. In fact, duodenal atresia as an isolated malformation has been reported to occur in fewer than 50% of cases.[35,97,118] In addition, as many as one third of the cases of duodenal atresia also have trisomy 21.

Duodenal atresia is characterized by hydramnios in utero and confirmed by the observation of the "double-bubble" sign on ultrasound. Fogel et al.[34] reported a 27% incidence of congenital heart malformations in a series of 15 fetuses diagnosed with duodenal atresia prenatally. The most common cardiac lesion was a ventricular septal defect and two of the fetuses with CHD had coexisting trisomy 21. On the other hand, in a series of infants undergoing surgical evaluation for bowel obstruction, only 5.2% of those identified with jejunal or ileal atresia had congenital cardiac anomalies.[28] Again, this is probably due to the difference in pathogenesis between duodenal and jejunal or ileal lesions.

The reported association of congenital heart defects with anorectal anomalies varies widely. Accounts of imperforate anus in patients with CHD range from 0.8% to 2.2%.[43,114] In a series of 222 patients with imperforate anus, Greenwood et al.[40] reported a 12% incidence of cardiac anomalies. The majority of these were ventricular septal defects with or without tetralogy of Fallot. In a series of 68 cases of anorectal malformations, 22% had cardiac malformations.[108] However, 3 of the 15 cases were of isolated patent ductus arteriosus. If corrected for this, the overall incidence of CHD was 17%. In contrast, Touloukian found that only 5.6% of patients with anorectal anomalies had coexisting congenital heart defects.[110]

Heterotaxy syndromes, characterized by a lack of normal symmetry of the visceral organs, involve abnormalities of the spleen as well as the heart. Heterotaxy syndromes, also known as cardiosplenic syndromes, can be divided into asplenia syndrome and polysplenia syndrome. Asplenia syndrome is characterized by an absent spleen, trilobed lungs bilaterally, a symmetrical liver centrally positioned within the abdominal cavity, and intestinal malrotation. In contrast to their normal anatomic position, the aorta and inferior vena cava are found on the same side of the spine. Some form of cardiac anomaly is found in essentially all patients with asplenia syndrome. In a review of 145 cases of asplenia syndrome, the most common cardiac malformations noted included total anomalous pulmonary venous return, atrioventricular septal defects, pulmonary stenosis, and transposition of the great arteries.[113] As many as 42% of the cases are also complicated by dextrocardia. In contrast, with polysplenia syndrome, there are two or more spleens and bilateral morphologic left lungs, and as many as 80% of cases also have intestinal malrotation. In approximately 70% of the patients the inferior vena cava is absent. Although less common in asplenia syndrome, CHD is frequently reported in polysplenia syndrome. The most frequent cardiac malformations include total anomalous pulmonary venous return, atrioventricular septal defects, double-outlet right ventricle, and transposition of the great arteries.[107,113] Extracardia has been reported in approximately 37% of the cases of polysplenia syndrome.

Ventral Wall Defects

In general, defects in the anterior abdominal wall occur during embryogenesis and are due to (1) failure to fuse of one or more of the ectomesodermic folds, (2) failure of the protruded small bowel to return to its normal intraabdominal position by the 12th week of gestation, or (3) vascular compromise of either the umbilical vein or the right omphalomesenteric artery. Ventral wall defects are usually categorized according to their pathogenesis and for that reason the association of CHD varies accordingly.

Omphalocele occurs in approximately 1 in 5000 live births and is characterized by herniation of the intraabdominal contents into the base of the umbilical cord. The defect is located centrally and is the result of the failed fusion of the lateral ectomesodermic folds. Thus, the herniated intraabdominal contents are covered by an amnioperitoneal membrane. In contrast, if infolding and fusion of the caudal ectomesenteric fold fails, bladder extrophy exists. On the other hand, if the defect involves the cephalic ectomesenteric fold, thoracic ectopic cordis can result.

There is a well-established relationship between omphalocele and cardiac, noncardiac, as well as chromosome abnormalities.[14,77] Aneuploidy, especially trisomies 13 and 18, has been identified in 35% to 58% of cases of omphalocele.[47,69,71,81] The frequency of congenital heart malformations coexisting with omphalocele varies from 20% to 47%.[18,25,39,81] In addition, the relationship between CHD and omphalocele appears to be related to embryogenesis. For example, if the caudal ectomesenteric fold is predominantly involved, then the risk of cardiac anomalies is extremely low. On the other hand, Greenwood et al.[39] reported a 10% incidence of congenital heart disease if the lateral mesenteric folds were involved and a 100% incidence of cardiac defects if the cephalic ectomesenteric fold was involved in the defect. The most common cardiac lesion appears to be tetralogy of Fallot, although atrial ventricular defects were not uncommon.[57]

The prenatal diagnosis of omphalocele relies on the ultrasound identification of a centrally located mass protruding through a defect in the anterior abdominal wall. In the vast majority of cases the herniated mass is covered with a thin amnioperitoneal membrane. The frequency of CHD in prenatally diagnosed cases of omphalocele is similar to those identified postnatally. In a study of 37 fetuses diagnosed prenatally with omphalocele, Fogel et al.[34] detected 13 cases of cardiac malformations. Of those with CHD, 31% had chromosome abnormalities. In a similar series of 46 prenatally diagnosed cases of omphalocele, 12 were also complicated by congenital cardiac malformations.[57]

Beckwith-Wiedemann syndrome, characterized by omphalocele, macroglossia, and gigantism, occurs in approximately 1 in 13,000 live births. It has also been associated with cardiac anomalies.[44,92,96] Greenwood et al.[44] described a 32% frequency of congenital cardiac abnormalities among 13 cases of Beckwith-Wiedemann syndrome. Only 7 of the 12 had truly structural cardiac anomalies, with the remaining 5 having only isolated cardiomegaly. In a review of Beckwith-Wiedemann syndrome, Pettenati et al.[92] noted an 18% incidence of CHD in 22 new cases, with an overall frequency of 34% when combined with 226 previously reported cases. No preponderance of a specific congenital heart malformation was described.

A rare syndrome in which there is an anterior abdominal wall defect is pentalogy of Cantrell. It is characterized by (1) a midline supraumbilical abdominal defect, (2) a defect of the lower sternum, (3) deficiency of the diaphragmatic pericardium, (4) an anterior diaphragmatic hernia, and (5) CHD. By definition, all patients with this rare syndrome will have some form of cardiac malformation. In a review of 36 cases of pentalogy of Cantrell, atrioventricular septal defects were the most common cardiac malformation, occurring in 50% of the cases.[111] Ventricular septal defects and

tetralogy of Fallot were observed in 18% and 11% of the cases, respectively.

Unlike the ventral wall defects previously described, gastroschisis is less frequently associated with CHD or aneuploidy.[14,77] The incidence of gastroschisis ranges from 1 in 10,000 to 1 in 15,000 live births. It is characterized by a full-thickness paraumbilical defect, usually on the right side, with evisceration of abdominal organs, predominantly loops of bowel. The defect is believed to be the result of vascular compromise to the right omphalomesenteric artery. The prenatal diagnosis is made with ultrasound, demonstrating a defect in the anterior abdominal wall to the right of the umbilical cord insertion with herniation of intraabdominal organs that are not covered by a membrane.

Although the risk of cardiac anomalies associated with gastroschisis is very low, it is not zero. In a series of 13 infants born with gastroschisis, 1 was complicated by transposition of the great arteries.[18] In another series in which gastroschisis was diagnosed prenatally, 2 of 17 fetuses also had cardiac malformations.[34] One case involved an atrioventricular septal defect in conjunction with trisomy 18, and the other had a ventricular septal defect.

Genitourinary System

Numerous abnormalities of the renal and genitourinary system exist, several of which are associated with cardiac and extracardiac malformations. In a series of 1000 patients with CHD, 131 had coexisting genitourinary anomalies.[114] Common findings included 23% with hydronephrosis, 21% with genital malformations, 18% with renal agenesis, and 11% with horseshoe kidney. Of 108 infants diagnosed with coarctation of the aorta, 26 (24%) had coexisting genitourinary malformations.[114] Similarly, of 126 patients with ventricular septal defect, 26 (21%) had a genitourinary anomaly.[114] Other series report the frequency of genitourinary malformations associated with congenital heart defects to range from 5.3% to 8.1%.[36,43]

In an investigation involving 453 infants with genitourinary anomalies, 34 had coexisting congenital cardiac malformations.[41] The association between bilateral renal agenesis and CHD was striking with 71% of the patients having a cardiac malformation. However, when excluding those cases of isolated patent ductus arteriosus, which is not uncommon in neonates with pulmonary hypoplasia, the incidence of CHD fell to 43%. Others have not found as strong an association and describe a cardiovascular anomaly rate of only 14% in patients with renal agenesis.[115] Horseshoe kidney has also been associated with congenital cardiac malformations and has been identified in as many as 44% of the cases.[41] A relationship between other genitourinary anomalies and congenital heart defects is uncommon. However, CHD has been described in 2% to 5% of patients with ureteral obstruction or renal dysplasia.[48] No patterns between variety of genitourinary anomaly and specific cardiovascular malformation have been demonstrated.

Skeletal System

The nomenclature used for the classification of skeletal dysplasias is often confusing. This is mainly because most systems that categorize skeletal anomalies are descriptive and lack uniform diagnostic criteria. Even so, the frequency of skeletal dysplasias reported in a series of over 200,000 deliveries was 2.4 per 10,000 and the incidence among perinatal deaths was 9.1 per 1000.[15] With more than 200 skeletal dysplasias described, the frequency of each individual syndrome is relatively rare. Therefore, information regarding associated cardiac malformations in many of these skeletal dysplasias is limited by the reporting of small series or the lack of data altogether.

Although the incidence varies, congenital cardiac defects are known to coexist in patients with skeletal dysplasia. Greenwood et al.[43] noted an 8.8% incidence of skeletal malformations in infants with congenital heart disease. Wallgren et al.[114] identified skeletal anomalies in 16.1% of infants with congenital heart disease, one third of whom had tetralogy of Fallot. Skeletal malformations were reported in 4.6% of those in another series of infants with congenital heart disease.[36]

Short-ribbed polydactyly syndromes are a group of skeletal disorders characterized by short limbs and constricted thorax, with or without postaxial polydactyly. They are autosomal recessively inherited and are universally lethal. The risk of cardiac anomalies has been reported to be as high as 40%.[48] A variety of cardiac malformations have been described in cases of short-ribbed polydactyly syndromes, but the predominant anomaly is transposition of the great vessels.[79,106]

As the name implies, thrombocytopenia with absent radius (TAR syndrome) is characterized by a platelet count <100,000/mm^3 and bilateral absence of the radius. In addition, the ulna and humerus can be unilaterally or bilaterally absent or hypoplastic. Cardiac defects have been noted in 33% of patients with TAR syndrome.[33] The most frequent abnormalities were tetralogy of Fallot and atrial septal defect. The inheritance pattern is autosomal recessive.

Fanconi's syndrome, an autosomal-recessive disorder, is occasionally manifest by absence of the radius. Unlike TAR syndrome, patients with Fanconi's syndrome, in which the radius is missing, also have absence of the thumb. These patients are at increased risk

of having congenital heart disease. The risk of cardiac malformation was 14% in one study.[72]

Apert's syndrome is an autosomal-dominant disorder in which the majority of cases are new mutations. It is characterized by irregular craniosynostosis predominantly involving the coronal sutures with flat facies, hypertelorism, and syndactyly. Cardiac as well as noncardiac malformations have been described in patients with Apert's syndrome. Cardiac defects occur in approximately 10% of patients and include pulmonic stenosis, overriding aorta, ventricular septal defect, and endocardial fibroelastosis.[61]

Similar to Apert's syndrome, Carpenter's syndrome is characterized by brachycephaly with variable synostosis of the coronal, sagittal, and lambdoid sutures. In addition, there is brachydactyly of the hands with clinodactyly, partial syndactyly, or camptodactyly. Although the risk of congenital heart disease in these patients was originally reported to be rare (<5%) it now appears that as many as 50% of cases are complicated by cardiovascular defects.[22] The most common cardiac malformations reported include ventricular septal defect, atrial septal defect, pulmonic stenosis, tetralogy of Fallot, and transposition of great vessels. This syndrome is inherited in an autosomal-recessive manner.

Robin's anomalad (Pierre Robin syndrome) is a developmental facial abnormality of varying degrees in which there is micrognathia, glossoptosis, and cleft soft palate. In general, this disorder is sporadic, although familial tendencies have been noted.[83] Approximately one third of infants with this syndrome have other associated anomalies. Cardiac defects are more commonly seen in severe cases of Robin's anomalad with an overall frequency of 9%.[29]

Arthrogryposis multiplex congenita is a group of disorders in which multiple joint contractures are present at birth. The etiology for joint contractures is usually secondary to either intrinsic factors such as neurologic, muscular, or joint problems, or to extrinsic factors such as fetal crowding and constraint. Most cases are sporadic, however; depending on the etiology, autosomal-dominant as well as autosomal-recessive patterns of inheritance have been described.[10,66] Numerous congenital anomalies have been associated with arthrogryposis and the incidence of congenital heart defects ranges from 25% to 30%.[48,66] The majority of CHDs are found in those cases which are familial.

Holt-Oram syndrome involves anomalies of the upper limb, shoulder girdle, and cardiovascular system. It is inherited in an autosomal-dominant fashion, with variable expression. In these patients, the thumbs may be bifid, hypoplastic, or absent. Hypoplasia or absence of the first metacarpal and radius is not uncommon. Defects of the ulna, humerus, clavicle, scapula, and sternum have also been noted. Overall, approximately 50% of patients have some vascular disease. A large family, in which 19 members were affected with Holt-Oram syndrome, all had moderate to severe congenital cardiac anomalies.[8] The most common congenital heart disease described was atrial or ventricular septal defect.

Ellis-van Creveld syndrome (chondroectodermal dysplasia), an autosomal-recessive disorder, is characterized by irregular shortening of the forearm and lower leg associated with postaxial polydactyly. Approximately 50% of patients with Ellis-van Creveld syndrome will have a coexisting congenital heart defect. The most common cardiac anomaly noted is atrial septal defect.[60]

Twin Gestation

Many twin studies have noted an increased incidence of congenital anomalies when compared to singleton gestations.[78,101,105] Malformations tend to be higher in monozygotic twins than in dizygotic twins, but the risk of structural abnormalities is increased in dizygotic twins of like sex.[16,101] This probably holds true for congenital cardiac anomalies as well. In a retrospective study of 109 multiple gestations complicated by cardiac malformations, 63% were monozygotic.[5] The most common cardiac lesions were ventricular septal defect and tetralogy of Fallot, which occurred in 21% and in 15% of the cases, respectively. Among a large series of 1195 twins, 18.3% had congenital anomalies of which 14.9% were single malformations and 3.4% were multiple malformations.[78] In addition, there was more than a twofold increase in cardiovascular malformations (17.5 in 1000) when compared to singleton gestations, the majority of which were septal defects. Again, a significant proportion of the cases complicated by cardiac anomalies were monozygotic gestations.

Conjoined twins are a rare form of monozygotic twins whose bodies are connected to varying degrees. The incidence ranges from 1 in 33,000 to 1 in 165,000 births.[95] The most common types of conjoined twins reported in a review of 81 sets were thoracoomphalopagus (28%) and thoracopagus (18%).[31] Because the chest wall is shared in these types of conjoined twins, cardiac defects were common. In a similar report, 75% of twin gestations had cardiac malformations when a fused chest wall existed.[80] In a series of 14 cases of conjoined twins, all pairs had cardiac anomalies when the chest wall was involved.[7] Interestingly, it has been reported that as many as 25% of conjoined twins with no thoracic structures in common will have cardiac defects.[46] The prenatal diagnosis of conjoined twins can be done with ultrasound. Because the prognosis for conjoined twins depends to a large extent on which organs are shared, prenatal identification of major anomalies, especially cardiac, can be beneficial in the obstetric as well as the neonatal management of these unique pregnancies.[62]

SUMMARY

In this chapter, we have emphasized the association of cardiac and extracardiac malformations. In so doing,

TABLE 8–7. ANTENATAL ULTRASONOGRAPHIC DIAGNOSES AND THE INCIDENCE OF CONGENITAL CARDIAC DISEASE

Diagnosis	Percentage Associated
CNS	
Hydrocephalus	12
Dandy-Walker syndrome	3
Agenesis of corpus callosum	15
Meckel-Gruber syndrome	14
Mediastinum and/or chest	
Tracheoesophageal fistula	33
Esophageal atresia	30
Abnormalities of cardiac position	60
Diaphragmatic hernia	15
Gastrointestinal	
Duodenal atresia	17
Jejunal atresia	5
Anorectal anomalies	22
Imperforate anus	11
Ventral wall defects	
Omphalocele	30
Gastroschisis	5
Genitourinary	
Renal agenesis, bilateral	43
Horseshoe kidney	40
Renal dysplasia	5
Ureteral obstruction	2
Other	2
Skeletal	
Short-rib polydactyly	40
Thrombocytopenia with absent radius	33
Fanconi's	14
Apert's	10
Carpenter	4
Robin's sequence	9
Arthrogryposis multiplex congenita	30
Holt-Oram	50
Ellis-van Creveld	50
Twins	
Conjoined	25
Monoamniotic	3

Adapted, with permission, from Hess LW, Hess DB, McCaul JF, et al. Fetal echocardiography. In: Morrison JC (ed). Antepartal Fetal Surveillance. Obstet Gynecol Clin North Am: 1990; 17:41–79.

we have offered a review of those extracardiac anomalies that have a higher probability of coexisting with a cardiac defect. Though not all, the majority of these congenital anomalies are accessible to ultrasonographic prenatal diagnosis. Table 8–7 summarizes those fetal abnormalities that have been associated with congenital heart disease. In addition, we have reviewed the more common chromosomal abnormalities that are often found in conjunction with fetal cardiac as well as extracardiac malformations. Because of this increased risk of CHD, fetuses in which an extracardiac anomaly or chromosome abnormality is diagnosed deserve a complete evaluation with full fetal echocardiography. The opposite holds true as well. Fetuses with prenatally diagnosed cardiac malformations need to have other structural abnormalities ruled out. In addition, fetal karyotype analysis should be performed utilizing chorionic villus sampling, amniocentesis, or percutaneous umbilical blood sampling since the risk of aneuploidy approaches 40% in cases of prenatally diagnosed cardiac malformations.[21,116] This added information can influence counseling as well as obstetric management. Prenatal management of these patients requires a cooperative multidisciplinary team approach in which the diagnosis, prognosis, treatment options, and alternatives are discussed openly with family members in a supportive environment.

Acknowledgment

This chapter was supported in part by the Vicksburg Hospital Medical Foundation. The authors also wish to thank R. Preston McGehee, M.D., for the illustrations used in this chapter.

REFERENCES

1. Allan L, Tynan MJ, Campbell S, et al.: Echocardiographic and anatomical correlates in the fetus. *Br Heart J.* 44:444, 1980.

2. Allan LD, Crawford DC, Anderson RH, et al.: Echocardiographic and anatomical correlates in fetal congenital heart disease. *Br Heart J.* 52:542, 1984.

3. American Institute of Ultrasound in Medicine: Guidelines for performance of the antepartum obstetric ultrasound examination. *J Ultrasound Med.* 10:576, 1991.

4. American College of Obstetricians and Gynecologists: *Ultrasound in Pregnancy.* ACOG technical bulletin No. 187. Washington, DC: American College of Obstetricians and Gynecologists, 1993.

5. Anderson RC: Congenital cardiac malformations in 109 sets of twins and triplets. *Am J Cardiol.* 39:1045, 1977.

6. Azar GB, Snijders RJM, Gosden C, et al.: Fetal nuchal cystic hygroma: Associated malformations and chromosomal defects. *Fetal Diagn Ther.* 6:46, 1991.

7. Barth RA, Filly RA, Goldberg JD, et al.: Conjoined twins: Prenatal diagnosis and assessment of associated malformations. *Radiology.* 177:201, 1990.

8. Basson CT, Cowley GS, Solomon SD, et al.: The clinical and gentic spectrum of the Holt-Oram syndrome (heart-hand syndrome). *N Engl J Med.* 330:885, 1994.

9. Benacerraf BR, Harlow B, Frigoletto FD: Are choroid plexus cysts an indication for second-trimester amniocentesis? *Am J Obstet Gynecol.* 162:1001, 1990.

10. Bhatnagar DP, Sidhu LS, Aggarwal ND: Family studies for the mode of inheritance in arthrogryposis multiplex congenita. *Z Morphol Anthropol.* 68:233, 1977.

11. Bogart MH, Pandiani MR, Jones OW: Abnormal maternal serum chorionic gonadotropin levels in pregnancies with fetal chromosomal abnormalities. *Prenat Diagn.* 7:623, 1987.

12. Bromley B, Frigoletto FD, Benacerraf BR: Mild fetal lateral cerebral ventriculomegaly. Clinical course and outcome. *Am J Obstet Gynecol.* 164:863, 1991.

13. Burton BK: Recurrence risks for congenital hydrocephalus. *Clin Genet.* 16:47, 1979.

14. Calzolari E, Bianchi F, Dolk H, et al.: Omphalocele and gastroschisis in Europe: A survey of 3 million births 1980-1990. *Am J Med Genet.* 58:187, 1995.

15. Camera G, Mastroiacovo P: Birth prevalence of skeletal dysplasias in the Italian multicentrica monitoring system for birth defects. In: Papadatos CJ, Bartsocas CS, eds. *Skeletal Dysplasias.* NY: Alan R. Liss; 1982: p. 441.

16. Cameron AH, et al.: The value of twin surveys in the study of malformations. *Eur J Obstet Gynecol Reprod Biol.* 14:347, 1983.

17. Cannon C, Dildy GA, Ward R, et al.: A population-based study of congenital diaphragmatic hernia in Utah: 1988-1994. *Obstet Gynecol.* 87:959, 1996.

18. Carpenter MW, Curci MR, Dibbins AW, et al.: Perinatal management of ventral wall defects. *Obstet Gynecol.* 64:646, 1984.

19. Chervenak FA, Berkowitz RL, Romero RJ, et al.: The diagnosis of fetal hydrocephalus. *Am J Obstet Gynecol.* 147:703, 1983.

20. Chervenak FA, Isaacson C, Hobbins JC, et al.: Diagnosis and management of fetal holoprosencephaly. *Obstet Gynecol.* 66:322, 1985.

21. Claussen U, Ulmer R, Beinder E, et al.: Six year's experience with rapid karyotyping in prenatal diagnosis: Correlations between phenotype detected by ultrasound and fetal karyotype. *Prenat Diagn.* 14:113, 1994.

22. Cohen DM, Green JG, Miller J, et al.: Acrocephalopolysyndactyly type II–Carpenter syndrome: Clinical spectrum and an attempt at unification with Goodman and Summit syndromes. *Am J Med Genet.* 28:311, 1987.

23. Copel JA, Pilu G, Green J, et al.: Fetal echocardiography screening for congenital heart disease: The importance of the four-chamber view. *Am J Obstet Gynecol.* 157:648, 1987.

24. Copel JA, Pilu G, Kleinman CS: Congenital heart disease and extracardiac anomalies: Associations and indications for fetal echocardiography. *Am J Obstet Gynecol.* 154:1121, 1986.

25. Crawford DC, Chapman MG, Allan LD: Echocardiography in the investigation of anterior abdominal wall defects in the fetus. *Br J Obstet Gynaecol.* 92:1034, 1985.

26. Crawford DC, Chita SK, Allan DL: Prenatal detection of

congenital heart disease: Factors affecting obstetric management and survival. *Am J Obstet Gynecol.* 159: 352, 1988.

27. Crawford DC, Wright VM, Drake DP, et al.: Fetal diaphragmatic hernia: The value of fetal echocardiography in the prediction of postnatal outcome. *Br J Obstet Gynaecol.* 96:705, 1989.

28. DeLorimier AA, Fonkalsrud EW, Hays DM: Congenital atresia and stenosis of the jejunum and ileum. *Surgery.* 65:819, 1969.

29. Dennison WM: The Pierre-Robin syndrome. *Pediatrics.* 36:336, 1965.

30. DeVore GR: The prenatal diagnosis of congenital heart disease—A practical approach for the fetal sonographer. *J Clin Ultrasound.* 13:229, 1985.

31. Edmonds LD, Layde PM: Conjoined twins in the United States, 1970-1977. *Teratology.* 25:301, 1982.

32. Ferencz C, Rubin JD, McCarter RJ, et al.: Cardiac and noncardiac malformations: Observations in a population-based study. *Teratology.* 35:367, 1987.

33. Filkins K, Russo J, Bilinki I, et al.: Prenatal diagnosis of thrombocytopenia absent radius syndrome using ultrasound and fetoscopy. *Prenat Diagn.* 4:139, 1984.

34. Fogel M, Copel JA, Cullen MT, et al.: Congenital heart disease and fetal thoracoabdominal anomalies: Associations in utero and the importance of cytogenetic analysis. *Am J Perinatol.* 6:411, 1991.

35. Fonkalsrud EW, de Lorimer AA, Hayes DM: Congenital atresia and stenosis of the duodenum. A review compiled from the members of the surgical section of the American Academy of Pediatrics. *Pediatrics.* 43:79, 1969.

36. Gallo P, Nardi F, Marinozzi V: Congenital extracardial malformations accompanying congenital heart disease. *G Ital Cardiol.* 6:450, 1976.

37. Goldstein RB, LaPidus AS, Filly RA, et al.: Mild lateral cerebral ventricular dilation in utero. Clinical significance and prognosis. *Radiology.* 176:237, 1990.

38. Greenwood RD, Rosenthal A: Cardiovascular malformations associated with tracheoesophageal fistula and esophageal atresia. *Pediatrics.* 57:87, 1976.

39. Greenwood RD, Rosenthal A, Nadas AS: Cardiovascular malformations associated with omphalocele. *J Pediatr.* 85:818, 1974.

40. Greenwood RD, Rosenthal A, Nadas AS: Cardiovascular malformations associated with imperforate anus. *J Pediatr.* 86:576, 1975.

41. Greenwood RD, Rosenthal A, Nadas AS: Cardiovascular malformations associated with congenital anomalies of the urinary system. *Clin Pediatr.* 15:1101, 1976.

42. Greenwood RD, Rosenthal A, Nadas AS: Cardiovascular abnormalities associated with congenital diaphragmatic hernia. *Pediatrics.* 57:92, 1976.

43. Greenwood RD, Rosenthal A, Parisi L, et al.: Extracardiac abnormalities in infants with congenital heart disease. *Pediatrics.* 55:485, 1975.

44. Greenwood RD, Sommer A, Rosenthal A, et al.: Cardiovascular abnormalities in the Beckwith-Wiedemann syndrome. *Am J Dis Child.* 131:293, 1977.

45. Gupta JK, Lilford RJ: Assessment and management of fetal agenesis of the corpus callosum. *Prenat Diagn.* 15:301, 1995.

46. Harper RG, Kenigsberg K, Sia CG, et al.: Xiphopagus conjoined twins: A 300-year review of the obstetric, morphopathologic, neonatal, and surgical parameters. *Am J Obstet Gynecol.* 137:617, 1980.

47. Hauge M, Bugge M, Nielsen J: Early pre-natal diagnosis of omphalocele constitutes indication for amniocentesis. *Lancet.* 2:507, 1983.

48. Hess LW, Hess DB, McCaul JF, et al.: Fetal echocardiography. In Morrison JC, ed. *Antepartal Fetal Surveillance. Obstet Gynecol Clin N Am.* 17:41, 1990.

49. Hirsch JF, Pierre KA, Renier D, et al.: The Dandy-Walker malformation: A review of 40 cases. *J Neurosurg.* 61:515, 1984.

50. Hoffman JIE. Congenital heart disease: Incidence and inheritance. *Pediatr Clin North Am.* 37:25, 1990.

51. Hoffman JI, Christian R: Congenital heart disease in a cohort of 19,502 births with long-term follow up. *Am J Cardiol.* 42:641, 1978.

52. Holzgreve W, Feil R, Louwen F, et al.: Prenatal diagnosis and management of fetal hydrocephaly and lissencephaly. *Child's Nerv Syst.* 9:408, 1993.

53. Hook EB: Rates of 47, +13 and 46 translocation D/13 Patau syndrome in live births and comparison with rates in fetal deaths and at amniocentesis. *Am J Hum Genet.* 32:849, 1980.

54. Hook EB: Chromosome abnormalities and spontaneous fetal death following amniocentesis: Further data and associations with maternal age. *Am J Hum Genet.* 35: 110, 1983.

55. Hook EB, Woodbury DF, Albright SG: Rates of trisomy 18 in livebirths, stillbirths, and at amniocentesis. *Birth Defects.* 15:81, 1979.

56. Hsu LY, Kaffe S, Jenkins EC, et al.: Proposed guidelines for diagnosis of chromosome mosaicism in amniocenteses based on data derived from chromosome mosaicism and pseudomosaicism studies. *Prenat Diagn.* 12:555, 1992.

57. Hughes MD, Nyberg DA, Mack LA, et al.: Fetal omphalocele: Prenatal US detection of concurrent anomalies and other predictors of outcome. *Radiology.* 173:371, 1989.

58. Hyett JA, Moscoso G, Nicolaides KH: Cardiac defects in lst-trimester fetuses with trisomy 18. *Fetal Diagn Ther.* 10:381, 1995.

59. Hyett JA, Moscoso G, Nicolaides KH: First-trimester nuchal translucency and cardiac septal defects in fetuses with trisomy 21. *Am J Obstet Gynecol.* 172:1411, 1995.

60. Jones KL (Ed): Osteochondrdysplasias: Chondroectodermal dysplasia. In: *Smith's Recognizable Patterns of Human Malformations*, 5th ed. Philadelphia: WB Saunders; 1997: pp. 374–394.

61. Jones KL (Ed.): Craniosynostosis syndromes: Apert syndrome. In: *Smith's Recognizable Patterns of Human Malformation*, 5th ed. Philadelphia: WB Saunders; 1997, pp. 418–424.

62. Kato T, Yoshino H, Hebiguchi T, et al.: Experience with treatment of three pairs of conjoined twins. *Am J Perinatol.* 14:25, 1997.

63. Keith JD, Rowe RD, Vlad P: *Heart Disease in Infancy and Childhood*, 3rd ed. New York: MacMillan; 1978: pp. 9–174.

64. Kloster FF, Roelandt J, Ten Cate EJ, et al.: Multiscan echocardiography. II. Technique and initial clinical results. *Circulation.* 48:1075, 1973.

65. Landing BH: Syndromes of congenital heart disease with tracheobronchial anomalies. *Am J Roentgenol.* 123:679, 1975.

66. Lebenthal E, Schochet SB, Adam A, et al.: Arthrogryposis multiplex congenita: 23 cases in an Arab kindred. *Pediatrics.* 46:891, 1970.

67. Lian ZH, Zack MM, Erickson JD: Paternal age and the occurrence of birth defects. *Am J Hum Genet.* 39:648, 1986.

68. Machado MV, Crawford DC, Anderson RH, et al.: Atrioventricular septal defect in prenatal life. *Br Heart J.* 59: 352, 1988.

69. Mann L, Ferguson-Smith MA, Desai M, et al.: Prenatal assessment of anterior abdominal wall defects and their prognosis. *Prenat Diagn.* 4:427, 1984.

70. Martin GR, Ruckman RN: Fetal echocardiography: A large clinical experience and follow-up. *J Am Soc Echocardiogr.* 3:4, 1990.

71. Mayer T, Black R, Matlak ME, et al.: Gastroschisis and omphalocele. An eight-year review. *Ann Surg.* 192:783, 1980.

72. McDonald R, Goldschmidt B: Pancytopenia with congenital defects (Fanconi's anemia). *Arch Dis Child.* 35:367, 1965.

73. Mehrizi A, Folger GM, Rowe RD: Tracheoesophageal fistula associated with congenital cardiovascular malformations. *Bull Johns Hopkins Hosp.* 118:246, 1966.

74. Mellins RB, Blumenthal S: Cardiovascular anomalies and esophageal atresia. *Am J Dis Child.* 107:160, 1964.

75. Moe DG, Guntheroth WG: Spontaneous closure of uncomplicated ventricular septal defect. *Am J Cardiol.* 60:674, 1987.

76. Moller JH: Incidence of cardiac malformations. In Moller JH, Neal WA, eds. *Fetal, Neonatal, and Infant Cardiac Disease.* Norwalk, CT: Appleton; 1990: pp. 361–69.

77. Morrow RJ, Shittle MJ, McNay MB, et al.: Prenatal diagnosis and management of anterior abdominal wall defects in the west of Scotland. *Prenat Diagn.* 13:111, 1993.

78. Myrianthopoulos NC: Congenital malformations in twins: Epidemiologic survey. In: Bergsma D, ed. *Birth Defects*; Original Article Series, The National Foundation March of Dimes. Miami: Symposia Specialists; 1975: 11:1–39.

79. Naumoff P, Young LW, Mazer J, et al.: Short rib-polydactyly syndrome type 3. *Radiology.* 122:443, 1977.

80. Nichols BL, Blattner RJ, Rudolph AJ: General clinical management of thoracopagus twins. *Birth Defects.* 3:38, 1967.

81. Nivelon-Chevallier A, Mavel A, Michiels R, et al.: Familial Beckwith-Wiedemann syndrome: Prenatal echography diagnosis and histologic confirmation. *J Genet Hum.* 5:397, 1983.

82. Nora JJ, Nora AH: The evolution of special genetic and environmental counseling in congenital heart disease. *Circulation.* 57:205, 1978.

83. Nora JJ, Nora AH: *Genetics and Counseling in Cardiovascular Diseases.* Springfield, IL: Charles C Thomas; 1978.

84. Nora JJ, Nora AH: Maternal transmission of congenital heart disease: New recurrence risk figures and the questions of cytoplasmic inheritance and vulnerability to teratogens. *Am J Cardiol.* 59:459, 1987.

85. Nora JJ, Nora AH: Update on counseling the family with a first-degree relative with a congenital heart defect. *Am J Med Genet.* 29:137, 1988.

86. Nyberg DA, Kramer D, Resta RG, et al.: Prenatal sonographic findings of trisomy 18: A review of 47 cases. *J Ultrasound Med.* 12:103, 1993.

87. Nyberg DA, Hallesy D, Mahony BS, et al.: Meckel-Gruber syndrome. Importance of prenatal diagnosis. *J Ultrasound Med.* 9:691, 1990.

88. Olson GS, Halpe DCE, Kaplan AM, et al.: Dandy-Walker malformation and associated cardiac anomalies. *Child's Brain.* 8:173, 1981.

89. Opitz JM, Howe JJ: The Meckel syndrome (dysencephalia splanchnocystica, the Gruber syndrome). *Birth Defects.* 5:167, 1969.

90. Pandya PP, Kondylius A, Hilbert L, et al.: Chromosomal defects and outcome in 1015 fetuses with increased nuchal translucency. *Ultrasound Obstet Gynecol.* 5:15, 1995.

91. Parrish ML, Roessmann U, Levinsohn MW: Agenesis of the corpus callosum: A study of the frequency of associated malformations. *Ann Neurol.* 6:349, 1979.

92. Pettenati MJ, Haines JL, Higgins RR, et al.: Wiedemann-Beckwith syndrome: Presentation of clinical and cytogenetic data on 22 new cases and review of the literature. *Hum Genet.* 74:143, 1986.

93. Pilu G, Rizzo N, Orsini LF, et al.: Antenatal recognition of cerebral anomalies. *Ultrasound Med Biol.* 12:319, 1985.

94. Pilu G, Sandri F, Perolo A, et al.: Sonography of fetal agenesis of the corpus callosum: A survey of 35 cases. *Ultrasound Obstet Gynecol.* 3:318, 1993.

95. Ramadani HM, Johnshrud N, Nasser MA, et al.: The antenatal diagnosis of cephalothoracopagus janiceps conjoined twins. *Aust NZ J Obstet Gynaecol.* 34:113, 1994.

96. Ranzini AC, Day-Salvatore D, Turner T, et al.: Intrauterine growth and ultrasound findings in fetuses with Beckwith-Wiedemann syndrome. *Obstet Gynecol.* 89: 538, 1997.

97. Robertson FM, Crombleholme TM, Paidas M, et al.: Prenatal diagnosis and management of gastrointestinal anomalies. *Semin Perinatol.* 18:182, 1994.

98. Russ PD, Pretorius DH, Johnson MJ: Dandy-Walker syndrome: A review of fifteen cases evaluated by prenatal sonography. *Am J Obstet Gynecol.* 161:401, 1989.

99. Sahn DJ, Terry R, O'Rourke R, et al.: Multiple crystal cross-sectional echocardiography in the diagnosis of cyanotic congenital heart disease. *Circulation.* 50:230, 1974.

100. Sawaya R, McLaurin RL: Dandy-Walker syndrome: Clinical analysis of 23 cases. *J Neurosurg.* 55:89, 1981.

101. Schinzel AAGL, Smith DW, Miller JR: Monozygotic twinning and structural defects. *J Pediatr.* 95:921, 1979.

102. Seoud MA, Alley DC, Smith DL, et al.: Prenatal sonographic findings in trisomy 13, 18, 21 and 22. *J Reprod Med.* 39:781, 1994.

103. Smythe JF, Copel JA, Kleinman CS: Outcome of prenatally detected cardiac malformations. *Am J Cardiol.* 69:1471, 1992.

104. Snijders RJ, Shawwa L, Nicolaides KH: Fetal choroid plexus cysts and trisomy 18: Assessment of risk based on ultrasound findings and maternal age. *Prenat Diagn.* 14:1119, 1994.

105. Spellacy WN, Handler H, Ferre CD: A case control study of 1253 twin pregnancies from a 1982-1987 perinatal data base. *Obstet Gynecol.* 75:168, 1990.

106. Spranger J, Grimm B, Weller M, et al.: Short rib-polydactyly (SRP) syndromes, types Majewski and Saldino-Noonan. *Z Kinderheilk.* 116:73, 1974.

107. Stanger P, Rudolph AM, Edwards JE: Cardiac malpositions: An overview based on study of sixty–five necropsy specimens. *Circulation.* 56:159, 1977.

108. Teixeira OH, Malhotra K, Sellers J, et al.: Cardiovascular anomalies with imperforate anus. *Arch Dis Child.* 58:747, 1983.

109. Thorpe-Beeston JG, Gosden CM, Nicolaides KH: Prenatal diagnosis of congenital diaphragmatic hernia: Associated malformations and chromosomal defects. *Fetal Ther.* 4:21, 1989.

110. Touloukian RJ: Anorectal malformations. In: Bergsma D, ed. *Birth Defects Compendium,* 2nd ed. New York: Alan R Liss; 1979: p. 99.

111. Toyama WM: Combined congenital defects of the anterior abdominal wall, sternum, diaphragm, pericardium and heart: A case report and review of the syndrome. *Pediatrics.* 50:778, 1972.

112. Tulloh RMR, Tansey SP, Parashar K, et al.: Echocardiographic screening in neonates undergoing surgery for selected gastrointestinal malformations. *Arch Dis Child.* 70:F206, 1994.

113. Van Mierop LHS, Gessner IH, Schiebler GL: Asplenia and polysplenia syndrome. *Birth Defects.* 8:36, 1972.

114. Wallgren EI, Landtman B, Rapola J: Extracardiac malformation associated with congenital heart disease. *Eur J Cardiol.* 7:15, 1978.

115. Wilson RD, Baird PA: Renal agenesis in British Columbia. *Am J Med Genet.* 21:153, 1985.

116. Wladimiroff JW, Stewart PA, Sachs ES, et al.: Prenatal diagnosis and management of congenital heart defect: Significance of associated fetal anomalies and prenatal chromosome studies. *Am J Med Genet.* 21:285, 1985.

117. Wladimiroff JW, Stewart PA, Vosters RPL: Fetal cardiac structure and function as studied by ultrasound. A review. *Clin Cardiol.* 7:239, 1984.

118. Young DG, Eilkinson AW: Abnormalities associated with neonatal duodenal obstruction. *Surgery.* 63:832, 1968.

CHAPTER NINE

Accuracy and Utilization of Fetal Echocardiography

William J. Ott

One of the most common reasons that patients are referred for detailed fetal cardiac evaluation is the presence of a previous child or family member with a congenital heart disease (CHD). Depending on the type of lesion, the recurrence risk for CHD with the history of one previous child with CHD ranges from 1% to 4%. The risk increases three- to fourfold if there are additional siblings with CHD. The anomalies with the highest risk of recurrence are ventricular septal defects, endocardial cushion defects, and fibroelastosis.[1,2] In general, congenital heart disease follows a multifactorial inheritance pattern.

With the improving survival rates for CHD over the last few decades, an additional indication for fetal echocardiography is a parent with CHD.[1,2] A mother with a history of CHD appears to have a slightly higher risk of conceiving an offspring with CHD (5.8%, with a range of 2% to 12%) than does the father (3.1%, with a range of 1.5% to 4.5%). Studies by Buskens et al.[3] and Whittemore et al.[4] have suggested a higher relative risk of CHD in fetuses when the father rather than the mother has a CHD, but in a meta-analysis of the recent literature, Nora[1] has confirmed that there is a greater risk when the mother has CHD. Data for specific lesions are shown in Table 9–1.

Additional risks for CHD may be related to medical disease or environmental influences on the mother. Some series have reported that maternal *alcoholism* is associated with a 25% to 30% risk of cardiac disease in the neonate. Many *drugs* used by the mother in pregnancy, such as lithium, which may cause Ebstein's anomaly or tricuspid atresia; hydantoin; or trimethadione, have been associated with the development of CHD in the mother's offspring. *Infectious agents,* such as

rubella, are also associated with the development of CHD or other birth defects. *Diabetes mellitis* in the mother is also a risk factor for CHD. There have been some reports of poorly controlled insulin-dependent diabetes patients having a 30% to 50% risk of delivering an infant with CHD; but in general, the risks are only moderately increased over the background risk of 0.8%. The association of maternal lupus or other collagen vascular diseases and fetal heart block is also well known. Table 9–2, from a study by Nora and Nora,[5] summarizes some of the environmental risk factors associated with CHD.

Additional indications for a detailed fetal echocardiographic examination include: (1) fetal arrhythmias, (2) fetal hydrops, (3) intrauterine growth retardation, and (4) the presence of any other structural anomaly seen on ultrasound examination.

Fetal Cardiac Arrhythmias

Irregularities in the fetal heart rate are a common finding and one of the frequent indications for fetal echocardiography. Table 9–3, taken from the work of Friedman et al.,[6] shows the types of arrhythmias seen at the Yale Cardiovascular Center.

Isolated extrasystole is usually benign and self-limiting, but approximately 1% of these patients may have concomitant structural heart disease or may develop reentrant tachycardia later in the mother's pregnancy. A careful fetal cardiac evaluation and follow-up of the arrythmia is, therefore, necessary.

Bradyarrhythmias in the fetus (<60 bpm) are most commonly associated with complete heart block. Almost half of fetuses with complete heart block also

TABLE 9–1. CONGENITAL HEART DISEASE OCCURRENCE RISKS IN OFFSPRING WITH ONE AFFECTED PARENT

Defect	Risk when Mother Affected (%)	Risk when Father Affected (%)
Aortic stenosis	8.0	3.8
Atrial septal defect	6.1	3.5
Atrioventricular canal	11.6	4.3
Coarctation of the aorta	6.3	3.0
Patent ductus arteriosus	4.1	2.0
Pulmonary stenosis	5.3	3.5
Tetralogy of Fallot	2.0	1.4
Ventricular septal defect	6.0	3.6
TOTAL	5.8	3.1

Data from Nora JN. From generational studies to a multilevel genetic-environmental interaction. J Am Coll Cardiol: 1994; 23: 1468–71.

have structural abnormalities. Of the remaining group with a structurally normal heart, 50% are associated with maternal autoimmune diseases.

Structural Heart Disease and Extracardiac Anomalies

There is a strong association between structural anomalies of the fetal heart and other, extracardiac structural anomalies. Table 9–4 shows the incidence and type of cardiac anomaly frequently found when other structural

anomalies are present. Friedman et al.[7] found 11 cardiac structural abnormalities among 73 fetuses undergoing fetal echocardiography because of the presence of extracardiac malformations (15%). Since between 5% and 50% of various extracardiac structural anomalies are associated with CHD a detailed fetal echocardiographic examination should be obtained whenever *any* structural anomaly is found on ultrasound examination.

Routine Cardiac Screening

Since cardiac defects are the most common structural abnormalities seen in liveborn infants, many authors have recommended that routine fetal cardiac screening be used in all obstetric patients.[29,30] Copel et al.[31] found an abnormal four-chamber view in 71 of 74 structurally abnormal fetal hearts (96%) seen in a group of high-risk fetuses undergoing detailed fetal echocardiographic evaluation, whereas Wigton et al.[32] found that the four-chamber view was abnormal in only 11 of 33 (33.3%) similar patients. Two prospective studies in low-risk populations, one by Achiron et al.,[33] using an extended fetal echocardiographic examination, and one by Vergani et al.,[34] using only the four-chamber view, showed a sensitivity of 86% and 43%, respectively. A sensitivity of 48% for the four-chamber view alone was found in the study by Achiron et al.[33] The addition of the aortic and pulmonary outflow tracts to the four chamber view has also been suggested.[35]

Ott performed a randomized, prospective outcome study of routine fetal cardiac screening over a two year period using the four chamber and left ventricular out-

TABLE 9–2. ENVIRONMENTAL FACTORS AND CONGENITAL HEART DISEASE

	Frequency of CHD (%)	Most Common Lesions[a]
(1) Maternal alcoholism	25–30	VSD, PDA, ASD
(2) Drugs		
Amphetamines	5–10 (?)	VSD, PDA, TGA
Hydantoin	2–3	PS, ASD, coarc, PDA
Trimethadione	15–30	TGA, Tet
Lithium	10	Ebstein's, tricuspid atresia, ASD
Thalidomide	5–10	Tet, VSD, ASD, truncus
(3) Infections		
Rubella	35	Peripheral pulmonary stenosis, PS, PDA, VSD, ASD
(4) Maternal conditions		
Diabetes	3–5	TGA, VSD, coarc
	(30–50)	(For cardiomegaly and cardiomyopathy)
Lupus erythematosus	?	Heart block
Phenylketonuria	25–50	Tet, VSD, ASD

[a]VSD, ventricular septal defect; PDA, patent ductus arteriosus; ASD, atrial septal defect; TGA, transposition of the great arteries; PS, pulmonary stenosis; coarc, coarctation of the aorta; Tet, tetralogy of Fallot; truncus, truncus arteriosus.
Data from Nora JN, Nora AH. Maternal transmission of congenital heart diseases: New recurrence risk figures and the question of cytoplasmic inheritance and vulnerability to teratogens. Am J Cardiol: 1987;59:459–63.

TABLE 9–3. DISTRIBUTION OF FETAL CARDIAC ARRHYTHMIAS SEEN AT THE YALE FETAL ECHOCARDIOGRAPHY CENTER

Isoated extrasystole	826
Supraventricular tachycardia	41
Atrial flutter	9
Atrial fibrillation	2
Sinus tachycardia	6
Junctional tachycardia	1
Ventricular tachycardia	4
Second-degree atrioventricular block	6
Complete heart block	26

Data from Friedman AH, Copel JA, Kleinman CS. Fetal echocardiography and fetal cardiology: Indications, diagnosis and management. Semin Perinatol: *1993;17:76–88.*

flow tract views in 1136 low-risk patients and compared it to detailed fetal echocardiographic evaluation in 886 high-risk patients seen during the same time period.[36]

Adequate four-chamber views were obtained in 87.7% (80% to 95%; 95% confidence intervals) of the patients examined, and adequate four-chamber and left ventricular outflow tract views were obtained in 66.4% (62.7% to 70.1%; 95% confidence intervals) of the patients.

The ability to obtain adequate views was uniformly distributed across gestational ages. The incidence of CHD in the low-risk group was 1.23% (14 of 1136) and in the high-risk group was 1.8% (16 of 886), not a statistically significant difference ($p = .2899$).

The accuracy and predictive values for the antenatal diagnosis of CHD using the four-chamber and left ventricular outflow views in the low-risk group and the detailed fetal echocardiographic examination in the high-risk group are shown in Table 9–5. In the low-risk group, only 2 of the 14 patients with congenital heart disease were correctly identified (sensitivity of 14.3%), whereas initially there were 12 patients with false positive diagnosis. When these patients were rescanned, all 12 were correctly reclassified as being without CHD. In the high-risk group, 10 of 16 patients with CHD were correctly identified (sensitivity of 62.5%). There were two false positive diagnoses: a small ventricular septal defect and a diagnosis of transposition of the great vessels, both of which were not present at birth.

In addition, the high-risk group was separated into two subgroups based on the presence or absence of specific risk factors for CHD. These factors are listed in Table 9–6. The incidence of CHD in the subgroup with risk factors for CHD was 12.5% (11 of 88), significantly greater than the 0.7% (5 of 798) incidence in the subgroup without risk factors for CHD ($p = .0001$). These findings are somewhat different from the study by

TABLE 9–4. EXTRACARDIAC ANOMALIES AND CONGENITAL HEART DISEASE: COMBINED FETAL AND NEONATAL SERIES

Extracardiac Anomalies	Seen with CHD (%)	CJD Frequently Seen[a]	References
Central nervous system			
Hydrocephaly	6	VSD, Tet	7
Holoprosencephaly (with trisomy 13)	7	Complex	8
Agenesis of corpus callosum	14	Nonspecific	9
Mild ventriculomegaly	7	VSD, AV canal	8, 10
Respiratory			
Tracheo-esophageal fistula	21	ASD, VSD, coarc	11, 12
Gastrointestinal			
Duodenal atresia (with trisomy 21)	21 (55)	VSD, AV canal	13, 14
Jejunal–iliac atresia	5	Nonspecific	15
Anal–rectal atresia	15	Tet, VSD	16–18
Abdominal wall			
Gastroschisis	5	TGA, AV canal, VSD	14, 19, 20
Omphalocele	27	Tet	14, 20, 21
(Beckwith-Wiedeman)	(50)	(Nonspecific)	22
Diaphragmatic hernia	12	Tet	14, 23–25
Genitourinary	8	VSD, coarc	26–28

[a] VSD, ventricular septal defect; Tet, tetralogy of Fallot; AV, atrioventricular; ASD, atrial septal defect; coarc, coarctation of the aorta; TGA, transposition of the great arteries.

TABLE 9–5. ACCURACY OF FETAL CARDIAC EXAMINATION

Four-chamber and Left Ventricular Outflow Views for the Diagnosis of CHD in the Low-risk Group (N = 1136)

	Anomaly	No Anomaly	
Abnormal ultrasound	2	12 (0)	14
Normal ultrasound	12	1110 (1122)	1122
Total	14	1122 (1122)	1136

Sensitivity: 14.3%
Specificity: 99.0% (100%)
Positive predictive value: 14.3% (100%)
Negative predictive value: 99.0% (99%)
(Figures in parenthesis are after rescanning the false positive cases.)

Detailed Fetal Echocardiographic Studies for the Diagnosis of CHD in the High-risk Group (N = 1136)

	Anomaly	No Anomaly	
Abnormal ultrasound	10	2	12
Normal ultrasound	6	868	874
	16	870	886

Sensitivity: 62.5%
Specificity: 99.8%
Positive predictive value: 83.3%
Negative predictive value: 99.3%

TABLE 9–6. HIGH-RISK PATIENTS THOUGHT TO BE AT INCREASED RISK FOR CONGENITAL HEART DISEASE

Risk Factor	Number of Patients
Questionable anomaly seen on outside ultrasound	25
Insulin-dependent diabetic	13
Maternal drug exposure	10
Fetal heart arrhythmia	10
History of structural anomaly associated with congenital heart disease	8
Previous child with heart defect	8
Collagen vascular disease	6
Viral infection in early pregnancy	5
History of relative with heart defect	3
Mother with heart defect	2
TOTAL	88

Data from Ott WJ. The accuracy of antenatal fetal echocardiography screening in high and low risk patients. Am J Obstet Gynecol: 1995;172:1741–9.

TABLE 9–7. HIGH-RISK INDICATIONS FOR FETAL ECHOCARDIOGRAPHY

Indications	Percentage of Total
History of previous child with CHD	37
Epileptic medication	14
Maternal diabetes	13
Maternal CHD	11
Paternal CHD	6.5
Abnormal morphometries, Hx drug abuse	5.5
Relative with CHD	5
OTHER[a]	8

[a]Includes alcohol abuse, collagen vascular disease, etc.
Data from Buskens E, Stewart PA, Hess LW, et al. Efficiency of fetal echocardiography and yield by risk category. Obstet Gynecol: 1996; 87:423–8.

Buskens et al.,[3] who evaluated 3223 patients with risk factors for CHD. Buskens et al.'s high-risk factors are listed in Table 9–7. They found an incidence of CHD in this high-risk group of 1.58%, markedly lower than the 12.5% incidence in the study by Ott.[36] Both studies, however, indicate a significant increase in the incidence of CHD in patients with risk factors when compared to patients without risk factors.

Cooper et al.[37] reviewed the literature and reported their own experience with patients referred for fetal echocardiographic examination because of risk factors for CHD. They found 43 defects and missed 25 defects in 915 fetuses studied, an incidence of CHD of 7.7% in their high-risk population; this is intermediate between the studies by Buskens et al. and Ott. Table 9–8 shows

TABLE 9–8. INCIDENCE OF CHD BY INDICATION

Indication	Total Number of Patients	Percentage CHD	Range %
Family Hx of CHD	2993	1.67	(.07–3.3)
Diabetes mellitus	782	2.94	(1.2–8.0)
Lithium exposure	46	2.17	(0–8.3)
Ultrasound anomaly[a]	802	14.21	(9.5–25)
Chromosomal anomaly	197	15.74	(13–50)
Suspected CHD on outside ultrasound	256	42.97	(29–69)

[a]Any anomaly seen on ultrasound, excluding CHD.
Data from Cooper MJ, Enderlein MA, Dyson DC, et al. Fetal echocardiography: Retrospective review of clinical experience and an evaluation of indications. Obstet Gynecol: 1995;86:577–82.

TABLE 9–9. ACCURACY OF DETAILED ANTENATAL CARDIAC EXAMINATIONS

Population	Sensitivity	Specificity	Positive Predictive Value	Negative Predictive Value	Number of Anomalies	Number of Patients	Reference
High risk	51	99	95	100	47	3223	3
High risk	92	99	96	99	75	1022	31
High risk	63	99	83	99	16	886	36
Low risk	82	100	95	99	21	5347	38
High risk	81	NA	99	NA	91	989	39
High risk	62	100	100	96	13	124	40
High risk	57	NA	100	NA	49	NA	41
High risk	91	99	84	99	23	303	42

the indications for fetal echocardiography and the incidence of CHD in their own patients and their review of the literature.[37]

The difference in incidence of CHD in these studies of high-risk patients reflects the differences in the risk factors and the patient populations studied.

Accuracy of Fetal Echocardiography

A wide range of accuracy for detailed fetal echocardiography has been reported in the literature. Table 9–9 lists some of the recent studies reporting the accuracy of detailed fetal echocardiography for the diagnosis of CHD. Sensitivities range from 51% to 91%, with an average of approximately 70%. Even in the best of hands, detailed fetal echocardiography cannot identify all structural heart lesions. Small ventricular septal and atrial septal defects and anomalies of the outflow tracts are lesions that are most commonly missed.

Most of studies that have evaluated the accuracy of a simple four-chamber view for the diagnosis of congenital heart disease are retrospective in nature, evaluating the presence or absence of an abnormal four-chamber view in patients that have had detailed echocardiography later in their pregnancies.[30-32,38] One prospective study by Vergani et al.[34] identified 26 of 32 congenital heart lesions (sensitivity of 81%) in a mixed high- and low-risk population. The incidence of congenital heart disease in their population was 0.52%, suggesting a possibility of population bias. Stoll et al.[43] published their experience with routine ultrasound screening in over 100,000 unselected patients in France from 1979 to 1988. They were able to identify only 9.2% of the fetuses with congenital heart disease. The recently published RADIUS study[44] was able to identify only 16% of fetuses with cardiac anomalies using the four-chamber view, whereas Kirk et al.[45] identified 78% of fetuses with structural heart defects using both the four-chamber and the left ventricular

outflow views. However, since all infants scanned in the Kirk et al. study were not included in the outcome statistics, their high sensitivity may be an overestimation. The sensitivity of 14.3% reported by Ott in the prospective study of the four-chamber and left ventricular track views in low-risk patients is similar to the RADIUS and the French study by Stoll et al.

Sensitivities of between 10% and 20% reported by prospective studies of the four-chamber view indicate that all patients with *any risk factor* for CHD should be referred for more detailed fetal echocardiographic studies at centers experienced in the technique.

SUMMARY

Many conditions exist that necessitate referral for detailed fetal echocardiography. A family history of CHD, maternal medical disease such as diabetes mellitus or collagen vascular disease, or maternal exposure to teratogens or viral agents in the first trimester are all strong risk factors for CHD in the fetus and should indicate the need for fetal echocardiography. The highest incidence of CHD will be seen in fetuses with suspected CHD on a basic ultrasound examination or fetuses with *any other structural anomaly* seen on ultrasound examination. In addition, fetuses with inadequate growth (small for gestational age), even if there is no evidence of structural anomalies, are also at risk for CHD.

All these fetuses should be referred to a tertiary center for detailed fetal echocardiographic studies and any additional evaluation that may be necessary.

REFERENCES

1. Nora JN: From generational studies to a multilevel genetic-environmental interaction. *J Am Coll Cardiol.* 23:1468–71, 1994.

2. Nora JN: Causes of congenital heart diseases: Old and new modes, mechanisms, and models. *Am Heart J.* 125:1409–19, 1993.

3. Buskens E, Stewart PA, Hess LW, et al.: Efficiency of fetal echocardiography and yield by risk category. *Obstet Gynecol.* 87:423–8, 1996.

4. Whittemore R, Wells JA, Castellsague X: A second-generation study of 427 probands with congenital heart defects and their 837 children. *J Am Coll Cardiol.* 23:1459–67, 1994.

5. Nora JN, Nora AH: Maternal transmission of congenital heart diseases: New recurrence risk figures and the question of cytoplasmic inheritance and vulnerability to teratogens. *Am J Cardiol.* 59:459–63, 1987.

6. Friedman AH, Copel JA, Kleinman CS: Fetal echocardiography and fetal cardiology: Indications, diagnosis and management. *Semin Perinatol.* 17:76–88, 1993.

7. Burton BK: Recurrence risks for congenital hydrocephalus. *Clin Genet.* 16:47–53, 1979.

8. Bromley B, Frigoletto FD, Benacerraf BR: Mild fetal lateral cerebral ventriculomegaly. Clinical course and outcome. *Am J Obstet Gynecol.* 164:863–7, 1991.

9. Parrish ML, Roessmann U, Levinsohn MW: Agenesis of the corpus callosum: A study of the frequency of associated malformations. *Ann Neurol.* 6:349, 1979.

10. Goldstein RB, LaPidus AS, Filly RA, et al.: Mild lateral cerebral ventricular dilatation in utero. Clinical significance and prognosis. *Radiology.* 176:237–42, 1990.

11. Chervenak FA, Berkowitz RL, Romero RJ, et al.: The diagnosis of fetal hydrocephalus. *Am J Obstet Gynecol.* 147:703–16, 1983.

12. Pilu G, Rizzo N, Orsini LF, et al.: Antenatal recognition of cerebral anomalies. *Ultrasound Med Biol.* 12:319–25, 1985.

13. Fonkalsrud EW, DeLorimier AA, Hays DM: Congenital atresia and stenosis of the duodenum. A review compiled from the members of the Surgical Section of the America Academy of Pediatrics. *Pediatrics.* 43:79–83, 1969.

14. Fogel M, Copel JA, Cullen MT, et al.: Congenital heart disease and fetal thoracoabdominal anomalies: Associations in utero and the importance of cytogenetic analysis. *Am J Perinatol.* 8:411–6, 1991.

15. DeLorimier AA, Fonkalsrud EW, Hays DM: Congenital atresia and stenosis of the jejunum and ileum. *Surgery.* 65:819–27, 1969.

16. Greenwood RD, Rosenthal A, Nadas AS: Cardiovascular malformations associated with imperforate anus. *J Pediatr.* 86:576–9, 1975.

17. Teixeira OH, Malhotra K, Sellers J, et al.: Cardiovascular anomalies with imperforate anus. *Arch Dis Child.* 58:747–9, 1983.

18. Touloukian RJ: Anorectal malformations. In: Bergsma D, ed. *Birth Defects Compendium*, 2nd ed. New York: Alan R. Liss; 1979: pp. 99–100.

19. Seashore JH: Congenital abdominal wall defects. *Clin Perinatol.* 5:61–77, 1978.

20. Carpenter MW, Curci MR, Dibbins AW, et al.: Perinatal management of ventral wall defects. *Obstet Gynecol.* 64:644–51, 1984.

21. Greenwood RD, Rosenthal A, Nadas AS: Cardiovascular malformations associated with omphalocele. *J Pediatr.* 85:818–21, 1974.

22. Greenwood RD, Sommer A, Rosenthal A, et al.: Cardiovascular abnormalities in the Beckwith-Wiedemann syndrome. *Am J Dis Child.* 131:293–4, 1977.

23. Greenwood RD, Rosenthal A, Nadas AS: Cardiovascular abnormalities associated with congenital diaphragmatic hernia. *Pediatrics.* 57:92–7, 1976.

24. Thorpe-Beeston JG, Gosden CM, Nicolaides KH: Prenatal diagnosis of congenital diaphragmatic hernia: Associated malformations and chromosomal defects. *Fetal Ther.* 4:21–8, 1989.

25. Crawford DC, Wright VM, Drake DP, et al.: Fetal diaphragmatic hernia: The value of fetal echocardiography in the prediction of postnatal outcome. *Br J Obstet Gynaecol.* 96:705–10, 1989.

26. Greenwood RD, Rosenthal A, Parisi L, et al.: Extracardiac abnormalities in infants with congenital heart disease. *Pediatrics.* 55:485–92, 1975.

27. Wallgren EL, Landtman B, Rapola J: Extracardiac malformations associated with congenital heart disease. *Eur J Cardiol.* 7:15–24, 1978.

28. Gallo P, Nardi F, Marinozzi V: Congenital extracardiac malformations accompanying congenital heart disease. *G Ital Cardiol.* 6:450–9, 1976.

29. DeVore GR: The prenatal diagnosis of congenital heart disease—A practical approach for the fetal sonographer. *J Clin Ultrasound.* 13:229–45, 1985.

30. Allan LD, Crawford DC, Chita SK, et al.: Prenatal screening for congenital heart disease. *Br Med J.* 292:1717–9, 1986.

31. Copel JA, Pilu G, Green J, et al.: Fetal echocardiographic screening for congenital heart disease: The importance of the four-chamber view. *Am J Obstet Gynecol.* 157:648–55, 1987.

32. Wigton TR, Sabbagha RE, Tamura RK, et al.: Sonographic diagnosis of congenital heart disease: Comparison between the four-chamber view and multiple cardiac views. *Obstet Gynecol.* 82:219–24, 1993.

33. Achiron R, Glaser J, Gelernter I, et al.: Extended fetal echocardiographic examination for detecting cardiac malformations in low risk pregnancies. *Br Med J.* 304:671–4, 1992.

34. Vergani P, Mariani S, Ghidini A, et al.: Screening for congenital heart disease with the four-chamber view of the fetal heart. *Am J Obstet Gynecol.* 167:1000–3, 1992.

35. DeVore GR: The aortic and pulmonary outflow tract screening examination in the human fetus. *J Ultrasound Med.* 11:345–8, 1992.

36. Ott WJ: The accuracy of antenatal fetal echocardiography screening in high and low risk patients. *Am J Obstet Gynecol.* 172:1741–9, 1995.

37. Cooper MJ, Enderlein MA, Dyson DC, et al.: Fetal echocardiography: Retrospective review of clinical experience and an evaluation of indications. *Obstet Gyencol.* 86:577–82, 1995.

38. Achiron R, Glaser J, Gelernter I, et al.: Extended fetal echocardiographic examination for detecting cardiac malformations in low risk pregnancies. *Br Med J.* 304:671–4, 1992.

39. Crawford DC, Chita SK, Allan LD: Prenatal detection of congenital heart disease: Factors affecting obstetrical

management and survival. *Am J Obstet Gynecol.* 159:
352–6, 1988.

40. Sandor GG, Farquarson D, Wittmann B, et al.: Fetal
echocardiography: Results in high-risk patients. *Obstet
Gynecol.* 67:358–64, 1986.

41. Benacerraf BR, Pober BR, Sanders SP: Accuracy of fetal
echocardiography. *Radiology.* 165:847–9, 1987.

42. Callan NA, Maggio M, Steger S, et al.: Fetal echocardiography: Indications for referral, prenatal diagnoses, and
outcomes. *Am J Perinatol.* 8:390–4, 1991.

43. Stoll C, Alembik Y, Dott PM, et al.: Evaluation of prenatal

diagnosis of congenital heart disease. *Prenat Diagn.* 13:
453–61, 1993.

44. Crane JP, LeFever ML, Winborn RC, et al.: A randomized
trial of prenatal ultrasonographic screening: Impact on
the detection, management, and outcome of anomalous
fetuses. *Am J Obstet Gynecol.* 171:392–9, 1994.

45. Kirk JS, Riggs TW, Comstock CH: Prenatal screening for
cardiac anomalies: The value of routine addition of the
aortic root to the four-chamber view. *Obstet Gynecol.* 84:
427–31, 1994.

CHAPTER TEN

Fetal Cardiac Imaging

Darla B. Hess, Greg Flaker, Kul B. Aggarwal, Linda C. Buchheit, and L. Wayne Hess

Congenital heart disease (CHD) accounts for approximately 50% of all deaths attributed to lethal malformations in children.[1] Defects of fetal cardiac anatomy and function are four times as common as neural tube defects and over six times more common than serious chromosomal defects.[2] Obstetric health care providers in the United States either offer or provide screening for neural tube defects and Down syndrome (trisomy 21) for 100% of obstetric patients under currently recognized national standards.[3] The four most common CHDs occurring in the first year of life are ventricular septal defects, coarctation of the aorta, transposition of the great arteries, and tetralogy of Fallot.[4] When a sonogram is performed during pregnancy for defined clinical reasons, a four-chamber view of the fetal heart is routinely performed. Approximately 60% of all pregnant women in the United States undergo an ultrasound examination for clinically established reasons.[5] However, a four-chamber view of the fetal heart does not reliably detect the four most common CHDs listed above.[6] Therefore, the vast majority of fetuses with CHD go undetected even in those women who have undergone an obstetric ultrasound. A screening program for fetal CHD would require 100% of pregnant women to undergo a targeted ultrasound and fetal echocardiogram, since fewer than 50% of fetuses with CHD have a risk factor for its development. This would require a major commitment of financial resources. No study has been performed to determine whether this would be a cost-effective utilization of medical financial resources. Therefore, it is currently recommended that only those fetuses with significant risk factors be referred for a targeted sonogram and fetal echocardiogram.[7]

In 1997 the American College of Cardiology (ACC) and American Heart Association (AHA), in collaboration with the American Society of Echocardiography, presented recommendations and an executive summary concerning the performance of fetal echocardiography.[8] They recommended that fetal echocardiography be performed only by trained fetal echocardiographers. Such experts may be cardiologists, perinatologists (obstetricians), or radiologists with special training. Table 10–1 lists clear-cut indications for referral of a patient for a fetal echocardiogram. Table 10–2 lists possible indications (ACC and AHA guidelines) for a fetal echocardiogram. Table 10–3 lists patients who should not be referred for a fetal echocardiogram (ACC and AHA guidelines). Expanding on the ACC and AHA guidelines, Tables 10–4 through 10–6 list commonly accepted indications for a fetal echocardiogram. Table 10–7 lists cardiac defects reported with selected medications. Tables 10–8 through 10–13 expand further on these indications for a fetal echocardiogram. Table 10–14 outlines goals for the fetal echocardiogram examination. Table 10–15 reviews the most common reasons for referral to our fetal echocardiography laboratory at the University of Missouri–Columbia.

HISTORICAL PERSPECTIVE

Successful management of congenital heart disease is a late 20th century accomplishment that has paralleled advanced technology development. The natural history of the disease was well established early because of a lack of effective therapy. The first successful operation for congenital heart disease occurred just before the onset of World War II in 1939,

TABLE 10–1. INDICATIONS FOR A FETAL ECHOCARDIOGRAM

Abnormal appearing heart on general fetal ultrasound examination.

Fetal tachycardia, bradycardia, or persistent irregular rhythm on clinical or screening ultrasound examination.

Maternal or family risk factors for cardiovascular disease, such as parent, sibling, or first-degree relative with congenital heart disease.

Maternal diabetes mellitus (TGA, VSD, CA risk for fetus).[a]

Maternal systemic lupus erythematosus (heart block risk for fetus).

Teratogen exposure during a vulnerable period.

Other fetal organ system anomalies (including chromosomal).

Performance of transplacental therapy or presence of a history of significant but intermittent arrhythmia. Reevaluation examinations are required in these conditions.

Fetal distress or dysfunction of unclear etiology.

[a]TGA, Transposition of the great vessels; VSD, ventricular septal defect; CA, coarctation of the aorta.

when a patent ductus arteriosus was successfully ligated.[9] Open heart surgery was first performed in 1957 using a cardiopulmonary bypass to support the circulation.[10] Invasive catheter intervention began with the Rashkind[11] balloon atrial septostomy in 1966. Closure of a patent ductus arteriosus was achieved by Porstmann[12] in 1967. Most older congenital cardiac repairs or palliations were introduced in the 1960s.[13] The Fontan[14] operation was performed at the Mayo Clinic in 1970 (Table 10–16). The Norwood[15] operation, arterial switch operation,[16] and neonatal heart transplant[17] became practical realities in the late 1980s. Survival of neonates and subsequent pregnancy with congenital heart disease has also became a reality (Table 10–17).

Fetal echocardiography is a recent development with practical development beginning approximately 15 years ago. Winsburg,[18] in 1972, was the first investigator to quantitate fetal cardiac anatomy with blind M-mode echocardiography. Thereafter Ianniruberto et al.,[19] DeLuca et al.,[20] Wladimiroff and McGhia,[21] Sahn et al.,[22] Silverman and Golbus,[23] Kleinman et al.,[24] DeVore et

TABLE 10–2. POSSIBLE INDICATIONS FOR A FETAL ECHOCARDIOGRAM

Previous history of multiple fetal losses

Multiple gestation

TABLE 10–3. PATIENTS WHO SHOULD NOT UNDERGO A FETAL ECHOCARDIOGRAM

Low-risk pregnancies with normal anatomic findings on ultrasound examinations

Occasional premature contractions without sustained tachycardia or signs of dysfunction or distress

Presence of a noncardiovascular system abnormality when evaluation of the cardiovascular system will alter neither medical management decisions nor fetal outcome

al.,[25] and others evaluated fetal cardiac anatomy and function with two-dimensional (2D), M-mode, and Doppler technology. With further advances in ultrasound technology Reed et al.,[26] Huhta et al.,[27] and others furthered knowledge in fetal echocardiography.

TIMING OF THE FETAL ECHOCARDIOGRAM

In our fetal echocardiography laboratory we prefer to perform the examination at 18 to 20 weeks' gestation. As outlined by Dr. Castillo in his chapter on transvagi-

TABLE 10–4. FETAL INDICATIONS FOR FETAL ECHOCARDIOGRAPHY

Intrauterine growth retardation

Fetal cardiac dysrhythmia

Fetal aneuploidy or other malformation

Polyhydramnios (AFI[a]> 25)

Oligohydramnios (AFI[a]< 5)

Abnormal four-chamber view, cardiac axis, or abnormal screening sonogram

Documented maternal viral or other infection known to affect fetal heart

Twin–twin transfusion or multifetal gestation with discordance of fetal growth

Fetal macrosomia (estimated fetal weight of > 4500 g) with evidence of cardiac compromise

Two-vessel umbilical cord

Cardiac teratogen exposure

Before extensive fetal therapy such as fetal blood transfusion, fetal surgery

Marked abnormalities with Doppler interrogation of the fetal circulation

Decreased perfusion of vital organs during power Doppler evaluation or color flow mapping

Nonimmune hydrops fetalis

[a]AFI, amniotic fluid index.

TABLE 10–5. MATERNAL INDICATIONS FOR FETAL ECHOCARDIOGRAPHY

Insulin-dependent diabetes mellitus

Collagen vascular disease

Viral, bacterial, parasitic, or other infection known to affect fetal or maternal heart
  Rubella (PPAS, PDA, VSD, ASD risk for the fetus)[a]
  Toxoplasmosis
  Coxsackie virus
  Cytomegalovirus
  Mumps virus

Drug or teratogen exposure known to affect fetal heart
  Lithium
  Amphetamines
  Alcohol
  Anticonvulsant
  Phenytoin
  Trimethadione
  Isoretinoin

Heavy metal toxicity

Maternal congenital or hereditary heart disease

Severe renal dysfunction uncorrected by dialysis or renal transplant

Advanced maternal age refusing chorionic villus sampling, genetic amniocentesis, or triple screening

Phenylketonuria (tetrology of Fallot, ventricular septal defect, atrial septal defect risk for the fetus)

[a]PPAS = peripheral pulmonary artery stenosis; PDA = patent ductus arteriosis; VSD = ventricular septal defect; ASD = atrial septal defect.

TABLE 10–6. FAMILIAL INDICATIONS FOR FETAL ECHOCARDIOGRAPHY

Congenital heart disease in first degree relative

Genetic or strongly familial syndromes associated with fetal heart disease
  Marfan's syndrome
  Noonan's syndrome
  Tuberous sclerosis
  Velocardiofacial syndrome

nal echocardiography (Chapter 11), fetal echo can be successfully performed as early as 8 to 10 weeks' gestation. However, the sensitivity and specificity of the examination appears maximal at 18 to 20 weeks' gestation.[28] This timing also allows repetition of fetal echo examinations when the first examination is incomplete before 22 weeks' gestation (the time limit for pregnancy termination in our state). In those patients with suspected lesions that may progress or occur later in gestation (i.e., fetal aortic stenosis or other flow lesions) we usually repeat the fetal echo again at 28 to 30 weeks' gestation. However, fetal echo is technically possible from 8 to 10 weeks' gestation until term.

EQUIPMENT

Full fetal cardiac evaluation necessitates the presence of a high-resolution, real-time ultrasound machine with duplex, M-mode, color M-mode, pulse, continuous wave, power, and color flow Doppler capability (Doppler ultrasonic energy should be kept at or below 100 mW/cm^2—spatial peak temporal average for the shortest necessary time). High-resolution imaging requires high transducer frequency (5 to 7.5 MHz) independent image expansion capabilities, cine-loop, machine-assisted presets for fetal echo optimization, and depth selection. However, lower frequency (2 to 4 MHz) transducers must be available for patients who are difficult to image. Additionally, a computer-assisted analysis (and digital image storage) system with a full package of obstetrical, cardiac, and Doppler programs is essential to make appropriate measurements and calculations. Video recording for later playback is also essential. The VCR should have slow motion, forward and reverse playing, and single-frame advance capabilities.

Recent technological breakthroughs of parallel processing and the use of higher interrogation and line density triangulation have allowed for better resolution at any given depth and have improved Doppler imaging. This has permitted low flow velocities at high frame rates and detection of higher flow at any depth with the same line density. It has permitted higher Nyquist limits at a given depth to reduce aliasing and larger sequential packet size for improved velocity accuracy. Thus, increased sensitivity is obtained with decreased ambiguity. With new transducer models using six to eight planes on array transducers, dynamic range focusing has been further developed and expanded.[29]

In the past, the need for high-resolution images obtainable with high-frequency transducers allowed successful performance of quality fetal echocardiography in only 50% of gravidas who exceeded 150 lb.[30] With the new equipment breakthroughs, the successful percentage is much higher (>95% in our experience).

Two-Dimensional Imaging

The following is a suggested practical approach to beginning fetal echocardiography: First, the fetal

TABLE 10–7. SELECTED MEDICATIONS AND REPORTED CARDIAC DEFECTS[a, b]

Drug	Cardiac Defect
Amantadine	VSD
Amobarbital	VSD, ASD, limb deformities, cleft lip and/or palate, club foot, polydactyly, NTD
Carbamazepine	VSD, ASD, NTD
Chlorambucil	VSD, ASD, renal agenesis
Chlordiazepoxide	VSD, ASD, microcephaly, duodenal atresia
Chloroquine	TF, Wilms' tumor, hemihypertrophy
Chlorothiazide	Fetal bradycardia
Clomiphene	VSD, ASD, microcephaly, NTD, cleft lip and/or palate, syndactyly, club foot
Cocaine	Cardiac dysrhythmia, VSD, ASD, valvular stenosis, urinary and limb defects, bowel atresia
Coumadin	VSD, ASD, NTD, scoliosis, limb hypoplasia, cleft palate
Cyclophosphamide	VSD, ASD, cleft palate, hand abnormalities
Diphenhydramine	VSD, ASD, cleft lip (palate, club foot, GU anomalies)
Ethanol	PDA, ASD, VSD, TGA, micropthalmia, microcephaly, GU defects, diaphragmatic hernia
Ethosuximide	PDA, cleft lip and/or palate, hydrocephalus
Haloperidol	Aortic valve defect, limb reduction
Ibuprofen	Premature closure of ductus arteriosus
Indomethacin	Premature closure of ductus arteriosus, penile agenesis, phocomelia, oligohydramnios
Lithium	Ebstein's anomaly, ASD, VSD, coarctation of the aorta, mitral atresia, TGA, NTD
Lysergic acid diethylamide	VSD, ASD, coarctation
Meclizine	Hypoplastic left heart, ear and eye defects
Meprobamate	VSD, ASD, omphalocele
Methotrexate	Dextroposition of the heart, absent digits, hypertelorism
Metronidazole	VSD, ASD, limb, urinary and fascial anomalies
Minoxidil	VSD, transposition, clinodactyly, omphalocele
Paramethadione	VSD, ASD, oligodactyly, malformed kidneys
Procarbazine	VSD, ASD, oligodactyly, malformed kidneys
Prochlorperazine	VSD, cleft palate, skeletal defects
Quinine	VSD, ASD, NTD, hydrocephalus, limb and fascial defects, urogenital, vertebral, and GI anomalies
Retinoic acid	VSD, ASD, hydrocephalus, NTD, micropthalmia, microcephaly, limb abnormalities, cleft palate
Tolbutamide	VSD, ASD, syndactyly
Trimethadione	TGA, TF, HLHS, microcephaly, cleft lip, malformed hands, club foot, ambiguous genitalia, esophageal atresia, TE fistula
Valproic acid	VSD, ASD, NTD, fascial dysmorphism, hydrocephalus, cleft lip, microcephaly, scoliosis, limb reduction, renal hypoplasia, duodenal atresia, hand deformity

[a]See Table 10–12 for abbreviations; HLHS, hypoplastic left heart syndrome; NTD, neural tube defects; PDA, patent ductus arteriosus; TGA, transposition of the great arteries.
[b] Many of the listed associations are based on case reports. Many of these associations may be coincidental rather than causative.

position should be determined. Understanding the views of the fetal heart requires understanding the three-dimensional arrangements of both the mother and the fetus. The fetal position within the uterus and its relationship to maternal head, feet, and spine must be understood. Once these orientations are estab-lished, the orientation of the fetal heart within the fetal body is determined. The fetal heart lies transversely in the fetal chest since the fetal lungs are not aerated. The heart lies superiorly to the fetal liver and stomach. The apex of the fetal heart is against the anterior chest wall. The pulmonary outflow tract

TABLE 10–8. RECURRENCE RISKS FOR CARDIOVASCULAR ANOMALIES

Anomaly	Mother Affected (%)	Father Affected (%)	Prior Sibling Affected (%)
Ventricular septal defects	6.0	1.0	3.0
Patent ductus arteriosis	4.0	2.5	3.0
Atrial septal defect	4.0	1.5	2.5
Tetralogy of Fallot	7.5	1.5	2.5
Pulmonary stenosis	6.0	2.0	2.0
Coarctation of the aorta	4.0	2.0	2.0
Aortic stenosis[a]	15.0	3.0	2.0
Transposition of the great arteries	5.0	2.0	1.5
Atrioventricular canal	14.0	1.0	2.0
Truncus arteriosis	5.0	2.0	1.0
Endocardial fibroelastosis[b]	–	–	4.0
Tricuspid atresia	–	–	1.0
Ebstein's anomaly	–	–	1.0
Pulmonary atresia	–	–	1.0
Hypoplastic left or right heart[c]	–	–	9.0

[a] Some cases of subaortic stenosis are autosomal dominant; supravalvular aortic stenosis is autosomal recessive.
[b] Both autosomal and X-linked recessive forms have been reported.
[c] Autosomal recessive forms of hypoplastic left heart and autosomal dominant forms of hypoplastic right heart have been reported.
Adapted, with permission, from Hess LW, Hess DB, McCaul JF, et al. Fetal echocardiography. Obstet Gynecol Clin N Am:*1980; 17:41–79.*

TABLE 10–9. CARDIAC MALFORMATIONS CAUSED BY TERATOGENS

Potential Teratogen	Frequency of Heart Defects (%)	Most Common Malformations[a]
Drugs		
Alcohol	30	VSD, PDA, ASD
Amphetamines	5	VSD, PDA, ASD, TGA
Anticonvulsants		
Hydantoin	3	PS, AS, CA, PDA
Trimethadione	30	TGA, TF, HLHS
Lithium	10	Ebstein's, TA, ASD
Thalidomide	10	TF, VSD, ASD, truncus arteriosus
Retinoic acid	10	VSD
Infections		
Rubella	35	Peripheral pulmonary artery stenosis, PDA, VSD, ASD
Maternal conditions		
Diabetes	5	TGA, VSD, CA
Lupus	40	Heart block
Phenylketonuria	10	TF, VSD, ASD

[a]VSD, ventricular septal defect; PDA, patent ductus arteriosus; ASD, atrial septal defect; TGA, transposition of the great arteries; PS, pulmonary valve stenosis; AS, aortic valve stenosis; CA, coarctation of the aorta; TF, tetralogy of Fallot; HLHS, hypoplastic left heart syndrome; TA, tricuspid valve atresia.
Adapted, with permission, from Hess LW, Hess DB, McCaul JF, et al. Fetal echocardiography. Obstet Gynecol Clin N Am:*1990; 17:41–79.*

(pulmonary valve) is superior and anterior to the aortic outflow tract (aortic valve). The great arteries are perpendicular to one another at their origins. Availability of a detailed model of the fetal heart helps maintain these special arrangements at the sonographer's recall. Once the sonographer is oriented, a targeted ultrasound examination should be performed with the primary intent of the examination directed toward detecting unsuspected noncardiac fetal anomalies. Approximately 70% of noncardiac fetal anomalies should be detected by this sonogram when performed in a tertiary referral center. The targeted study should include measurements of biparietal diameter (BPD), femur length (FL), abdominal circumference (AC), estimated fetal weight (EFW), chest circumference (CC) at the level of

TABLE 10–10. VULNERABLE PERIODS FOR TERATOGENIC INFLUENCES ON FETAL CARDIOVASCULAR DEVELOPMENT

Abnormality	Embryonic Event Completed (Days)	Limits of Vulnerable Period (Days)
Conotruncal septation	34	14–34
Endocardial cushions	38	14–38
Ventricular septum	44	14–44
Atrial septum	55	14–55
Semilunar valves	55	14–55
Patent ductus arteriosus	–	14–60
Coarctation of aorta	–	14–60

Adapted, with permission, from Hess LW, Hess DB, McCaul JF, et al. Fetal echocardiography. Obstet Gynecol Clin N Am:*1990; 17:41–79.*

TABLE 10–11. TYPES OF CONGENITAL HEART DISEASE (CHD) ASSOCIATED WITH CHROMOSOMAL ANEUPLOIDY

Population	Incidence of CHD (%)	Most Common Cardiac Defects[a]
Normal karyotype	0.8	VSD, PDA, ASD
Trisomy 22	65	ASD, VSD, PDA
Trisomy 21	50	ECD, VSD, ASD, PDA
Trisomy 18	99	VSD, DORV, PS
Trisomy 13	90	VSD, PDA, Dext
Trisomy 8	50	VSD, ASD, PDA
Trisomy 9	50	VSD, CA, DORV
4p−	40	VSD, ASD, PDA
5p −	25	VSD, PDA, ASD
13q −	25	VSD
14q −	50	PDA, ASD, Tet
18q −	50	VSD
45X	35	CA, AS, ASD
XXXXY	14	PDA, ASD, ARC
Triploidy	50	VSD
Cat-eye syndrome	40	TAPVR, VSD, ASD

[a]VSD, ventricular septal defect; PDA, patent ductus arteriosus; ASD, atrial septal defect; TAPVR, total anomalous pulmonary venous return; Dext, dextrocardia; DORV, double-outlet right ventricle; PS, pulmonary valve stenosis; ECD, endocardial cushion defect; CA, coarctation of the aorta; AS, aortic valve stenosis; ARC, anomalous right coronary artery; Tet, tetralogy of Fallot.

Adapted, with permission, from Hess LW, Hess DB, McCaul JF, et al. Fetal echocardiography. Obstet Gynecol Clin N Am:1990; 17:41–79.

TABLE 10–12. GENETIC SYNDROMES WITH CARDIOVASCULAR ABNORMALITIES POTENTIALLY DETECTABLE UTILIZING FETAL ECHOCARDIOGRAPHY

	Cardiac Abnormality
Autosomal recessive	
Adrenogenital (21 and 3)	Arrhythmias
Conradi	VSD
Cutis laxa	Pulmonary hypertension, peripheral pulmonary artery stenosis
Ellis-van Creveld	ASD, single atrium
Friedreich's ataxia	Myocardiopathy
Glycogenosis IIa, IIIa, and IV	Myocardiopathy
Ivemark's	Atrial isomerism
Laurence-Moon-Biedl	VSD
Mucolipidosis III	Aortic valve disease
Mucopolysaccharidosis (MPS) IH (Hurler's)	AI and MI
MPS IS (Scheie), MPS IV (Morquio), MPS VI (Maroteaux-Lamy)	Aortic valve disease
Osteogeneis imperfecta	Aortic valve disease
Pseudoxanthoma elasticum	MI
Refsum's	Atrioventricular conduction defects
Seckel's	VSD
Smith-Lemli-Opitz	VSD
Thalassemia major	ASD, TF, dextrocardia
Thrombocytopenia and absent radii (TAR)	Myocardiopathy
Autosomal dominant	
Apert's	VSD, TF
Complete heart block	Third-degree heart block
Crouzon's	CA
Familial periodic paralysis	Supraventricular tachycardia
Forney	MI
Holt-Oram	ASD, VSD
Idiopathic hypertrophic subaortic stenosis (IHSS)	Subaortic muscular hypertrophy
LEOPARD	PS
Marfan's	AI, MI
Myotonic dystrophy (Steinert)	Myocardiopathy
Neurofibromatosis	PS, CA
Noonan's	PS, ASD, IHSS
Osteogenesis imperfecta	AI
Treacher-Collins	VSD, ASD
Tuberous scleroses	Myocardial rhabdomyoma, supraventricular tachycardia
Wolfe-Parkinson-White	Supraventricular tachycardia
X-linked recessive	
Muscular dystrophy (Duchenne)	Myocardiopathy
Muscular dystrophy (Dreifuss)	Myocardiopathy

VSD, ventricular septal defect; ASD, atrial septal defect; AI, aortic insufficiency; MI, mitral insufficiency; CA, coarctation of the aorta; PS, pulmonic valve stenosis; TF, tetralogy of Fallot.

Adapted, with permission, from Hess LW, Hess DB, McCaul JF, et al. Fetal echocardiography. Obstet Gynecol Clin N Am:1990; 17:41–79.

the fetal heart, cardic/thoracic ratio, head circumference (HC), etc., as outlined by the American Institute of Ultrasound in Medicine guidelines. The fetal stomach bubble is then identified. At the level of the stomach, the cross section of the aorta and vena cava should also be identified (no vena cava and azygous hypertrophy are frequent with anomalous pulmonary venous return). When the transducer is moved cephalad, the fetal heart should be seen. The stomach bubble and the heart should be located on the same side. Situs solitus is the normal position of the heart (heart in the left chest). Abnormalities of cardiac situs (situs inversus or situs ambiguous) are frequently associated with other defects such as anomalous pulmonary venous return and atrial isomerism, asplenic, and Ivemark's syndromes, etc.

TABLE 10–13. ANTENATAL SONOGRAPHIC DIAGNOSES THAT SHOULD PROMPT FETAL CARDIAC EVALUATION WITH INCIDENCE OF ASSOCIATED CONGENITAL HEART DISEASE

System or Diagnosis	Incidence of Congenital Heart Disease (%)
Central nervous system	
Hydrocephalus	12
Dandy-Walker syndrome	3
Agenesis of corpus callosum	15
Meckel-Gruber syndrome	14
Mediastinum	
Tracheoesophageal fistula	33
Esophageal atresia–tracheoesophageal fistula	30
Abnormalities of cardiac position (situs abnormality)	60
Gastrointestinal	
Duodenal atresia	17
Jejunal atresia	5
Anorectal anomalies	22
Imperforate anus	11
Omphalocele	30
Gastroschisis	5
Diaphragmatic hernia	15
Genitourinary	
Renal agenesis	
Bilateral	43
Unilateral	17
Horseshoe kidney	40
Renal dysplasia	5
Ureteral obstruction	2
Others	2
Twins	
Conjoined	25
Monoamniotic	3
Skeletal anomalies	
Short rib–polydactyly (three types)	40
Thrombocytopenia–absent radii	33
Fanconi's	14
Apert's	10
Carpenter's	4
Robin's	9
Arthrogryposis	30
Holt-Oram	50
Ellis-van Creveld	50

Adapted, with permission, from Hess LW, Hess DB, McCaul JF, et al. Fetal echocardiography. Obstet Gynecol Clin N Am:1990; 17:41–79.

TABLE 10–14. GOALS OF A FETAL ECHOCARDIOGRAM

To define the morphology of the fetal heart on a segmental basis
  Situs
  Atrial segments
  Pulmonary veins
  Atrioventricular connections
  Ventricular morphology
  Ventricular atrial connections
  Right atrial great vein connections
  Great artery morphology
  Atrial septum
  Ventricular septum
  Foramen ovale
  Cardiac axis within chest

To determine the presence of flow disturbances and determine the velocity of flow in all cardiac chambers, arteries, veins, foramen ovale, and ductus arteriosus

To measure chamber and vessel sizes and wall thicknesses when an abnormality is detected

To define fetal heart rate and abnormalities of rhythm

To evaluate both systolic and diastolic function of the fetal heart

TABLE 10–15. INDICATIONS FOR FETAL ECHOCARDIOGRAPHY AT THE UNIVERSITY OF MISSOURI—COLUMBIA

	Percentage of Referrals	Percentage of Scanned Fetuses with Heart Disease
Family history of congenital heart disease	42.7	1.9
Fetal arrhythmia	22.1	1.3
Fetal abnormalities (anatomy or growth)	11.7	33.7
Maternal disease (diabetes, PKU)[a]	8.9	3.7
Drug or teratogen exposure	7.3	1.0
Abnormal amniotic fluid	2.7	4.3
Other (second opinion, nonimmune hydrops, etc.)	4.6	71.0

[a]PKU, phenylketonuria.

TABLE 10–16. COMMON SURGICAL PROCEDURES FOR CONGENITAL HEART DISEASE

Surgical Procedure	Description[a]
Blalock-Hanlon	Surgical removal of the atrial septum for TGA
Blalock-Taussig	Subclavian artery to pulmonary artery anastomosis (for complete transposition of great arteries palliation)
Brock	Closed pulmonary valvotomy and infundibulectomy
Central shunt (Cooley)	Conduit or anastomosis between aorta and pulmonary artery
Damus-Kaye-Stansel	Pulmonary artery end-to-side anastomosis to aorta, valved conduit between right ventricle and main pulmonary artery (for complete TGA correction)
Fontan	Anastomosis or conduit between right atrium and pulmonary artery (for pulmonary artresia and ventricular septal defect or where there is effectively only one ventricle)
Glenn	Superior vena cava to pulmonary artery anastomosis (most commonly in conjunction with Fontan)
Great arterial switch (Jatene)	Aorta and pulmonary moved to the proper ventricles in TGA, coronary arteries reimplanted, corrects TGA
Kono	Replacement of aortic valve with aortic valve annular enlargement (for aortic outflow obstruction)
Mustard	Atrial switch with intraatrial baffle made of pericardium (for complete TGA)
Norwood	Pulmonary artery anastomosis to aorta, conduit from aorta to main pulmonary artery (for hypoplastic left heart)
Park	Atrial septostomy with catheter blade
Patch	Closure of a hole or surgical incision
PDA ligation	PDA is ligated
Potts	Descending aorta to left pulmonary artery shunt
Pulmonary artery band (Dammann-Muller)	Constrictive band placed around main pulmonary artery
Rashkind	Atrial septostomy with catheter balloon for complete TGA
Rastelli	Valved conduit from right ventricle to pulmonary artery, ventricular septal defect closure with aortic valve incorporated into left ventricle (correction of double-outlet right ventricle)
Senning	Atrial switch with intraatrial baffle made of atrial wall flaps
Subclavian flap	Subclavian artery is sacrificed and brought down to form aortic wall in coarctation repair
Valvectomy	Valve excision
Valvotomy (surgical or balloon)	Surgical opening of an obstructed valve
Valve replacement	Valve excised and replaced with prosthesis
Valvuloplasty	Repair of valve
Waterson	Ascending aorta anastomosis to right pulmonary artery

[a]Abbreviations: TGA, transposition of great arteries; PDA, patent ductus arteriosus.

Adapted, with permission, from Hess DB, Hess LW: Management of cardiovascular disease in pregnancy. Obstet Gynecol Clin N Am:1992; 19:679–695.

Four-Chamber Heart

The four-chamber view of the fetal heart is obtained once situs is identified (Figures 10–1, 10–2, 10–3, 10–3A, 10–4, and 10–4A). In a plane perpendicular to the fetal spine (Figure 10–1) the view is obtained cephalad from the abdominal circumference. A complete fetal rib should be imaged to verify the proper plane. If the four-chamber view of the fetal heart is normal, it should reveal the following findings:

1. There are four cardiac chambers, which are all approximately the same size. Right and left

TABLE 10–17. MORTALITY RISKS IN THE PREGNANT CARDIAC PATIENT

Mortality < 1%
  New York Heart Association class I or II
    Atrial septal defect
    Ventricular septal defect
    Patent ductus arteriosus
    Pulmonic and/or tricuspid disease
    Corrected tetralogy of Fallot
    Mitral stenosis
    Porcine cardiac valve
Mortality 5% to 15%
  New York Heart Association class II or IV
    Mitral stenosis with atrial fibrillation
    Aortic stenosis
    Metallic prosthetic valve
    Coarctation of aorta
    Uncorrected tetralogy of Fallot
    Marfan's syndrome with normal aorta on echo
    Prior myocardial infarction

Adapted, with permission, from Hess DB, Hess LW: Management of cardiovascular disease in pregnancy. Obstet Gynecol Clin N Am: 1992; 19:679–695.

ventricles, right and left atria, mitral and tricuspid valves, intraventricular septum, intraatrial septum, and a patent foramen ovale are identified. The septae and atrioventricular (AV) valves will meet in the center of the heart.

2. The left atrium has four pulmonary veins entering it. At least two of these can be identified by minor cephalad to caudad rotation of the transducer in the same plane.

3. Opening into the left atrium is the flap valve of the foramen ovale. The foramen ovale occupies the middle third of the atrial septum.

4. The atrial septum extends approximately 3 mm above the level of the atrioventricular valves.

5. The eustachian valve can frequently be seen in the right atrium as the pulmonary veins are identified in the left atrium when the transducer is rotated.

6. The descending aorta pulsates behind the left atrium.

7. Compared to the mitral valve, the tricuspid valve is about 3 mm apically placed.

8. The left ventricle is smooth in appearance compared to the rough right ventricle. The shape of the fetal ventricles is more round than in the adult heart.

9. The moderator band (portion of the trabecula septomarginalis) can be visualized in the right ventricle.

10. The fetal heart should occupy approximately one third of the chest cavity.

11. The thicknesses of the ventricular walls and septum are approximately equal [in the adult the left ventricular (LV) free wall is thicker than the right ventricular (RV) free wall].

12. The cardiac axis is $43° \pm 7°$ (Figure 10–5).[31]

The last chamber crossed by drawing a line from the fetal spine anteriorly to the fetal chest wall is the right ventricle (Figure 10–5). A line drawn directly down the ventricular septum intersecting this line (i.e., cardiac axis) will have an angle of $43° \pm 7°$. The entire right atrium and only a small portion of the left atrium and right ventricle (which contains the tricuspid valve) are located on the pulmonary side of this line.

If the four-chamber view of the heart is entirely normal, 4% to 40% of fetal CHDs can be excluded. Table 10–18 lists fetal cardiac defects that can possibly be detected with a four-chamber view of the fetal heart. Utilizing quantitative M-mode and Doppler evaluation of the four-chamber view should markedly improve sensitivity and specificity of the four-chamber view. However, the cardiac physiology of the fetal heart (different from the adult) must be remembered when using this technology (Table 10–19).

The Five-Chamber View

By angling the transducer cephalad while maintaining the four-chamber view location anteriorly, the five-chamber view of the fetal heart is imaged. This view is a slight variation of the four-chamber view. The ascending aorta makes the "fifth" chamber, which separates the left and right atria. The aortic valve is clearly visualized in this view. The ventricular septum smoothly connects with the right wall of the ascending aorta (Figures 10–6 and 10–7).

Right Ventricular Outflow Tract

Further rotating the transducer cephalad while maintaining and slightly shifting 5° superiorly from the four-chamber location allows the right ventricular outflow tract to be imaged. This view demonstrates the right ventricle, pulmonary valve, and pulmonary artery (Figure 10–8). Further twisting (angling) and rotating from this view allows the appreciation that the great arteries exit the heart perpendicular to one another (Figure 10–9). In D-transposition of the great vessels the great arteries exit parallel to one another).

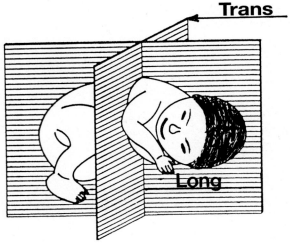

Figure 10–1. The four-chamber view of the fetal heart is imaged in the plane transverse to the fetal spine cephalad from the fetal stomach bubble. Trans, transverse fetal plane; Long, longitudinal fetal plane.

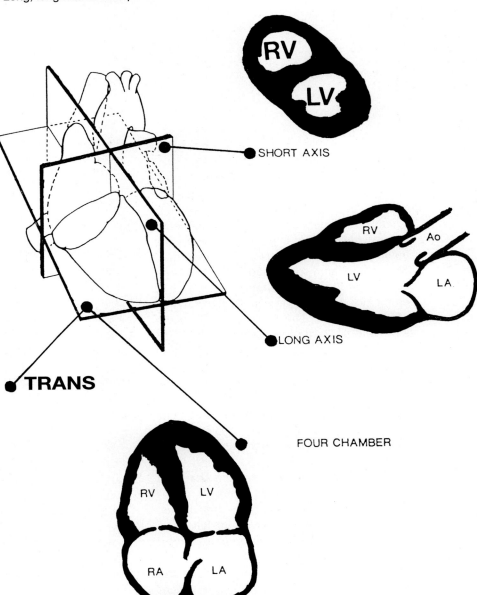

Figure 10–2. The three scanning planes for the fetal heart to visualize the four chambers, long axis (of left ventricle) and short axis (of the LV and RV). Trans, transverse fetal plane from Figure 10–1; RV, right ventricle; LV, left ventricle; RA, right atrium; LA, left atrium; Ao, aorta.

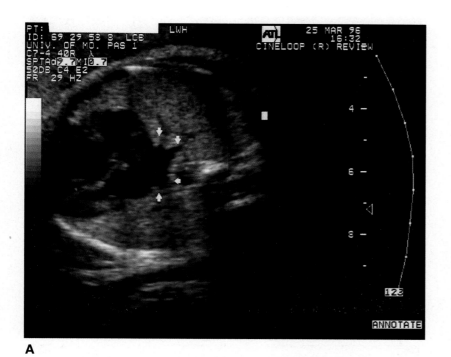

A

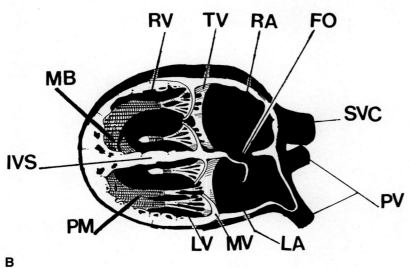

B

Figure 10–3. A. Sonographic four-chamber view of the fetal heart. Arrows mark pulmonary veins entering the left atrium. **B.** Graphic four-chamber heart as noted in Figure 10–3A. MB, moderator band; RV, right ventricle; TV, tricuspid valve; RA, right atrium; FO, foramen ovale; SVC, superior vena cava; PV, pulmonary veins; LA, left atrium; MV, mitral valve; LV, left ventricle; PM, papillary muscle, IVS = Interventricular septum.

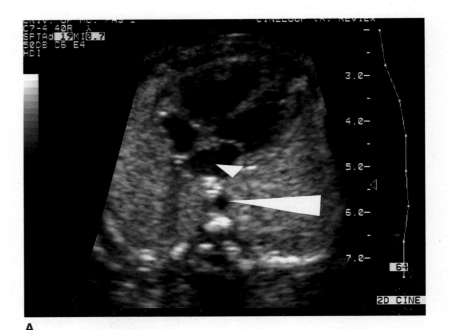

A

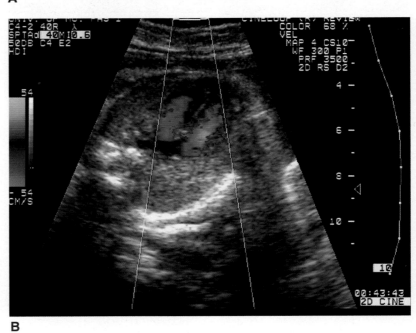

Figure 10–4. A. Four-chamber view of the fetal heart. Note aorta (long arrow) behind the left atrium (small arrow). **B.** Color flow four-chamber view of the fetal heart.

B

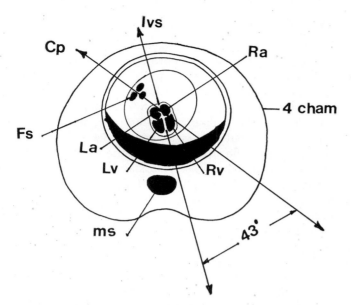

Figure 10–5. Four-chamber heart plane (4 cham). Note the line (Cp, central plane) drawn from the three ossification centers of the fetal spine (Fs) through the center of the fetal chest. The last cavity crossed regardless of fetal position in utero is always the right ventricle (Rv). A second line (Ivs, interventricular septum plane) is drawn down the center of the interventricular septum. The cardiac axis (angle between these lines) is 43° ± 7°. La, left atrium; Lv, left ventricle; Ra, right atrium; ms, maternal spine.

TABLE 10–18. FETAL CARDIAC ANOMALIES POSSIBLY EXCLUDED WITH A FOUR-CHAMBER VIEW OF THE HEART[a]

Hypoplasia of RV or LV

Single ventricle

Large ASD (primary) or VSD

Atrioventricular canal defect

Coarctation of the aorta (right and/or left ventricular disproportion on four-chamber view)

Premature closure of foramen ovale

AV valve atresia or stenosis

Ebstein's anomaly

Pericardial effusion

Cardiac situs abnormalities

Cardiac hypertrophy

Cardiomyopathy

Ectopic cordis

Cardiac tumors

[a]RV, right ventricle; LV, left ventricle; ASD, atrial septal defect; VSD, ventricular septal defect; AV, atrioventricular.

TABLE 10–19. FETAL CARDIAC PHYSIOLOGY

Two umbilical arteries exit from the iliac arteries to take venous blood to the placenta, which has a low vascular resistance.

One umbilical vein returns oxygenated blood to the fetus; the blood is then shunted past the liver via the ductus venosus.

Oxygenated and venous blood is mixed in the inferior vena cava.

Venous blood returns from the superior vena cava.

The eustachian valve in the right atrium shunts oxygenated blood from the inferior vena cava across the patient's foramen ovale into the left atrium.

The fetal ventricles work in parallel rather than in series as in the adult.

The right ventricle has greater flow in the fetus than the left ventricle (60% to 40% ratio).

Seven to eight percent of right ventricular flow is circulated to the fetal lungs; the remainder is shunted to the systemic circulation via the ductus arteriosus.

All left ventricular output is pushed into the ascending aorta. The right ventricle ejects blood into the pulmonary artery, ductus arteriosus, and descending aorta.

Ventricular compliance is decreased in the fetus. The fetal heart rate is 120 to 160 beats per minute (BPM). Increases of heart rate to compensate for cardiovascular abnormalities are not common in the fetus.

Ventricular filling in the fetus is more dependent on active atrial pumping that it is in the adult. Filling pressures in the fetal left and right ventricles are approximately equal.

Fetal cardiac myosin structure and function change throughout gestation.

po_2 in umbilical artery 20 to 22 mm Hg with 46% to 51% oxygen saturation; umbilical veins 30 to 35 mm Hg with 85% oxygen saturation.

Fetal systemic blood pressure 60/30 mm Hg.

Hemoglobin F is present with a hemoglobin of 16 g/dL.

The ductus venosus and arteriosus close following birth and the ventricles shift to series operation.

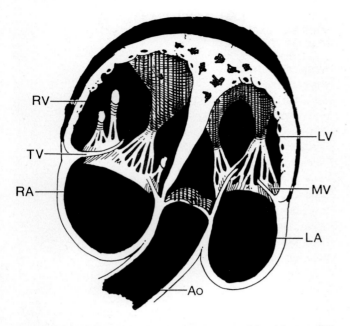

Figure 10–6. Graphic five-chamber view of fetal heart. RV, right ventricle; TV, tricuspid valve; RA, right atrium; Ao, aorta; LA, left atrium; MV, mitral valve; LV, left ventricle.

Long-Axis View of Left Ventricle

The long-axis view of the left ventrical is obtained by rotating the transducer approximately 90° from the four-chamber view with the plane of insonation from the right shoulder to the left hip of the fetus (Figures 10–10 and 10–11). This view allows visualization of the left atrium, the pulmonary veins entering the left atrium, the mitral valve, the ventricular septum, the right ventricle, the aorta arising from the left ventricle, and the aortic valve. Three papillary muscles support the mitral valve. The septal leaflet of the mitral valve is supported by a separate papillary muscle. A papillary muscle also originates from the left ventricular (LV) free wall. Rocking the transducer in this view frequently reveals these relationships. Large ventricular septal defects are seen as an interruption of the ventricular septum before it joins the anterior wall of the aorta. Table 10–20 lists congenital cardiac defects detectable with a long-axis view of the left ventricle.

Short-axis View

The short-axis view of the fetal heart is obtained in a plane approximately perpendicular to the long-axis view of the left ventricle. The transducer plane is from the left shoulder to the right hip of the fetus. The short-axis view varies as the plane of intersection extends from the apex of the fetal heart to the base of the heart (Figure 10–12). Figure 10–13 shows the visi-

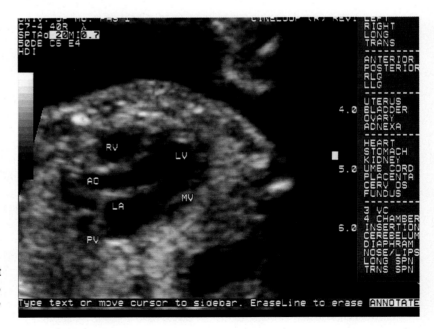

Figure 10–7. Five-chamber view of fetal heart sonographically. RV, right ventricle; Ao, aorta; LV, left ventricle; MV, mitral valve; LA, left atrium; PV, pulmonary vein.

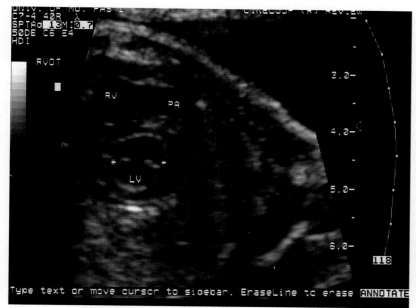

Figure 10–8. Right ventricular outflow tract (RVOT) with short-axis view (cross section) of the left ventricle (LV) at the level of the papillary muscles (marked with asterisks). RV, right ventricle; PA, pulmonary artery.

ble anatomy of the short-axis view at the level of the aortic valve leaflets. Figure 10–14A shows the corresponding sonogram of the same view. Figure 10–14B shows the bifurcation of the left and right pulmonary arteries at the short-axis level. Also at this level, the right atrium, tricuspid valve, right ventricle, pulmonary valve, main pulmonary artery, cross section of the aorta with three cusps of the aortic valve, coronary artery ostia and aortic valve cusps (Figures 10–15 and 10–16), left pulmonary artery, right pulmonary artery, right pulmonary artery wrapping around the cross section of the aorta, and ductus arteriosus are clearly visualized. This view also demonstrates that the pulmonary artery diameter is approximately 20% larger than the ascending aorta. This is the "doughnut" view of the heart, with the pulmonary artery wrapping around the cross section of the aorta. It should also be noted that the pulmonary artery is in the long-axis and the aorta is in a short-axis presentation. Since these vessels are perpendicular to one another, any view of the aorta in the long axis would present the pulmonary artery (or branches) on cross section (short axis), and vice versa.

Long-Axis View of the Great Veins

The long-axis view of the great veins is through the long axis of the fetus to the right and parallel to the fe-

tal spine (Figure 10–17). The connections of the inferior and the superior vena cava to the right atrium are clearly demonstrated in the view. Structures visible in this view include the inferior and superior vena cavae, the right atrium, possibly the right atrial appendage and eustachian valve, the tricuspid valve, the right ventricle, and possibly the aortic and pulmonary valves (Figures 10–18 and 10–19). The inferior vena cava enters the lower aspect of the right atrium and is separated from the tricuspid valve by the triangle of Koch.

Aortic Arch View

The ascending aorta crosses initially from left to right and passes behind the pulmonary artery. It then bends right to left and moves anteriorly as it becomes the transverse arch, adjacent and superior to the ductus arteriosus. It then moves right to left, moves posteriorly, and becomes the descending aorta. Three vessels arise from the top of the aorta: (1) the brachiocephalic, (2) the left common carotid, and (3) the left subclavian arteries. The right pulmonary artery (cross section) is found within the curve of the aortic arch. The segment of the aorta between the left subclavian artery and the ductus arteriosus is the "isthmus."

The aortic arch (Figures 10–20 and 10–21) is best imaged in a longitudinal plane of the fetus to the left of the spine. The scan plane should transect the left pos-

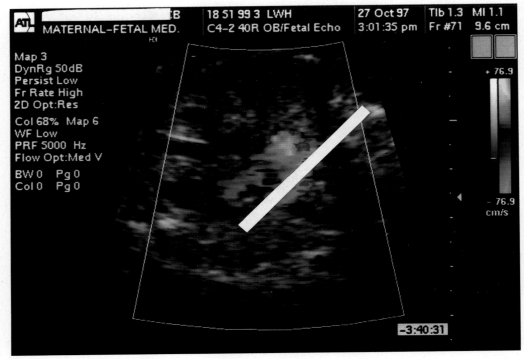

A

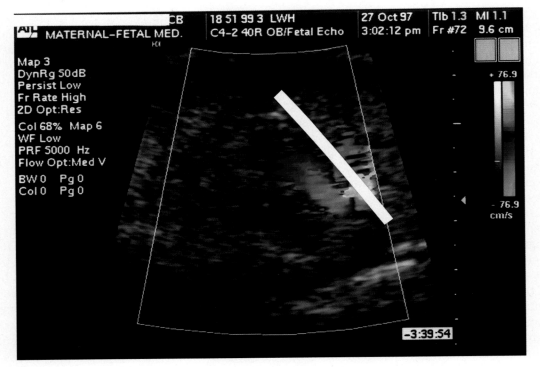

B

Figure 10–9. A. Aortic outflow tract with color flow mapping revealing blood flow toward the transducer (red) parallel to and above the plane marked by the white line. **B.** Pulmonary outflow trace on the same patient as in **A** obtained by leaving the transducer on the same spot on the maternal abdomen and rocking it from side to side. Note the blood flow is away from the transducer (blue) inferior to and in the same direction as the white line. It should also be noted that the aorta and pulmonary arteries are perpendicular to one another as demonstrated in **A** and **B**.

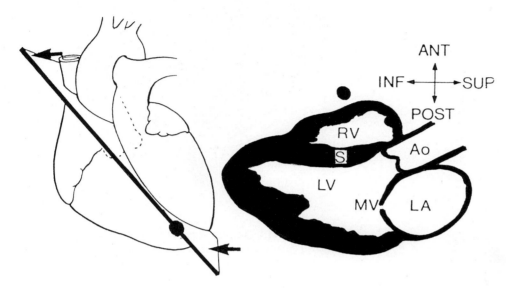

Figure 10–10. Graphic representation of long-axis view of left ventricle in plane shown in Figure 10–2. Large dot shows plane of section. RV, right ventricle; LV, left ventricle; S, interventricular septum; MV, mitral valve; Ao, aorta; LA, left atrium; ANT, ventral surface; POST, dorsal surface; INF, caudad; SUP, cephalad.

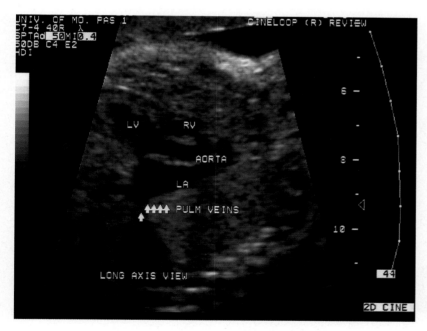

Figure 10–11. Sonogram of the long axis of the left ventricle.

TABLE 10–20. CONGENITAL CARDIAC DEFECTS POTENTIALLY DETECTABLE WITH A LONG-AXIS VIEW OF THE LEFT VENTRICLE

Hypoplastic left ventricle
Hypoplastic right ventricle
Ventricular septal defect
Aortic stenosis or regurgitation (with Doppler)
Transposition of the great arteries
Truncus arteriosus
Tetralogy of Fallot
Anomalous pulmonary venous return
Atrial isomerism
Mitral stenosis or regurgitation (with Doppler)
Left ventricular systolic or diastolic dysfunction

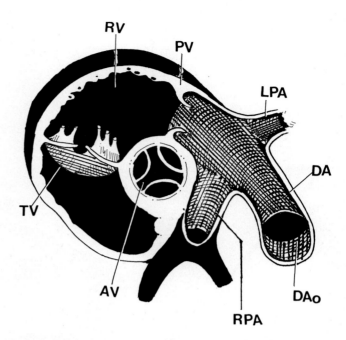

Figure 10–13. Graphic short axis of great arteries. Abbreviations as in Figure 10–12. AV, aortic valve.

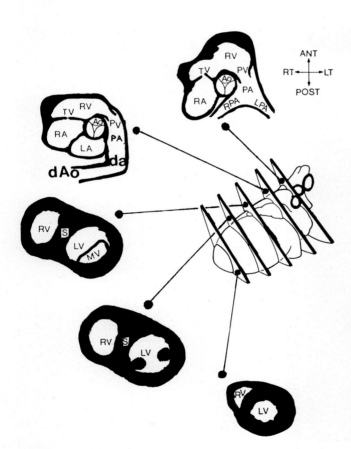

Figure 10–12. Short-axis views of the fetal heart at various short-axis planes. Abbreviations as in Figure 10–10. RA, right atrium; TV, tricuspid valve; PV, pulmonary valve; PA, pulmonary artery; da, ductus anteriosus; dAo, descending aorta; RPA, right pulmonary artery; LPA, left pulmonary artery, ANT, anterior; S, septum; RT, right; LT, left; POST, posterior.

terior chest wall and exit the right lateral chest wall. The aorta appears as a "candy cane" with three vessels exiting from the tight curve of the cane. This view is particularly important to exclude interrupted aortic arch and document coarctation of the aorta.

Ductal Arch View

The ductus arteriosus originates anterior to the aorta and has a broader curve than the aortic arch. It does not have any vessels originating from it. The ductus arteriosus enters the descending aorta superior to the point at which the transverse arch becomes the descending aorta. The ductus arteriosus is best imaged from the ventral surface of the fetus, with the transducer parallel to the fetal spine angled slightly in a plane from the left shoulder to the right hip. It has a "hockey stick" appearance (Figures 10–22 and 10–23). The ductus arteriosus is difficult to image from the dorsal side of the fetus because the fetal spine limits the resolution of images.

Three-Dimensional Fetal Cardiac Ultrasound

Three-dimensional (3D) evaluation of the fetal heart remains in its infancy at present. Several investiga-

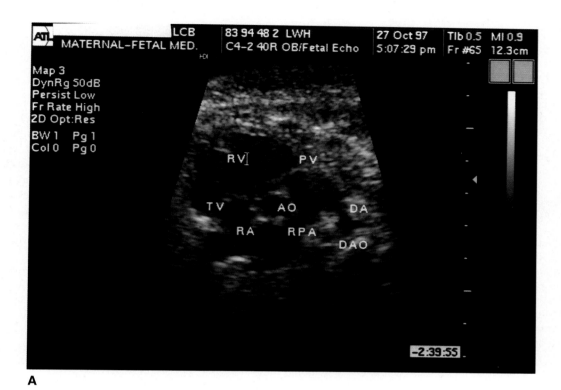

A

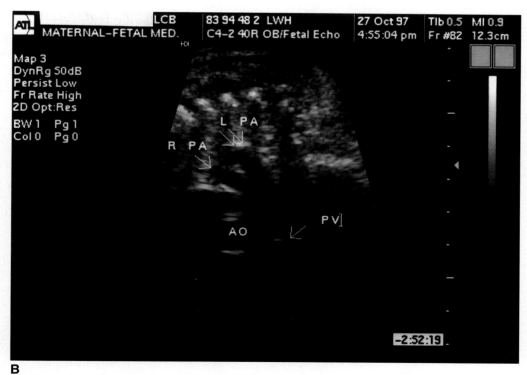

B

Figure 10–14. A. Sonogram—short axis of the great vessels. Abbreviations as in Figure 10–12. **B.** Short-axis view showing bifurcation of pulmonary artery into the right pulmonary artery (RPA) and left pulmonary artery (LPA).

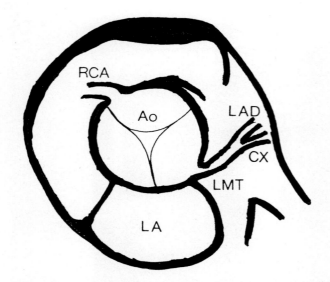

Figure 10–15. Right coronary artery (RCA) and left main trunk coronary artery (LMT) exiting from the two coronary cusps of the aortic valve (Ao). Note there is a third, noncoronary cusp in the aortic valve. The left coronary trunk branches into the left anterior descending and circumflex coronary arteries. Cx, circumflex artery; LAD, left anterior descending artery.

tors have attempted 3D evaluation of the fetal heart.[32,33] This technique is presently limited by current computer technology but is evolving rapidly. Within the next 5 years this will almost certainly come to practical utility.

M-Mode Echocardiography

Duplex-directed M-mode and color M-mode echocardiography can help quantitate fetal cardiac anatomy in real time. Because of advances in 2D echocardiographic technology, M mode is not as helpful in the practical evaluation of lesions as it has been in the past. It does, however, have a unique use in the assessment of fetal arrhythmias, pericardial effusions (Figure 10–24), and in cardiac measurements. Cardiac activity plotted against time can be revealed by M-mode tracings. M-mode combined with color flow Doppler can be useful with M mode imparting temporal resolution to the color flow information.

M-mode echocardiography provides an "icepick" view of the heart with high sampling rates; it also allows clear visualization of valve motion, which is missed by real-time scanning that has a frame rate of 20 to 60 Hz. Thus, M mode does truly add another dimension to cardiac scanning, although its utility has limits.

Figures 10–25 through 10–28 demonstrate methods of measuring the four-chamber, long-axis, and

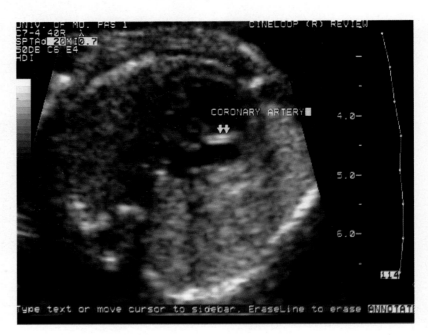

Figure 10–16. Sonogram of left coronary artery.

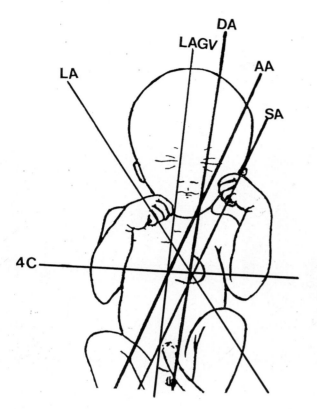

Figure 10–17. Image planes for the various cardiac views. 4C, four-chamber plane; LA, long-axis left ventricle plane; LAGV, long-axis great veins plane; DA, ductal arch plane; AA, aortic arch plane; SA, short-axis left ventricle plane.

short-axis views of the fetal heart with M mode. Figures 10–29 through 10–36 demonstrate septal, chamber, and wall thickness and aortic diameter throughout pregnancy as reported by Allan et al.[34] and DeVore et al.[35] Table 10–21 demonstrates calculation of fractional cardiac changes based on Figure 10–25. Figures 10–37 through 10–40 demonstrate methods of calculating ventricular volumes.[36] The technique that has proved most useful is Simpson's rule. Chapter 14, Congenital Cardiac Defects in the Fetus, provides regressing equations for cardiac dimensions from Tan et al.[37] The chapter also provides aortic arch ratios from Hornberger et al.[38] However, the limitations of all these M-mode measurements must be understood. A discussion of these limitations is beyond the scope of this book.

Doppler Echocardiography

The basic physics of Doppler frequency shift analysis by Chirp Z or fast Fourier transform is beyond the scope of this book. Additionally, basic fluid mechanics of blood flow is also beyond the scope of this book. We

therefore limit our discussion to the clinical application of Doppler to the fetal heart. Basic principles of Doppler interrogation are discussed in depth in Chapter 4.

Doppler modes of operation are either continuous or pulsed wave. Color Doppler is pulsed wave Doppler emitted in multiple planes and color coded in an entire 2D image plane (see section on color Doppler). All Doppler is governed by the following Doppler equation:

$$v = \frac{c \times f_d}{df_o \times \cos \theta}$$

where v = velocity of measured flow, c = speed of sound in tissues (1540 m/s), f_d = Doppler shift frequency, f_o = insonation frequency, and θ = angle of insonation in degrees. Table 10–22 demonstrates $\cos \theta$ at various angles of insonation. It should be noted that $\cos 0° = 1$ and $\cos 90° = 0$. Therefore, the best Doppler velocity will be obtained parallel to flow, and velocity cannot be recorded by Doppler shift perpendicular to flow. Additionally, there is an approximate 6% decrease in measured velocity with insonation at an angle of 20° off parallel. It should also be noted that the insonation frequency (2 to 10 MHz) is in the "ultrasound" frequency and cannot be heard. However, the Doppler shift frequency is in the audible range and can be heard by the human ear. This allows the examiner to have a "stethoscope" to examine the heart with Doppler. The Doppler shift velocity displayed visually and audible sound are both valuable for use in diagnosis.

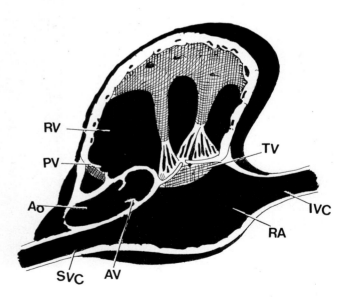

Figure 10–18. Graphic long axis of great veins. TV, tricuspid valve; IVC, inferior vena cava; RA, right atrium; AV, aortic valve; SVC, superior vena cava; Ao, aorta; PV, pulmonary valve; RV, right ventricle.

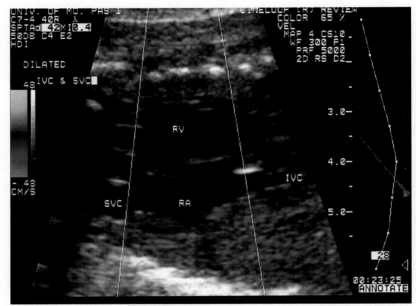

A

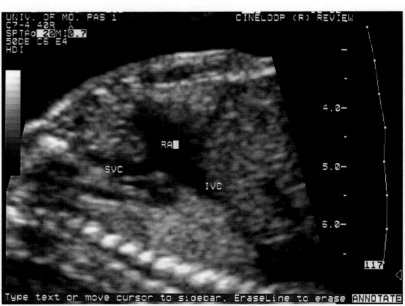

B

Figure 10–19. A. Long axis of the great veins showing enlarged right ventricle (RV) and dilated superior vena cava (SVC) and inferior vena cava (IVC). **B.** Long axis of the great veins showing right atrium and right atrial appendage.

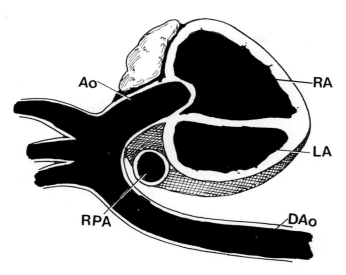

Figure 10–20. Aortic arch. Ao, aorta; RA, right atrium; LA, left atrium; DAo, descending aorta; RPA, right pulmonary artery.

In continuous wave Doppler the transducer has two piezoelectric crystals. One of those crystals is constantly emitting sound and the other crystal is constantly listening to the reflected (returning) sound. Practically, this means that there is no limit to velocities that can be measured within the human body with continuous wave Doppler. However, this technology suffers from range ambiguity, and any velocity or vessel in the "icepick" plane of insonation is measured. Continuous wave Doppler is "steerable" in newer ultrasound machines but cannot be depth controlled.

Pulse Doppler transducers have only one piezoelectric crystal that both emits and listens for the reflected (returning) sound. The crystal emits a burst of sound and does not emit it again until the reflected sound returns and is "heard." Pulsed Doppler, therefore, allows range gating (setting a specific depth at which to measure velocities). This technology also allows setting a "target volume" and pulse repetition frequency. However, this technology suffers from both depth and velocity limits. The pulse repetition frequency imposes a limit on the maximum Doppler shift frequency (velocity) that can be measured. The maximum measurable frequency is limited to half the pulse repetition frequency. Higher frequency shift velocities result in a phenomena called "aliasing."

This imposes the following relationships:

1. The greater the depth selection, the lower the pulse repetition frequency.
2. The lower the pulse repetition frequency, the lower the velocity that can be measured.
3. The greater the depth, the lower the velocity that can be measured.

The pulses of sound emitted and sampled over time and sampling frequency limit the maximum observable frequency shift. This limit is called the

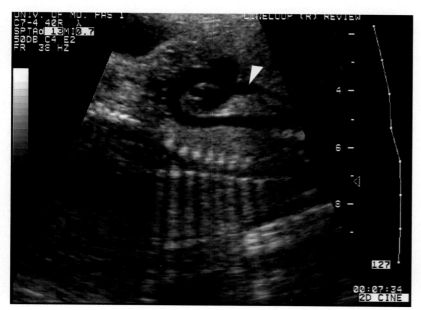

Figure 10–21. Sonogram of the aortic arch. Note the right branch of the pulmonary artery (RPA) on cross-sectional view. Also note the inferior vena cava (arrow) entering the right atrium (RA).

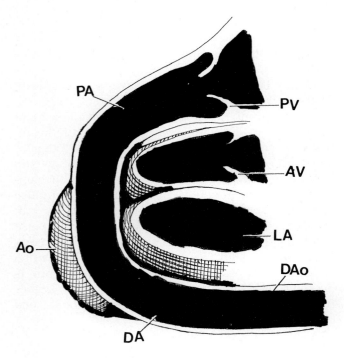

Figure 10–22. Ductal arch.

"Nyquist limit" and is equal to half the sampling frequency. This leads to several points to remember with pulse Doppler:

1. If the (Doppler) frequency shift is less than the Nyquist limit, it can be accurately recorded.
2. If the (Doppler) frequency shift is equal to the Nyquist limit, it is not possible to determine the direction of flow reliably.
3. If the true (Doppler) frequency is greater than 1 but less than twice the Nyquist limit, the frequency shift (velocity) appears in a reverse fashion.
4. If the (Doppler) frequency shift is exactly twice the Nyquist limit the frequency shift (velocity) appears to be zero.

Modern ultrasound equipment attempts to bypass these limits by using high-pulse repetition frequency, pulsed multigate, and multiple sample volume techniques.

The physics of blood flow must also be remembered when using Doppler evaluations. The flow velocity profile is generally considered laminar (parabolic) rather than turbulent when velocities are measured. This allows use of the Bernoulli equation of fluid mechanics.

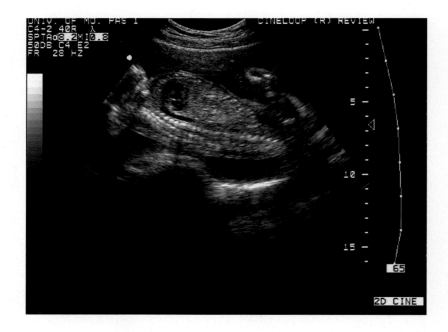

Figure 10–23. Sonogram of ductal arch.

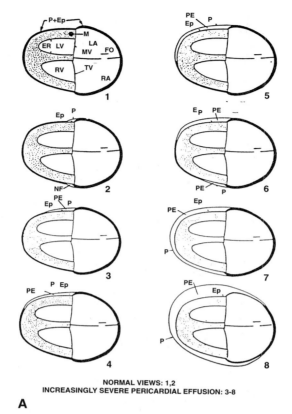

NORMAL VIEWS: 1,2
INCREASINGLY SEVERE PERICARDIAL EFFUSION: 3-8

A

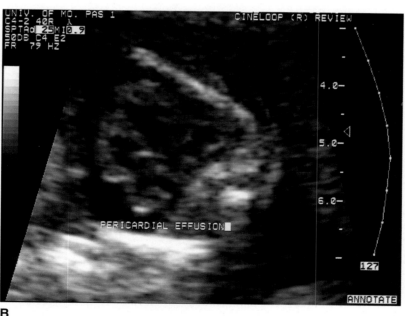

B

Figure 10–24. A. Documentation of pericardial effusion by two-dimensional echocardiography. P, pericardium; Ep, epicardium; PE, pericardial effusion; LV, left ventricle; RV, right ventricle; LA, left atrium; RA, right atrium; MV, mitral valve; TV, tricuspid valve; Fo, foramen ovale. (*Courtesy of Greggory R. DeVore, MD.*) **B.** Four-chamber view of fetal heart with severe pericardial effusion.

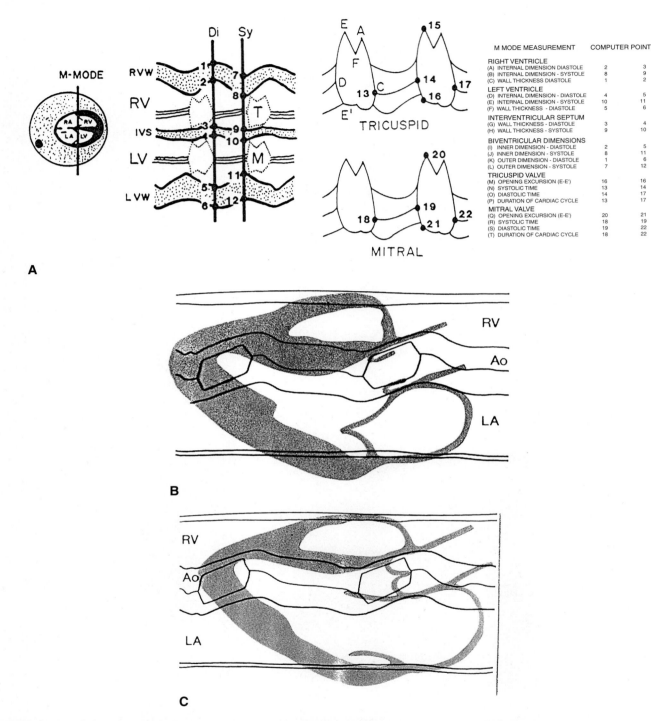

Figure 10–25. A. Schematic of M mode from which measurements are computed. The M mode is recorded perpendicular to the interventricular septum at the level of the mitral and tricuspid valves. The numbers indicate the sequence in which the indicated points are digitized and the measurements subsequently computed. RA, right atrium; RV, right ventricle; LA, left atrium; LV, left ventricle; RVW, right ventricular wall; IVS, interventricular septum; LVW, left ventricular wall; T, tricuspid valve; M, mitral valve; D, beginning of diastole; E–E¹, maximal excursion of leaflets in early diastole; A, atrial systole; C, closure of the leaflet at end-diastole. **B.** M mode of aortic valve excursion superimposed on 2D long-axis view where pattern is obtained with aortic valve open. **C.** M Mode of aortic valve excursion superimposed on 2D long-axis view where pattern is obtained with aortic valve closed. *(Reprinted, with permission, from DeVore GR, Siassi B, Platt LD. Fetal echocardiography IV. M-Mode assessment of ventricular size and contractility during the second and third trimesters of pregnancy in the normal fetus. Am J Obstet Gynecol:1984;150:983.)*

TABLE 10–21. CALCULATION OF FRACTIONAL CHANGES OF THE VENTRICLES BASED ON MEASUREMENTS OBTAINED IN FIGURE 10–25

Right ventricle	
Fractional shortening	$[(A - B)/A](100)$
Mean circumferential shortening	$(A - B)/AN$
Left Ventricle	
Fractional shortening	$[D - E)/D](100)$
Mean circumferential shortening	$D - E/DR$
Biventricular	
Inner fractional change	$[(I - J)/I](100)$
Outer fractional change	$[(K - L)/K](100)$

Adapted, with permission, from DeVore GR, Siassi B, Platt LD. Fetal echocardiography IV. Normal anatomy as determined by real time-directed M-mode ultrasound. Am J Obstet Gynecol:1984; 150:981.

The Bernoulli equation is:

$$P_1 + \tfrac{1}{2} M v_1^2 = P_2 + \tfrac{1}{2} M v_2^2$$

where P_1 = pressure in one area of flow, M = mass density of fluid, v_1 = velocity in one area of flow; P_2 = pressure in another area of flow in a parallel circuit, and v_2 = velocity of flow in another area of flow in a parallel circuit. This equation can be simplified via several assumptions (beyond the scope of this book) to:

$$P_1 - P_2 = 4 v_2^2$$

This allows the calculation of a pressure change across an obstructed area of flow when the velocity distal to the obstruction is known.

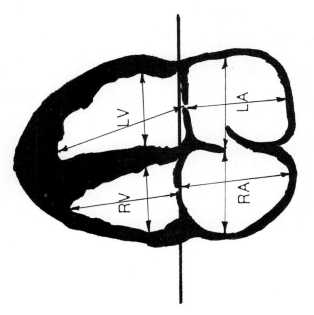

Figure 10–26. Plane of M-mode measurement on a four-chamber view of the heart.

Doppler measurements in the fetus include velocities across the mitral, tricuspid, pulmonic, aortic valves and various venus flows. Flow is also measured in the inferior vena cava, across the foramen ovale, and in the ductus arteriosus. Pulmonary vein flow is measured rarely. Flow across the AV valves is biphasic with E and A peaks (Figure 10–41). The A peak in early gestation is higher than the E peak. These peaks begin to equalize at term. Following birth, the E wave is higher than the A wave. The E wave represents rapid ventricular filling by gravity. The A wave represents ventricular filling via atrial contraction. Table 10–23 demonstrates measurement sites for the AV valves. It should be noted that the E and A peaks are also used to evaluate diastolic function in the fetus (Table 10–24 and Figures 10–42 and 10–43). The semilunar valves have a uniphasic flow peak (Figures 10–44 and 10–45). The maximum velocity acceleration time (slope of the upward curve) is generally measured. Table 10–25 lists expected velocities across these various valves.[39,40] Flow is always forward across the AV and semilunar valves in the normal fetus. Flow across the foramen ovale is biphasic (Figure 10–46) and always in a forward direction from right atrium to left atrium in the normal fetus. Flow across the ductus arteriosus[41–43] is always forward (pulmonary artery to aorta) in the normal fetus (Figures 10–47 and 10–48). This flow is forward both in systole and in diastole. Flow in the superior and inferior vena cava is triphasic. The A wave results from right atrial contraction. The S wave represents right atrial relaxation. The D wave represents rapid ventricular filling.

Doppler can be used to calculate the cardiac output of the left and right ventricles of the fetus. Cardiac output is:

$$CO = A \times v \times HR$$

Where CO = cardiac output; $A = \pi d$, where d is the diameter of the pulmonary or aortic arteries; and HR = heart rate. The critical area of an obstruction can be calculated by:

$$A_2 = \frac{A_1 \times v_1}{v_2}$$

where A_2 = cross-sectional area of obstruction, A_1 = cross-sectional area proximal to an obstruction, v_1 = velocity proximal to obstruction, and v_2 = velocity distal to the obstruction.

COLOR FLOW MAPPING

Color flow Doppler suffers from the same limits as pulse Doppler. As a general rule, forward (toward the transducer) blood flow is colored red, and reverse (away from the transducer) blood flow is colored blue.

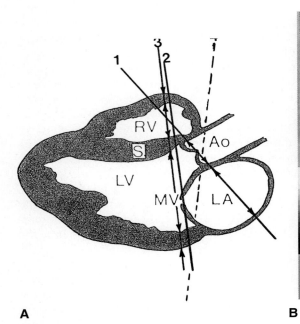

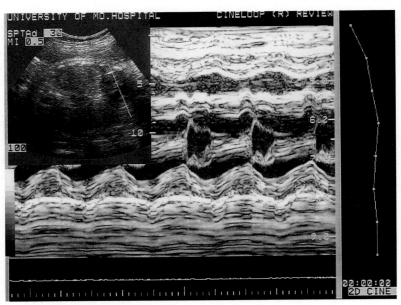

A

B

Figure 10–27. A. Planes of M-mode measurement on the long-axis view of the left ventricle. Plane 1: Aortic leaflet excursion, left atrial interval dimension, and aortic diameter. Plane 2: Mitral valve leaflet excursion. Plane 3: Just past mitral valve leaflets. Plane 4: Evaluation of mitral valve prolapse. **B.** Mitral valve leaflet excursion on M-mode echocardiography. **C.** Color M-mode echocardiography shows complete AV block with atrial rate of 152 and ventricular rate of 72.

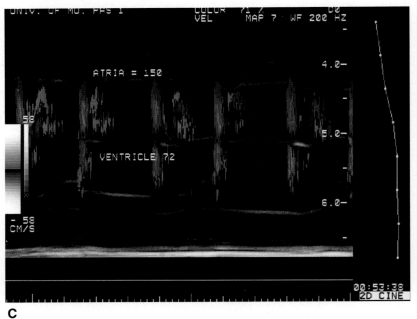

C

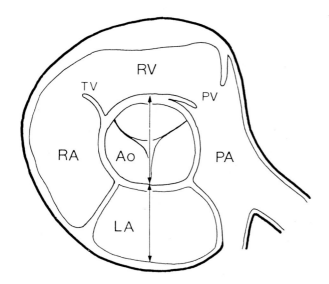

Figure 10–28. M-Mode plane of measurement on the short-axis view. Ao, aorta; LA, left atrium; RA, right atrium; TV, tricuspid valve; RV, right ventricle; PA, pulmonary artery; PV, pulmonary valve.

Aliasing brightens and reverses the color map despite the true direction of flow. In our experience, color flow mapping is essential to determine the exact congenital cardiac lesion which is present. Figure 10–49 shows color flow mapping of the fetal aorta.

POWER DOPPLER (ANGIOGRAPHY)

Power Doppler (PD) is a new technique[44] that displays the strength (rather than the speed and direction, as with color flow) of the Doppler signal in color. PD is based on the integrated power of the Doppler spectrum. PD is able to use more of the available dynamic range of the Doppler signal when producing images and is much less angle dependent. PD does not alias because the integral of the PD spectrum is the same whether the signal wraps around or not. PD has greater sensitivity than color Doppler for flow in small vessels and those with low-velocity flow. This potentially gives PD the ability to detect ischemia or hyperemia in organs with small vessels. PD also has a greater ability to define flow boundaries sharply compared to color flow mapping. The major disadvantages of PD are flush artifact with moving organs and its inability to detect direction and velocity of flow. Figure 10–50 demonstrates power Doppler imaging of the aorta.

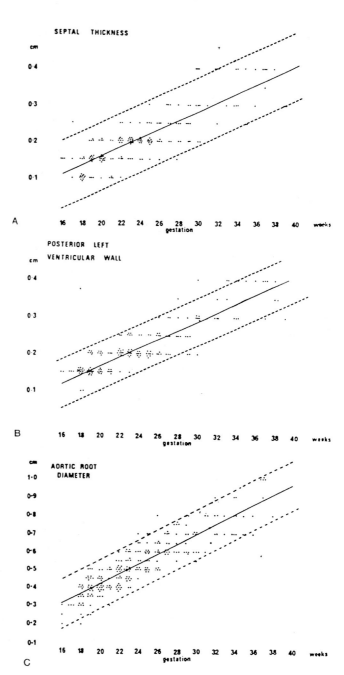

Figure 10–29. Graphic display of normal M-mode measurements of septal thickness **(A)**, posterior left ventricular wall thickness **(B)**, and aortic root diameter **(C)** in fetuses from 16 weeks' gestation to term. Values in centimeters (*y* axis) are plotted against gestational age (*x* axis); the dotted lines represent two standard deviations from the standard error of the mean (straight line). *(Reprinted, with permission, from Allan LD, Joseph MC, Boyd EGC, et al. M-mode echocardiography in the developing human fetus. Br Heart J:1982; 47:573.)*

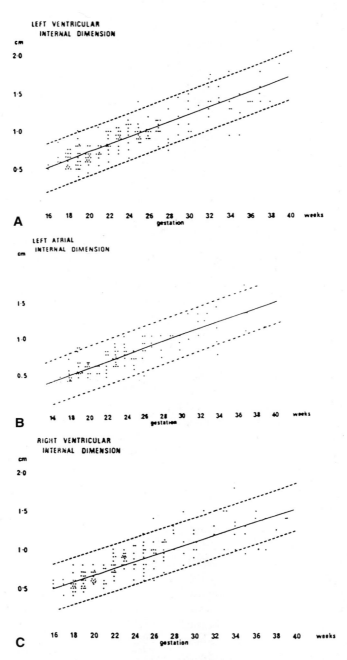

Figure 10–30. Graphic display of normal M-mode measurements of left ventricular **(A)**, left atrial **(B)**, and right ventricular **(C)** internal diameters in fetuses from 16 weeks' gestation to term. *(Reprinted, with permission, from Allan LD, Joseph MC, Boyd EGC, et al. M-mode echocardiography in the developing human fetus. Br Heart J:1982; 47:573.)*

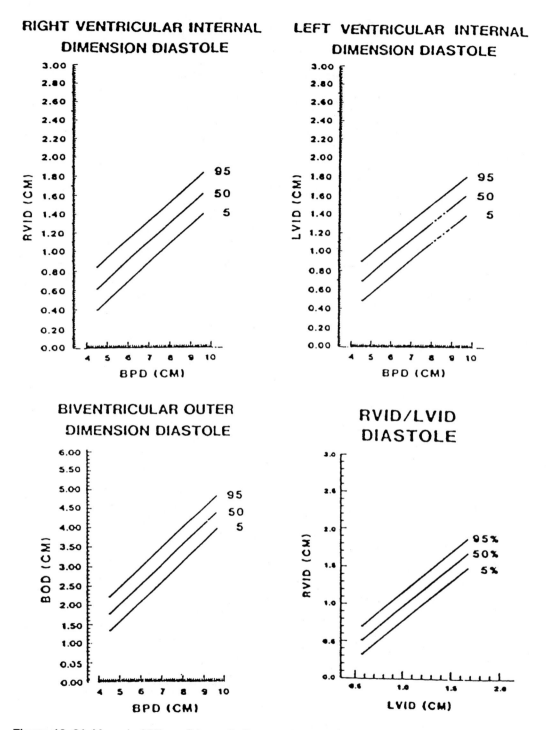

Figure 10–31. M-mode 95% confidence limit measurements for ventricular chambers and biparietal diameter (BPD). *(Reprinted, with permission, from DeVore GR. Cardiac imaging. In Sabbagha RE, ed.* Diagnostic Ultrasound Applied to Obstetrics and Gynecology. *Philadelphia: JB Lippincott, 1987.)*

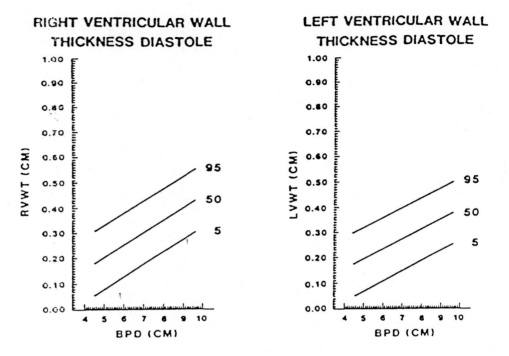

RIGHT VENTRICULAR WALL THICKNESS DIASTOLE

LEFT VENTRICULAR WALL THICKNESS DIASTOLE

INTERVENTRICULAR SEPTAL WALL THICKNESS DIASTOLE

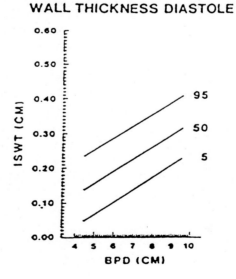

Figure 10–32. M-mode 95% confidence limit measurements for ventricular walls and biparietal diameter (BPD). *(Reprinted, with permission, from DeVore GR, Siassi B, Platt LD. Fetal echocardiography IV. M-mode assessment of ventricular size and contractility during the second and third trimesters of pregnancy in the normal fetus. Am J Obstet Gynecol:1984; 150:986.)*

TRICUSPID VALVE EXCURSION

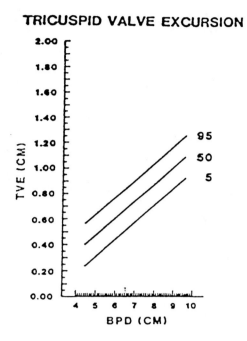

MITRAL VALVE EXCURSION

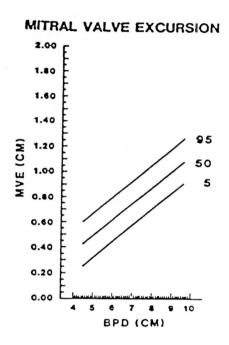

AORTIC ROOT DIMENSION
DIASTOLE

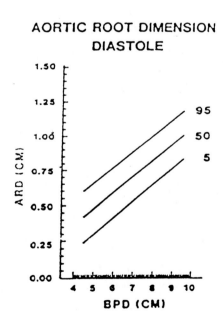

AORTIC VALVE EXCURSION

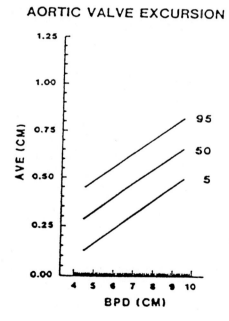

Figure 10–33. M-mode 95% confidence limit measurements for valve excursion and biparietal diameter (BPD). *(Reprinted, with permission, from DeVore GR. Cardiac imaging. In Sabbagha RE, ed.* Diagnostic Ultrasound Applied to Obstetrics and Gynecology. *Philadelphia: JB Lippincott, 1987.)*

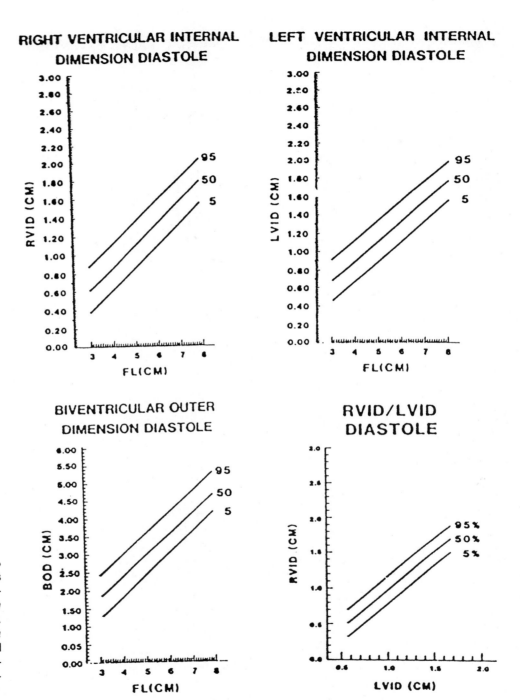

Figure 10–34. M-mode 95% confidence limit measurements for ventricular chambers and femur length (FL). *(Reprinted, with permission, from DeVore GR. Cardiac imaging. In Sabbagha RE, ed.* Diagnostic Ultrasound Applied to Obstetrics and Gynecology. *Philadelphia: JB Lippincott, 1987.)*

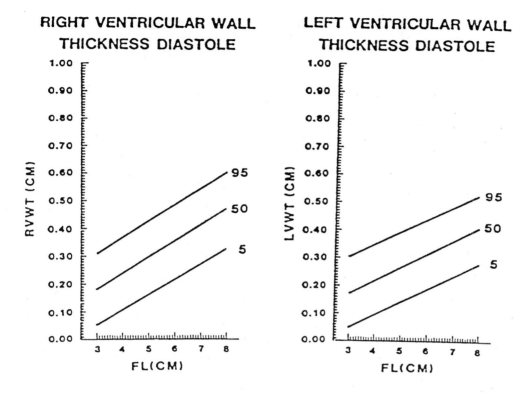

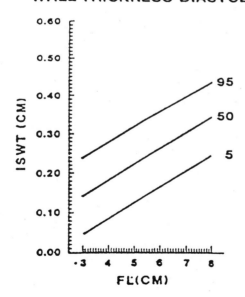

Figure 10–35. M-mode 95% confidence limit measurements for ventricular walls and femur length (FL). *(Reprinted, with permission, from DeVore GR. Cardiac imaging. In Sabbagha RE, ed. Diagnostic Ultrasound Applied to Obstetrics and Gynecology. Philadelphia: JB Lippincott, 1987.)*

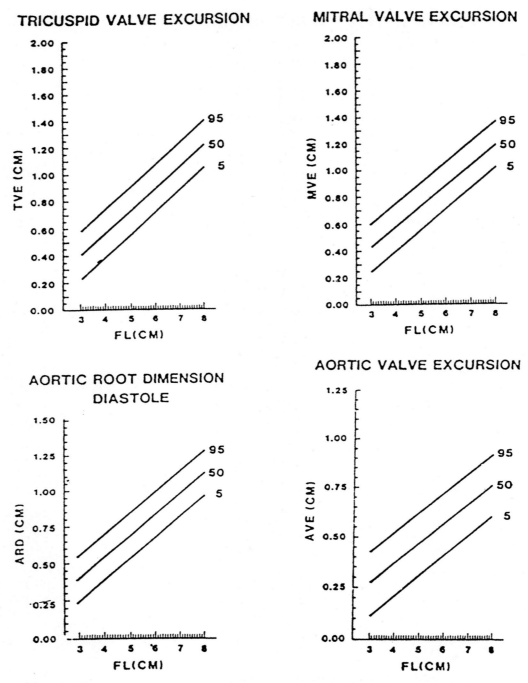

Figure 10–36. M-mode 95% confidence limit measurements for valve excursion and femur length (FL). *(Reprinted, with permission, from DeVore GR. Cardiac imaging. In Sabbagha RE, ed. Diagnostic Ultrasound Applied to Obstetrics and Gynecology. Philadelphia: JB Lippincott, 1987.)*

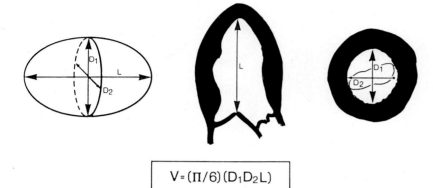

$$V = (\Pi/6)(D_1 D_2 L)$$

Figure 10–37. Long diameter method to calculate left ventricular volume. D_1 and D_2 are measured at the mitral valve level of the short axis.

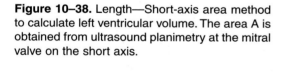

Figure 10–38. Length—Short-axis area method to calculate left ventricular volume. The area A is obtained from ultrasound planimetry at the mitral valve on the short axis.

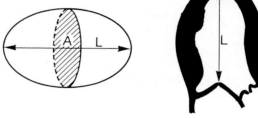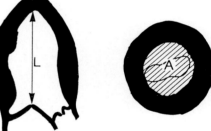

$$V = 2/3\ AL$$

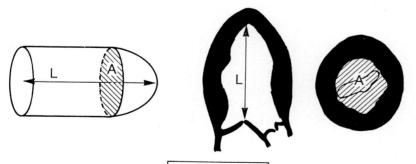

$$V = 5/6\ AL$$

Figure 10–39. "Bullet" method to calculate left ventricular volume. The area is obtained via planimetry as in Figure 10–38.

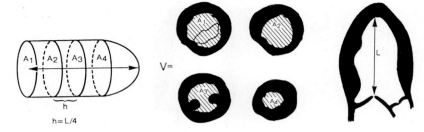

Figure 10–40. Simpson's rule method for left ventricular volume. Areas are again obtained via planimetry on the ultrasound machine. This is the most used volume method. Most ultrasound machines have software within them to make these calculations.

$$V = \left[(A_1 + A_2 + A_3)h\right] + \left[(A_4 h/2) + (\Pi/6)(h^3)\right]$$

TABLE 10–22. VALUES FOR COSINE OF ANGLE θ

Angle θ (°)	Cosine
0	+1.00
1	+1.00
2	+1.00
3	+1.00
4	+1.00
5	+1.00
6	+0.99
7	+0.99
8	+0.99
9	+0.99
10	+0.98
20	+0.94
30	+0.87
40	+0.77
50	+0.64
60	+0.50
70	+0.34
80	+0.17
90	0.00
100	−0.17
120	−0.50
140	−0.77
160	−0.94
180	−1.00

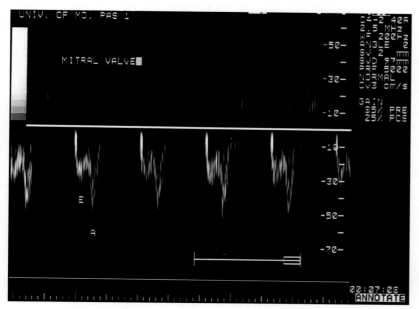

Figure 10–41. Biphasic flow across the mitral valve with Doppler interrogation. E and A peaks are clearly seen.

TABLE 10–23. AV INFLOW VELOCITY MEASUREMENTS

Measurement	Sampling Site
Peak E wave	Valve annulus
Peak A wave	Valve annulus
E/A ratio	Valve annulus
Acceleration time (AT)[a]	Valve tips
Deceleration time (DT)[b]	Valve tips

[a]Acceleration time is the upward slope of the E wave.
[b]Deceleration time is the downward slope of the E wave.

TABLE 10–24. DETERMINANTS OF DIASTOLIC FUNCTION

Active relaxation
Chamber stiffness
  Myocardium
    Myocardial fibers
    Extracellular component
  Wall thickness
  Left ventricular geometry
  Right ventricular–left ventricular interaction
  Pericardial forces
Mitral valve orifice
Atrioventricular coupling
Intrathoracic pressure

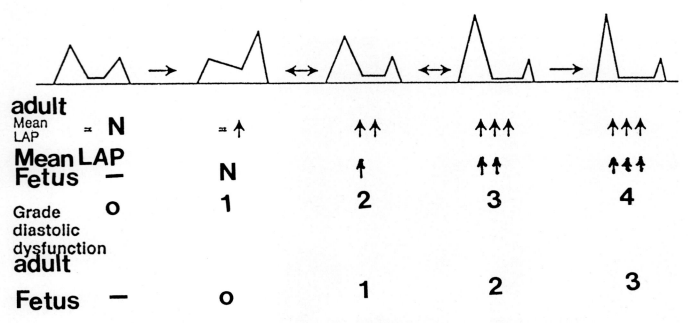

	Normal	Abnormal Relaxation	Pseudo-normalization	Restriction (reversible)	Restriction (irreversible)
adult Mean LAP	= N	= ↑	↑↑	↑↑↑	↑↑↑
Mean LAP Fetus	—	N	↑	↑↑	↑↑↑
Grade diastolic dysfunction adult	o	1	2	3	4
Fetus	—	o	1	2	3

Figure 10–42. E to A peak evaluation for diastolic dysfunction in the fetus. The fetus has a "stiff" ventricle compared to the adult and normally has a "grade 1" diastolic dysfunction compared to the adult. LAP, Left atrial pressure; N, normal.

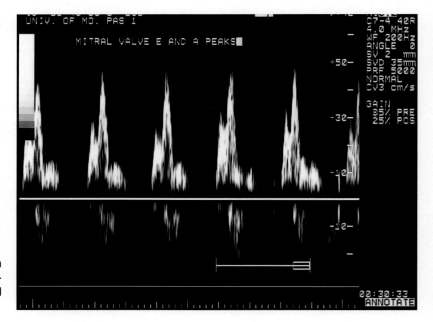

Figure 10–43. E to A wave of the mitral valve in a fetus with hydrops fetalis and diastolic dysfunction. Compare Figures 10–41, 10–42, and 10–43 to note the degree of dysfunction.

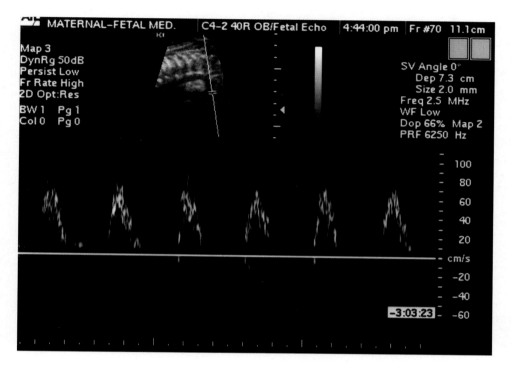

Figure 10–44. Uniphasic Doppler flow in the fetal aorta at a velocity of 68 cm/s.

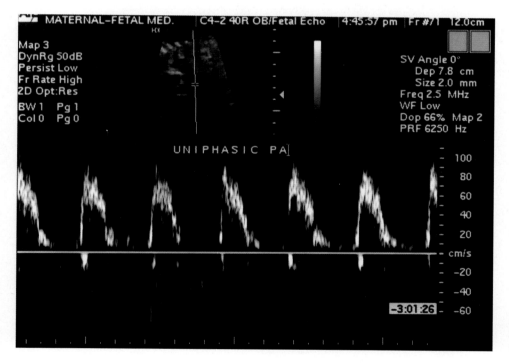

Figure 10–45. Uniphasic flow in the pulmonary artery at a velocity of 70 cm/s.

**TABLE 10–25. FLOW MEASUREMENT
IN THE NORMAL FETAL HEART**

	Peak Velocity (cm/s)	Mean Temporal Velocity (cm/s)
Tricuspid valve[a]	51 ± 9.1	11.8 ± 3.1
Mitral valve[a]	47 ± 8.3	11.2 ± 2.3
Pulmonary valve[a]	60 ± 12.9	16 ± 4.1
Aortic valve[a]	70 ± 12.2	18 ± 3.3
Right ventricular output[b]	307 ± 127 mL/kg/min	
Left ventricular output[b]	232 ± 106 mL/kg/min	

[a]Angle-corrected maximal and mean temporal flow velocities across the cardiac valves are expressed as mean ± SD.
[b]Cardiac output derived from tricuspid and mitral valve area and mean velocities (mean ± SD).
Adapted from Reed KL, Meijboom EJ, Sahn DJ, et al. Cardiac Doppler flow velocities in human fetuses. Circulation:1986;73:41.

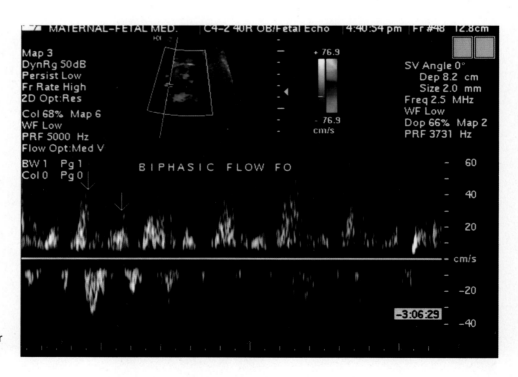

Figure 10–46. Biphasic Doppler flow across the foramen ovale.

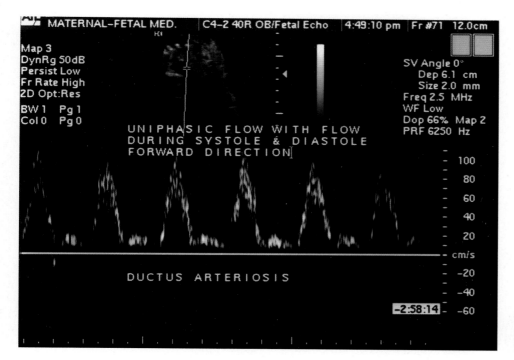

Figure 10–47. Uniphasic flow in the ductus arteriosus with forward flow in both systole and diastole.

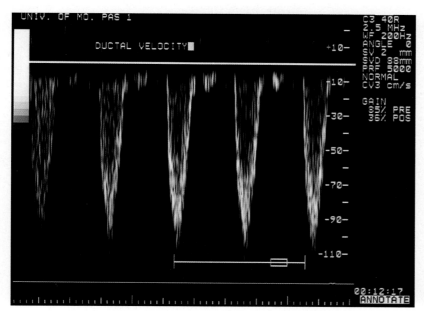

Figure 10–48. Ductal velocity at 110 cm/s. This is the fastest flow in the body of the normal fetus.

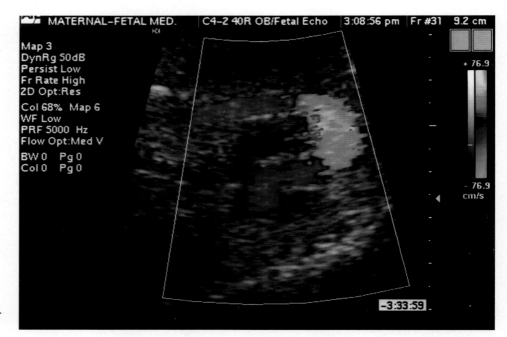

Figure 10–49. Color flow mapping of the fetal aorta.

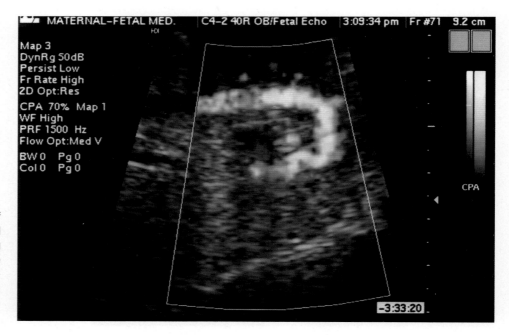

Figure 10–50. Power Doppler of the aorta in the same patient and at the same time of color mapping shown in Figure 10–49. Notice there is far better edge enhancement in the arch of the aorta with power Doppler compared to the color flow map.

REFERENCES

1. Hofman JI, Christian R: Congenital heart disease in a cohort of 19,502 births with long term follow-up. *Am J Cardiol.* 42:641–7, 1987.
2. Lian ZH, Zach MM, Erickson JD: Paternal age and occurrence of birth defects. *Am J Hum Genet.* 39:648–60, 1986.
3. Rose NC, Palomaki GE, Haddow JE, et al.: Maternal serum alpha fetoprotein screening for chromosomal abnormalities: A prospective study in women aged 35 and older. *Am J Obstet Gynecol.* 170:1073–80, 1994.
4. Mitchell SC, Korones SB, Berendes HW: Congenital heart disease in 56,109 births. *Circulation.* 43:323–32, 1971.
5. Ewigman BG, Crane JP, Frigoletto, et al.: Effect of prenatal ultrasound screening on perinatal outcome. *N Engl J Med.* 329:821–7, 1993.
6. Vergani P, Mariani S, Ghidini A, et al.: Screening for congenital heart disease with the four-chamber view of the fetal heart. *Am J Obstet Gynecol.* 167:1000–3, 1992.
7. Hess DB, Hess LW: Fetal echocardiography. *The Female Patient.* 21:17–34, 1996.
8. ACC/AHA guidelines for the clinical application of echocardiography: Executive summary. *J Am Coll Cardiol.* 29:862–79, 1997.
9. Hess DB, Hess LW: Management of cardiovascular disease in pregnancy. *Obstet Gynecol Clin N Am.* 19:679–95, 1992.
10. Becker RN: Intracardiac surgery in pregnancy. *Ann Thorac Surg.* 36:453–63, 1983.
11. Chew PC, Chew SC, Lee YK, et al.: Congenital heart disease in pregnancy. *Singapore Med J.* 16:97–106, 1975.
12. Engle MA: The adult with congenital heart disease. *Dis Mon.* 27:1–68, 1981.
13. Etheridge MJ, Pepperall RJ: Heart disease and pregnancy at the Royal Women's Hospital. *Med J Australia.* 2: 277–84, 1971.
14. Lutz DJ, Noller KL, Spittell JA, et al.: Pregnancy and its complications following cardiac valve prosthesis. *Am J Obstet Gynecol.* 131:460–5, 1978.
15. Kahler RL: Cardiac disease. In Burrow GN, Ferris, TF, eds. *Medical Complications During Pregnancy.* Philadelphia: WB Saunders; 1975: p. 105.
16. Czeizel A, Pornoi A, Peterfly E: Study of children of parents operated on for congenital cardiovascular malformations. *Br Heart J.* 47:290–8, 1982.
17. Kaplan S: Congenital heart disease. In Wyngarder JB, Smith LA, eds. *Cecil Textbook of Medicine,* 18th ed. Philadelphia: WB Saunders; 1988: pp. 98–122.
18. Winsberg F: Echocardiography of the fetal and newborn heart. *Invest Radiol.* 7:152–7, 1972.
19. Ianniruberto A, Iaccarino M, Deluca I, et al.: Analisi delle strutture cardiac fetal: Mediante ecografia. Nota technica. In Colagrande C, Ianniruberto A, Talia B, eds. *Proceedings of the Third National Congress of the SISUM.* Terlizzi, Italy: 1977 Sept.: pp. 285–90.
20. Deluca I, Ianniruberto A, Colonna L: Aspatti ecografici del cuore fetal. *G Ital Cardiol.* 8:778–83, 1978.
21. Wladimiroff JW, McGhie JS: M-mode ultrasonic assessment of fetal cardiovascular dynamics. *Br J Obstet Gynaecol.* 88:1241–7, 1981.
22. Sahn DJ, Lange LW, Allen HD, et al.: Quantitative real-time cross-sectional echocardiograpy in the developing normal human fetus and newborn. *Circulation.* 62:588–97, 1980.
23. Silverman NH, Golbus M: Echocardiographic techniques for assessing normal and abnormal fetal cardiac anatomy. *J Am Coll Cardiol.* 5:208–95, 1982.
24. Kleinman CS, Hobbins JC, Jaffe CC, et al.: Echocardiographic studies of the human fetus: Prenatal diagnosis of congenital heart disease and cardiac dysrhythmia. *Pediatrics.* 65:1059–67, 1980.
25. Devore GR, Siassi B, Platt L: Fetal echocardiography IV: M-mode assessment of ventricular size and contractility during the second and third trimesters of pregnancy in the normal fetus. *Am J Obstet Gynecol.* 150:981–91, 1984.
26. Reed K, Meijboom EJ, Sahn DJ, et al.: Cardiac Doppler flow velocities in human fetuses. *Circulation.* 73:41, 1986.
27. Huhta JC, Moise KJ, Fisher DJ, et al.: Detection and quantitation of constriction of the fetal ductus arteriosus by Doppler echocardiography. *Circulation.* 75:406–10, 1987.
28. Yagel S, Weissman A, Rotstein Z, et al.: Congenital heart defects—Natural course and in utero development. *Circulation.* 96:550–5, 1997.
29. Sahn, D. Echocardiography 1) Case studies demonstrating state of the art, 2) Recent Advances Lecture CME meeting sponsored by Division of Continuing Medical Education, University of Alabama. Nov 8th and 9th, 1996.
30. Devore GR, Medearis AL, Bear MB, et al.: Fetal echocardiography: Factors that influence imaging of the fetal heart during the second trimester of pregnancy. *J Ultrasound Med.* 12:659–63, 1993.
31. Shipp TD, Bromley B, Hornberger L, et al.: Levorotation of the fetal cardiac axis: A clue for congenital heart disease. *Obstet Gynecol.* 85:97–102, 1995.
32. Nelson T, Pretorius D, Sklansky M, et al.: Three-dimensional echocardiographic evaluation of fetal heart anatomy and function: Acquisition, analysis, and display. *J Ultrasound Med.* 15:1–9, 1996.
33. Zosmer N, Jurkovic D, Jauniaux E, et al.: Selection and identification of standard cardiac views from three-dimensional volume scans of the fetal thorax. *J Ultrasound Med.* 15:25–32, 1996.
34. Allan LD, Joseph MC, Boyd EGC, et al.: M-mode echocardiography in the developing human fetus. *Br Heart J.* 47:573–81, 1982.
35. DeVore GR: Cardiac imaging. In Sabbagha RE, ed. *Diagnostic Ultrasound Applied to Obstetrics and Gynecology.* Philadelphia: JB Lippincott; 1987.
36. Schmidt KG, Silverman NH, Hoffman JI: Determination of ventricular volumes in human fetal hearts by two dimensional echocardiography. *Am J Cardiol.* 76:1313–6, 1995.
37. Tan J, Silverman NH, Hoffman J, et al.: Cardiac dimensions determined by cross-sectional echocardiography in the normal human fetus from 18 weeks to term. *Am J Cardiol.* 70:1459–67, 1992.
38. Hornberger LK, Weintraub RG, Pesonen E, et al.: Echocardiographic study of the morphology and growth of the aortic arch in the human fetus. *Circulation.* 86:741–7, 1992.
39. Reed KL, Meijboom EJ, Scagnelli SA, et al.: Cardiac Doppler flow velocities in human fetuses. *Circulation.* 73:41–6, 1986.

40. Wladimiroff JW, Stewart PA, Burghouwt MT, et al.: Normal fetal cardiac flow velocity waveforms between 11 and 16 weeks gestation. *Am J Obstet Gynecol.* 167:736–9, 1992.

41. Berning RA, Silverman NH, Villegas M, et al.: Reversed shunting across the ductus arteriosus or atrial septum in utero heralds severe congenital heart disease. *J Am Coll Cardiol.* 27:481–6, 1996.

42. Huhta JC, Moise KJ, Fisher DJ, et al.: Detection and quantitation of constriction of the fetal ductus arteriosus by Doppler echocardiography. *Circulation.* 75:406–12, 1987.

43. Sherer DM, Fromberg RA, Divon MY: Prenatal ultrasonographic assessment of the ductus venosus: A review. *Obstet Gynecol.* 88:626–32, 1996.

44. Murphy KJ, Rubin JM: Power Doppler: It's a good thing. *Semin Ultrasound CT MRI.* 18:13–21, 1997.

CHAPTER ELEVEN

Transvaginal Fetal Echocardiography in the First and Second Trimester

Ramon A. Castillo

Congenital heart disease (CHD) is one of the most common abnormalities affecting newborns, with a prevalence of 0.2% to 1%.[1] Accurate prenatal diagnosis has been reported in 92% of patients studied using the four-chamber view after 18 weeks' gestation.[2] This finding has been disputed by other echocardiographers, who currently recommend that the evaluation of the right and left outflow tracts be included when a fetal echocardiogram is performed.[3] Other sonographers suggest that a comprehensive cardiac evaluation is not complete without measurements of the dimensions of the heart utilizing a gestational age-dependent nomogram as well as visualization of the intracardiac structures in the so-called long-axis and short-axis views. Utilizing the combined evaluation of four chambers and outflow tracts, 83% of fetuses with cardiac abnormalities were detected in a large series of low-risk patients.[4] The differences in detection rates as well as the problems associated with accurate prenatal diagnosis of CHD are further discussed in an excellent review by Buskens et al.[5] The authors expand on the methodologic problems encountered in the literature and therefore the reader is referred to this article for further discussion.

A detailed evaluation of the first trimester heart can be performed using the transvaginal approach. High-frequency transducers provide the necessary resolution because structures are small. Views obtained during routine second-trimester echocardiography can be reproduced using the transvaginal approach in the first trimester of pregnancy. However, lack of transducer mobility and orientation, as well as the size of the structures, may limit the information obtainable. A comparison of fetal echocardiograms performed dur-

ing the first trimester of pregnancy using the transvaginal and the transabdominal approach demonstrated that the cardiac structures were better visualized using the transvaginal approach. During this time period, all of the ultrasound modalities aid in the evaluation of the fetal heart. Table 11–1 lists the ultrasound modalities that aid in the evaluation of the heart using the transvaginal approach.

Table 11–2 lists the percentage of cardiac structures visualized as reported by Dolkart and Reimers.[6] The cardiac structures that apparently can be defined earliest are the mitral and tricuspid valves, which are highly echogenic by the 10th week. Whereas the four-chamber heart could be seen as early as 11 weeks, it was not visualized in all cases studied until 13 weeks' gestation. The optimal time for evaluation appears to be at 14 to 15 weeks' gestation. In this gestational age range, the percentage of cardiac structures that can be visualized is highest and the probability of the fetal chest being out of the maternal pelvis is the lowest. Using the transvaginal approach, gestational age is one of the most critical factors in allowing for proper evaluation of cardiac structures.[7] If the evaluation is performed too early, proper visualization may not be possible. Before the 10th week of gestation, most structures, although present, are not yet amenable to evaluation with most commercially available transducers.

Several factors have been found to influence the yield of positive findings in deciding which approach is best suited to a particular patient. Maternal adipose tissue thickness or previous lower abdominal surgery have been demonstrated to impair the ability to visualize the fetal heart adequately.[8] These two variables are

TABLE 11–1. ULTRASOUND MODALITIES USED IN TRANSVAGINAL SONOGRAPHY

Real time
M mode
Doppler ultrasound
Color Doppler
Chromomapping

specific to transabdominal sonography and may be circumvented with the use of the transvaginal approach. At the same time, high-frequency transducers can be used since the depth of penetration required is usually less.

CARDIAC ACTIVITY

Contractions of the human heart become apparent by day 22 following conception.[9] Ultrasonographic detection of motion in the primitive heart has been documented as early as day 25 after fertilization. There is adequate documentation of a change in fetal heart rate from 90 beats per minute (BPM) at initial detection to a peak of 140 to 160 BPM between 8 and 9 weeks menstrual age.[10] Some investigators have shown a peak at 9 weeks of approximately 160 BPM with a decline to 140 BPM, whereas others have found not such a marked increase but a plateau at 140 BPM.[11] Documentation of the early embryonic heart motion is possible with two-dimensional echocardiography. In order to record and archive the presence of cardiac activity, both M mode and Doppler ultrasound can be utilized (Figures 11–1 and 11–2).

The association between low fetal heart rates and an increase in the incidence of fetal loss has been demonstrated.[12,13] Rates of 80 to 85 BPM or less are of concern and should be followed with serial ultrasonographic evaluation. It is important that maternal pulsations not be confused with fetal heart motion. M mode is useful in discriminating the cardiac tube movement from pulsations of maternal blood vessels. If the fetal pole lies adjacent to the wall of the uterus, it may be difficult to establish the origin of the pulsations. Changing the orientation of the transducer as well as approaching the embryo at a different angle may be useful to establish the difference. Parameters that have been correlated to the presence of cardiac activity as well as to mean heart rate include the size of the yolk sac, the crown–rump length and the gestational sac diameter as well as the level of human chorionic gonadotropin.[14,15] Although there appears to be a linear relationship between these variables, definitive conclusions cannot be drawn. Serial ultrasounds may be necessary before an accurate diagnosis of viability can be made.

The demonstration of normal ultrasonographic findings, including cardiac activity, does offer some degree of reassurance even in the presence of symptoms suggestive of an impending fetal loss. According to Frates et al.,[16] there is no difference in outcome when a normal heart rate is detected even in the presence of

TABLE 11–2. PERCENTAGE OF CARDIAC STRUCTURES VISUALIZED AT EACH GESTATIONAL AGE.

View	10–10.9 weeks (n = 8)	11–11.9 weeks (n = 10)	12–12.9 weeks (n = 10)	13–13.9 weeks (n = 13)	14–14.9 weeks (n = 11)
Four chamber	0	30	90	100	100
Five chamber	0	0	10	54	64
Aortic arch	0	0	20	23	73
Short-axis aorta	0	10	70	62	82
Short-axis ventricles	0	10	40	31	27
Long-axis left ventricle	0	20	40	46	55
Inferior vena cava	0	10	10	54	91
Superior vena cava	0	10	10	23	36
Pulmonary trunk	0	0	40	38	82
Mitral valve	25	60	90	100	100
Tricuspid valve	25	60	90	100	100
Aortic valve	0	0	20	46	64
Pulmonary valve	0	0	20	15	36
Ductus arteriosus	0	0	50	23	73
Short-axis base	0	10	30	46	73

Reprinted, with permission, from Dolkart LA, Reimers FT. Transvaginal fetal echocardiography in early pregnancy: Normative data. Am J Obstet Gynecol: 1991;165: 688–91.

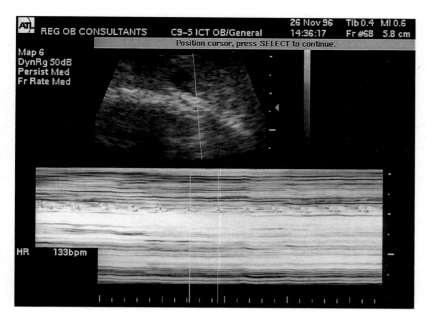

Figure 11–1. M-mode recording of heart rate at 6 weeks' gestation.

bleeding and cramping, signs that when present before the advent of fetal ultrasonography were suggestive of impending miscarriage.

CARDIAC ANATOMY

To perform an adequate evaluation of the fetal heart, all of the previously described ultrasonographic modalities are utilized. The size of the heart relative to the fetal chest must be evaluated. The position of the heart must also be established at the onset of the study. Ex-

tracardiac landmarks are used for this purpose, such as the fetal stomach, which is visible at an early gestational age. Detailed examination of intracardiac structures should be performed emphasizing the size of the ventricles and the appearance of the septum, the valves, and the outflow tracts.[17] Fluid collections surrounding the heart should be excluded at this time.

Figure 11–3 demonstrates an apical four-chamber view of the heart at 13 weeks. The ventricular septum can be visualized through its entire length. At this gestational age, the membranous portion is usually less

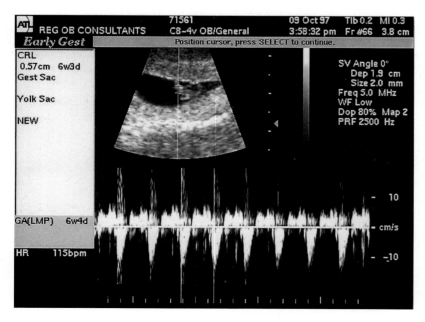

Figure 11–2. Doppler recording of a 6-week heart.

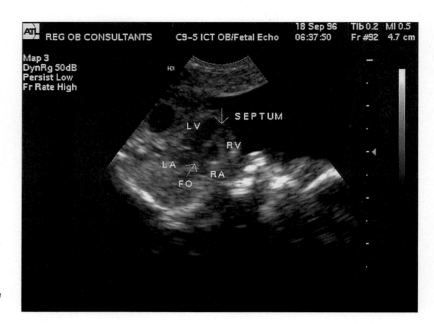

Figure 11–3. Apical four-chamber view of the heart.

echogenic but its proper evaluation is necessary since most septal defects are localized here. The interventricular valves can also be demonstrated. Real-time visualization allows for the recognition of the foramen ovale.

Figure 11–4 demonstrates a long-axis view of the heart. The right ventricle, pulmonary artery, and thoracic aorta are visualized in the corresponding anatomic position.

Color Doppler sonography has improved our ability to evaluate the fetal heart. It can aid in the identifi-

cation of small structures and therefore delineate the small vessels arising from the heart. Figure 11–5 shows a typical four-chamber view with color juxtaposed. All four chambers are seen with flow demonstrated through the foramen ovale. Careful application of this technique is recommended because small movements of the transducer may create false images, as seen in Figure 11–6. Here a ventricular septal defect (VSD) is suggested in a 13-week fetus who, at 20 weeks' gestation, was shown to have a completely normal heart.

Figures 11–7 and 11–8 depict the main outflow

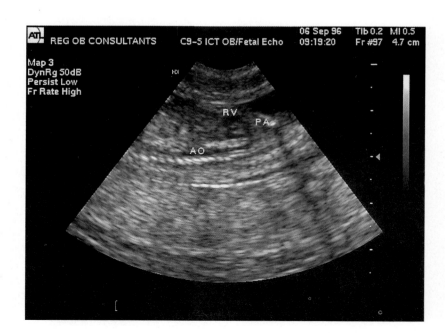

Figure 11–4. Long-axis view of the heart.

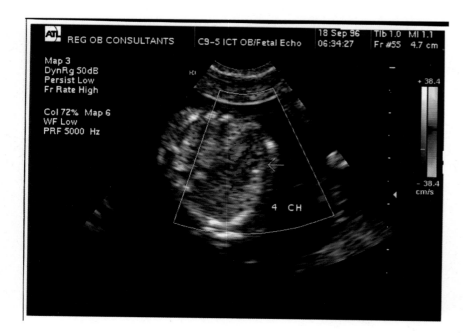

Figure 11–5. Four-chamber heart view with color at 14 weeks' gestation.

tracts in their anatomic positions. Color superimposition helps in localizing the small vessels as well as identifying their position. Fetal cardiac flow velocities can also be obtained during this gestational period.[18] Figures 11–9 and 11–10 demonstrate the flow velocity profile through the ascending aorta and pulmonary artery. Whereas the peak systolic velocities in the aorta appear to be higher than those of the pulmonary artery, this value has been determined to be statistically insignifi-

cant.[19] Clinical application of this modality is limited at this time.

M-mode echocardiography, useful in characterizing arrhythmias, can also be utilized to evaluate the young heart. Figure 11–11 shows the wall motion at the level of the atrium and can be compared to that of the ventricles as well. This modality may be used to demonstrate the presence of abnormal fluid collections as seen in cases of pericardial effusions.

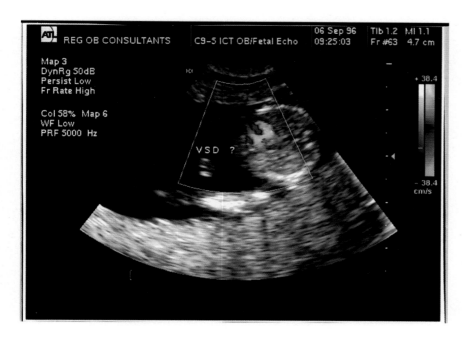

Figure 11–6. Color falsely representing a VSD in a 13-week heart.

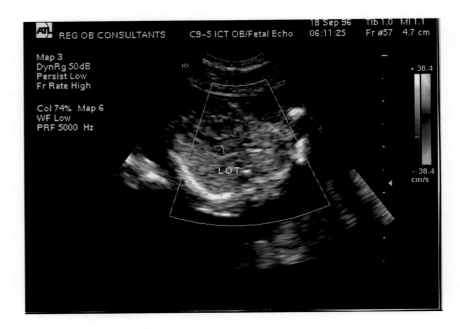

Figure 11–7. Left outflow tract at 15 weeks.

Another tool available to improve the resolution of early cardiac structures is chromomapping. This feature allows for the assignment of color to gray-scale echo intensities. Figure 11–12 demonstrates this technique in a 10-week heart. At this early stage of development, this special resolution provides significant enhancement to the appropriate visualization of intracardiac structures. The human eye is apparently able to discriminate color differences better than shades of gray.

CARDIAC ABNORMALITIES

Available information on the types of cardiac abnormalities that can be identified in early pregnancy is limited to case reports. Table 11–3 presents information about 13 cases in which a diagnosis of CHD was made before 14 weeks' gestation.[20–23] Transducers of frequency greater than 5 MHz were utilized and the examinations performed in centers of high volume with significant expertise in this type of evaluation. Significantly, in all

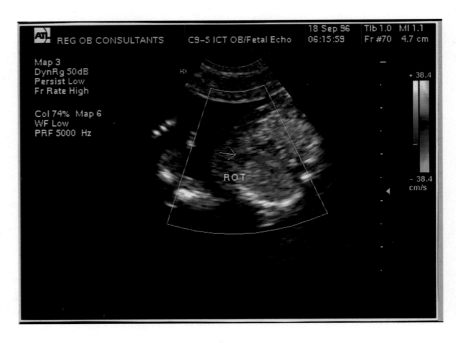

Figure 11–8. Right outflow tracts at 15 weeks.

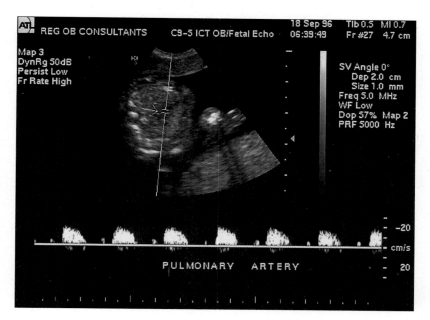

Figure 11–9. Velocity flow profile of the aorta at 15 weeks.

cases, there were extracardiac abnormalities present, of which hygromas and hydrops were the most common.

Two studies involving populations at high and low risk for fetal heart defects, but performed at different gestational ages, are available for comparison.[3,24] Although both studies have similar sensitivities and false positive rates, they differ in two significant aspects. In the population diagnosed at an early gestational age, there were twice the number of extracardiac anomalies and karyotypic abnormalities. This comparison suggests that the populations may not be entirely the same and that testing at different intervals may be complementary (Table 11–4).

Utilizing the transvaginal approach with the aid of color flow mapping, a VSD was seen in a 15-week fetus (Figure 11–13). Chromosomes obtained by amniocentesis demonstrated a trisomy 21.

SUMMARY

The current techniques for the transvaginal evaluation of the fetal heart have been presented. It has been demonstrated that by the 13th week of gestation, most

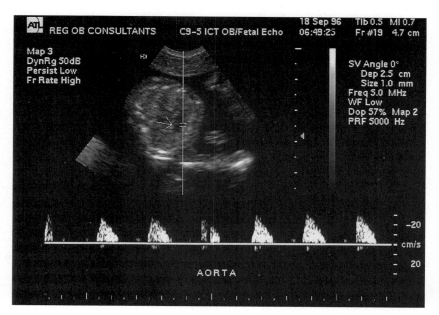

Figure 11–10. Velocity flow profile of the pulmonary artery at 15 weeks.

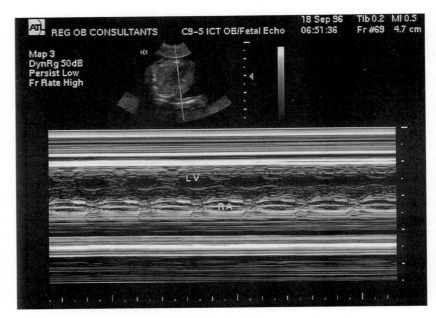

Figure 11–11. M-mode recording of atrial and ventricular wall motion.

of the cardiac structures can be visualized and, in some cases, significant structural abnormalities have been identified. Until several major issues regarding transvaginal fetal echocardiography are elucidated, several points need to be taken into consideration before widespread use is advocated in early pregnancy.

The first issue is the equipment to be used and technical expertise of the sonographer. Ultrasound equipment refinements and developments require constant updating of techniques utilized for evalua-

tion of the fetal heart. Optimal results are usually achieved in large centers where a diverse population is seen and the sonographers have expertise in both the transvaginal approach and early fetal heart evaluation.

The second issue is the importance of an understanding of fetal cardiac development, as well as appreciation of the natural history of most abnormalities seen with ultrasound. It is important to remember that although some anomalies, such as the atrioventricular

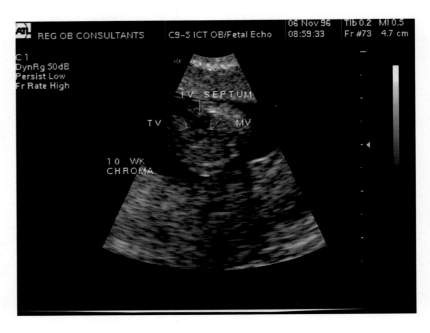

Figure 11–12. Transvaginal apical view of a 10-week heart using chromomapping.

TABLE 11–3. TYPES OF ANOMALIES THAT CAN BE IDENTIFIED BEFORE 14 WEEKS' GESTATION

Case	Gestational Age	Anomaly	Associated Findings	Karyotype[a]
1	10	Tachycardia	Effusion	Normal
2	11	Ectopia cordis, VSD	Omphalocele, hygroma	Normal
3	11	AVSD	Hydrops	45X
4	12	Large right atrium	Hygroma	Normal
5	12	VSD, truncus	Hygroma	Normal
6	11	AVSD, large right atrium and ventricle	Hygroma, effusion	Normal
7	11	VSD, large aortic root	Agenesis of kidneys	Normal
8	12	VSD, large atrium and ventricle	Hydrops	Normal
9	12	VSD, pericardial effusion, large left ventricle	Hydrocephalus, club feet	Normal
10	11	Small left ventricle, pericardial effusion	Cystic hygroma	Triploidy
11	13	VSD, overriding aorta	Oligohydramnios, no bladder	N/A
12	12	Ectopia cordis	Omphalocele, hygroma	Normal
13	11	Bradycardia, AVSD	Skin edema	N/A

[a]N/A, not available.

(AV) canal and ectopia cordis, may be identified at early stages of fetal development, others, such as ventricular septal defects, may not be evident until the fetus has achieved a certain gestation. It is also relevant to understand that some abnormalities such as hypoplastic left heart and tumors of the heart are progressive and may not be evident until the second or third trimester.

The third issue is the acquisition of appropriate images of the cardiac anatomy as seen through the vagina. Using the transvaginal approach, the examiner is limited in the number of views that can be obtained. Furthermore, fetal position is of great importance as transducer mobility is impaired. Patience in allowing the fetus to move to a better position may be required to achieve greater visibility of the cardiac structures.

The fourth issue is the occurrence of false negative and false positive findings. Because fetal karyotyping is recommended in cases of congenital heart disease, some patients may have had this invasive procedure recommended unnecessarily, with its corresponding increase in morbidity. At the same time, other patients may be falsely reassured of a normal outcome.

The fifth issue is cost effectiveness of ultrasound at this time. Several large studies, including the RADIUS[25] and Helsinski[26] trials offer contradictory information regarding the usefulness and cost effectiveness of routine ultrasound screening for anomalies. If we add a first trimester cardiac evaluation to the prenatal testing routinely offered, the cost may increase significantly.

With the information available at the current state of technology, early transvaginal fetal cardiac evaluation should be performed by well-trained echocardiographers utilizing high-resolution equipment. It may be useful in the high-risk fetus or the obese mother, who may benefit from the transvaginal approach, and where the yield of positive cases may justify the cost. Finally, a study performed in the first trimester should not replace a thorough evaluation during the second trimester.

TABLE 11–4. COMPARISON OF POPULATIONS AT HIGH RISK AND LOW RISK FOR CARDIAC ANOMALIES

Gestational Age	Overall Sensitivity (%)	False Positives	Four-chamber Sensitivity (%)	Associated Anomalies (%)	Karyotype (%)
Bromley et al.[4] ≥ 18 weeks	83	2	63	36	17
Bronshtein et al.[23] 12–16 weeks	77	3	59	62	36

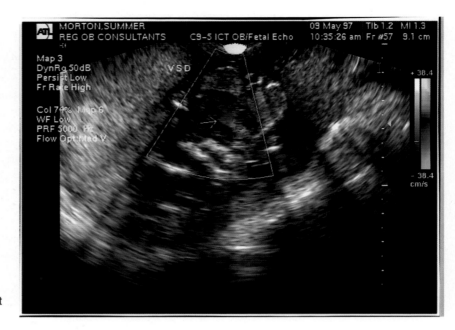

Figure 11–13. Ventricular septal defect at 15 weeks' gestation.

In the second trimester, other anomalies may be recognized as well, and additional evaluation such as fetal karyotyping may be performed.

REFERENCES

1. Hoffman JIE: Congenital heart disease: Incident and inheritance. *Pediatr Clin N Am.* 37:25–43, 1990.
2. Copel J, Pilu G, Green J, et al.: Fetal echocardiographic screening for congenital heart disease: The importance of the four-chamber view. *Am J Obstet Gynecol.* 157:648–55, 1987.
3. Wigton T, Sabbagha R, Tamura R, et al.: Sonographic diagnosis of congenital heart disease: Comparison between the four-chamber view and multiple cardiac views. *Obstet Gynecol.* 82:219–24, 1993.
4. Bromley B, Estroff J, Sanders S, et al.: Fetal echocardiography: Accuracy and limitations in a population at high and low risk for heart defects. *Am J Obstet Gynecol.* 166: 1473–81, 1992.
5. Buskens E, Grobbee D, Hess J, et al.: Prenatal diagnosis of congenital heart disease—Prospects and problems. *Eur J Obstet Gynecol Reprod Biol.* 60:5–11, 1995.
6. Dolkart L, Reimers F: Transvaginal fetal echocardiography in early pregnancy: Normative data. *Am J Obstet Gynecol.* 165 (Sept): 688–91, 1991.
7. D'Amelio R, Giorlandino C, Masala L, et al.: Fetal echocardiography using transvaginal and transabdominal probes during the first period of pregnancy: A comparative study. *Prenat Diagn.* 11: 69–75, 1991.
8. DeVore G, Medearis A, Bear M, et al.: Fetal echocardiography: Factors that influence imaging of the fetal heart

during the second trimester of pregnancy. *J Ultrasound Med.* 12:659–63, 1993.
9. Moore, K: *The Developing Human: Clinically Oriented Embryology.* Philadelphia:WB Saunders; 1982.
10. Schats R, Jansen C, Wladimiroff J: Embroyonic heart activity: Appearance and development in early human pregnancy. *Br J Obstet Gynaecol.* 97:989–94, 1990.
11. Hertzberg B, Mahony B, Bowie J: First trimester fetal cardiac activity: Sonographic documentation of a progressive early rise in heart rate. *J Ultrasound Med.* 7:573–5, 1988.
12. May D, Sturtevant N: Embryonal heart rate as a predictor of pregnancy outcome: A prospective analysis. *J Ultrasound Med.* 10:591–3, 1991.
13. Laboda L, Estroff J, Benacerraf B: First trimester bradycardia: A sign of impending fetal loss. *J Ultrasound Med.* 8:561–3, 1989.
14. Cacciatore B, Tiitinen A, Stenman U, et al.: Normal early pregnancy: Serum hCG levels and vaginal ultrasound findings. *Br J Obstet Gynaecol.* 97:899–903, 1990.
15. Zimmer E, Chao C, Santos R: Amniotic sac, fetal heart area, fetal curvature and other morphometrics using first trimester vaginal ultrasonography and color Doppler imaging. *J Ultrasound Med.* 13:685–90, 1993.
16. Frates M, Benson C, Doubilet P: Pregnancy outcome after a first trimester sonogram demonstrating fetal cardiac activity. *J Ultrasound Med.* 12:383–6, 1993.
17. Bronshtein M, Siegler E, Eshcoli Z, et al.: Transvaginal ultrasound measurements of the fetal heart at 11 to 17 weeks of gestation. *Am J Perinatol.* 9:38-42, 1992.
18. Wladimiroff J, Huisman T, Stewart P, et al.: Normal fetal Doppler inferior vena cava, transtricuspid and umbilical artery flow velocity waveforms between 11 and 16 weeks gestation. *Am J Obstet Gynecol.* 166:921–4, 1992.

19. Wladimiroff J, Huisman T, Stewart P: Fetal cardiac flow velocities in the late 1st trimester of pregnancy: a transvaginal Doppler study. *J Am Coll Cardio.* 17:1357–9, 1991.

20. Achiron R, Rotstein Z, Lipitz S, et al.: First trimester diagnosis of fetal congenital heart disease by transvaginal ultrasonography. *Obstet Gynecol.* 84:69-72, 1994.

21. Gembruch U, Knopfle G, Chatterjee M, et al.: First trimester diagnosis of fetal congenital heart disease by transvaginal two-dimensional and Doppler echocardiography. *Obstet Gynecol.* 75:496–8, 1990.

22. Bennett T, Burlbaw J, Drake C, et al.: Diagnosis of ectopia cordis at 12 weeks gestation using transabdominal ultrasonography with color flow Doppler. *J Ultrasound Med.* 10:695–6, 1991.

23. Bronshtein M, Zimmer E, Milo S, et al.: Fetal cardiac abnormalities detected by transvaginal sonography at 12–16 weeks gestation. *Obstet Gynecol.* 78:374–8, 1991.

24. Bronshtein M, Zimmer E, Gerlis L, et al.: Early ultrasound diagnosis of fetal congenital heart defects in high-risk and low-risk pregnancies. *Obstet Gynecol.* 82:225–9, 1993.

25. Crane J, LeFevre M, Winborn R, et al.: A randomized trial of prenatal ultrasonographic screening: Impact on the detection, management and outcome of anomalous fetuses. *Am J Obstet Gynecol.* 171:392–9, 1994.

26. Saari-Kemppainen A, Karjalaninen O, Ylostalo P, et al.: Ultrasound screening and perinatal mortality: Controlled trial of systematic one-stage screening in pregnancy. *Lancet.* 336:387–91, 1990.

CHAPTER TWELVE

Fetal Anatomic Imaging

John W. Seeds

It is entirely appropriate to begin a comprehensive examination of the technique and utility of fetal echocardiography with an introduction to the technique and utility of antepartum diagnostic ultrasound generally. A brief discussion of the nature of ultrasound, the nature of the images produced, and the utility of ultrasound applied to fetal anatomy other than cardiac will enable the reader to more fully understand the benefits and limitations of the technique when applied to the fetal heart. Diagnostic antepartum ultrasound, perhaps more so than many other diagnostic imaging modalities, is intensely dependent on the skill and methodology of the examiner not only in the interpretation of the images produced but, more importantly, in the very production of those images. A review of the broader subject of ultrasound in obstetrics will provide the reader with the overall context within which fetal echocardiography represents a distinct and critically important area of focused specialization.

Images of fetal anatomy are used to determine fetal number and presentation, to assess fetal growth, to monitor fetal condition, and to diagnose a wide but limited range of fetal congenital anomalies.[1-3] Fetal anatomic imaging may be accomplished using any of several current technologies that demonstrate widely variable clarity, utility, and inherent risk, including plain radiography, computed tomography, magnetic resonance imaging (MRI), and ultrasound. Plain radiography does not provide fetal soft tissue detail and has been associated with an increased risk of childhood malignancy. Magnetic resonance imaging is capable of considerable soft tissue detail, but the time interval necessary to accumulate the image data results in degradation of image clarity in the case of fetal movement, and the possibility of adverse fetal effects from MRI has not yet been clearly excluded.[1] Real-time ultrasound provides high-resolution images of fetal soft tissue anatomy largely immune to loss of clarity from fetal movement and without known risk to the fetus or the mother, despite decades of careful study.[1] Ultrasound images, as with computerized tomography and MRI, are two-dimensional anatomic depictions, typically in black, white and shades of gray, that may be anatomically interpreted and form the basis of biometric assessments of the size of fetal organs and structures. Ultrasound has become the preferred method of fetal anatomic imaging largely because of its ease of application, the relatively inexpensive equipment available, and the lack of any apparent adverse side effects.

THE NATURE OF ULTRASOUND

Sound is a rhythmic distortion of the normal spatial relationships between the molecules of a medium that is propagated through that medium from the source.[1] Loudspeaker cones vibrate, creating alternate zones of high and low pressure or density in the adjacent air molecules that are propagated through the air by virtue of the springlike qualities of the normal electromagnetic intermolecular forces, always seeking to reestablish the norm. These rhythmic distortions may be described using an analogy to a sine wave, with wavelength, frequency, and amplitude. Any sound with a frequency above 20,000 cps, or cycles per second (20 kHz), is called *ultrasound*. In medical imaging applications, the frequencies used are generally between 3 and 10 million cps (3 and 10 MHz).

Images are computer depictions of anatomy based on sound reflections or echos from tissue surfaces. A brief sound pulse, often no more than a microsecond in duration, is generated by a crystal element built into a transducer, propagates through a medium such as the human body and encounters surfaces between tissues. An echo may be produced at such a surface and is reflected back to the transducer. The same transducer that has generated the pulse of sound detects the reflected echo. A computer uses the time of pulse generation, the time of echo reception, and an assumed 1540-m/s average speed of sound in soft tissue to estimate the distance from transducer surface of the tissue generating the echo. Sound pulses are repeatedly and sequentially generated along the surface of the transducer and result in sufficient echos to allow the construction of a compound image of soft tissue based on these echos (Figure 12–1).[1] The displayed image is updated so rapidly that movement in real time is depicted on screen. Any given crystal element is active for only a microsecond every millisecond interval, or 0.1% of any exposure period.

Ultrasound imaging systems are designed to show the relative strength of the echos by showing the appropriate pixel on the display screen in various shades of gray, or *grayscale*. The stronger a particular echo, the brighter the respective pixel at the appropriate location on screen. The visual clarity of each image is maximized through the design of the instrument to optimize clarity for the likely clinical application based on the estimated depth of the anatomy of interest. Higher frequency, for instance a 5-MHz transducer (5 million cps sound frequency) compared to a 3.5-MHz transducer (3.5 million cps), provides improved image sharpness in some ways but does not penetrate tissue as deeply as lower-frequency transducers. Maternal habitus also impacts on image clarity. Heavy patients suffer reduced image clarity because of reverberation artifact intro-

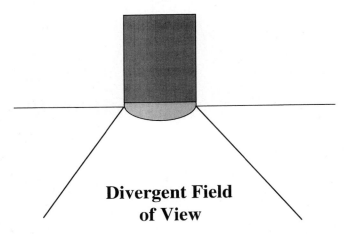

Convex Array Transducer

Divergent Field of View

Figure 12–2. The curved surface of the convex array transducer produces a divergent field of view, allowing the imaging of a wide, deep field of anatomy through a relatively narrow observation aperture.

duced into the images as a result of maternal tissue compartments. This typically takes the form of a "snowstorm"-like overlay artifact that makes fetal imaging more difficult in the case of the heavy patient.

The ultrasound image may be rectangular, as in the case of the older style linear array, or pie shaped, as in the convex array (Figure 12–2) or the endovaginal transducers. The advantage of the latter array is its convex curved surface, which provides a broader deep field of view from a more limited contact area because of the pie-shaped divergent field of view. The divergent field facilitates examination of the late term pregnancy or the very early gestation, where a smaller imaging win-

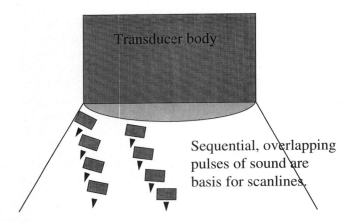

Transducer body

Sequential, overlapping pulses of sound are basis for scanlines.

Figure 12–1. Brief pulses of sound are generated at the surface of the transducer. These pulses are produced in rapid overlapping sequence along the surface of the transducer. Echos from tissue surfaces within the subject return to the transducer, are detected, are catalogued by the instrument, and form the basis for the on-screen images.

Endovaginal Transducer

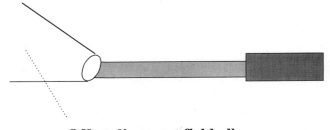

Offset divergent field allows greater lateral pelvic visualization

Figure 12–3. The endovaginal phased array transducer is necessarily compact and generally produces its divergent field of view at a slight offset from the axis of the instrument to allow greater lateral visualization using a rotational movement.

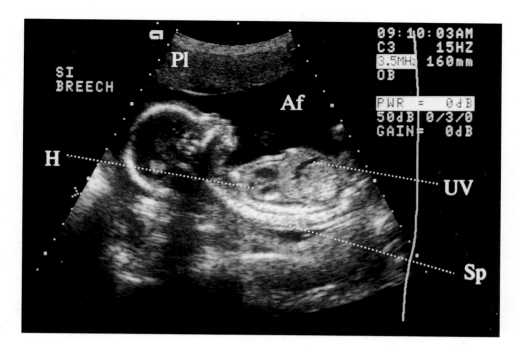

Figure 12–4. This is a saggital sonogram of a midtrimester fetus demonstrating the visual characteristics of ultrasound. Echos are apparent from both skeletal and soft tissue elements. The brighter the echo, the brighter the image. The placenta (Pl) is seen; amniotic fluid (Af) appears black or anechoic; the umbilical vein (UV) may be seen; and the fetal spine (Sp) and heart (H) are apparent. This fetus is in breech position.

dow may be available. Also, endovaginal transducers must of necessity be small and the divergent field of view provides for the greatest anatomic examination from the smallest physical transducer (Figure 12–3).

Fetal anatomic visualization with ultrasound is based on the visual quality of the echo contrast of tissues compared to adjacent fluids and between adjacent tissues that demonstrate contrasting echo textures. Complex tissues generate many echos and produce a bright on-screen image, whereas homogeneous substances, such as fluid of any kind, generate few echos and appear dark or black (Figure 12–4). Amniotic fluid, ovarian cyst fluid, fetal urine or blood, cerebrospinal fluid, all produce few if any echos and, therefore, appear black on screen. This black appearance of fluids or other homogeneous tissues is called "anechoic," "echopenic," "echospared," or "echopoor." Tissue adjacent to fluid creates maximum visual contrast and allows for anatomic examination of tissue surface architecture. Each specific tissue at each specific gestational age produces a characteristic echo pattern or texture visually and, contrasted with adjacent tissues, allows for fetal soft tissue diagnosis.

IMAGE PRODUCTION

Placement of an ultrasound transducer in contact with a patient through a transmission medium such as acoustic gel or mineral oil, either of which provides direct coupling between surfaces, results in an image on screen. The inherent two-dimensional nature of any ultrasound

image may be deceptive to the neophyte and imposes a burden on the examiner to visualize each and every area of anatomic interest methodically by deliberately directing the scanplane at that area of interest. Remote review of selected bidimensional images does not provide the opportunity to be more complete at a later time. With ultrasound, what you see is what you get. To see a specific area of anatomic interest, the examiner must deliberately look at it. Basic transducer movements are used that include angling, sliding, and rotation (Figure 12–5). Generally, most transducer movements are a combination of one or more of these basic movements. The examiner must identify the current image and then determine what part of anatomy is desired and the type of movement necessary to produce the desired image.

Clinical Ultrasound Imaging

Fetal ultrasound examination provides a wide variety of information that often facilitates optimal obstetrical care.[1,2] Sonography may confirm or establish fetal number (Figure 12–6),[4] and gestational age within reasonable limits,[5] may establish fetal viability (Figure 12–7) and presentation, may estimate fetal weight and monitor growth, may locate the placenta (Figure 12–8), and may detect a wide range of fetal malformations.[1,2] Whereas the most likely obstetrical benefit from sonography is confirmation of gestational age, the most important function of antenatal ultrasound to the prospective mother is, arguably, the examination of fetal anatomy and the confirmation of a "normal" baby.

Basic Transducer Movements

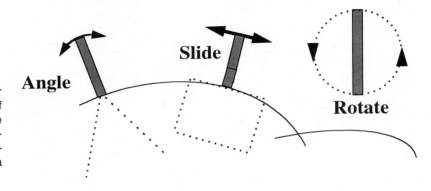

Figure 12–5. Each of the basic transducer movements is illustrated here with the field of view produced by each movement. Changing the angle of entry allows examination of a pie-shaped field; sliding produces more of a rectangular field; and rotation allows examination of a cylindrical field.

The majority of pregnancies present no clinical abnormality. The majority of pregnancies have a known last menstrual period (LMP), and do not suffer comorbid medical conditions that may adversely affect fetal development; most pregnancies show normal clinical progress toward a term delivery of a normal living child. Routine ultrasound examination of such a presumed low-risk population may provide benefit, however, from correction of erroneous dates, detection of a low-lying placenta, and provision of baseline data that can facilitate the later diagnosis of growth abnormalities, early detection of multiple gestation, or detection of the unexpected fetal malformation.[6] The detection of the unexpected malformation remains, however, the least probable benefit compared to the others simply because

only 3% to 5% of human progeny demonstrate malformation, half are relatively minor, many congenital conditions are functional rather than structural, and, of the unexpected serious structural abnormalities, only a portion are detectable with ultrasound.[7] In contrast, gestational age errors may affect up to 10% of gravidas with a sure menstrual history[2,6]; growth abnormalities affect up to 20% of fetuses (10% growth restriction and 10% growth augmentation[8,9]); twins complicate 1% of pregnancies; and placenta previa complicates 0.5% of pregnancies.

Ultrasound may be used in either of two clinical circumstances, including *routine* use in all pregnancies, regardless of indications, or *selective* use based on clinical indications for the examination. Clinical indi-

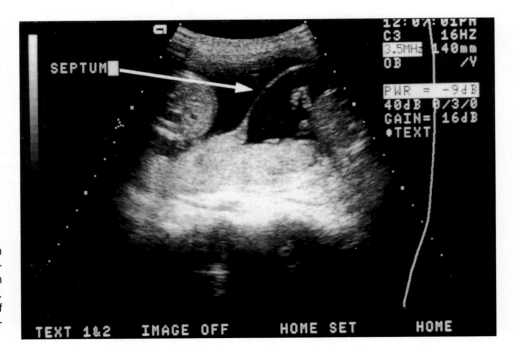

Figure 12–6. The identification of twins may facilitate optimal obstetrical care. Here, the septum between twins is clearly shown. Identification of the septum is of major significance since it excludes monoamniotic twins.

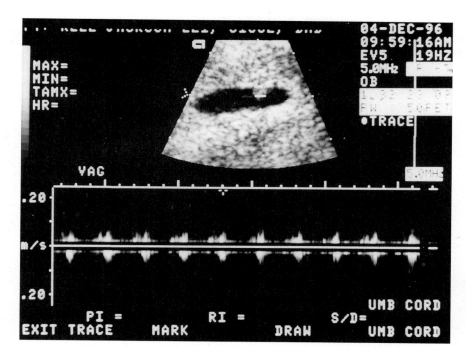

Figure 12–7. Here pulse Doppler documents fetal viability by showing a pulsatile frequency shift across the lower portion of this image, caused by movement of the fetal heart in this very early gestation.

cations for antepartum ultrasound were compiled and reported by a Consensus Development Conference convened by the National Institutes of Health (NIH) in 1984 (Table 12–1).[2] Ultrasound examination because of one of these indications is called an *indicated or selective* ultrasound examination. Many practitioners, however, believe that ultrasound examination of the obstetrical

patient is of benefit regardless of indications and recommend *routine* ultrasound examination. It remains unclear whether routine ultrasound provides benefits to the low-risk population that justify the cost.

Obstetric ultrasound may be either a definitive diagnostic test or a screening test. The role depends on the indication for testing, the objectives of testing, and

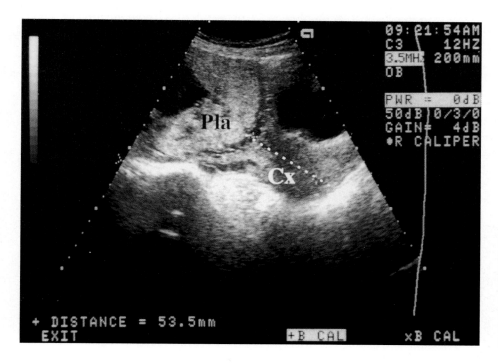

Figure 12–8. Ultrasound is the technique of choice to establish placental location. Here, the placenta (Pla) is clearly seen to overlie the internal os of the cervix (Cx). The dashed line overlies the endocervical canal. Measurement of cervical length may be useful in predicting risk of premature labor.

TABLE 12–1. INDICATIONS FOR OBSTETRIC ULTRASOUND—NIH CONSENSUS CONFERENCE

Assignment of gestational age
Evaluation of fetal growth
Evaluation of vaginal bleeding
Determination of presentation
Suspected multiple gestation
Adjuct to amniocentesis
Resolution of fundal height discrepancy
Evaluation of pelvic mass
Suspected hydatidiform mole
Adjunct to cerclage
Suspected ectopic pregnancy
Guidance of invasive procedures
Suspected fetal death
Suspected uterine anomaly
Intrauterine device (IUD) localization
Ovarian follical surveillance
Biophysical profile
Observation of peripartal events
Suspected amniotic fluid abnormalities
Suspected abruption
Adjunct to external version
Estimation of fetal weight
Abnormal maternal serum α-fetoprotein
Fetal anomaly surveillance
Follow-up of placentation
History of previous anomaly
Serial evaluation of growth of twins
Evaluation of late registrants

From the Department of Health and Human Services. Diagnostic Ultrasound Imaging in Pregnancy. Washington, DC: U.S. Government Printing Office, February 1984.

the skill and training of the examiner. For instance, an ultrasound examination performed because of possible inaccuracy of the clinical gestational age in a woman at no known risk for congenital malformation is diagnostic for the confirmation of gestational age but screening for fetal congenital malformation. On the other hand, an ultrasound examination being performed in the case of a woman with a prior child with an open neural tube defect is diagnostic for a recurrence of an open neural tube defect, but screening for confirmation of gestational age.[10]

The Normal Population

An issue of interest in any discussion of the routine screening ultrasound examination is the size of the "normal" population of obstetric patients with no known medical or historical risk factor and a known LMP. The RADIUS (*r*outine *a*ntenatal *d*iagnostic *i*maging with *ul-*

trasound) study was a multicenter study intended to establish the potential clinical benefit of routine ultrasound in a low-risk population using defined criteria to identify low-risk patients.[11] Patients were recruited from 109 practices that included family practice, obstetrics and gynecology, private, academic, and HMO practices that used a total of 28 different ultrasound units. Entry criteria included a known LMP, gestational age under 18 weeks, and no plans to move from the area. Of an initial registry of 53,867 patients, 32,317 were excluded for one or more predefined exclusion factors (Table 12–2). Their results suggest that the truly low-risk group constitutes only about 39% of an antenatal population. Furthermore, over 40% of the "low-risk" patients underwent selective ultrasound based on clinical indications. Since up to 40% of obstetrical patients are not sure of their LMP, and since anyone not sure of their LMP was excluded at the outset of the RADIUS study, the true proportion of low-risk antenatal patients may be even smaller. Since 3163 patients declined participation, and 2357 were lost to follow-up, only 15,530 patients, or 29% of the initial registrant group, were ultimately randomized to routine versus selective ultrasound in this study.

LEVELS AND LIABILITY

Level I or Level II?

The nomenclature surrounding obstetric ultrasound examinations is not uniform. In 1977, the Scarborough Conference established a two-level scheme of ultrasound examinations specifically and only to complement a maternal serum alphafetoprotein (MSAFP) screening pilot project.[12] The nomenclature created has often been used and/or misused but never accepted by any professional or regulatory organization. *Level I*

TABLE 12–2. RADIUS STUDY EXCLUSION CRITERIA

Prior ultrasound	Pelvic mass
Prior stillbirth	Fetal death
Irregular menses	Ectopic pregnancy
LMP contraceptive induced	Molar gestation
Ovulation induction	Multiple gestation
Size discrepancy	Planned abortion
Prior growth-restricted infant	Planned amniocentesis
Diabetes	Planned cerclage
Chronic hypertension	Planned ultrasound

Adapted, with permission, from Ewigman BG, Crane JP, Frigoletto FD, et al. Effect of prenatal ultrasound screening on perinatal outcome. N Engl J Med: 1993; 329:821–7; and Crane JP, LeFevre ML, Winborn RC, et al. A randomized trial of prenatal ultrasonographic screening: Impact on the detection, management, and outcome of anomalous fetuses. 1994; 171:392–9.

ultrasound examination in the context of the Scarborough Conference was intended only to establish fetal viability, gestational age, and to detect multiple gestation. No recognized standard of obstetrical ultrasound content today is limited to these few findings. *Level II* ultrasound was an examination that included the findings of Level I, but in addition recorded a search for fetal anomalies known to be associated with elevated MSAFP.[10,13] Other terms have been applied to the level I ultrasound such as "basic," "office," "low risk," "screening," and the level II examination has been referred to variously as "targeted," "high detail," "genetic," "referral," or "fetal." Many individual centers have created their own "levels," indicating specific types of sonographic examination such as a designated level to indicate fetal cardiac echography, but these nomenclatures are not universally accepted.

The American College of Obstetricians and Gynecologists (ACOG) has recognized two levels of acuity in obstetric ultrasound in technical bulletins since 1987; it has called the office low-risk screening exam the "basic" ultrasound, and the indicated search for fetal abnormalities the "targeted" examination.[14] Guidelines for content do not differ between the basic and the targeted examinations, but the skill, training, and experience of the examiner, as well as the detail of the anatomic imaging, are considered to be higher for the targeted exam (Table 12–3). The American College of Radiology (ACR) and the American Institute of Ultrasound in Medicine (AIUM) have collaborated to produce guidelines that are similar to those of ACOG but do not recognize two levels of obstetric ultrasound examination.[15] The specified diagnostic content recommended for the examination is similar to that defined by the ACOG, but specific recommendations regarding image documentation are included (Table 12–3). The recognition of two levels of obstetric ultrasound by ACOG assumes that every obstetric patient will undergo historical screening for risk factors intended to identify an increased risk for either medical complications or fetal abnormalities and that those pregnancies which are associated with risk factors are candidates for an examination targeting that specific risk possibility while screening for most others. This two-tiered ultrasound system is analogous to the general concept of health care regionalization. The single level AIUM/ACR guidelines suggest that all patients should receive an examination meeting certain criteria for content and quality, a position not in dispute, but one that does not recognize differences in disease prevalence between primary care and referral practices. Furthermore, the volume demands and the expense of a standard that all obstetric ultrasound be done in referral centers are unreasonable and impractical burdens.

Obstetric Ultrasound and Medical Liability

Liability must be considered in any discussion of obstetrical ultrasound.[16–18] Liability exposure is associated with every clinical service. Ultrasound is no exception. Although the low-risk population presents a low prob-

TABLE 12–3. GUIDELINES FOR TARGETED EXAMINATION CONTENT

Equipment	AIUM/ACR, Real Time	ACOG, Real Time
Documentation	Permanent, labeled images of biometry, anatomy; written report.	Not specified.
Levels	Limited sonography; may be performed only in clinical emergency.	*Limited* scan for specific circumstances or under urgent conditions.
		Basic ultrasound: Primarily biometric; should include fetal and maternal anatomy.
		Comprehensive: Examination for high risk for abnormal physiology or anatomy.
First trimester	Location of gestational sac, fetal life, fetal number, crown–rump length.	Sac location, embryonic identification, life, crown–rump length, fetal number, uterine–adnexal anatomy.
Second and/or third trimester	Fetal life, fetal number, fetal presentation, amniotic fluid volume, placental location, estimated gestational age with BPD, femur interval growth, uterus–adnexae. Anatomic survey: Cerebral ventricles, four-chamber heart, spine, stomach, bladder, cord insertion, kidneys.	Fetal life, fetal number, fetal presentation, amniotic fluid volume, placental location, assessment of gestational age. Maternal pelvis anatomic survey: Cerebral ventricles, four-chamber heart, spine, stomach, bladder, cord insertion, kidneys.

Adapted, with permission, from American Institute of Ultrasound in Medicine. Guidelines for the performance of the antepartum obstetrical examination. Rockville, MD: 1991; and American College of Obstetricians and Gynecologists. Ultrasonography in pregnancy. ACOG Technical Bulletin Number 187. Washington, DC: December 1993.

ability for adverse outcome, the risk is not zero. An adverse outcome that may be associated with the failure to perform an ultrasound when indicated, the performance of an incomplete ultrasound, or the inappropriate interpretation of an ultrasound may lead to legal action to recover alleged damages.[18] The four basic elements of tort litigation include *damages, duty, negligence,* and *causation.*[16] An adverse outcome may be related to an ultrasound examination that is alleged to have been improperly done or improperly interpreted when that error may have directly or indirectly caused the adverse outcome. The plaintiff must show that there was a *professional relationship* between the defendant and the plaintiff that imposed a *duty* on the defendant to provide an ultrasound examination that was within the *standard of care.* If it is shown that the examination provided was below the standard of care, then *negligence,* or a *breech of professional duty* is the expected conclusion. *Damages* must be established, and it must be shown that the damages were *caused* by the negligence.

Fetal structural or cytogenetic abnormalities are a reality of human reproduction. Up to 3% of human progeny demonstrate a serious abnormality and many, but by no means all, of these have been shown to be detectable by ultrasound over the past 20 years.[1,7,18-23] The majority of these abnormalities occur with no family history. The unexpected birth of a baby with a major anomaly to a woman who had undergone an ultrasound examination that failed to detect the abnormality may appear to her to constitute a basis for litigation.

Liability exposure may be minimized by providing optimal service, by creating appropriate patient expectations, by adequate documentation of the performance of a standard service, and by the liberal use of referral resources.[1,17] The sonographer or sonologist should attempt to optimize the quality of the service. He or she can and should document every major facet of the examination in order to provide for a defense, but the most effective tool in the defense against liability exposure is clear communication of realistic expectations to the patient. The patient should understand the goals and the limitations of the examination provided. Written, informed consent that includes a reasonable and clear statement of clinical goals and limits may be useful.[1] This consent should not be written in medical jargon or legalese but should be straightforward in normal English and attempt to avoid producing a suspicious result. It has been shown that it is the quality of communication between the patient and the physician that governs the liklihood of lawsuit in the face of adverse clinical outcome. The majority of medical malpractice lawsuits do not arise from objective negligence, whereas the majority of objective medical negligence does not result in malpractice action.[17]

Successful defense of an allegation of negligence should include clear documentation that a standard of care of ultrasound examination was performed and is, therefore, typically based either on the ACOG guidelines or the AIUM/ACR guidelines. If the defendant can show that the examination in question has included appropriate imaging and interpretation by showing that the examination has followed accepted guidelines, then an allegation of negligence may be defended. If, however, the examination has not been complete, or the documentation is not complete, the defense is weaker despite any questions of damages, causation, or duty. Documented efforts to screen the patient for historical risk factors that may indicate the possibility of an abnormality and the possible benefit of a targeted or referral examination are also useful since it can be argued that the examination in the case of the low-risk patient may be held to a different diagnostic sensitivity standard than the examination of the patient with known risk factors examined in a referral facility. This standard of sensitivity also varies between specific anomalies. For instance, anencephaly should never be missed by any examiner, but hypoplastic left heart syndrome may be missed in early gestation by any examiner. The most important behaviors to limit liability are clear communication of realistic expectations to the patient, the performance of a complete examination, and the careful documentation of that examination.[1,16,17]

Written documentation should include not only the general findings of fetal number, position, placentation, fluid volume, cardiac activity, and fetal biometry, but also a statement that specific fetal anatomic areas were seen or not seen and appeared normal or not.[1]

OBSTETRICAL ULTRASOUND CONTENT

Each obstetrical ultrasound examination in the second and third trimester should provide information regarding the general contents of the uterus, growth parameters of the fetus, and an anatomic survey of fetal anatomy. Failure to provide a complete examination may significantly increase liability exposure. These categories of information should be included regardless of the indication for the examination. Abbreviated examinations are defensible in certain limited situations, including emergent circumstances, physical limitations imposed by the habitus of the patient, or previous complete examination by skilled examiners. The circumstances on which a limited or abbreviated examination is based should be documented in the record.

SURVEY OF UTERINE CONTENTS

Fetal number, viability, position, amniotic fluid volume, along with location of the placenta, are considered basic findings of the examination. Evaluation of maternal adnexae should also be accomplished.

Viability may be confirmed by videotape of fetal or cardiac movement, or by still films of an M-mode echocardiogram or a Doppler signal demonstrating fetal cardiac movement (see Figure 12–7). If the fetus is in breech position near term, efforts should be made to establish the type of breech, i.e., frank or complete. If twins are discovered, a separating membrane should be sought (see Figure 12–6). The location of the placenta relative to the cervical os should be evaluated.

Amniotic fluid is a physiologic extension of the fetal urinary tract.[1,23] No obstetric ultrasound examination is complete without an observation of the amount of amniotic fluid. Amniotic fluid volume may be estimated subjectively by an experienced examiner or semiquantitated through the use of the amniotic fluid index (AFI). The AFI is the sum total, in centimeters, of the greatest vertical pockets of amniotic fluid in each of the four frontal quadrants of the uterus. An AFI below 5 cm is considered oligohydramnios, whereas an AFI over 30 cm is polyhydramnios.

Biometry

Accurate fetal biometry satisfies at least three goals, the first of which is to establish or confirm gestational age. Second, estimation of fetal weight is often a clinically helpful derivative of fetal biometry. Finally, the detection of significant fetal asymmetry may lead to the suspicion and diagnosis of anomalies that cause asymmetry, such as hydrocephalus in the case of an unusually large head, or dwarfism in the case of an unusually small femur length.

The standard fetal dimensions include crown–rump length (CRL) in the first trimester, and biparietal diameter (BPD), head circumference (HC), abdominal circumference (AC), and femur length (FL) after the first trimester.[1,5] The precision (95% confidence limits) of the estimate of gestational age from individual dimensions or combinations of dimensions before 20 weeks' gestation is about ±1 week (Table 12–4).[5]

Gestational age should always be based on the average estimated gestational age from two or more dimensions if there is no more than a week's discrepancy between them. If a greater discrepancy is found, an explanation is needed. Using multiple fetal dimensions improves precision of the estimate and offers the opportunity for technical quality control as well as the possibility of the identification of significant asymme-

TABLE 12–4. PRECISION OF FETAL BIOMETRY

Dimension[a]	Mean Error (Weeks)	95% CI ±[b]
BPD	−0.35	0.94
AC	−0.29	1.04
FL	−0.05	0.96
BPD and/or FL avg	−0.16	0.80
HC and/or FL avg	−0.11	0.76
BPD and/or AC and/or FL avg	−0.15	0.78
BPD and/or HC and/or AC and/or FL avg	−0.24	0.74

[a]For abbreviations, see text.
[b]CI, confidence interval.
Reprinted, with permission, from Hadlock FP, Harris RB, Martinez-Poyer J. How accurate is second trimester fetal dating? J Ultrasound Med: 1991; 10:557–61.

try's leading to the detection of a fetal growth abnormality associated with congenital abnormality. If asymmetries are detected, the measurements should be repeated to establish their technical accuracy and, if accurate, then efforts should be turned to an appropriate developmental explanation for the asymmetry.

Estimated fetal weight may be a clinically useful derivative of fetal biometry through the use of any of a number of regression equations that have been developed and reported.[8,9,24] Often, one or more of these weight estimation systems is incorporated into contemporary ultrasound machines and a weight estimate is automatically provided once all the necessary variables are recorded. Virtually all of the weight estimate systems provide an estimated weight that has 95% confidence limits of ±20%. (That is, 95% of the estimates will be within 20% of the actual birthweight if birth occurs within a defined interval of time, most often 3 days.[1]) Often, accuracy of ±10% is attributed to these techniques, but this level of variance relates to a single standard deviation (SD) and in a practical sense means that only 67% of the estimates (±1 SD) will be within 10% of the actual birthweight. This level of confidence may not be sufficient for many clinical decisions.

Fetal biometry, including the specific dimensions measured, the gestational age derived from the dimensions, and the estimated fetal weight, if appropriate, should be recorded in the formal report as well as documented in image format. The precision of the estimate of age or weight should be clearly indicated. Clinical decisions based on inaccurate biometry or on inappropriate confidence in the accuracy of the estimates may result in adverse outcomes and can lead to liability exposure.

Fetal Anatomic Survey

The fetal anatomic survey should be methodical and complete. From central nervous system to extremities, each major fetal system should be examined and specific screening images saved for documentation. This examination should include an occipitofrontal cranial view; an evaluation of intracranial contents, including the size of the ventricular atrium at the choroid; a posterior fossa view; longitudinal and transverse images of the fetal spine; a chest and four-chamber view; a transverse upper abdomen view to include fetal stomach; a transverse abdomen at the umbilicus; a transverse abdomen at the kidneys; a transverse pelvis at the bladder; and at least a femur if no increased risk of long-bone displasia is known.[1,6,7,13,10,19,20]

Documentation of Anatomic Images

Specific anatomic image documentation may take many forms, including Polaroid pictures, thermal prints, multiformat transparencies, digital image files on floppy or magnetooptical discs, or videotape recording of the examination. Some clinicians may argue against prolific image documentation as a liability danger rather than a protection, and it is certainly possible that the image documentation may contain an image of a missed diagnosis; but it is far more likely that complete documentation will establish that a standard examination has been performed and therefore assist in the defense of an allegation of negligence. Whatever image format is chosen, the images from a basic or low-risk or screening examination that can support a standard of care service should include images of major anatomic landmarks most likely to be affected by significant abnormalities (Table 12–5).

TABLE 12–5. RECOMMENDED DOCUMENTED IMAGES

Occipitofrontal cranial (BPD)
Posterior fossa
Coronal longitudinal spine
Four-chamber heart
Stomach
Kidneys
Cord insertion
Bladder
Femur

The Images

The following recommended standard images are most relevant to the ultrasound examination of a fetus between 16 and 22 weeks gestational age, but most should be included in any obstetrical ultrasound examination past 14 weeks' gestation.

Occipitofrontal Cranial View

The cranial image typically used for measurement of the biparietal diameter (BPD) is transverse to the cranial midline and extends between the occiput and the frontum (Figure 12–9). It should demonstrate a midline, mirror image symmetry of parietal curvature (Figure 12–10), uniform oval cranial contour, ventricular atria under 10 mm in diameter, and a cavum septum pellucidi; the head size should be consistent with other fetal dimensions, such as FL and AC. The easiest approach to the development of this view is to align the transducer with the fetal spine, slide up to the fetal head, and then turn the transducer 90°. Minor adjustments may be needed to center the midline and produce the ideal image. Failure to appreciate the expected anatomic features should result in suspicion of abnormality. The cranial contour should be smooth and oval, the midline should be in the midline, and the atria should measure under 10 mm in diameter, measured perpendicular to the axis of the ventricle and not including the ventricular sidewalls.[1]

Absence of midline membranes may indicate holoprosencephaly (Figure 12–11); absence of cavum is seen with agenesis of the corpus callosum; dilation of the atrium may be seen with hydrocephalus (Figure 12–12) or spina bifida (Figure 12–13); and a small BPD is seen with spina bifida and a large BPD with hydrocephalus.[10,13]

The BPD is the largest transverse diameter of the fetal head. The BPD is correctly measured from the outer edge of one skull table to the inner edge of the opposite skull table. The HC is measured at the outer edge of the skull table throughout the perimeter of the head.[5]

Posterior Fossa View

From the previous occipitofrontal plane, slight caudal rotation of the occipital heel of the transducer will bring the posterior fossa and the cerebellar hemispheres into view (Figure 12–14).

The proper posterior fossa image contains the cisterna magna, the cerebellar hemispheres, and the brainstem. Obliteration of the cistern and deformities of the cerebellar hemispheres are seen in cases of spina bifida (Figure 12–15).[13] An enlarged cistern has been asso-

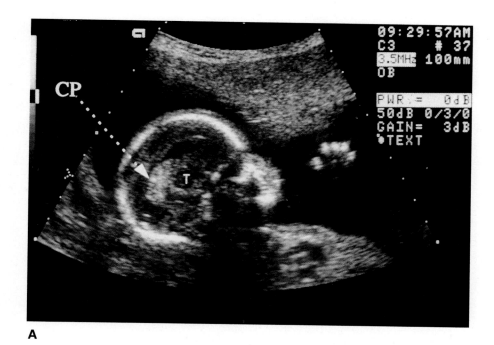

A

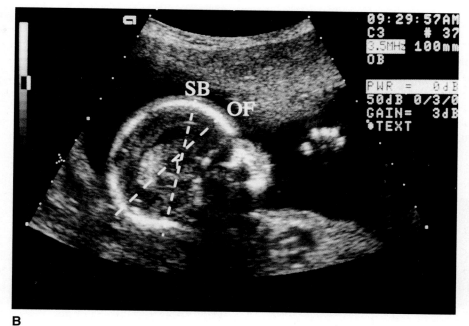

B

Figure 12–9. A. This slightly parasagittal cranial view shows the fetal cranium and the choroid plexus (CP) arising from above the thalamus (T), filling the atrium of the lateral ventricle. **B.** Reorienting the scanplane to align with the occipito-frontal plane (dashed line OF) produces an image appropriate for measuring the biparietal diameter and assessing the size of the atrium. Alignment with the sub-occipitobregmatic plane (dashed line SB) produces an image of the posterior fossa.

ciated with cerebellar hypoplasia in trisomy 18.[10] Dilatation of the fourth ventricle, which normally lies unseen between the cerebellar hemispheres, indicates a Dandy-Walker malformation, and increased nuchal skin thickness outside of the occipital skull table has been shown to be a useful marker for fetal Down syndrome.[25–27]

Fetal Spine
Historically, the most popular view of the fetal spine was an oblique plane (Figure 12–16) because the

oblique view is likely to include virtually all of the gently flexed fetal spine in one image. However, small dysraphic lesions are not easily detected from the oblique view, and a series of two or three coronal views is recommended for optimal sensitivity. Divergence of the normally parallel echocenters indicates the presence of spina bifida.[13] Transverse views of the fetal spine are also considered important and are included in each of the following transverse fetal trunk echocenter images. While the transverse spine must be evaluated in each

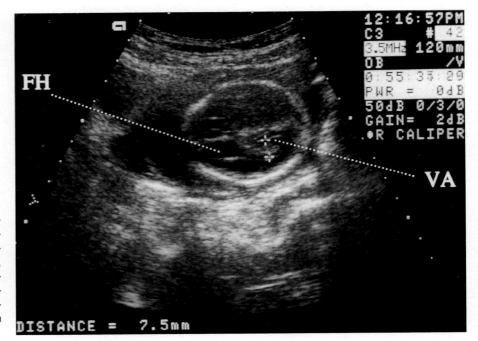

Figure 12–10. This occipitofrontal cranial image shows a uniform oval curvature, frontal horns of the lateral ventricles (FH), the ventricular atrium (VA), and the midline. Anechoic immature fetal brain, not fluid, surrounds the ventricle. The atrium is measured as indicated and should remain below 10 mm in the normal case.

trunk view, it need not be separately documented. The transverse fetal spine appears as three echocenters, one ventral midline and two dorsal paramedian echocenters, that assume the points of an equilateral triangle. These three echocenters should maintain a consistent relationship to one another at each level.

Four-Chamber Heart

A detailed examination of the fetal heart is the focus of the remainder of this text, but a brief review of the minimal screening examination is included here for completeness. A normal four-chamber heart view provides adequate screening of the fetal chest in the low-risk pa-

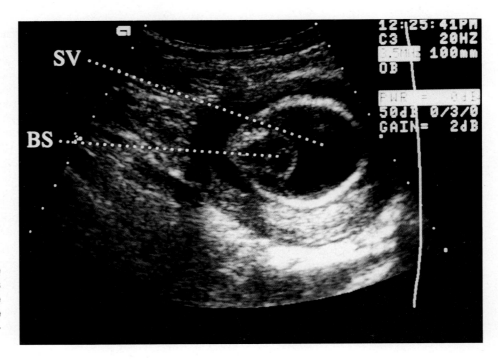

Figure 12–11. This is an oblique coronal view of the cranium of a fetus with holoprosencephaly. Notice there is no midline margination within the single ventricle (SV) above the brainstem (BS).

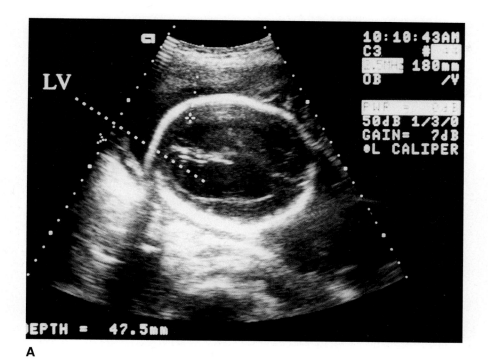

A

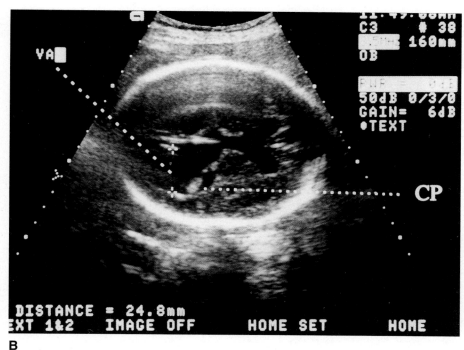

B

Figure 12–12. A. The dilated lateral ventricle (LV) of this fetus with hydrocephalus is apparent. **B.** Another fetus with hydrocephalus is shown here. The ventricular atrium (VA) is clearly dilated, and the choroid plexus (CP) is seen to droop dependently to the lateral margin of the ventricle.

tient (Figure 12–17).[1,6,19-21] Development of this image may be accomplished by aligning the scanplane with the fetal spine, then sliding to the level of the fetal chest, and then turning the transducer 90°. Optimal images will result from minor adjustments that align the scanplane with a fetal rib, then slide very slightly above or below the rib into an interspace.

The heart should occupy about one third of the area of the chest, with the sagittal midline passing through the left atrium, the base of the interventricular septum, and exiting the right ventricle. The long axis of the heart should intersect the sagittal midline at about 45°. The cardiac ventricles should be symmetrical at their base and synchronous in their activity on real-

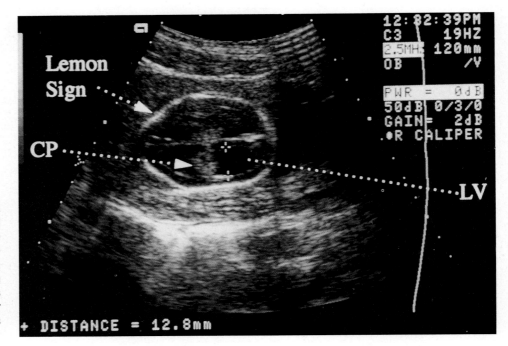

Figure 12–13. Open spina bifida causes tethering of the spinal cord and alters intracranial anatomy to result in ventriculomegaly, frontoparietal indentations (lemon sign), and a biparietal diameter less than expected. Here, the lemon sign is illustrated, and the ventricular atrium (LV) is mildly dilated in this fetus with spina bifida.

time examination. The lung fields should be homogeneous, with the exception of the anechoic great vessels.

The heart may be shifted to one side or the other in the presence of a diaphragmatic hernia (shifted away from the hernia) (Figure 12–18), asymmetric pleural effusions (Figure 12–19), or mass lesions such as cystic adenomatoid malformation of the lung or sequestration of the lung. Asymmetries of the cardiac ventricles may indicate hypoplastic syndromes of the right or left, or valvular stenosis. Abnormalities of the axis have been associated with conotruncal abnormalities such as tetralogy of Fallot or truncus arteriosus.

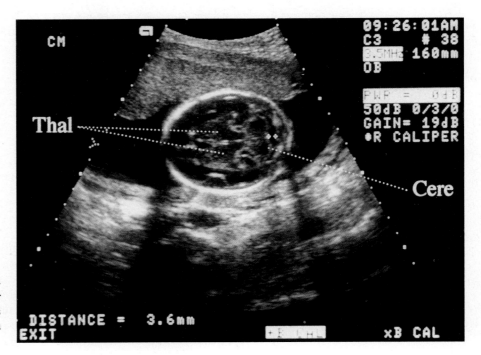

Figure 12–14. The suboccipitobregmatic scanplane shows the posterior fossa, with cerebellar hemispheres (Cere), thalami (Thal), and cisterna magna (cursors).

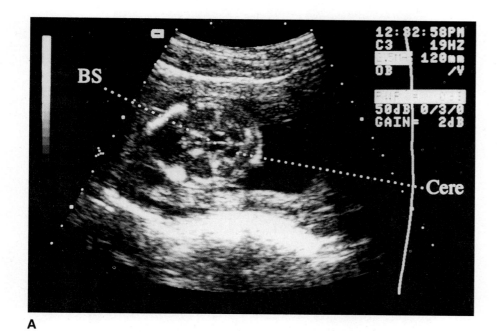

A

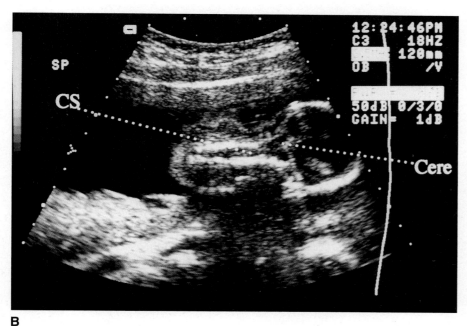

B

Figure 12–15. A. The suboccipito-bregmatic plane in a fetus with spina bifida demonstrates the compression deformity of the cerebellar hemispheres (Cere) typical with spina bifida. Notice the obliteration of the cisterna magna. BS = brainstem. **B.** A coronal view of the posterior fossa clearly shows the displacement of the cerebellar hemispheres (Cere) down into the upper cervical spinal canal (CS).

Stomach

Sliding the transducer (already transverse to the fetal trunk for the four-chamber heart view) caudally below the diaphragm should show the stomach below the diaphragm on the left side of the abdomen (Figure 12–20). Certainly persistent failure to image a stomach after 16 weeks should be suspicious, perhaps for esophageal atresia.[1] Likewise, two anechoic upper abdominal structures should raise suspicion for duodenal atresia.[21] In the case of duodenal atresia, the sagittal midline should pass between the twin upper abdominal anechoic masses.

Near the level of the fetal stomach, a transverse view of the abdomen, adjusted for optimal symmetry, provides the image from which to measure the abdominal circumference. The AC is measured at the perimeter of the abdomen at the outer skin edge.

Kidneys

The kidneys may be detected in the same transverse abdominal scanplane as the stomach, or they may be slightly caudal to it. The kidneys are seen as circular, slightly hypoechoic relative to the surrounding tissue, and located in the paraspinal areas of the dorsal ab-

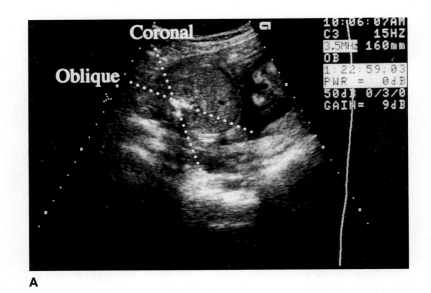

A

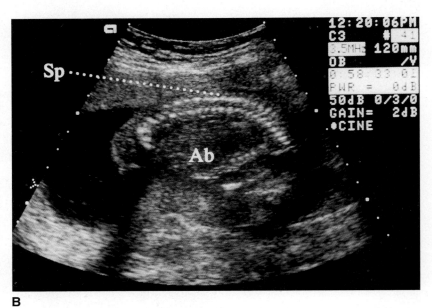

B

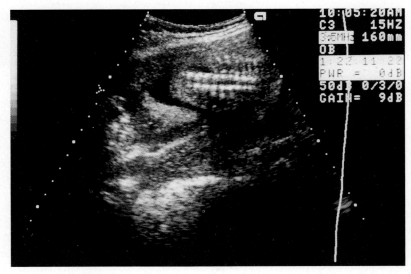

C

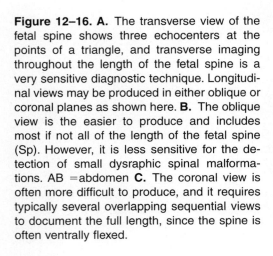

Figure 12–16. A. The transverse view of the fetal spine shows three echocenters at the points of a triangle, and transverse imaging throughout the length of the fetal spine is a very sensitive diagnostic technique. Longitudinal views may be produced in either oblique or coronal planes as shown here. **B.** The oblique view is the easier to produce and includes most if not all of the length of the fetal spine (Sp). However, it is less sensitive for the detection of small dysraphic spinal malformations. AB =abdomen **C.** The coronal view is often more difficult to produce, and it requires typically several overlapping sequential views to document the full length, since the spine is often ventrally flexed.

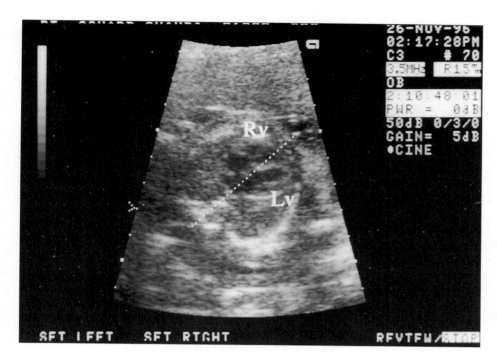

Figure 12–17. A transverse view of the fetal chest at the level of the heart shows the heart centered in the chest. The midline indicated by the dotted line crosses the left atrium, the base of the interventricular septum, and the right ventricle (Rv). The left ventricle (Lv) is the more posterior of the ventricles.

domen (Figure 12–21).[23,28] The renal pelvis may or may not be distinct, and when seen it should measure no more than 5 mm in AP (anterior–posterior) diameter.[28] The kidney circumference to abdominal circumference ratio (KC/AC) in early pregnancy is typically about 0.29.

Longitudinal parasagittal or coronal imaging may be accomplished, and kidney dimensions indexed to gestational age are available but of limited value. If the kidneys are seen and appear normal with normal amniotic fluid and normal bladder filling, the probability of major urinary tract abnormalities is slight. Absence of

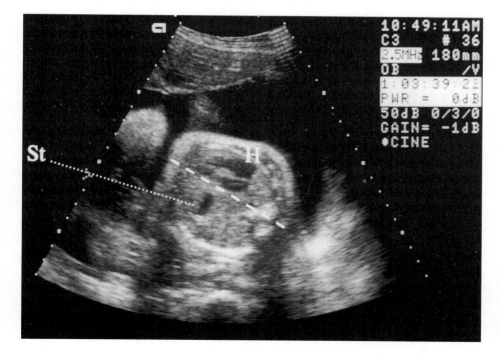

Figure 12–18. A four-chamber view of a fetus with diaphragmatic hernia clearly shows the heart (H) displaced to the left of the midline (dashed line), and the stomach (St) abnormally located in the left side of the chest.

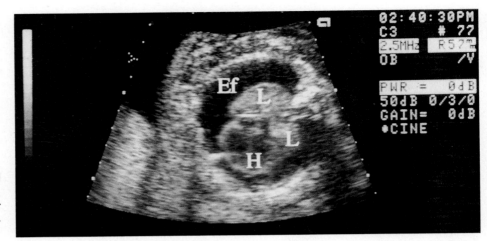

Figure 12–19. Congenital pleural effusions (Ef) are demonstrated here. Effusions are seen as anechoic or hypoechoic accumulations surrounding the lungs (L) and the heart (H).

one or both kidneys, dilatation of one or both pelves, or cystic changes (Figure 12–22) in either renal parenchyma should raise suspicion, as should severe oligohydramnios or absent bladder filling.[23]

Cord Insertion

Transverse imaging further caudally should allow evaluation of the cord insertion (Figure 12–23), although later in gestation this becomes more difficult to visualize because of flexion of the fetal thighs and crowding. Carefully following the abdominal wall around should show the break at the entry of the umbilical vein and arteries. Both omphalocele and gastroschisis (Figure 12–24) should be detected by careful examination of the cord insertion.[22]

Bladder

The fetal bladder should be detected with careful imaging in every fetus after 16 weeks (see Figure 12–23).[23] Located in the retropubic midline, this anechoid structure may be absent in the case of renal agenesis or enlarged in the case of obstructive uropathy. The umbilical arteries may be found along each side of the fetal bladder.

Femur

The combined incidence of short limb dysplasias in the general population in the absence of prior history is less than 1 per 1000.[1] Short-limb dysplasias not causing significantly diminished FL are rare among this family of anomalies. Therefore, FL measurement for gestational age assessment, if normal and consistent with

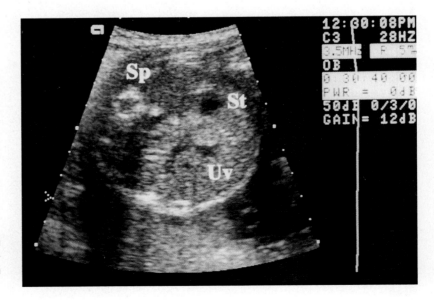

Figure 12–20. The transverse upper abdominal scan shows stomach (St), spine (Sp), and umbilical vein (Uv). This is an appropriate image from which to measure abdominal circumference.

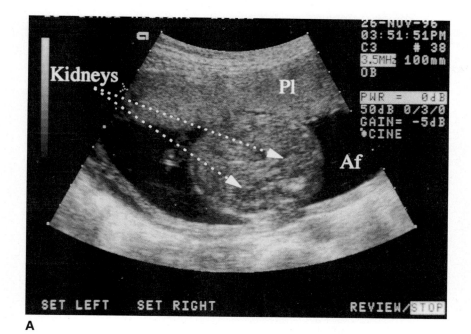

A

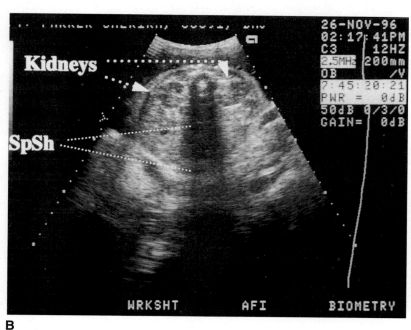

B

Figure 12–21. A. The kidneys are relatively hypoechoic and not sharply outlined in the second trimester, as illustrated here. The placenta (Pl) is seen and the anechoic amniotic fluid (Af) surrounding the fetus. **B.** In the third trimester, the deposition of perinephric fat outlines the kidneys more clearly, as seen here. Calcification of the fetal spine results in a dense acoustic shadow (SpSh).

expected age and other fetal dimensions, is considered adequate screening for short-limb dysplasias in a patient with no history of risk factors (Figure 12–25). The FL is measured from blunt end to blunt end, parallel to the shaft.

Bowing or angulation of one or both femurs combined with less than expected dimensions is strong evidence of abnormality and should prompt further evaluation.

In summary, a relatively limited set of observations

made from a discrete set of images (Table 12–5) included in the basic (office, level I, obstetrical, etc.) examination of the low-risk patient constitutes the basis for fetal anatomic diagnosis through the detection of dysmorphology associated with specific fetal malformations (Table 12–6). The detection of one or more of these features should result in the referral of the patient for a targeted (level II, referral, high detail, genetic, fetal, etc.) examination. Failure to examine these anatomic areas, failure to interpret them accurately, or

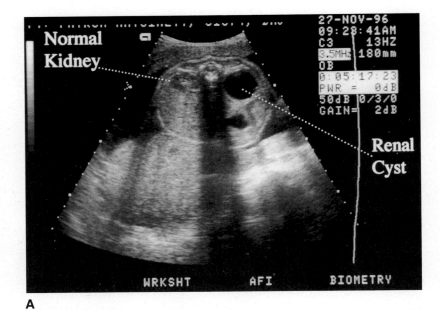

A

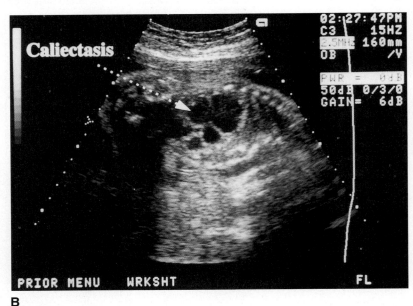

B

Figure 12–22. A. Ureteropelvic junction obstruction leads to hydronephrosis and often the growth of a renal cyst, as seen here. This represents the dilatation of a segment of the ureter or renal pelvis as a result of the obstruction. **B.** A sagittal view of a kidney with severe hydronephrosis and caliectasis is seen here. The anechoic areas are dilated renal calices that are seen to interconnect.

failure to document either the images or the interpretation may provide support for an allegation of negligence.

Qualitative or quantitative observations that should raise suspicion of abnormality include abnormalities of fluid volume, fetal malpresentation, unusual fetal posturing, or biometric asymmetries. Significant *oligohydramnios* may result from fetal urinary tract abnormalities such as *renal agenesis, dysplasia,* or *obstructive uropathies.*[23] *Polyhydramnios* may result from severe central nervous system abnormalities, including *anencephaly, hydrocephalus,* and *hydranencephalus,* or gas-

trointestinal abnormalities, such as *esophageal atresia, duodenal atresia, jejunal atresia,* fetal abdominal masses of variable origin, or even fetal aneuploidy. Fetal malformation is a significant etiologic factor in fetal malpresentation. Any noncephalic presentation should be evaluated for fetal malformation. Unusual head, hand, or limb posturing may result from fetal malformation or aneuploidy. Biometric asymmetries such as a large BPD with *hydrocephalus,* a small BPD with *holoprosencephaly,* or short femurs with *long-bone dysplasias* or fetal aneuploidy should produce suspicion and consideration of referral.

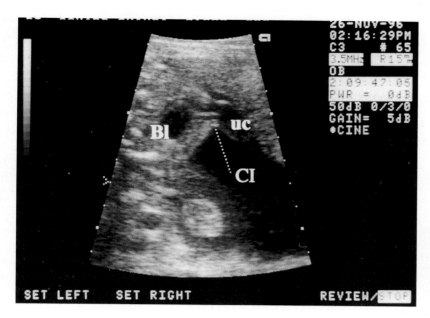

Figure 12–23. Transverse imaging of the fetal abdomen at the level of the cord insertion (CI) shows the typical abrupt attachment of the umbilical cord (uc). The bladder (Bl) is often seen in such a view. This view excludes omphalocele or gastroschisis, both of which occur at this level.

DIAGNOSTIC SENSITIVITY OF ULTRASOUND

The sensitivity of the obstetric ultrasound examination for the detection of fetal malformation logically varies with experience and training, with the nature and severity of the malformation, with the gestational age of the fetus, and with the focal acuity of the examination. For example, spina bifida is found more often and more reliably if the examiner is trained and experienced with its detection and/or if the examiner is specifically searching for spina bifida, as in the case of elevated MSAFP.[13] Furthermore, diagnostic sensitivity is enhanced if the fetus is 30 weeks' gestation instead of 14 weeks' gestation and/or if the lesion is five segments long with a large sac instead of one or two segments and very low. Diagnostic sensitivity is enhanced if the fetus is cephalic and back up in a thin woman with adequate amniotic fluid and impaired in a deeply engaged breech in an obese woman with oligohydramnios.

The diagnostic sensitivity of ultrasound in the detection of fetal congenital malformation among low-risk patients cannot be easily evaluated since sensitivity is higher for major malformations than for minor, higher for later gestational ages than for earlier, higher for the more highly trained and focused examiner than for the less experienced, and higher for the high-risk patient than for the low-risk patient. Most importantly, it is precisely the lowest risk patient who is more often examined by the least experienced examiner.

Fetal Anatomic Imaging and Aneuploidy

Minor Dysmorphology and Fetal Aneuploidy

Recent interest has grown in the use of ultrasound for the detection of minor fetal dysmorphic features as a *screen* for aneuploidy.[25,26,29-41] The incorporation of several of these subtle observations into scoring systems has been promoted for use in both the screening and the detection of fetal aneuploidy in low-risk populations, and most recently such a scoring system has been examined for the reduction of risk in high-risk populations (advanced maternal age) if none of the specified suspicious features are detected.[39-41] Clearly, however, it may be argued that these subtle observations are not reasonable diagnostic goals for the basic ultrasound examination performed in the low-risk patient for primarily obstetrical purposes since the sensitivity is not optimal in the hands of the less experienced examiner.

The RADIUS Study and Major Anomaly Sensitivity

The RADIUS study may provide useful experience with regard to the screening sensitivity for fetal malformation in a low-risk group, but the results at first appear disappointing.[42] Among the routinely screened patients, anomalies occurred in 2.4% compared to 2.1% of the selectively scanned patients.[11,42] Of the anomalies present, only 35% were detected antenatally, and only 17% of these before 24 weeks' gestation. However, closer examination of the data shows that ventriculoseptal de-

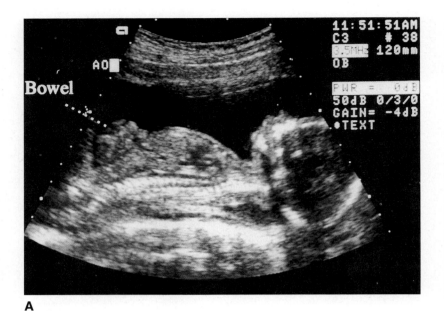

A

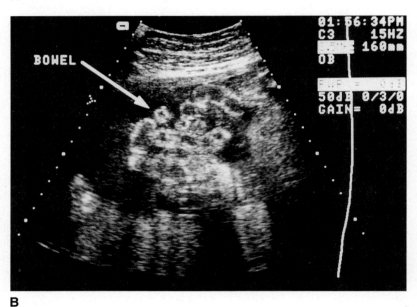

B

Figure 12–24. A. This sagittal view of a fetus with gastroschisis clearly shows bowel loops resting anteriorly and inferiorly to the cord insertion. **B.** The bowel loops float freely in amniotic fluid in the case of gastroschisis as seen here. Later in gestation, inflammatory reaction results in bowel wall thickening and increased echogenicity associated, on occasion, with matting together and even obstruction.

fects of unspecified clinical significance, cleft lip, and clubbed foot are included in the missed diagnoses. Although these are not insignificant, they are not often considered in the same context as more serious or disabling malformations, such as anencephaly or omphalocele.

Among more serious malformations the detection rate reported in the RADIUS study was 78% (62 of 80 detected).[42] These included neural tube defects (7 of 8 detected), other central nervous system (CNS) anomalies (2 of 2 detected), hygroma (2 of 2 detected), complex cardiac malformations (9 of 21 detected), diaphragmatic hernia (1 of 1 detected), duodenal atresia (1 of 1 detected), omphalocele (1 of 1 detected), hydronephrosis

(28 of 29 detected), limb reduction defects (2 of 5 detected), and other miscellaneous anomalies (3 of 4 detected). The anomalies deleted from this analysis that resulted in the lower overall rate also included cleft lip (3 of 10 detected), ventriculoseptal defect (0 of 16 detected of unspecified significance), atrioseptal defect (0 of 5 detected), clubbed foot (2 of 24 detected), and esophageal atresia (0 of 3 detected), an anomaly that may not produce any anatomic findings under 20 weeks' gestation.

It may effectively be argued that a 78% detection rate for serious anomalies among low-risk patients during examinations performed in 28 different ultrasound laboratories is really a fairly successful result.[42]

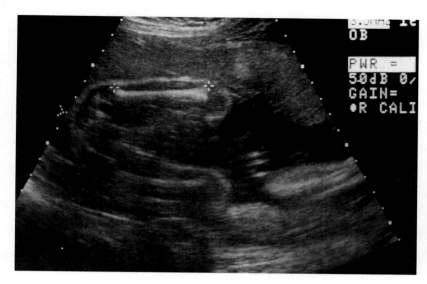

Figure 12–25. The femur is easily imaged in its entirety from metaphyseal plate to metaphyseal plate. Femur length is measured from end to end parallel to the shaft, as illustrated here, and excludes the epiphyses as these are not visualized with ultrasound. The femur should present a relatively straight and uniform shape as seen here.

Other Investigators and Ultrasound Anomaly Sensitivity

Campbell and Pearce,[19] in 1984, reported the detection of 34 of 38 (89%) possible anomalies among 11,664 low-risk patients. Their reported sensitivity with a high-risk group of patients was similar, with 96% for anomalies of the CNS, 95% for genitourinary and limb anomalies, 91% for gastrointestinal anomalies, and 80% for cardiac malformations.

Hill et al.,[20] in 1985, reported an ultrasound detection rate of 10 of 11, or 90%, for anomalies of the CNS; 12 of 13, or 92%, for the genitourinary system; 4 of 8, or 50%, for anomalies of the skeletal system; 3 of 15, or 20%, for the gastrointestinal system; and 0 of 13 for the heart. Sabbagha et al.,[21] in 1985, reported diagnostic sensitivity of 94% for the CNS, 92% for the genitourinary system, and 100% for gastrointestinal and limb abnormalities, for an overall sensitivity of 96%.

Levi et al.,[6] in 1991, in reviewing an experience with 16,370 low-risk patients, reported a diagnostic sensitivity of 79% for anomalies of the CNS, 79% for the genitourinary system, and 51% for the gastrointestinal tract, but only 23% sensitivity for malformations of the limbs or the heart. Bromley et al.,[43] in 1992, looked at the sensitivity with both low- and high-risk patients and found an overall sensitivity of 83% for major malformations and essentially no difference in diagnostic sensitivity between the two groups.

Multiple investigators in recent years have documented an overall sensitivity for ultrasound of 92% for spina bifida.[13] Many MSAFP screening programs include this information about sensitivity in counseling and the result is a lower rate of invasive testing after a normal ultrasound examination.

These levels of sensitivity of ultrasound for the detection of anomalies in a high-risk patient when the examination is performed by subspecialists with extensive experience do not likely apply to the case of the low-risk patient in the office but instead probably represent the highest expected technical sensitivity under optimal circumstances.

Sonographic Screening for Aneuploidy

A large number of dysmorphic observations have been associated with an increased risk of fetal aneuploidy and some have been combined and studied as screening markers (Table 12–7).[25,26,29–41] Most of these, individually and in combination, have been evaluated for sensitivity and predictive value by investigators with extensive training, experience, and focus, and this diagnostic performance is not likely to be duplicated in low-risk patients undergoing basic or routine obstetrical ultrasound examinations.

Biometric Asymmetry and Aneuploidy

Both Lockwood et al.[30] and Benacceraf et al.[29] described the use of short femur length as a screen for Down syndrome in 1987. Humeral length as well has been examined as a screening marker for Down syndrome.[36,37] Other investigators, however, using the same or similar criteria, found much lower sensitivities (Table 12–8).

Minor Dysmorphology

Benacerraf et al.[25,27] first reported *increased fetal nuchal skin thickness* in Down syndrome. Crane and Gray[26] reported increased nuchal thickness in 12 of 16 fetuses with Down syndrome, while finding the same thing in only 1.05% of nonaneuploid fetuses. Benacerraf

TABLE 12–6. DYSMORPHIC CLUES TO FETAL ANOMALIES

Observation	Possible Association
CNS	
Frontal notching	Spina bifida
Mild ventriculomegaly	Spina bifida
	Down syndrome
	Hydrocephalus
Absent cavum	Agenesis of corpus callosum
Cerebellar compression	Spina bifida
Absent cisterna magna	Spina bifida
Nuchal skin >5 mm thick	Down syndrome
Spinal dysraphism	Spina bifida
Chest	
Mediastinal displacement	Diaphragmatic hernia
	Cystic adenomatoid malformation
	Pulmonary sequestration
Pleural effusion	Chylothorax
Cardiac axis deviation	Conotruncal anomalies
Ventricular asymmetry	Hypoplastic heart syndrome
Single ventricle	Atrioventricular canal defect
Atriomegaly	Ebstein's anomaly
	Ventricular outflow obstruction
Abdomen	
Absent stomach	Esophageal atresia
Dual anechoic masses	Duodenal obstruction
Eccentric anechoic mass	Renal
	Ureteropelvic junction UPJ obstruction
	Retroperitoneal urinoma
	Intestinal atresia
	Ovarian cysts
	Lymphatic cysts
Renal pyelectasis	Ureteropelvic junction obstruction
	Ureteral reflux
	Down syndrome
Hyperechoic gut (bone equivalency)	Down syndrome
	Cystic fibrosis
Megacystis	Urethral obstruction
	Urethral valves
	Urethral atresia
	Cloacal plate syndrome
	Prune belly syndrome
Tissue at cord insertion	Omphalocele
	Gastroschisis
Extremities	
Short limbs	Familial variation
	Short-limb dysplasia
	Teratogen
Fractures	Osteogenesis imperfecta
Clubbed foot	Fetal aneuploidy

Reprinted, with permission, from Seeds JW, Chescheir NC, Wade RV. Practical Sonography in Obstetrics and Gynecology. Philadelphia: Lippincott-Raven; 1996.

TABLE 12–7. MINOR DYSMORPHIC MARKERS OF FETAL ANEUPLOIDY

Short femur
Short humerus
Nuchal skin thickening
Mild ventriculomegaly
Small ears
Facial clefting
Echogenic bowel
Mild pyelectasis
Isolated choroid plexus cyst
Digital hypoplasia
Abnormal hand posturing
Clubbed foot
Cisterna magna over 10 mm
Cerebellar hypoplasia
First-trimester hygroma
Echogenic cardiac moderator band

Adapted from references 25, 26, and 29–41.

et al.[35] found *renal pyelectasis* of 4 mm or greater in 210 of 7400 (2.8%) of fetuses examined, with Down syndrome occurring in 3.3% of these examined fetuses, or 25% of the fetuses with Down syndrome. *Hyperechoic fetal bowel* was reported by Dicke and Crane[38] and Dubinsky et al.[44] to be associated with fetal aneuploidy.

MULTIPLE MARKER SCORING SYSTEMS

Benacerraf et al.[39] examined major and minor dysmorphology as well as growth asymmetry detected in 43 aneuploid fetuses from among 5000 referred for examination because of advanced maternal age or abnormal

TABLE 12–8. LIMB LENGTH AND DOWN SYNDROME

Senior Author	Marker[a]	Sensitivity (%)	False Positive (%)
Benacceraf	Femur < 0.91 Exp	68	2
Nyberg	Femur < 0.91 Exp	24	4.7
Perella	Femur < 0.91 Exp	28	23
Lockwood	BPD/FL >+1.5 SD	70	7
Shah	BPD/FL >+1.5 SD	18	6
Dicke	BPD/FL >+1.5 SD	18	4
Benacerraf	Hum < 0.9 Exp	50	6
Rotmensch	Hum < 0.9 Exp	28	9
Nyberg	hum < 0.9 Exp	24	4.5

[a]Exp, expected; BPD/FL, biparietal diameter divided by femur length; Hum, humerus.
Data from References 30, 31–34, 36, and 37.

MSAFP. They found that 17 of 32 (53%) of the Down syndrome fetuses were identified by limb asymmetries and 69% had nuchal skin thickness over 6 mm and/or a major anomaly. Using a scoring system awarding 1 point for short femur or renal pyelectasis and 2 points for nuchal skin thickness over 6 mm or a major anomaly, and considering 2 points as the cutoff, 81% of the Down fetuses and 100% of the trisomy 13 and 18 pregnancies would be identified with a 4.4% false positive rate.[39] The predictive value for the system was estimated to be 6.87%, 3.75%, and 1.91% for risk populations of 1 of 250, 1 of 500, and 1 of 1000, respectively.

More recently, this same group reviewed a larger experience from the converse point of view. They concluded that in the case of the pregnancy at risk for fetal aneuploidy because of advanced maternal age, a sonographic search for these multiple markers that resulted in the detection of none of them could be used to substantially reduce the probability of fetal aneuploidy.[41] This attempt to reduce quantitatively the empiric age-based risk of fetal aneuploidy through the use of ultrasound requires further study and confirmation before universal application but appears very promising.

The sonographic identification of these minor dysmorphic features of fetal aneuploidy is not currently a reasonable goal for the office obstetrical ultrasound examination performed on a low-risk patient for obstetrical indications. On the other hand, limb asymmetries, nuchal skin thickening, renal pyelectasis, and echogenic bowel may be identified from the standard views of the basic screening ultrasound examination. Awareness of the implications of these observations and a commitment to methodical examination of the standard scanplanes will increase sensitivity for such findings.

SUMMARY

The most likely benefits of routine ultrasound in the low-risk patient are obstetrical, with confirmation of dates, detection of multiple gestation, and baseline growth data, and location of the placenta being primary advantages gained from such an examination. The detection of the unexpected major fetal malformation is the least likely benefit of routine ultrasound. The RADIUS study was intended to solve these problems but applied such intense selection that the final population for study may have had little relevance to the average population. The rate of adverse outcomes among the control group was so low that few interventions would have appeared useful.

Diagnostic sensitivity of the screening obstetrical ultrasound examination appears to be highest in high-risk patients examined by highly specialized and experienced personnel that may be of limited availability. Diagnostic sensitivity may be quite good,

however, even in low-risk patients with a basic or routine examination if recognized guidelines for content are followed and referral to experienced referral resources for unclear or suspicious images is liberally practiced.

Optimal service and minimum liability exposure will result if the following guidelines are followed:

1. The obstetric population should be carefully screened for historical or clinical risk factors that may indicate increased probability of fetal abnormality. Identification of such increased risk should cause consideration of referral.
2. The screening ultrasound examination should be methodical and complete and include examination of each of several recommended scanplane views to maximize diagnostic sensitivity.
3. The performance of a complete and methodical examination should be carefully documented with both descriptive text and image records to show that a standard of care service was provided.
4. Referral for second opinion should be easily considered and easily obtained in the case of any suspicious finding.

Should every obstetrical patient have an ultrasound examination? Only if it is competently performed and properly recorded and the patient is aware of appropriate goals and limitations. The ideal gestational age is between 18 and 22 completed weeks.

REFERENCES

1. Seeds JW, Chescheir NC, & Wade RV: *Practical Sonography in Obstetrics and Gynecology.* Philadelphia: Lippincott-Raven; 1996.
2. *Diagnostic Ultrasound Imaging in Pregnancy.* Published by The Department of Health and Human Services. Washington, DC, 20402: U.S. Government Printing Office; February, 1984.
3. Chervenak FA, et al.: Advances in the diagnosis of fetal defects. *N Engl J Med.* 315:305–9, 1986.
4. Hughey MJ, Olive DL: Routine ultrasound scanning for the detection and management of twin pregnancies. *J Reprod Med.* 30:427, 1985.
5. Hadlock FP, Harris RB, Martinez-Poyer J: How accurate is second trimester fetal dating? *J Ultrasound Med.* 10:557–61, 1991.
6. Levi S, Hyjazi Y, Schaaps JP, et al.: Sensitivity and specificity of routine antenatal screening for congenital anomalies by ultrasound: The Belgian multicentric study. *Ultrasound Obstet Gynecol.* 1:102–8, 1991.
7. Vintzileos AM, et al.: Antenatal evaluation and management of ultrasonically detected fetal anomalies. *Obstet Gynecol.* 69:640, 1987.

8. Seeds JW: Impaired fetal growth: Ultrasonic evaluation and clinical management. *Obstet Gynecol.* 64:577, 1984.

9. Ott WJ, Doyle S: Ultrasonic diagnosis of altered fetal growth by use of a normal ultrasonic fetal weight curve. *Obstet Gynecol.* 63:201, 1984.

10. Main DM, Mennuti MT: Neural tube defects: Issues in prenatal diagnosis and counseling. *Obstet Gynecol.* 67:1, 1986.

11. Ewigman BG, Crane JP, Frigoletto FD, et al.: Effect of prenatal ultrasound screening on perinatal outcome. *N Engl J Med.* 329:821–7, 1993.

12. Macri JN, Haddow JE, Weiss RR: Screening for neural tube defects in the United States: A summary of the Scarborough Conference. *Am J Obstet Gynecol.* 133:119–21, 1979.

13. Watson WJ, Chescheir NC, Katz VL, et al.: The role of ultrasound in evaluation of patients with elevated maternal serum alpha-fetoprotein: A review. *Obstet Gynecol.* 78:123–30, 1991.

14. *Ultrasonography in Pregnancy.* ACOG Technical Bulletin Number 187, December, 1993. Published by the American College of Obstetricians and Gynecologists, 409 12th Street SW, Washington, DC, 20024-2188.

15. Americal Institute of Ultrasound in Medicine. *Guidelines for the Performance of the Antepartum Obstetrical Examination.* Rockville, MD: AIUM; 1991.

16. *Professional Liability for Residents.* Published in 1993 by Council on Resident Education in Obstetrics and Gynecology, 409 12th Street SW, Washington, DC, 20024-2188.

17. Kravitz RL, Rolph JE, McGuigan K: Malpractice claims data as a quality improvement tool: I. Epidemiology of error in four specialties. *JAMA.* 266(15):2087–92, 1991.

18. Perone N, Carpenter RJ, Robertson JA: Legal liability in the use of ultrasound by office-based obstetricians. *Am J Obstet Gynecol.* 150:801, 1984.

19. Campbell S, Pearce JMF: The prenatal diagnosis of fetal structural anomalies by ultrasound. *Clin Obstet Gynaecol.* 10:475–506, 1985.

20. Hill LM, Breckle R, Gehrking RT: Prenatal detection of congenital malformations by ultrasonography. *Am J Obstet Gynecol.* 151:44–51, 1985.

21. Sabbagha RE, Sheikh Z, Tamura RK, et al.: Predictive value, sensitivity, and specificity of ultrasonic targeted imaging for fetal anomalies in gravid women at high risk for birth defects. *Am J Obstet Gynecol.* 152:822–8, 1985.

22. Carpenter MW, et al.: Perinatal management of ventral wall defects. *Obstet Gynecol.* 64:646, 1984.

23. Hobbins J, Romero R, Grannum P, et al.: Antenatal diagnosis of renal anomalies with ultrasound. *Am J Obstet Gynecol.* 148:868–77, 1984.

24. Bracero LA, Baxi LV, Rey HR, et al.: Use of ultrasound in antenatal diagnosis of large for gestational age infants in diabetic gravid patients. *Am J Obstet Gynecol.* 152:43, 1985.

25. Benacerraf BR, Barss VA, Laboda LA: A sonographic sign for the detection in the second trimester of the fetus with Down's syndrome. *Am J Obstet Gynecol.* 151:1078–83, 1985.

26. Crane JP, Gray DL: Sonographically measured nuchal skinfold thickness as a screening tool for Down syndrome: Results of a prospective clinical trial. *Obstet Gynecol.* 77:533–8, 1991.

27. Benacerraf BR, Gelman R, Frigoletto FD: Sonographic identification of second-trimester fetuses with Down's syndrome. *N Engl J Med.* 317:1371–6, 1987.

28. Arger P, Coleman B, Mintz M, et al.: Routine fetal genitourinary tract screening. *Radiology.* 156:485–9, 1985.

29. Benacerraf BR, Frigoletto FD, Laboda LA: Sonographic diagnosis of Down syndrome in the second trimester. *Am J Obstet Gynecol.* 153:49–54, 1985.

30. Lockwood C, Benacerraf B, Krinsky A, et al.: A sonographic screening method for Down syndrome. *Am J Obstet Gynecol.* 157:803–9, 1987.

31. Perrella R, Duerinckx AJ, Grant EG, et al.: Second-trimester sonographic diagnosis of Down syndrome: Role of femur-length shortening and nuchal-fold thickening. *AJR.* 151:981–5, 1988.

32. Dicke JM, Gray DL, Songster GS, et al.: Fetal biometry as a screening tool for the detection of chromosomally abnormal pregnancies. *Obstet Gynecol.* 74:26–31, 1989.

33. Shah YG, Eckl CJ, Stinson SK, et al.: Biparietal diameter/femur length ratio, cephalic index and femur length measurements: Not reliable screening techniques for Down syndrome. *Obstet Gynecol.* 75:186–91, 1990.

34. Benacerraf BR, Neuberg D, Frigoletto FD: Humeral shortening in second-trimester fetuses with Down syndrome. *Obstet Gynecol.* 77:223–8, 1991.

35. Benacerraf BR, Mandell J, Estroff JA, et al.: Fetal pyelectasis: A possible association with Down syndrome. *Obstet Gynecol.* 76:58–63, 1990.

36. Rotmensch S, Luo JS, Liberati M, et al.: Fetal humeral length to detect Down syndrome. *Am J Obstet Gynecol.* 166:1330–5, 1992.

37. Nyberg DA, Resta RG, Luthy DA, et al.: Humerus and femur length shortening in the detection of Down's syndrome. *Am J Obstet Gynecol.* 168:534–9, 1993.

38. Dicke JM, Crane JP: Sonographically detected hyperechoic fetal bowel: Significance and implications for pregnancy management. *Obstet Gynecol.* 80:778–83, 1992.

39. Benacerraf BR, Neuberg D, Bromley B, et al.: Sonographic scoring index for prenatal detection of chromosomal abnormalities. *J Ultrasound Med.* 11:449–54, 1992.

40. Benacerraf BR, Nadel A, Pergament E, et al.: Ultrasonographic detection of the second-trimester fetus with autosomal trisomies using a sonographic scoring index. *Radiology.* 193:135–41, 1994.

41. Nadel AS, Bromley B, Frigoletto FD, et al.: Can the presumed risk of autosomal trisomy be decreased in fetuses of older women following a normal sonogram? *J Ultrasound Med.* 14:297–302, 1995.

42. Crane JP, LeFevre ML, Winborn RC, et al.: A randomized trial of prenatal ultrasonographic screening: Impact on the detection, management and outcome of anomalous fetuses. *New Engl J Med.* 171:392–9, 1994.

43. Bromley B, Estroff JA, Sanders SP, et al.: Fetal echocardiography: Accuracy and limitations in a population at high and low risk for heart defects. *Am J Obstet Gynecol.* 166:1473–9, 1992.

44. Dubinsky TJ, Nyberg DA, Mahony BS, et al.: Hyperechogenic fetal bowel: Clinical significance. *J Ultrasound Med.* 12:S55, 1993.

CHAPTER
THIRTEEN

Operating a Fetal Echocardiography Laboratory

Gina Harris

This book contains an enormous amount of information about the performance of fetal echocardiography. When preparing to write this particular chapter on operating a fetal echocardiography laboratory, I made the assumption that there would be ample information in the literature about managing an ultrasound suite. I quickly learned that I was mistaken. After a thorough search, I found a scarcity of such information. There is an abundance of information about the physics of ultrasound and how to perform ultrasound studies, but there is essentially nothing available to guide those of us who manage these units.

This chapter outlines issues to consider when establishing and operating a fetal echocardiography laboratory. General recommendations are discussed. It is impossible to provide specific rules to adhere to, because all health care systems are different and have their own unique strengths and barriers to overcome. Each institution must decide for itself how priorities are to be set regarding equipment purchases, staffing levels, space allocations, and the like. These priorities must change from system to system depending on such factors as the institution's mission, the population served, the location of the facility, obligations for education and research, and availability of resources.

The reader may finish this chapter with more questions than answers. However, those questions and the process of answering them form the foundation for planning and implementing a fetal echocardiography unit. To date, this chapter contains the entirety of information that this author is aware of that relates to the subject of operating a laboratory for fetal echocardiography, or perinatal ultrasound in general. As with any

emerging specialty area, the pool of information is sure to expand as that specialty is practiced on a larger scale. This is likely to be true for fetal echocardiography. It is my hope that this chapter serves as a stimulus for future authors to share their expertise in managing these units.

PHYSICAL FACILITIES

Space, specifically the amount, organization, and location of that space, is a fundamental factor in establishing a fetal echocardiography laboratory. "The physical facilities in which perinatal care is provided should be conducive to care that meets the unique needs of mothers . . . , fathers, and families" (p. 26).[1] If you have the luxury of planning the space for the perinatal ultrasound unit rather than making the unit fit a predetermined space, you should take advantage of your opportunity by planning early and carefully. Planning the physical facilities is best handled by utilizing a team approach. It is essential to involve representatives from the following areas:

- Physicians (including Maternal–Fetal Medicine and Cardiology)
- Ultrasonographers
- Nurses
- Plant engineering
- Clinical engineering
- Facilities design
- Information services
- Administration

Each institution has limitations that must be accounted for, and "provisions for individual units should be consistent with a regional perinatal care system and state and local public health regulations" (p. 26).[1] Resources that should be consulted in planning the ultrasound unit include the following:

- American Institute of Ultrasound in Medicine (AIUM)
- Association of Registered Diagnostic Medical Sonographers (ARDMS)
- Joint Commission on the Accreditation of Healthcare Organizations (JCAHO)
- American College of Obstetricians and Gynecologists (ACOG)
- American Academy of Pediatrics (AAP)

Utilizing an interdisciplinary approach helps ensure that such regulations are adhered to and that the needs of the patients and staff are met.

Location of the Ultrasound Unit

Ideally, the ultrasound unit should be located in close proximity to the other obstetric services that patients must access. For ultimate patient convenience, it is desirable to be close to the prenatal clinic, but it is not absolutely essential. At the University of Missouri, the Perinatal Assessment Suite is located in an ambulatory care building adjacent to University Hospital. However, the prenatal clinics are both located off site, approximately 2 miles from the hospital. To minimize difficulties that patients may have in attending appointments in separate sites, the staff makes a point of coordinating appointments to allow adequate travel time. In the future, there are plans to relocate all of the prenatal clinics to the same ambulatory care building as the Perinatal Assessment Suite.

If invasive fetal surveillance procedures are to be performed on patients who are past the point of viability (defined at University Hospital as 24 weeks' gestation), it is essential that the ultrasound unit be in close proximity to Labor and Delivery. In the event that the fetal status becomes nonreassuring (e.g., fetal distress, placental bleeding), it is critical that the delivery be accomplished quickly. If it is impossible to locate the ultrasound unit in close proximity to Labor and Delivery, it becomes necessary to make arrangements to perform such invasive procedures within Labor and Delivery or in an area that is in close proximity. In addition, mechanisms must be put into place by which patients with nonreassuring fetal status (e.g., preterm labor, cervical incompetence, fetal distress) can be transported to Labor and Delivery. When such an event occurs at University Hospital, the Emergency Services staff are contacted, and the patient is transported to the inpatient facility via ambulance. Invasive procedures that must be performed after 24 weeks' gestation are scheduled and performed in one of the labor rooms.

Number of Rooms

In planning the optimal number of rooms in the fetal echocardiography laboratory, it is essential to analyze current patterns of care and give consideration to the following factors:

- Projected patient volume (including "peaks and valleys" in that volume)
- Projected exam time
- Potential other uses for the rooms (to allow for flexibility)
- Allowances for expansion of services

The following formula can be used to estimate the number of fetal echocardiography rooms needed.

$$\frac{\text{Number of projected exams per year}}{\left(\begin{array}{c}\text{Number of operating} \\ \text{days per year}\end{array}\right) \times \left(\begin{array}{c}\text{Number of examina-} \\ \text{tions per day}\end{array}\right)}$$

Example:

$$\frac{\text{5000 fetal echo examinations per year}}{\text{250 operating days} \times \text{6 examinations per day}}$$

$$\approx 3 \text{ ultrasound rooms}$$

If the ultrasound rooms in which fetal echocardiograms are performed are also used for other perinatal sonography, this must be factored into the equation.

Example: 5000 exams per year
- 1500 fetal echos (average = 6 examinations/day) = room used 30% of time
- 3500 perinatal ultrasounds (average = 10 examinations/day) = room used 70% of time

250 operating days × 0.3 (fetal echo time) = 75 days of fetal echos per year
250 operating days × 0.7 (perinatal scan time) = 175 days of perinatal scans per year

$$\frac{\text{5000 examinations per year}}{\left(\begin{array}{c}\text{75 fetal echo days} \\ \times \text{6 exams/day}\end{array}\right) + \left(\begin{array}{c}\text{175 perinatal ultrasound} \\ \text{days} \times \text{10 scans/day}\end{array}\right)}$$

$$\approx 2 \text{ scan rooms}$$

Size of Rooms

There are no national regulations regarding acceptable size of ultrasound rooms. At University Hospital's Perinatal Assessment Suite, the ultrasound rooms are 100 ft^2 (10 ft × 10 ft). This allows enough room for the ultrasound machine, an examination table, a small desk, a stand for the printer, and a tall filing cabinet. There is enough space to accommodate the sonographer, a physician, and one or two family members. This size room has been found to be adequate, but if it is possible to plan for a slightly larger room (e.g., 12 ft × 12 ft), this is preferable.

Organization of Space

To be cost effective, it is preferable to combine like areas into one unit. Fetal echocardiography is one aspect of fetal surveillance and perinatal subspecialty care. Patients requiring fetal echocardiography quite often require additional subspecialty services. As a result, it is logical that the fetal echocardiography laboratory be located within a fetal assessment unit. Additional services that should be considered for inclusion in the type of unit described are routine prenatal ultrasound, electronic fetal monitoring (i.e., nonstress testing), prenatal diagnostic procedures (i.e., genetic amniocentesis, chorionic villus sampling, amniocentesis for fetal blood typing), Maternal–Fetal Medicine consultation, and prenatal care for complex patients who are managed by the Maternal–Fetal Medicine specialist.

The configuration of the ultrasound rooms themselves should be considered carefully. It is preferable to have them in close proximity to each other within the unit to optimize traffic flow. If a computerized information management system is planned, either for image management or report production, proximity makes the networking process much simpler. In addition, work flow is optimized if the ultrasonographers are able to maintain close contact with each other. This contact facilitates collaboration among the sonographers, improving the quality of the work that is produced. It also allows the sonographers to assist each other when workload becomes unevenly distributed, such as when patients do not keep their appointments or studies take longer than originally planned, thus improving work efficiency.

This room estimate provides a starting point from which to refine the unit's space requirements. In addition to ultrasound rooms, space should be allocated for consultation before or following the examination. Information that is shared during consultation is sensitive. It focuses on such issues as paternity, family history of genetic disorders or malformations, use of illicit substances, and decisions regarding continuing versus terminating pregnancy. Often, information that is given to families is unfavorable and upsetting. For these reasons, all examination and consultation rooms must be single rooms, and extreme care must be taken to ensure privacy.

To facilitate the operation of the unit, the following areas must be planned:

- Storage area
- Utility areas (both clean and dirty)
- Clerical area
- Waiting area
- Physician work area
- Nursing work area

Areas that should be considered for inclusion in the plans for the ultrasound unit are examination rooms and a children's activity area. Examination rooms can be utilized for clinic visits, history taking, physical examination, or additional consultation space. If these are available, the unit can function as a private clinic as well as a fetal surveillance area. Because the population served by the ultrasound unit is families, one must consider the likelihood of patients needing to bring their children with them to their visits. It is optimal to plan an area in which the children can play during their parents' visit. At University Hospital, such an area exists within the general waiting area for the unit. Recommendations are made to patients before their visit that if children must attend, the patients should have another adult accompany them so they may supervise the child(ren) in the play area during the patient's visit.

Climate Control

One critical element that must be addressed early in the planning process is that of ventilation and temperature control of the ultrasound rooms. Ultrasound machines produce tremendous amounts of heat. In a 100 ft³ room like that described above, it takes only a few hours for the room temperature to rise to approximately 99°F when a standard air conditioning system is in place. These temperature extremes are not only uncomfortable, they can create a health hazard for patients and staff. In addition, they lead rapidly to ultrasound equipment malfunction and potentially permanent damage to the equipment.

To maintain optimal ultrasound room climate control, these rooms should be cooled separately from the remainder of the rooms in the unit. It is preferable to have the temperature of each room controlled by a separate thermostat. If separate control is not possible and the ventilation and air conditioning system must be set up in a zone format, this is another reason to ensure that the rooms are in close proximity to each other.

PERSONNEL

Qualifications

The quality of personnel selected to staff the fetal echocardiography laboratory is a critical element for the quality of the studies produced by the unit and for the satisfaction of patients cared for in the unit. Over the years, it has become clear that the one characteristic that is most important in a staff member is that of attitude. Most intelligent people can be trained to perform a number of skills, but no one can make another person have a positive attitude or a strong work ethic. When interviewing candidates for staffing positions, this is the characteristic on which I place the highest priority.

In addition to possessing positive personality characteristics, there are several qualifications that are preferable for the sonographers to meet. Sonographers should be RDMS certified or eligible for certification. In order to comply with the American Institute of Ultrasound in Medicine requirements for accreditation, sonography staff must be certified by the ARDMS or eligible for certification at the time of application for initial accreditation. Staff who are registry eligible must acquire certification before the next accreditation cycle. To maintain certification, staff must pursue continuing education activities. It is essential that the sonography staff take responsibility for their own continuing education. However, time and resources must be devoted to supporting the staff in these activities.

Sonographers in the fetal echocardiography laboratory should possess a thorough knowledge of fetal anatomy and have experience with perinatal ultrasound, especially morphology scans. In addition, they should have a thorough understanding of the clinical aspects (i.e., risk factors, expected outcomes, therapeutic interventions) of the fetal cardiovascular disease processes being studied. These characteristics allow the sonographer to function as an active member of the interdisciplinary team caring for the patient and her fetus. They also form the knowledge base from which the sonographer can participate in the education of students and resident physicians.

Staffing Guidelines

Just as there is minimal information in the literature about operating an ultrasound suite, there are no magic formulas available for calculating optimal staffing numbers. Time spent observing perinatal ultrasound and fetal echocardiography reveals that an anatomic survey (morphology scan) requires approximately 30 to 45 min to complete. Fetal echocardiography requires approximately 60 min to perform each study. This allows adequate time to review the rest of the fetal anatomy and conduct a full evaluation of the fetal heart. At University Hospital's Perinatal Assessment Suite, the sonographer begins the examination by performing the anatomic survey, including basic views of the fetal heart. The study is then finished by the Maternal–Fetal Medicine Specialist and an adult or pediatric cardiologist, who perform the complete fetal echocardiogram.

To calculate the necessary number of sonographers for the practice, the same formula that was used to calculate the number of ultrasound rooms can be utilized.

$$\frac{\text{Number of projected examinations per year}}{\left(\begin{array}{c}\text{Number of operating}\\\text{days per year}\end{array}\right) \times \left(\begin{array}{c}\text{Number of examina-}\\\text{tions per day}\end{array}\right)}$$

Example:

$$\frac{5000 \text{ fetal echo examinations per year}}{250 \text{ operating days} \times 6 \text{ examinations per day}}$$

$$\approx 3 \text{ ultrasonographers}$$

Scheduling Guidelines

To calculate the optimal number of fetal echo appointments available in a given day, the maximum available study hours in each day must be calculated. Fillinger and Zwolak[2] calculated the maximum number of hours available per vascular technologist for performance of studies by subtracting "time spent during each 8-hour day for equipment maintenance, physician consultation and discussions with referring physicians, breaks, coordinating emergent studies, supply purchases, continuing medical education, and 'non-study' clerical time" (p. 252). The following summarizes this calculation:

8.00 h possible work time per day
−0.75 h physician consultation per day
−0.50 h breaks per day
−0.75 h coordinating emergent studies, clerical time, etc.
6 h maximum available study hours per day

Once the maximum number of available study hours has been estimated, the schedule can be developed based on which days certain studies are performed and how long each of those types of studies take. Six hours maximum available study time per day can accommodate any of the following schedules:

- 6 fetal echos (at 1 h per study) per day
- 3 fetal echos (at 1 h per study)
  +4 anatomic surveys (at 45 min per study)
- 4 fetal echos (at 1 h per study)
  +2 anatomic surveys (at 45 min per study)
  +2 limited scans (at 15 min per study)

It is advisable to build into the schedule a number of "emergency" appointment slots. It is quite common for a referring provider to contact the perinatal ultrasound unit to schedule a patient who requires a study either the same day or the next day. By analyzing the patterns of referrals to your service, the optimal number of such slots can be determined so as to balance availability and cost effectiveness.

Support Staff

The care of the patient with pregnancy complications is accomplished by an interdisciplinary team. The ultrasonographer, the Maternal–Fetal Medicine Specialist and the cardiologist collaborate to perform the diagnostic procedures and outline the medical plan of care for the patient and her unborn child. However, the support staff are essential to patient care and unit functioning, as well.

Nursing staff assist in coordinating care, which is often complex and may involve numerous providers, such as Cardiothoracic Surgery, Anesthesiology, and Neonatology. Because the care is complex, there are often numerous information and education needs, and the nursing staff provides this education. In addition, the nurse often acts as a contact person for the patient and her family once they have left the unit. If the fetal echocardiography laboratory is part of a larger perinatal assessment unit, the nursing staff will establish its own relationship with the patient as they provide ongoing care, such as antenatal testing.

Social workers are a key component of the interdisciplinary team. Patients and families who find that their unborn child has a cardiac defect enter a grieving process. The social worker plays a critical role in patient and family support. The social worker can provide this support on an individual basis or assist the family in locating local or national support groups. The care that is required by the patient and the care that may be required by the infant are quite expensive, and the social worker can help these families identify resources that may provide some financial assistance.

The clerical staff are fundamental to the successful operation of any system, and the fetal echocardiography laboratory is no exception. These staff members perform scheduling, billing, and customer service functions that cannot be underestimated. Often, they develop a professional relationship with patients and families who are followed in the perinatal assessment unit, and they, too, are sources of ongoing care and support for these families. Because these staff members have a unique perspective on the "flow" of the unit, the planning and implementation of a fetal echocardiography laboratory should include them from the beginning.

EQUIPMENT

Equipment Selection

Selection of an ultrasound machine is a process that brings out the personal opinions of the staff who are to be using the equipment. There are a number of manufacturers of high-quality ultrasound machines, and each company produces several levels of machines. Each machine has features that are preferred by the sonography staff and others preferred by the medical staff. As with buying a car, a television, or a major appliance, people become loyal to certain manufacturers. Because of these factors, it is impossible to recommend a particular ultrasound machine for use in the fetal echocardiography laboratory. It is only possible to make suggestions about features that are preferable.

The machine that is selected should be at or near the top of the line produced by the manufacturer. To optimize the study, the ultrasound should have the following features:

- M-mode
- Color M-mode
- Steerable pulsed and continuous wave Doppler
- Color flow mapping
- Power angiography
- High-frequency, high-resolution transducers (5 to 7 MHz)
- Lower-frequency transducers (2 to 5 MHz) for patients who are difficult to image

Without these features, it may be difficult to determine the exact cardiac lesion that is present. Finally, it is optimal that the equipment have factory preset optimization packages for fetal echocardiography and Doppler exams along with the ability for the user to make adjustments.

Selection of the ultrasound equipment should be a group effort. It is essential to work with the sonography staff and the Maternal–Fetal Medicine and Cardiology physicians, who use the equipment to ensure that the equipment selected optimizes their clinical practice. Clinical engineering staff need to be involved early in the process because they are responsible for ensuring the safety of patient care equipment. Also, in many institutions, these are the staff that are on site to deal immediately with equipment malfunction. If ultrasound information (i.e., images, reports, correspondence) is to be shared with multiple areas or sites, it is critical to involve the Information Services staff from the very beginning. The level of desire to network ultrasound equipment and servers has a powerful impact on which machine should be selected and features that are required in that machine. For example, a number of ultrasound machines are now available with DICOM as a standard feature. DICOM is not a required feature, but it is preferable in that it can be connected more directly to information management systems without the need for additional computer hardware. These issues should be addressed early in the selection process, and forming an equipment acquisition team can facilitate the process.

Equipment Maintenance

As with any patient care equipment, care and maintenance of the ultrasound equipment is a key issue. Policies that address frequency of maintenance should be in place, and procedures that outline specifics for how the equipment is cared for must be developed. These policies should include the following topics:

- Cleaning the transducers, cables, housing, etc.
- Electrical safety checks
- Quality assurance audits

Cleaning the equipment is a fundamental activity, but it is crucial for ensuring patient and staff safety. The transducers and other parts that come in contact with patients must be cleaned and disinfected properly between patients in order to comply with infection control policies. Cleaning procedures and accepted products for disinfecting the equipment are outlined in the ultrasound equipment manuals. There are numerous options, and it is not difficult to identify an option that can fit any budget. It is critical, however, to adhere to these recommendations to avoid invalidating the equipment warranty. Ultrasound equipment is quite costly, and the importance of ongoing care to extend its life should not be minimized. Care in using the equipment and diligence in maintaining it will keep the ultrasound in service as long as possible and prevent unnecessary replacement costs.

Electrical safety checks are also important for patient and staff safety. The frequency of these checks is usually determined by the institution. Most institutions maintain a policy for performing electrical checks before use of the equipment for patient care and, then, ongoing checks either annually or semiannually. It is important to involve the clinical engineering staff early in the equipment acquisition process so they can plan for these checks and become familiar with the equipment if they are not already.

Quality assurance audits must be put into place to provide an ongoing evaluation of the technical performance of the ultrasound devices. The frequency of these audits is usually recommended by the ultrasound manufacturer, and they can range from audits every 3 months to annual audits. These audits consist of such assessments as equipment calibration and studies using phantom models. They are crucial to maintaining the diagnostic capability of the devices used in the fetal echocardiography laboratory, and they must be completed unfailingly to ensure the quality of the studies produced in that laboratory.

When developing an equipment maintenance plan, a key decision that must be made is whether to purchase a maintenance contract with the ultrasound manufacturer or to utilize internal resources (e.g., clinical engineering) for such maintenance. If the decision is made to enter into a maintenance contract, the equipment acquisition group must take the cost of this contract into consideration when the budget is prepared. These contracts usually cost approximately 8% to 10% of the original purchase price of the equipment. As such, they may range from $10,000 to $25,000 for 1 year of service. The decision regarding the cost effective-

ness of such a contract rests with the equipment acquisition group and the institution's administration. The alternative to purchasing maintenance contracts is to utilize internal resources for equipment maintenance. At University Hospital, the Clinical Engineering staff have received specialized education and training so that they are qualified to perform routine equipment checks and correct basic equipment malfunctions. Again, the decision remains one of institutional preference, but it is essential to determine a plan to ensure that equipment maintenance is completed.

INFORMATION MANAGEMENT

In the world of business in general, and in health care specifically, information management is critical to the success or failure of an organization. The same is true of the fetal echocardiography laboratory. In designing an information management system, the following components must be considered:

- Document storage and record keeping
- Image management
- Reporting
- Communication with referring providers

Document Storage and Record Keeping

In health care, the need to maintain patient records is well established, and entire departments are devoted to this process. The key issues regarding document storage center around patient confidentiality, accessibility of information to providers, and duration of record storage. Policies and procedures must be developed so that fetal echocardiography study results are stored in a manner that protects patient confidentiality but also allows easy accessibility to the information for comparison with future studies. It can be as simple as a group of locked files or as complex as a computerized information network. Regardless of the method utilized, it is prudent to plan the system at the same time the ultrasound equipment is being selected and space needs are being determined.

Image Management

Issues of accessibility and patient confidentiality must be addressed as policies and procedures are developed for image management. As with document storage, there are a number of ways to store ultrasound image information. These range from printing images on thermal paper and taping the images to the back of the ultrasound report to utilizing a computerized image management system. The type of system to use, one that uses film or one that is essentially paperless, is a decision that must be addressed at the time that the ultrasound machine is selected. The following are a number of factors to consider in making that decision between a film system or a filmless system:

- Cost of the hardware
- Cost of the disposables (i.e., paper, film, disks)
- Cost of personnel time handling images
- Quality and longevity of the images
- Available storage space
- Desire for hard copy of the images
- Need to network multiple sites
- Staff's comfort level with computers

At University Hospital, we are currently in the process of installing a filmless image management system. A cost comparison was completed, and the results revealed the potential for an annual cost savings of approximately $90,000, primarily in the cost of disposable items (i.e., film). Other cost savings are anticipated from the sonographers no longer needing to spend valuable time and energy handling the ultrasound images and preparing them for interpretation and storage.

Before we were able to move to such a system, however, a major practice change was necessary. The physicians and ultrasonographers had to agree that they would no longer print hard copy images of all ultrasound studies. The system is capable of producing prints of the ultrasound images, but the staff need only print those studies in which the actual images are to be sent to the referring provider. This type of system does not work in all settings, but the cost savings and potential for networking with multiple sites make it worth evaluating.

Reporting

The decision regarding whether or not to utilize a computerized reporting package is one of personal preference and budgetary freedom. The ultrasound devices have basic reporting packages as standard features, and these work well for producing written documentation of study findings. However, if the budget allows inclusion of a separate reporting package, this would be preferable. There are several effective and user-friendly reporting packages on the market, and more are rapidly being developed. These programs capture data from the ultrasound machine and put this information into a number of formats, such as a progress note or a letter. In addition, some packages are capable of compiling statistical information to create a database. Again, the decision to utilize a reporting package is one based on financial priorities. It is not an essential component of the ultrasound system, but it is preferable to include if it is financially possible.

Communication with Referring Providers

The patient population that is served by the fetal echocardiography laboratory is primarily that which is acquired from a strong referral base. Because the unit is part of a larger tertiary care system, the vast majority of patients seen in the fetal echocardiography laboratory are patients referred from other obstetric care providers. The success of the unit is dependent on a constant flow of referrals, and the satisfaction of the referring providers determines this. It is critical that the flow of information to those referring providers remain continuous, prompt, and as uninterrupted as possible. In planning an information management system, this ongoing communication with referring providers must be considered. A number of mechanisms for such communication exist, including the following:

- Dictating and mailing letters or progress notes
- Composing and faxing letters or progress notes via modem
- Calling the referring provider shortly after the visit
- Sending a copy of the written progress note with the patient to the referring provider
- Including the referring provider in an online medical record network

Each institution must decide for itself, based on its resources and the preferences of its physicians and referring providers, how information is to be communicated with those providers in the most efficient and effective manner.

ULTRASOUND ACCREDITATION

One of the issues that must be addressed when operating a perinatal ultrasound unit is whether or not to pursue accreditation of that laboratory. This is a question that is currently being debated by most providers of perinatal ultrasound services, and it is likely to receive more attention as time passes.

Rationale for Accreditation

According to the American Institute of Ultrasound in Medicine,[3] "with the rapidly expanding ultrasound technology and the increasing numbers of physicians utilizing ultrasound as a diagnostic tool, it is critical that standards and guidelines are established to ensure high quality patient care." This organization has developed guidelines for ultrasound practice and for the training of professionals who perform ultrasound, and in 1995 the group developed a process for ultrasound practice accreditation. Their rationale for pursuing accreditation is summarized as follows[3]:

> Applying for AIUM Ultrasound Practice Accreditation offers physicians and sonographers an opportunity to examine their standards and practices and compare them to nationally accepted ones. It fur-

ther allows a practice to gauge its strengths and weaknesses and to initiate changes for improving and strengthening the practice. The benefit of accreditation is that it will raise the awareness of quality ultrasound practice. It will increase patient confidence with the knowledge that the physician they have selected is in compliance with nationally accepted standards established by the profession to ensure quality patient care. (p. 2)

AIUM Accreditation Process

The process for applying for ultrasound accreditation is quite straightforward, and the AIUM has made the information easily accessible. A summary of the accreditation process and preliminary information is available from the American Institute of Ultrasound in Medicine's website at http://www.aium.org.

The first step in the process is to contact the AIUM and request an application packet. This can be accomplished at the AIUM's website or at the following address and phone:

American Institute of Ultrasound in Medicine
14750 Sweitzer Lane, Suite 100, Laurel, MD 20707
Phone: 301-498-4100   Fax: 301-498-4450

Assembling the application packet is a straightforward process, but adequate time should be allowed for gathering the information and completing the forms. If the necessary policies, procedures, and programs are in place, the packet itself can be completed in a few days. Completed application packets are accepted on a quarterly basis: March 1, June 1, September 1, and December 1. Once the application has been submitted, the review process takes approximately 4 months to finish. Although the process is not complicated, the following suggestions may help streamline it:

- Begin the application process early and allow adequate time to complete the packet.
- Acquire a set of AIUM standards and training guidelines to refer to as you complete the application.
- Review the application packet to assess your unit's compliance with the AIUM recommendations.
- If you determine that your unit is lacking any of the recommended policies or procedures, put these into place as soon as possible.
- If you determine that your unit is lacking a quality assurance program, begin the process to develop such a program.
- If your unit does not meet a recommendation, describe in detail your plan for coming into compliance.

Currently, the ultrasound accreditation process is voluntary. At the time of this writing, an issue of great debate is whether or not it will or should become a requirement for operating an ultrasound unit. In the current atmosphere of managed care, the other great debate is whether or not third-party payors will or should reimburse for studies performed in nonaccredited laboratories. Although the debates are far from finished, it is apparent that the prudent approach is to pursue voluntary ultrasound accreditation. The process itself is an eye-opening experience into the functioning of the ultrasound unit, and it allows the manager to put into place those mechanisms that ensure high-quality service.

QUALITY ASSURANCE

Rationale

Historically, ultrasound laboratories have not had formal quality assurance (QA) programs. The American Institute of Ultrasound in Medicine is just one of the factors that is encouraging the development of ongoing QA in the perinatal ultrasound and fetal echocardiography laboratory. Each year, the pressure of the Joint Commission on the Accreditation of Healthcare Organizations (JCAHO) for more widespread QA programs increases. As mentioned earlier, third-party payors are certain to increase their demand for proof of quality in determining reimbursement. As a result, a formal QA program is an essential component for the viability of the prenatal ultrasound unit.[4]

Components

The AIUM's description[3] of QA recommendations in its website summary is that "the ultrasound equipment specifications and performance must meet all state and federal requirements. Instrumentation used for diagnostic testing must be maintained in good operating condition and undergo periodic calibration. Evidence of proper maintenance must be documented." (p. 4) This provides a general overview of the AIUM's expectations, but a more thorough review of the application itself provides even clearer direction regarding recommended components for a QA program.

The application that the Perinatal Assessment Suite at University Hospital submitted outlined the following components for its Quality Assurance Program:

- Equipment maintenance and calibration: Our plan is to utilize a process similar to the QA audit format followed by the ultrasound manufacturer. It will address such issues as image quality, electrical power requirements and output, and mechanical integrity of the system.
- Correlation of ultrasound findings with other

diagnostic and clinical findings: This will be accomplished in a conference format in which ultrasound images will be reviewed and findings compared with clinical outcomes (e.g., infant physical examination data, description of pelvic anatomy at the time of cesarean section, pathology report information).

- Review of studies ordered for medical appropriateness: This component will be conducted at the conference just described. This type of practice review is essential to ensure proper utilization of technology and resources, and it is critical to the physician training process.
- Follow-up of abnormal ultrasound findings: This will be addressed in the conference format just described as well. These findings will also be discussed in a weekly multidisciplinary perinatal conference that is attended by obstetric and neonatal medical and nursing staff, pediatric medical subspecialty staff, pathology staff, perinatal ultrasound staff, social services staff, and medical students.
- Follow-up of complications: At University Hospital, there is already a process in place by which these types of variances are documented and tracked. These variances are reviewed and potential system issues and solutions are discussed at a monthly interdisciplinary QA meeting. Complications related to ultrasound procedures are included in this system.

By following the recommendations outlined in the AIUM applications, it is possible to establish a sound QA program for ultrasound. Like the accreditation process itself, formalized ultrasound QA is rapidly gaining support and popularity. It may take some time before it is mandatory, but it is prudent to begin formalizing the process before that time. Efforts to establish parameters for quality and maintain the highest level possible can only serve to improve the satisfaction of the customer, whether that is the patient and her family or the referring provider.

PHILOSOPHY OF THE UNIT

Family-Centered Approach

The fetal echocardiography unit is part of a larger perinatal subspecialty care system that provides services to patients experiencing complicated pregnancies. By definition, the population served is families. As such,[1] the "system should be oriented toward providing family-centered care, the underlying assumption of which is that the family is the primary source of support for anyone receiving health care services. Family-centered health care professionals engage parents as care givers and partners and seek to ensure that every encounter builds on the family's strengths, preserves their dignity, and enhances their confidence and competence. These health professionals strive to understand each family's priorities and needs, incorporating the family's perspectives into an individualized plan of care . . . ." (p. 9). This concept should be communicated and subscribed to from the administrative level to the bedside, and it should be reinforced often so that the family remains the focus of the department's efforts.

Service-Oriented Attitude

Most health professionals entered health care based on the desire to serve others, namely patients. However, service orientation focuses on service not only to our patients, but to those other individuals and systems that access our services. Entire texts have been written about customer focus and service orientation. Such an in-depth discussion is not necessary here. It is important, however, to communicate throughout the department that in the business of health care, customers will purchase services from businesses that meet their needs and treat them well. For the fetal echocardiography laboratory, this means that each physician's office that schedules a patient, each patient that inquires about results, and each hospital that requests records must be treated as if they were the first priority for the staff. A common misconception within some systems is that managed care contracts alone determine referral patterns, so service orientation is no longer essential. Contracts and affiliations do determine referral patterns, and an organization's service orientation is often a key factor in establishing those contracts and affiliations. Establishing and reinforcing a service-oriented attitude is critical to the survival of a fetal echocardiography laboratory, and this attitude must be conveyed throughout the staff.

Nonjudgmental Viewpoint

The need for fetal echocardiography is based on the risk for a congenital heart defect in the fetus. If the fetal echo confirms the existence of such a cardiac defect, the option of pregnancy termination is provided in many instances. If the patient and her family select this option, staff in the fetal echo unit must be supportive of their decision. Likewise, staff must support a family's decision to continue a pregnancy. The majority of staff who work in perinatal areas have confronted these issues early in their careers and have worked through their feelings regarding such dilemmas. It is because they are able to remain nonjudgmental that they can provide ongoing guidance and care to families faced with such difficult decisions.

SUMMARY

Ten years ago, the concept of an interdisciplinary team working together to manage a patient was relatively new. In 1998, this concept is central to the functioning of any perinatal subspecialty service, especially one that offers fetal echocardiography. Members of the interdisciplinary team, including Maternal–Fetal Medicine Specialists, Pediatric Cardiothoracic Subspecialists, Perinatal Sonographers, Advanced Practice Nurses for the subspecialties, staff nurses, social workers, and hospital chaplains pool their expertise to provide optimal care to families preparing for a child with a cardiac defect. In a similar fashion, these same professionals team up with financial staff, clerical staff, information specialists, and administrators to orchestrate the operation of the fetal echocardiography laboratory. Each individual brings a different perspective to the table in designing and operating the unit. When each member of the team recognizes these strengths and puts aside his or her personal agenda, the collaboration can provide the foundation for a strong and successful fetal echocardiography laboratory.

REFERENCES

1. Hauth JC, Merenstein GB (Eds.): *Guidelines for Perinatal Care*, 4th ed. Elk Grove Village, IL: American Academy of Pediatrics and The American College of Obstetricians and Gynecologists; 1997.
2. Fillinger MF, Zwolak RM: Will the vascular laboratory remain economically viable? Impact of the RBRVS payment system. *Semin Vasc Surg.* 7(4): 251–60, 1994.
3. American Institute of Ultrasound in Medicine: *Ultrasound Practice Accreditation*, http://www.aium.org.
4. Baker JD: Quality assurance in the vascular laboratory. *Semin Vasc Surg.* 7(4): 241–4, 1994.

CHAPTER Fourteen

Congenital Cardiac Defects in the Fetus

Guy A. Carter, Darla B. Hess, L. Wayne Hess, and Maria L. Evans

Congenital heart disease (CHD) accounts for almost half of all deaths attributed to lethal malformations in children.[1] These defects in cardiac anatomy and function are four times as common as neural tube defects and over six times as common as serious chromosomal defects.[2] The heart therefore has become a focus of investigation as developments in ultrasound technology have permitted physicians to spy on the previously cloistered fetus. With these investigations it is becoming increasingly apparent that CHD in the fetus, the newborn infant, and the growing child is a dynamic continuum of abnormal embryonic development resulting in deviant anatomic structure and resultant abnormal physiology and function. The intrauterine environment and the cardiac physiology are considerably different for the fetus compared to the newborn and the older infant, with major physiologic transitions required at birth. After birth, as the infant takes the first breath, pulmonary vascular resistance falls dramatically and pulmonary vascular flow correspondingly increases, resulting in functional closure of the foramen ovale; the ductus arteriosus closes as the Pao_2 (blood oxygen content) rises and circulating ductal maintenance prostaglandins fall.[3] Cardiac malformations that were present in utero become symptomatic as the defect compromises the infant's cardiac capabilities, with the presenting symptoms of congestive heart failure, cyanosis, or some combination of both. During fetal development, abnormalities in cardiac development may also become symptomatic, resulting in fetal congestive heart failure (expressed as nonimmune hydrops) or fetal death. Whether the defect presents clinically in the fetus before birth or in the neonate after birth, and the clinical features that are expressed, depend on the severity of the anatomic deviation and the resultant impact on the functional capability of the heart.

FREQUENCY AND DIAGNOSIS OF CONGENITAL HEART DEFECTS

The incidence of CHDs diagnosed in infants and children has typically been reported between 8 and 10 per 1000.[1–8] A wide variety of cardiac defects have been identified in infants and children (summarized in Table 14–1). Previous authors have noted that the incidence of cardiac defects is significantly higher in autopsy series of infants dying within the first month of life and the spectrum of defects seen differs, with more severe structural abnormalities (Table 14–2) more frequently identified in this group than in the more global population of infants and children. The incidence of structural cardiac defects identified in stillborn infants of over 20 weeks of gestation is even greater, with reported incidences of 23.5 to 63 per 1000.[1,5,9–11] These observations are consistent with the concept of congenital cardiac defects as a dynamic continuum: The more severe structural defects would be expected to produce a greater aberrancy of cardiovascular physiology with fetal distress and, when incompatible with continued growth and development, death of the individual fetus or neonate in early pregnancy or shortly following birth.

Cardiac defects in infants and children are typically first suspected and subsequently diagnosed as the physiologic changes in cardiac function and altered blood flow patterns induced by the structural defect become clinically evident. In the infant or older child this is most frequently found by the auscultation of a heart murmur, the appearance of cyanosis, or clinical congestive heart failure. For example, a ventricular septal defect (Figure 14–1) becomes evident within weeks after birth as the pulmonary vascular resistance

TABLE 14–1. CONGENITAL HEART DEFECTS IDENTIFIED IN INFANTS AND CHILDREN (PERCENTAGE OF ALL CHDS)

	Toronto[4]	Mitchell et al.[5]	Chicago[6]	California[1]
Ventricular septal defect	28.3	29.1	18	31.3
Atrial septal defect	10.3			
Secunduum	7.0	7.4	7.6	6.1
Primum	1.4	1.3		
AV canal	2.0	3.1	3.2	3.7
Pulmonary stenosis	9.9	10.5	8.5	13.5
Patent ductus arteriosus	9.8	7.7	11.1	5.5
Tetralogy of Fallot	9.7	3.5	13.1	3.7
Aortic stenosis	7.1	3.5	2.9	3.7
Coarctation of the aorta	5.1	6.6	6.3	5.5
Transposition of the great arteries	4.9	2.4	4.4	3.7
Common ventricle	1.5	0.9	1.0	0.6
Mitral and aortic atresia	1.5	3.3	1.4	0.6
Partial anomalous pulmonary venous drainage	1.4		0.5	
Total anomalous pulmonary venous drainage	1.4		0.8	0.6
Vascular ring	1.2	1.5	0.7	
Tricuspid atresia	1.2	1.1	2.4	
Endocardial fibroelastosis	0.9	0.7	1.6	
Pulmonary atresia	0.7	1.5	0.8	
Truncus arteriosus	0.7	1.9	1.7	2.5
Congenital aortic regurgitation	0.6		0.1	
Double-outlet right ventricle	0.5		0.3	0.6
Ebstein's anomaly	0.3		0.8	
Coronary artery anomalies	0.3	1.5	0.5	
Congenital mitral stenosis	0.2		0.1	
Interrupted aortic arch	0.2			
Primary pulmonary hypertension	0.2		0.3	
Aortopulmonary window	0.2		0.4	
Common atrium	0.2			
Tumor of the heart	0.1			
Cor triatriatum	0.1		0.2	
Miscellaneous		6.1	6.4	17.8

falls and the shunt flow correspondingly increases across the defect, producing turbulent flow and the appearance of an audible murmur. The other associated findings are defined by the extent of the physiologic alterations. With the increasing pulmonary vascular flow (systemic venous return plus the shunt volume) returning to the left ventricle, increasing the volume and resultant workload of the left ventricle, an enlarged and thickened left ventricle develops. This is identified by an increased heart size on chest x-ray examination and left ventricular hypertrophy on electrocardiography. The clinical signs associated with congestive heart failure begin to appear as the ventricular workload imposed on the heart begins to exceed cardiac capability.

Other structural defects may present earlier or later and may present with a different character of signs and symptoms depending on the degree and manner of alteration on cardiac hemodynamics resulting from the structural defect. An atrial septal defect (Figure 14–2) wherein the shunt dynamics produces a lesser degree of turbulence, and thus a softer murmur, and the shunt volume is better tolerated by the right ventricle and may not exceed cardiac capacity, may not be suspected or diagnosed for several years following birth. Defects with more severe alterations of function, as in transposition of the great arteries or critical aortic stenosis, are more likely to present with clinical symptoms shortly after birth.

Diagnostic accuracy and increased understanding of these cardiac defects have been augmented with the

TABLE 14–2. TYPES OF CONGENITAL HEART DEFECTS BY AUTOPSY DATA IN THE FIRST MONTH OF LIFE (PERCENTAGE OF TOTAL CASES)

	Toronto 111 Cases 1968–1970	Baltimore 83 Cases 1969–1971	Boston 350 Cases 1960–1969	Buffalo 165 Cases 1949–1964
Hypoplastic left heart syndrome	24.3	10	15	12
Coarctation of the aorta	17.1	13	14	13
Transposition of the great arteries	11.7	28	19	15
Truncus arteriosus	5.4	2	3	4
Tetralogy of Fallot	4.5	4	0.3	7
Ventricular septal defect	4.5	12	0.6	2
Pulmonary atresia	3.6	3	11	6
Pulmonary stenosis	3.6	2		
AV canal	3.6	1.4	0	4
Atrial septal defect	1.8	6	0	0
Total anomalous pulmonary venous drainage	1.8	1	4.9	0.6
Patent ductus arteriosus	0.9	2	0.6	2

Adapted, with permission, from Keith JD, Rowe RD, Vlad P: In Heart Disease in Infancy and Childhood. *New York: Macmillan Publishing Co., Inc.; 1978: p. 8.*

development of higher-resolution echocardiography and Doppler ultrasound systems. Real-time two-dimensional imaging of the heart enables direct noninvasive imaging. of the structural abnormalities that define the different cardiac defects. Equally important in formulating an accurate diagnosis of cardiac defects is the delineation of the changes in cardiac anatomy secondarily induced by the altered function associated with a structural defect. The enlargement of the left atrium and ventricle resulting from a left-to-right shunt at the ventricular or great vessel level is equally important in identifying a large ventricular septal defect, even before the defect is directly imaged, or in further differentiating a truncus arteriosus (Figure 14–3) from severe tetralogy of Fallot, both of which present anatomically with a large ventricular septal defect and an overriding aortic valve. The addition of Doppler (including color, continuous, and pulsed wave) ultrasound interrogation to the real-time sector scan will define the abnormal flow associated with a defect. This can aid in identifying a smaller muscular ventricular septal defect that may not have been definable by direct imaging, or by quantifying the velocity of flow to estimate the severity of a stenotic lesion as aortic or pulmonary stenosis.

The definition of cardiac defects during fetal development, where the examiner must deal with a patient who cannot be visualized directly and is within another individual, presents unique challenges. Other than changes in fetal heart rate or rhythm, or conditions apparent on obstetrical ultrasound that indicate probable fetal cardiac distress, such as nonimmune hydrops fetalis, the fetus frequently does not otherwise provide direct clinical clues to suggest the presence of

cardiac defects. Diagnosis during fetal development depends on the direct echocardiographic visualization of the defect, the changes in cardiac size or configuration secondary to the altered hemodynamics, and/or Doppler definition of aberrant flow patterns resulting from the functional aberrations. With contrasting cardiac function in utero compared to postpartum existence, the spectrum of diagnosed cardiac defects (see Table 14–3) and the echocardiographic and Doppler characteristics of these defects is similarly different. The most frequently diagnosed fetal cardiac defects are those that produce the more dramatic abnormalities of the intracardiac structure, such as atrioventricular canal, hypoplastic left heart syndrome, or common ventricle (univentricular heart), or that produce more severe deviation from normal cardiac function, such as critical aortic stenosis, Ebstein's anomaly of the tricuspid valve, or cardiomyopathy.[11–15] Extrapolating from the incidence of cardiac defects in stillborn fetuses, it is estimated that the incidence of cardiac defects in utero should be greater than the 8 to 10 per 1000 reported in newborns and children,[1,5] and that a greater incidence of more severe abnormalities should be seen. To evaluate the fetal heart more accurately and recognize the spectrum of structural aberrancies more completely, there must be an understanding of the differing cardiac function in the fetus contrasted to that in the infant and child.

FETAL CARDIOVASCULAR PHYSIOLOGY

The fetal heart functions within a very different environment in utero compared to postnatal demands. The

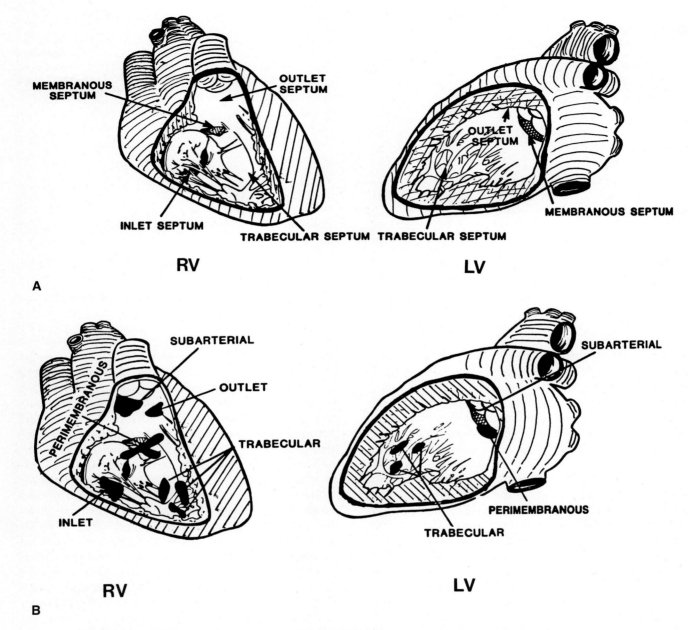

Figure 14–1. A. Cutaway views of the right ventricle (RV) and left ventricle (LV) showing the four portions of the ventricular septum: 1) outlet septum; 2) membranous septum; 3) inlet septum; and 4) trabecular septum. **B.** Cutaway views of the right ventricle (RV) and left ventricle (LV) showing the five types of ventricular septal defects (VSDs): 1) subarterial; 2) outlet; 3) perimembranous; 4) inlet; and 5) trabecular.

most obvious and important difference in the fetus is that the respiratory organ is the placenta, which receives its vascular flow in parallel with the systemic circulation (as branches of the iliac arteries) and returns the venous flow through the ductus venosus to the right atrium. During this time the ventricles function in parallel, sharing an equal pressure but not necessarily equal volume loads. Cardiovascular development must

progress such that at the moment of birth the infant has the capacity to abandon the placenta and begin using the lungs as the primary respiratory organ. As the lungs become the primary respiratory organ, the neonate must convert from the parallel circulatory pattern of the fetus to the adult series form of circulation, with the ventricles sharing equal volume loads but not necessarily equal pressure loads. The functional compro-

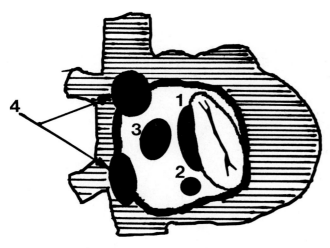

Figure 14–2. Cutaway view of the right atrium shows the four types of atrial septal defects: 1) primary; 2) coronary sinus; 3) secondary; and 4) sinus venosus.

mises that these divergent roles entail, along with the developmental changes of the cardiac structure and myocardial capabilities through pregnancy, define the nature of fetal cardiac physiology. In studies of fetal physiology, invasive studies have used the fetal lamb as an animal model, whereas the echo and Doppler studies have typically been of human in utero studies. The understanding of fetal cardiovascular hemodynamics has grown dramatically over the last three decades because of sophisticated animal studies and the progressive advent of diagnostic ultrasonography.

Before birth and after normal septation into a right and left ventricle, the fetal ventricles function in a parallel circulatory pattern rather than in the series fashion seen throughout the rest of the child's postnatal life

(Figure 14–4). To accommodate this there are alterations of cardiac anatomy that are functional and essential during fetal life but are normally discarded at birth. The left sixth aortic arch persists up to birth to provide a vascular communication between the pulmonary artery and the descending aorta (the ductus arteriosus), whereas the developing septa of the atrium (the septum primum and septum secundum) overlap to provide a valvelike function of the atrial septum that is permissive of flow from the right to the left atrium but prevents flow in a reverse direction.[16]

Blood distribution through the two parallel systems is not equal in either volume or oxygen content but is distributed with equal pressures by the ventricles. The orientation of the inferior vena cava (IVC) to the crista dividens of the foramen ovale divides the flow from the IVC into two streams that enter the right and left atria.[3,17,18] The eustachian valve, which extends from the anterior junction of the IVC with the right atrium toward the foramen ovale, aids in directing IVC return to the left atrium. Thus, oxygenated venous return from the placenta through the ductus venosus and IVC is preferentially directed into the left atrium, left ventricle, and ascending aorta. Of the total venous return to the heart, the inferior vena caval flow represents about two thirds of the total, and the flow across the foramen ovale about 25% of the total return. Superior vena caval flow, which comprises over one fifth of the total venous return, courses through the right atrium into the right ventricle. The right ventricle therefore pumps about 65% of the combined cardiac output, whereas the left ventricle pumps 35% (fetal cardiac output is customarily expressed as the combined output of both right and left ventricles).[17] The right ventricular output is divided between the lungs (5% to 10% of the combined output) and flows across the ductus arteriosus into the descending aorta (55% to 60% of the com-

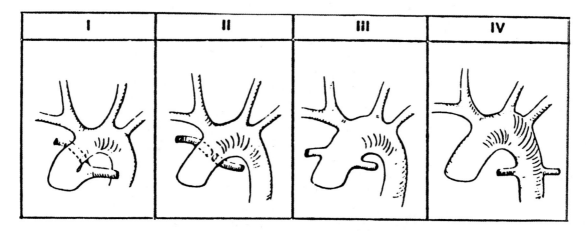

Figure 14–3. Types I–IV truncus arteriosus, after Collett and Edwards.

TABLE 14–3. CARDIAC DIAGNOSIS OF PRENATAL CONGENITAL HEART DEFECTS (PERCENTAGE OF TOTAL CASES)

	Connecticut[7] 170 Cases	London[8] 1009 Cases
Atrioventricular canal	21.8	17.5
Aortic valve atresia	12.9	16
Double-outlet right ventricle	8.8	3.3
Ventricular septal defect	8.2	5.9
Mitral atresia		5.9
Tetralogy of Fallot	6.5	4.6
Critical aortic stenosis	6.5	4.1
Cardiomyopathy		4.1
Univentricular heart	4.1	1.8
Ebstein's anomaly	4.1	7.4
Atrial isomerism	3.5	
Transposition of the great vessels	3.5	2
Coarctation of the aorta	2.9	11.2
Pulmonary atresia	2.9	5.5
Pulmonary stenosis	2.4	
Tricuspid atresia	2.4	4.5
Truncus arteriosus	1.8	1.4
Atrial septal defect	1.2	
Pulmonary atresia with ventricular septal defect	0.6	
Tumor		1.3
Absent pulmonary valve		1
Aoritic–left ventricular tunnel		0.4
Total anamalous pulmonary venous drainage		0.3
Other	5.9	0.5

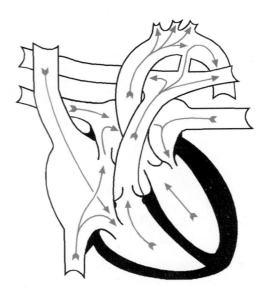

Figure 14–4. Normal fetal cardiac circulatory pattern. Arrows indicate direction of flow but do not reflect volume or velocity of flow. The foramen ovale functions as a valve, permitting right to left atrial flow but preventing reverse flow.

bined output), with the placenta eventually receiving 40% to 45% of the combined output. The left ventricular output is predominately directed into the coronary and brachiocephalic circulations, with only 10% of the combined output crossing the aortic isthmus.[17] The dominant axis of fetal ventricular output is thus: right ventricle > main pulmonary artery > ductus arteriosus > descending aorta.[18] With this parallel circulation and unrestricted communication between the systemic and pulmonary circulations across the ductus arteriosus, and pulmonary vascular resistance maintained at or above systemic vascular resistance during fetal development,[17] the pressures generated within the right and left ventricles are normally equal.

There is considerable change in the developing fetus throughout the gestational period. In order realistically to determine abnormalities at different times within normal gestation, normal changes in size and or configuration must be understood. Schmidt et al.,[19] us-

ing echocardiographic estimates previously validated in fetal sheep,[20] determined that ventricular volumes as calculated from two-dimensional echocardiography increased exponentially from 18 weeks of gestation to term. Calculated mean right ventricular volumes increased from 0.69 mL at 20 weeks to 2.86 mL at 30 weeks and 7.80 mL at 40 weeks of gestation, and left ventricular volume increased from 0.55 mL to 2.51 mL and 7.39 mL, respectively, over the same time intervals. The estimated mean combined cardiac output was 123 mL/min, 507 mL/min, and 1385 mL/min at 20, 30, and 40 weeks, respectively. Sahn et al.[21] measured the changing size of the cardiac structures by evaluating the diameters of the different chambers through pregnancy. In their study measurements were made just inferior to the atrioventricular (AV) valves from typical four-chamber views, timing diastole from valvular motion, and changing size was correlated to estimated fetal weight. Their data defined an increasing diameter of the ventricles equated to aWt^b, where Wt = fetal weight in grams; for the right ventricle, $a = 0.128$, and $b = 0.315$; for the left ventricle, $a = 0.099$ and $b = 0.329$; and for the total cardiac dimension, $a = 0.356$ and $b = 0.284$. In a more extensive evaluation of cardiac growth in the normal fetus, Tan et al.[22] measured dimensions for ventricular and atrial widths and lengths as well as diameters for the ductus arteriosus, great arteries, and superior and inferior vena cavae correlated to gestational age in weeks. Their data showed similar changes for ventricular size to those of Sahn et al.[21] (Table 14–4A).

Ursell et al.,[23] in an autopsy study of second-

TABLE 14–4A. REGRESSION EQUATIONS FOR CARDIAC SIZE RELATED TO FETAL AGE IN WEEKS

View and Chamber[a]	Equation (y = dimension, x = fetal age)
Four-chamber view	
LV width	$y = -0.9478 + 0.1090x - 0.001153x^2$
LV length	$y = -2.318 + 0.2356x - 0.002674x^2$
LA width	$y = -1.246 + 0.1305x - 0.001563x^2$
LA length	$y = -0.6508 + 0.0873x - 0.000674x^2$
RV width	$y = -0.9869 + 0.1075x - 0.001036x^2$
RV length	$y = -1.5082 + 0.1634x - 0.001514x^2$
RA width	$y = -1.4025 + 0.1410x - 0.001671x^2$
RV wall thickness	$y = -0.2315 + 0.02677x - 0.000316x^2$
Ventricular septum	$y = -0.1415 + 0.0200x - 0.000185x^2$
LV wall thickness	$y = -0.2135 + 0.2552x - 0.000295x^2$
Short-axis view	
Ductus arteriosus	$y = -0.01539 + 0.01325x$
Main pulmonary artery	$y = -0.1517 + 0.0279x$
Left pulmonary artery	$y = -0.0554 + 0.0136x$
Right pulmonary artery	$y = -0.0058 + 0.0117x$
Aortic width	$y = -0.4149 + 0.05327x - 0.000495x^2$
Aortic length	$y = -0.2770 + 0.03759x - 0.000174x^2$
RA width	$y = -2.145 + 0.1976x - 0.00273x^2$
RA length	$y = -1.2949 + 0.1406x - 0.001393x^2$
Long-axis view	
LV width	$y = -0.1739 + 0.0465x$
LV length	$y = -0.4990 + 0.0868x$
LA width	$y = -0.3422 + 0.0498x$
LA length	$y = -0.6408 + 0.0707x$
Sagittal view	
Inferior vena cava	$y = -0.09012 + 0.01883x$
Superior vena cava	$y = -0.004078 + 0.01673x$

[a]LV, left ventricle; RV, right ventricle; LA, left atrium; RA, right atrium.
Reprinted, with permission, from Tan J, Silverman NH, Hoffman JIE, Villagas M, Schmidt KG. Cardiac dimensions determined by cross-sectional echocardiography in the normal human fetus from 18 weeks to term. Am J Cardiol: 1992; 70:1459–67.

trimester fetuses, noted a linear increase in size of the arterial valvular diameters from 10 to 26 weeks. They also noted that the pulmonary valve was slightly larger than the aortic valve at all ages studied, and that the diameter of the aortic isthmus was slightly smaller than either the aortic valve or the descending aorta. These differences were ascribed to the differential in flow within these areas. Alterations of these values should be anticipated as a consequence of the changes in cardiac structure, function, and hemodynamics resulting from the developmental aberrations that define the CHDs.

Fetal cardiac mechanics continues to be an area of active investigation. To interpret prenatally diagnosed cardiac defects properly or to consider fetal cardiac in-terventions, it is essential to understand fetal cardiac mechanics and the mechanisms that can be recruited to optimize fetal cardiac function. In the fetus, as in the infant and child after birth, the major determinant variables for cardiac function are preload, after-load, inotropic state, coronary blood flow, and heart rate. Throughout gestation there are continuing changes in the structural and biochemical characteristics of the fetal heart. These changes include increases in the number and cross-sectional area of cardiac myocytes, increases in myofibrillar density, the development of sarcoplasmic reticulum, growth of the coronary arteries, an increase in myosin adenosine triphosphate activity, a change in myofilament sensitivity to calcium, and a decrease in glycogen levels,[24–27] which may suggest that there are major alterations in mechanical function associated with normal development. Studies to date have not correlated these structural changes with preload, after-load, or functional mechanics of the fetal heart.[27] In some studies little increase in cardiac output was observed with increasing preload.[28–33] Weil et al.[27] have speculated that although the fetal heart demonstrates a clear Starling mechanism, it may not be able to recruit reserve function because it functions near the peak of the curve at rest, and that the wall stress associated with working at the peak of the Starling curve may be a primary stimulus of fetal cardiac growth. Grant et al.[34] came to the conclusion that, in the fetus, pericardial pressure significantly limited left ventricular diastolic filling and stroke volume. They suggested that end-diastolic pressures did not accurately reflect increases in left ventricular volume if pericardial pressure increased concomitantly. They evaluated left ventricular end-diastolic diameter or left ventricular end-diastolic transmural pressure as indicators of preload and concluded that there was an increased cardiac function that could be attributed solely to an increased preload. They also concluded that ventricular interaction and pericardial pressure were interdependent and that an increase in right ventricular volume could decrease left ventricular volume and output by both displacing the septum to the left and simultaneously increasing the pericardial pressure over the left ventricular free wall. The current published data do not as yet conclusively define the correlation between the changes observed in the fetal heart and fetal cardiac functional mechanics.

As studies in animal models continue to define the correlates of fetal cardiac mechanics, the Doppler ultrasound evaluation of vascular flow characteristics is also being used to define the variations in flow characteristics and distribution in the normal and compromised human fetus.[35–38] Studies of atrioventricular valve flow velocities demonstrate that both early (E) and late (A) flow velocities (Figure 14–5) increase lin-

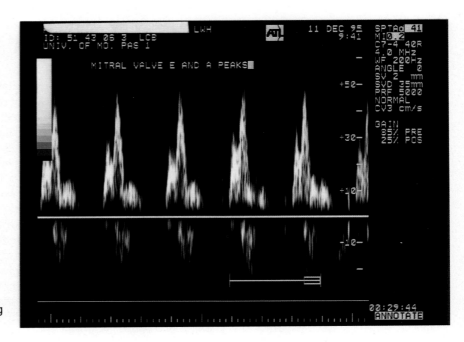

Figure 14–5. Doppler sonogram showing E and A peaks across mitral valve.

early with advancing fetal age; E velocities, however, increase more rapidly than A velocities, becoming nearly equal near term. A velocities remained higher than E velocities throughout gestation, suggesting that although fetal ventricular compliance increases throughout gestation, it remains lower than seen in the newborn and that fetal ventricular filling depends on atrial contraction. Tricuspid velocities were higher than mitral velocities at all ages before term[35–38] (Table 14–4B), with the ratio of the mitral valve to tricuspid valve E velocity of 0.96 (± 0.2) and an A velocity ratio of 0.93 (± 0.19).[36] These suggest that with the larger fetal right ventricular mass, right ventricular compliance is less than left ventricular compliance. Similarly, an age-related increase in peak flow velocity across the semilunar valves was as-

cribed to a reduction of after-load with decreasing vascular resistance in the umbilical, placental, and truncal levels; however, no age-related change was reported in the ascending aorta.[37] Fetal compromise is associated with significant alterations of both the arterial and the venous sides of the fetal circulation.[35] Compensatory arterial mechanisms are generated by fetal hypoxemia and mediated by arterial chemoreceptors.[39] Redistribution of blood with the highest oxygen saturation is designed to maintain oxygen delivery to the myocardium and the brain.[35] Hecher et al.[35] hypothesized that when the compensatory mechanisms of arterial redistribution reached their maximum limits, changes in the venous flow velocities occurred. In the human fetus it is currently not possible to measure volume flow (and redistribution) reliably by Doppler techniques (measurement errors of fetal vessel diameter, especially in a vessel with pulsating flow, limit the utility of Doppler techniques). Hecher et al.[35] described alterations in the peak systolic to peak diastolic (S/D) flow ratio and the percentage of reverse flow in the inferior vena cava in fetuses with cardiac defects and other causes of fetal compromise.

These reports indicate that diagnosis in the fetus of cardiac defects that result in fetal compromise can be improved with the understanding of fetal hemodynamics and the effective application of Doppler ultrasound techniques (utilizing not only color Doppler but also pulsed and continuous wave techniques) in addition to two-dimensional real-time imaging of fetal cardiac structure. The flow defect may present as reversed flow across a structure such as the ductus arteriosus

TABLE 14–4B. FLOW VELOCITIES AT 14 TO 16 WEEKS OF FETAL AGE

| | E Wave (cm/s) | | Peak A Wave (cm/s) |
	Mean	*Peak*	
Mitral valve	7.9 ± 1.6	20.3 ± 4.7	37.6 ± 6.3
Tricuspid valve	9.7 ± 2.1	23.1 ± 4.9	41.9 ± 5.3

	Mean	Peak
Ascending aorta	11.6 ± 1.7	38.7 ± 6.3
Pulmonary artery	11.2 ± 2.0	35.7 ± 6.7

Reprinted, with permission, from Wladimirhoff JW, Stewart PA, Burghouwt MT, Stijnen T. Normal fetal cardiac flow velocity waveforms between 11 and 16 weeks of gestation. Am J Obstet Gynecol: 1992; 167: 736–9.

(heralding severe right heart outflow obstruction) or the foramen ovale (frequent with variants of the hypoplastic left heart syndrome),[40] abnormal flow characteristics (such as the regurgitant flow of an aortic to left ventricle tunnel),[41,42] or more flow variations such as the changes in S/D ratio indicating associated changes in cardiac mechanics.[35] The appreciation of the hemodynamic compromise present is also of importance in counseling the parents regarding the likelihood of continuing the pregnancy to term and of potential problems that the infant may encounter after birth.

DIAGNOSTIC CHARACTERISTICS OF FETAL CONGENITAL HEART DEFECTS

Diagnostic echocardiographic visualization of cardiac structure by utilization of at minimum a four-chamber view should be possible in over 90% of all fetuses of 18 weeks' gestation or older.[43] The four-chamber view has become a standard component of obstetrical scans and is part of the obstetric ultrasound guidelines published by the American College of Obstetricians and Gynecologists (ACOG).[44] Indeed, in some series reporting congenital cardiac defects in the fetus, an abnormal four-chamber view has become the most common reason for referral for fetal echocardiography.[45] The four-chamber view identifies or suggests the presence of cardiac defects either directly by visualizing the structural aberration or indirectly by the changes in the cardiac structure induced by the deviant flow. This view alone should detect AV canal, hypoplastic left ventricle, single ventricle, mitral and/or tricuspid atresia, double-inlet right ventricle, Ebstein's anomaly, and large ventricular septal defects.[12]

Since the four-chamber view alone does not visualize the outflow tracts or the great vessels associated with either ventricle, there are a significant number of defects that typically are not identified by the four-chamber view alone. These include tetralogy of Fallot, truncus arteriosus, transposition of the great vessels, disease of the aortic or pulmonary valves, total or partial anomalous pulmonary venous drainage, coarctation of the aorta, and subaortic or subpulmonic ventricular septal defects.[46] Complete fetal echocardiography should consist of multiple views to define the structure and associations of the atria, ventricles, valvular components, great arteries, and venous inflow. The views should include the four-chamber view to show both atria and ventricles and the AV valves; a long-axis view to show the left ventricular outflow tract; sagittal views to show the pulmonary bifurcation, the aortic arch, and the ductal arch; short-axis views to show the right ventricular outflow tract; and apical short-axis views to show ventricular structure and the left ventricular papillary muscles.[15] Doppler ultrasound

should be used in addition to define blood flow patterns through the cardiac structure.

In a normal four-chamber view the heart should occupy about one third of the thorax; the two atria are of approximately equal size; the two ventricles are of approximately equal size and thickness and contract equally; the atrial and ventricular septa meet the two AV valves at the center of the heart in an offset cross; and two opening AV valves are seen.[13] With imaging of the great arteries using other views, two arterial valves can be seen; the aorta arises wholly from the left ventricle; the pulmonary trunk is slightly bigger than the aorta; the pulmonary valve is anterior and craniad to the aortic valve; at their origins the great arteries lie at right angles to and cross over each other; and the arch of the aorta is of similar diameter to the aorta and is complete.[13] In addition, the fetal position, the location (side) of the fetal stomach, and the relationship of the suprahepatic portion of the inferior vena cava to the right atrium should be noted to determine situs. Deviations from these criteria are the basis for the diagnosis of the cardiac defects.

Serial ultrasounds to assess the fetal heart and fetal condition are recommended when the pregnancy is continued. Recent evidence indicates that cardiac defects can be progressive in utero.[47,48] Pulmonary stenosis identified early in the second trimester may progress to pulmonary atresia or hypoplastic right ventricle.[46] Similarly, the development of nonimmune hydrops fetalis can develop later in the pregnancy from the presence of such severe structural cardiac defects as tricuspid insufficiency or Ebstein's anomaly of the tricuspid valve. Ventricular septal defects occurring as an isolated defect have shown spontaneous closure on subsequent examinations.[15]

Atrioventricular Canal

Although not the most common of congenital cardiac defects in the infant and child, an atrioventricular (AV) canal is generally described no more commonly than aortic stenosis or transposition of the great vessels (see Table 14–1). This cardiac defect (Figure 14–6) however, is the most frequently diagnosed of all cardiac defects identified in the fetus[13,15,46,49] (see Table 14–3). This defect is characterized by a large defect at the crux of the heart, involving the atrial and ventricular septa and the AV valves, producing an easily diagnosed malformation in the four-chamber view (Figure 14–7).[50] In the complete form of AV canal, the AV valve ring is not septated into a mitral and a tricuspid valve but exists as a common valve ring with five leaflets.[49] There is persistence of the foramen primum and failure of the developing ventricular septum to close with the endocardial cushions, resulting in a large common septal defect of the

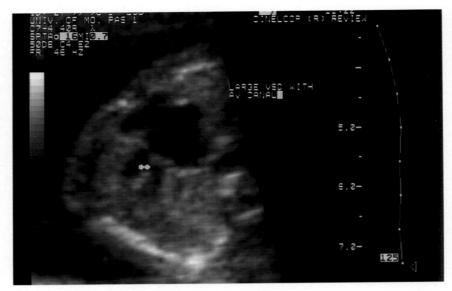

A

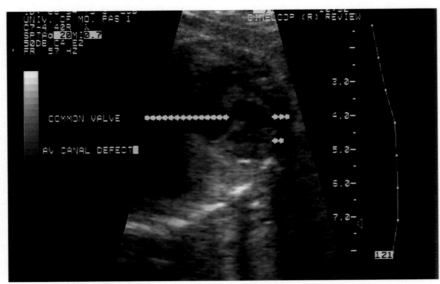

B

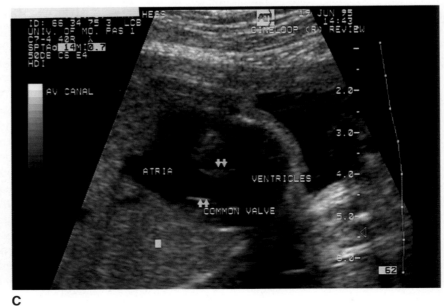

Figure 14–6. Atrioventricular (AV) canal defect. **A.** Double arrows show large VSD (ventricular septal defect). **B.** Triple arrows = left ventricle; double arrows = right ventricle; line of arrows points to common AV valve. **C.** Double arrows point to common AV valve leaflets.

C

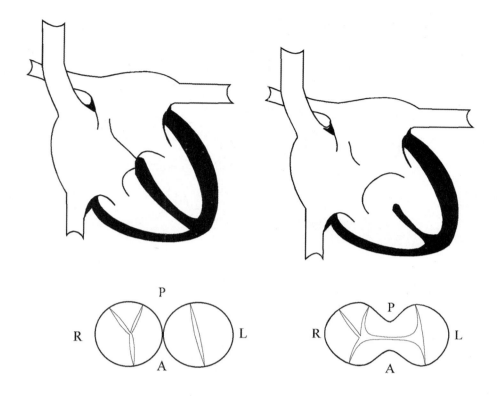

Figure 14–7. Normal four-chamber view (left) and the four-chamber view with complete AV canal defect. Note that in the normal heart the mitral valve resides slightly higher (toward the left atrium) than the tricuspid valve. With complete AV canal both valves lie at the same level and bridge across the defect in the central part of the heart. The valve configuration as viewed from above is diagramed below the heart diagrams.

lower atrial and upper ventricular septa. This defect is frequently associated with other complex cardiac defects or chromosomal defects, especially trisomy 21.[13,15]

Postnatally, the infant with an AV canal presents with increasing pulmonary vascular flow as pulmonary vascular resistance falls following initiation of pulmonary respirations and right ventricular compliance increases. These changes promote increasing left-to-right flows across both the atrial and the ventricular components of this defect. Additionally, the abnormal division of the AV valve results in valvular insufficiency, particularly of the mitral valve component. These abnormalities of function eventuate in congestive heart failure in the majority of infants with this defect.

Prenatally, with higher pulmonary vascular resistance and decreased right ventricular compliance with a thicker right ventricular wall, abnormal shunts at atrial and ventricular levels are not evident. Gembruch et al.[49] noted that, with all cases of identified complete AV canal, the diastolic blood flow interrogated with color flow or pulsed Doppler ultrasound did not show turbulence in either ventricle. However, significant AV valvular insufficiency may be present. Valvular insufficiency can be found by Doppler interrogation in nearly 75% of identified instances of complete AV canal. If there is pansystolic insufficiency (rather than limited to early systolic insufficiency only), nonimmune hydrops frequently develops.[49] Doppler interrogation usually does not show the presence of shunting at atrial or ventricular level but may demonstrate other abnormalities

of flow (such as reverse systolic flow in the ductus venosus and the hepatic vein), indicating the severity of cardiac dysfunction.

Complete AV canal defect can be readily diagnosed early in the second trimester by the characteristic anatomic changes in the cardiac configuration evident on two-dimensional fetal echocardiography. The large defect in the central portion of the heart includes the lower portion of the atrial septum (failure of the foramen primum to close) and the upper portion of the ventricular septum, with an apparently common AV valve. This AV valve spans the defect, which opens and has chordal attachments into the right and left ventricles, is difficult to miss, and is diagnostic of a complete AV canal defect. Because of the high incidence of associated chromosomal abnormalities (particularly trisomy 21) with this defect, when an AV canal malformation is evident karyotyping of the infant and screening for other noncardiac defects is important.[13,49,50]

Univentricular Heart

The univentricular heart category is used to describe all hearts in which both the systemic and pulmonary venous returns converge on a single ventricular chamber. The heart may be functionally univentricular because of failure of either the right or the left ventricle to grow normally (hypoplastic ventricle) or because of failure of embryologic development to progress normally through division of the early common ventricle into a true right and left ventricle (Figures 14–8 and

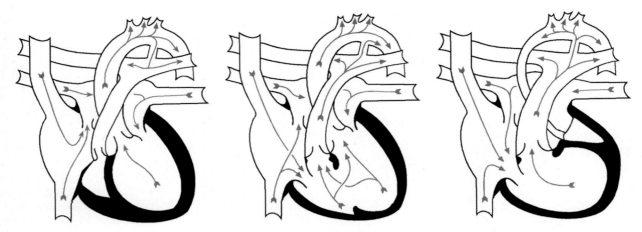

Figure 14–8. Variations of the univentricular heart. Tricuspid atresia with hypoplasia of the right ventricle, intact ventricular septum, and normal association of the great vessels are shown on the left. A common ventricle of indeterminate type and normal great vessel association is shown in the center diagram. The hypoplastic left heart syndrome with mitral and aortic valve atresia and hypoplasia of the ascending aorta are shown on the right.

14–9). Failure of growth may occur because of an absent atrioventricular communication (tricuspid or mitral atresia) or inadequate ventricular outflow development (pulmonary or aortic atresia). The diagnosis of univentricular heart is further described by defining the number of inflow valves, the anatomic character of the functioning ventricle, and the number and position of the outflow tracts. The hypoplastic left heart syndrome therefore would be a single-inlet univentricular heart

with right ventricular anatomy, and a single-outlet pulmonary artery without transposition. The common physiology of the univentricular heart is persistence of the parallel circulatory pattern with mixing of systemic and pulmonary circulations within the single pumping chamber. Cardiac output from the common ventricle is not typically divided evenly into the pulmonary and the systemic circulations. Blood flows are proportional to pulmonary and systemic vascular resistance if no

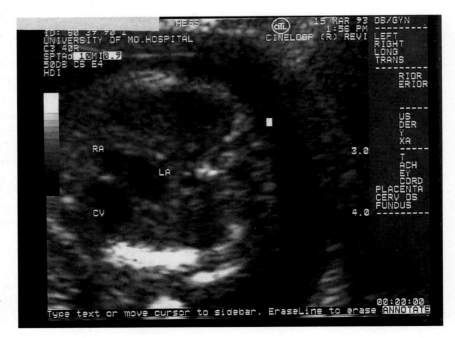

Figure 14–9. Sonogram of univentricular heart. RA = right atrium; LA = left atrium; CV = common ventricle.

other restrictions are present. With outflow atresia (either pulmonary or aortic) the blood flow into the circuit associated with the atretic valve will depend on the continued patency of the ductus arteriosus following birth. Before birth the total cardiac output is frequently maintained at nearly normal levels, and the pregnancy progresses normally. The aberrant intracardiac flows may, however, result in progressive changes in cardiac growth and development that can be visualized on serial echocardiograms. Following birth, the normal series type of circulation cannot be established and the neonate rapidly becomes progressively compromised by the aberrant hemodynamics. The clinical presentation will vary from severe cyanosis if the pulmonary circulation is compromised, shock if the systemic circulation is compromised, or congestive heart failure if both the pulmonary artery and the aorta communicate with the common ventricle without restrictions.

These defects produce a similar and recognizable two-dimensional echocardiographic picture with only one ventricle identified, or, if a rudimentary ventricle is present, marked discrepancy in ventricular sizes. The hypoplastic left heart syndrome is characterized by underdevelopment of the aorta, aortic valve, left ventricle, and mitral valve. Typically, both the aortic and mitral valves are atretic, and the ventricular septum is intact. The left ventricle can vary in size from essentially slitlike to smaller than normal.[51] All of the blood flow is carried by the right side of the heart, with resultant enlargement of the right atrium and ventricle.[51,52] Hypoplasia of the right ventricle (Figure 14–10) is typically

seen with and categorized by either pulmonary atresia, usually with an intact ventricular septum; hypoplasia of the right ventricular outflow tract and underdeveloped main pulmonary artery; or tricuspid atresia, either with or without a ventricular septal defect.[51] The right ventricle can vary from a slitlike ventricle (more typically seen with pulmonary atresia with intact septum) to more moderate hypoplasia (more consistent with tricuspid atresia with a ventricular septal defect).[51] Tricuspid atresia can be subdivided by the presence or absence of a ventricular septal defect, the presence of associated transposition of the great arteries (either d or l types), and the degree of pulmonary stenosis.[54] With atresia of either the pulmonary or the tricuspid valves, all of the blood flow is carried across the foramen ovale into the left atrium and via the mitral valve through the left ventricle. With a hypoplastic left heart or pulmonary atresia or with tricuspid atresia with an intact ventricular septum, the ductus arteriosus provides the only link for blood flow that would otherwise have traversed the atretic valve structure (the systemic or pulmonary circulation becomes dependent on ductal patency).

Traditional wisdom would maintain that the morphologic characteristics of the hypoplastic left heart are present from the time of early cardiac development (the first 6 to 8 weeks of fetal development). Allan et al.[53] have described serial ultrasound studies of a fetus that demonstrated aortic stenosis with a left ventricle of normal size at 22 weeks, but developing striking ventricular disproportion consistent with hypoplastic left ventricle by 32 weeks. Pulmonary atresia, particularly

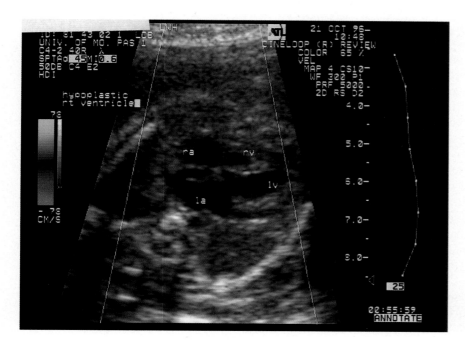

Figure 14–10. Hypoplastic right ventricle. RA = right atrium; LA = left atrium; RV = right ventricle; LV = left ventricle.

when gross tricuspid insufficiency is present, may present with a normal size right ventricle in early pregnancy but have a disproportionately small right ventricle by birth.[46,55]

The appearance of what has been described as the more classic single ventricle varies depending on the nature of the atrioventricular connection, the morphology of the dominant ventricle, and the nature of the ventricular–arterial connections. The AV valve connection may be double inlet, a single common AV valve, or an atretic AV valve; the dominant ventricle may be of right, left, or indeterminate character; and the arteries may be normally related, d transposed, or l transposed (d = dextrorotated; l = levorotated.)[56]

Postnatal mortality and morbidity for this group remains high and, untreated, may approach 100%. The clinical presentation depends on the variant anatomy; however, the final surgical intervention for all variants of this group is most frequently a modified Fontan procedure or cardiac transplantation.

With hypoplastic left heart syndrome the systemic flow is progressively decreased as the ductus arteriosus closes following birth, resulting in cardiogenic shock, metabolic acidosis, and death usually within the first week of life. Norwood et al.[57] developed a staged surgical approach for treatment of the hypoplastic left heart syndrome. The first stage is performed in the newborn period and consists of reconstructing the aortic arch using the main pulmonary artery and creating a Blalock-Taussig–type shunt to the pulmonary arteries now separated from the main pulmonary artery. Subsequent stages eventuate with a Fontan-type repair.

For the infant with pulmonary atresia or tricuspid atresia with an intact ventricular septum, pulmonary blood flow is progressively compromised as the ductus arteriosus constricts. This results in progressive hypoxemia, deep cyanosis, and death shortly after birth. The creation of an aorta-to-pulmonary artery shunt is undertaken shortly after birth to increase pulmonary blood flow as initial palliation, with eventual palliation afforded by a Fontan procedure.

The clinical presentation of other variations of the univentricular heart depends on the ventricular–arterial connections and the presence or absence of outflow obstruction into either the pulmonary or the systemic circulations. The Fontan procedure eventually separates the two combined vascular flows into a series circulation, provided that favorable anatomy and size of the distal pulmonary arteries and low pulmonary vascular resistance are present.

Fetal diagnosis of the univentricular heart can be made in the four-chamber view when only one ventricle can be imaged or where there is a marked discordance in the size of the two ventricles. Caution must be exercised to avoid confusion of enlarged papillary muscles as a ventricular septum.[51] This pitfall may be avoided by delineating the relationship of the muscles with the AV valve(s). Multiple imaging planes should be used to determine the relationship of the great arteries with the ventricles. With valvular atresia, motion of the atretic valve is minimal or absent. With the hypoplastic left heart syndrome, imaging of the aortic arch defines a diminutive ascending aorta with an enlarged pulmonary artery; with pulmonary atresia the right ventricular outflow tract is diminutive and a very small main pulmonary artery is visualized. Color Doppler mapping or pulsed wave Doppler imaging indicates absent forward flow across the atretic valve and may demonstrate retrograde flow in the aorta (with aortic atresia) or the ductus arteriosus or pulmonary artery (with pulmonary atresia).[13,46,51,58]

Tetralogy of Fallot

Tetralogy of Fallot is a relatively frequent CHD that is characterized anatomically in the infant by the presence of a large-malalignment ventricular septal defect, a large aortic root that overrides the crest of the ventricular septum (arising in part from the right ventricle as well as from the left ventricle), infundibular and frequently valvular pulmonary stenosis with a smaller than normal pulmonary artery, and subsequent right ventricular hypertrophy[59] (Figure 14–11). Following birth this combination of structural defects results in decreased pulmonary flow and cyanosis, with the severity of cyanosis and neonatal distress related to the severity of the right ventricular outflow tract obstruction. In the most severe form with effective pulmonary atresia the infant depends on the ductus arteriosus to provide blood flow into the pulmonary artery, and thus oxygenated pulmonary venous return to the heart. These infants have progressively worsening hemodynamics as the ductus closes, with rapidly increasing infant morbidity and mortality. With milder degrees of right ventricular outflow obstruction the infant is not as severely compromised and may not even be obviously cyanotic. Complete surgical repair with closure of the ventricular septal defect and relief of the right ventricular outflow obstruction is possible in the neonate in whom the pulmonary artery anatomy is favorable; likewise, a Blalock-Taussig shunt may be performed shortly after birth for palliation to relieve the cyanosis. In the absence of other major anomalies tetralogy of Fallot can have a favorable outcome.

In contrast to infants, the fetus with tetralogy of Fallot does not develop right ventricular hypertrophy greater than that usually seen in normal fetal development.[60] Other than the presence of a ventricular septal

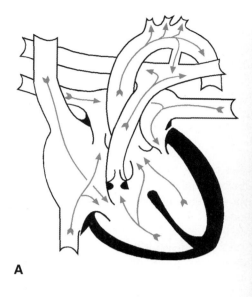

A

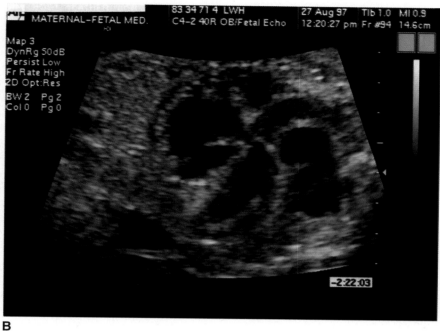

B

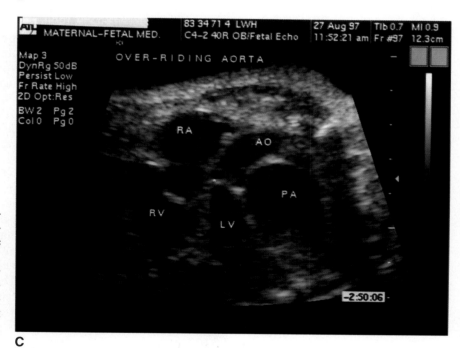

C

Figure 14–11. Tetralogy of Fallot. **A.** Characteristics include subvalvular (infundibular) pulmonary stenosis, a large sub-aortic (malalignment) ventricular septal defect, aortic root overriding the crest of the ventricular septum, and right ventricular hypertrophy. **B.** Tetralogy of Fallot. **C.** Tetralogy of Fallot. RA = right atrium; RV = right ventricle; LV = left ventricle; Ao = aorta; PA = dilated pulmonary artery.

defect, the ventricular and atrial chambers in the four-chamber view are generally normal in appearance, and the diagnosis of tetralogy of Fallot may not be apparent.[60–63] Kirk et al.[63] were able to diagnose only two of eight instances of tetralogy of Fallot prenatally with the four-chamber view alone. In the aortic-root view (five-chamber view) the overriding of the aorta and the ventricular septal defect may be demonstrated; however, the overriding is angle dependent and may be difficult to ap-

preciate.[60] Other important echocardiographic markers for the diagnosis of tetralogy of Fallot include an enlarged or dilated aortic root, a smaller than expected pulmonary artery diameter, an abnormal aorta-to-pulmonary artery ratio, and the demonstration of pulmonary stenosis. All of these findings can be progressive throughout the pregnancy, with measurements of vessel diameters near normal at 15 to 16 weeks, and may only be demonstrated on repeated evaluations as the fetus grows.[60–63] Doppler flow mapping may show retrograde flow into the pulmonary artery with increasing outflow obstruction where there is pulmonary atresia.[61,64]

Other diagnoses that may be confused with tetralogy include truncus arteriosus or double-outlet right ventricle. Truncus arteriosus has a single great artery that arises straddling the crest of the ventricular septum with a large subaortic (subtruncal) ventricular septal defect. The echocardiographic features are similar to tetralogy of Fallot with pulmonary atresia. The definitive diagnosis is made by visualizing the branched pulmonary artery arising from the aorta. The four-chamber view is most often normal. In double-outlet right ventricle both the aorta and the pulmonary artery arise from the right ventricular chamber. There is discontinuity of the aortic and mitral valves, with a ventricular septal defect beneath the crista supraventricularis.[59] Careful determination of the origin of the great vessels with multiple views assists in identification of this defect.

Coarctation of the Aorta

Coarctation is a CHD characterized by obstructive narrowing of the distal aortic arch or the proximal portion of the descending aorta. Rudolph et al.[65] classified coarctation as either localized (juxtaductal) or aortic isthmus narrowing. With juxtaductal coarctation the aorta is discretely narrowed opposite the ductus arteriosus by an eccentric shelf projecting into the lumen (Figure 14–12). The aortic arch is usually normal; how-

ever, there may be mild hypoplasia between the left subclavian artery and the coarctation site. With aortic isthmus narrowing there is a significant length of prominent tubular hypoplasia of the aortic arch at least between the left subclavian artery and the ductus arteriosus, with a localized constriction immediately adjacent to the ductus arteriosus. The ductus arteriosus is typically patent, with a diameter near that of the descending aorta, and a ventricular septal defect is usually also present.[59] A bicuspid aortic valve is typically present with either type. Coarctation of the aorta with associated cardiac anomalies [ventricular septal defect (VSD) and patent ductus arteriosus (PDA)] is the second leading cause of heart failure in the newborn, with the mortality rate for infants with complex coarctation highest in the first 2 months of life.[66]

The etiology and evolution of coarctation of the aorta are not completely defined.[8] Allan et al.[67] has suggested that coarctation is present as early as 21 weeks of gestation and that the resultant right ventricular dilatation may be evident by 26 weeks. Rudolph et al.[65] suggested that coarctation developed in response to altered hemodynamics and altered blood flow patterns, describing the contraductal shelf as an exaggeration of a normal slight indentation found in the posterior wall that became obstructive because of abnormal ductal flow diverted toward the posterior wall of the aorta. Others have suggested that there is extension of contractile ductal tissue into the aorta, which results in narrowing as the ductus closes following birth.[68] By this latter mechanism, the coarctation would not be obstructive until after birth, and another explanation for the prominent tubular hypoplasia would be necessary. With continuing studies utilizing serial fetal Doppler and two-dimensional echocardiography evaluations, Allen et al.[69] have suggested that there may be two forms of coarctation: one presenting with isthmal hypoplasia that is hemodynamically significant during fetal development, and the other only becoming apparent in postnatal life and dependent on ductal closure for its complete development. The possibility that milder forms of coarctation may be consistent with normal early fetal echocardiograms and some may not become evident until the ductus closes after birth must be considered when the diagnosis of coarctation in the fetus is contemplated. This may be a limitation to the prenatal diagnosis of this cardiac defect.

The diagnosis of coarctation of the aorta may be suspected when there is a prominent disparity between the right and the left heart structures, with the left ventricle and ascending aorta appearing smaller than the right ventricle and pulmonary artery, respectively.[70–72] Normally the right ventricular diameter is slightly larger than the left, and the diameter of the pulmonary artery is normally slightly greater than the aorta. When there is a coarctation of the aorta, the relative sizes of

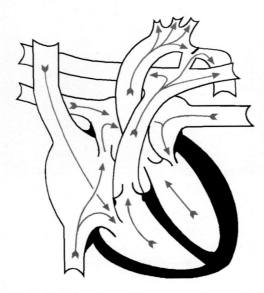

Figure 14–12. Coarctation of the aorta. The localized contraductal shelf may have a variable length of associated tubular hypoplasia of the aortic arch, a bicuspid aortic valve, and a ventricular septal defect. The ductus frequently remains patent following birth.

the right ventricle and pulmonary artery are increased. With coarctation of the aorta, the described mean ratio of the right-to-left ventricular diameters was 1.69 ± 0.16 compared to a normal ratio of 1.19 ± 0.08, and the ratio of the aorta-to-pulmonary artery diameters was 1.61 ± 0.35 compared to a normal ratio of 1.18 ± 0.06.[69,72] Although these differences were statistically significant, they represent only indirect cardiac changes resulting from the abnormal hemodynamics imposed by the developing defect. More direct evaluation of the aortic arch is also important in making a definitive diagnosis. The contraductal shelf is not visualized in a significant number of fetal echocardiographic studies even though coarctation of the aorta has been identified by other criteria.[70–72] Normal measurements of the aortic root, ascending aorta, transverse arch, isthmus, descending aorta, and left common carotid artery were reported by Hornberger et al.[70] They noted that the internal diameter of each segment increased linearly with fetal age throughout the second and third trimesters. A gradual tapering of the aorta was noted at all gestational ages, with the largest diameter at the aortic root and the smallest at the isthmus (derived ratios presented in Table 14–5). This is consistent with the normal flow dynamics in the aorta, with the least volume flowing across the isthmus from the ascending into the descending aorta. Hornberger et al.[72] concluded that quantitative distal arch hypoplasia was the most consistently identified abnormality signifying coarctation on the initial study. Diagnosis of coarctation of the aorta by two-dimensional echocardiography in the fetus requires multiple views other than the four-chamber view to visualize the aortic and ductal arches, with measurements of the aortic arch at selected levels to identify the variations from normal that define coarctation.

Doppler examination of blood flow patterns in the fetus has shown reduced flow in the aorta in 11 of 12 fetuses with confirmed coarctation.[69] Since the pressures within the ascending and descending aorta and the pulmonary artery are equal in the fetus, any increased velocity is unlikely to be identified at the site of obstruction.[72] With left heart obstructive lesions reversed flow across the foramen ovale (left to right flow) has been described.[73] Sharland et al.[71] noted that this was frequently but not uniformly found with coarctation and was occasionally found in the absence of any left heart obstruction. Similarly, they found that Doppler evaluation of flows across the arterial valves did not help in distinguishing abnormals from false positives.

Sharland et al.[71] decided that although the diagnosis of coarctation of the aorta was possible in the fetus, this defect did continue to evolve up to and perhaps after birth such that the prenatal diagnosis could be difficult to exclude definitively or impossible to predict in every case. In their institution from 1980 through 1990 they identified 78 cases of suspected coarctation or interruption of the aortic arch on fetal echocardiography. Of these, after birth 50 infants had coarctation of the aorta, 4 had an interrupted aortic arch, and 24 infants were reported to be normal. Their conclusions were that the most severe forms of coarctation were associated with relative hypoplasia of left heart structures relative to right heart structures and a correct diagnosis could be made. The false positives were a concern, and their review of the data suggested that discrimination of real and false positives may not always be possible. Milder forms of coarctation are consistent with normal fetal echocardiographic features, and the diagnosis may not be evident until after birth and the ductus closes. Since coarctation is commonly identified with Turner's syndrome (XO) and can be seen in trisomies 18 and 13, karyotyping should be done when this diagnosis is made or suspected.[71]

Transposition of the Great Arteries

The structural defect of complete transposition of the great arteries prevents the infant from achieving a normal series type circulation following birth, retaining instead two parallel and separate paths for the pulmonary and the systemic circulations (Figure 14–13). With the great arteries transposed, the aorta arises from the right ventricular infundibulum, placing the aortic root anterior and to the right of the pulmonary trunk, which arises from the left ventricle. For the fetus, however, where the respiratory organ is included in the systemic circulation, this does not significantly alter cardiac function, and the pregnancy progresses normally. In the postnatal environment the respiratory and systemic circulations are separated, and the child becomes severely cyanotic and hypoxemic. The current preferred surgical approach for transposition of the great arteries is the arterial switch procedure as first proposed by Jatene et al.[74] The results have improved until the hospital surgical mortality today is about 5%. Primary surgical repair must be accomplished within the first weeks of life for optimal results.[75]

This alteration of cardiac structures has no signifi-

TABLE 14–5. NORMAL RATIOS OF AORTIC SEGMENTS

Aortic root/ascending aorta	1.13 ± 0.09
Transverse arch/ascending aorta	0.94 ± 0.09
Isthmus/ascending aorta	0.81 ± 0.09
Descending aorta/ascending aorta	0.96 ± 0.09
Left common carotid artery/transverse aorta	0.48 ± 0.08

Reprinted, with permission, from Hornberger LK, Weintraub RG, Pesonen E, Murillo-Olivas A, Simpson IA, Sahn C, Hagen-Ansert S, Sahn DJ. Echocardiographic study of the morphology and growth of the aortic arch in the human fetus. Circulation: 1992; 86:741–7.

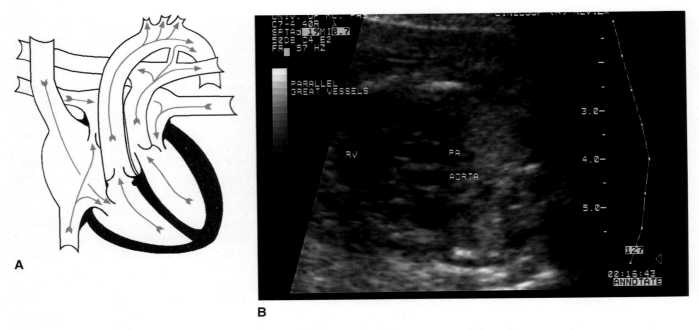

Figure 14–13. Transposition of the great vessels. **A.** With the aorta and the pulmon-ary artery reversed in their origin from the ventricles, parallel circulation is maintained following birth. **B.** Aorta and pulmonary artery (PA) coming off the right ventricle (RV) parallel to one another.

cant effect on fetal cardiac dynamics. The typical four-chamber view is usually normal, with no chamber enlargement or other alterations evident. Multiple views to identify the aorta and the pulmonary artery and define their ventricular associations are necessary for diagnosis. The anatomic landmarks that identify the right ventricle are a moderator band or trabecula septomarginalis near the apex and an outflow tract through an infundibular chamber beneath the semilunar valve.[18] Normally the inflow portion of the right ventricle is parallel to that of the left ventricle; the outflow path, however, crosses over and lies anterior and craniad to the left ventricular outflow path.[18] The main pulmonary artery quickly divides into a right and a left pulmonary artery and connects with the descending aorta by the ductus arteriosus (the ductal arch) during fetal development. The ascending aorta continues through the aortic arch from which the innominate, left common carotid, and left subclavian arteries arise directly into the descending aorta. Diagnosis of transposition of the great arteries relies on the identification of a parallel relationship of the great vessels rather than their normal right-angle crossing at the level of the aortic root.[13,62] Distal to the semilunar valves, however, at the level of the aortic arch, the aorta, and the pulmonary artery–ductus arteriosus do course in a parallel manner for a short segment and should not be mistaken for an abnormality. It is therefore important also to define the associations of the great vessels with the underlying

ventricle. Noting that the aorta arises anteriorly above the infundibulum of the right ventricle, and that the posterior vessel arising from the left ventricle has the typical branching pattern of the pulmonary artery, defines the diagnosis of transposition of the great arteries.[76] Doppler evaluation of intracardiac flow patterns will be normal.

Critical Aortic Stenosis

Aortic stenosis (Figure 14–14) is difficult to diagnose in the fetus before birth, with most reports identifying the fetus that has poor ventricular function or dimensions, or both.[77–79] In these situations it is difficult to distinguish between severe aortic stenosis and the hypoplastic left heart syndrome. Rudolph[3] noted that infants born with aortic stenosis appeared normal at birth, suggesting that a normal combined ventricular output and normal placental circulation were maintained in utero. He hypothesized that, with aortic stenosis, left ventricular hyperplasia would ensue, making the left ventricle less compliant than the right and promoting preferential filling of the right ventricle and decreasing the diastolic volume of the left ventricle. This decreased filling volume could mollify the elevation of the left ventricular pressure, which would otherwise be increased above that of the right ventricle and the aorta if normal left ventricular output were maintained.

After birth the clinical status of the infant depends

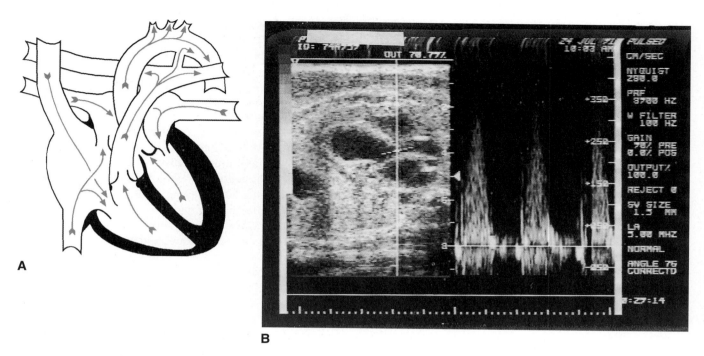

Figure 14–14. Critical aortic stenosis. **A.** Progressive obstruction to left ventricular outflow by the thickened aortic valve produces increasing hypertrophy of the left ventricle, with decreasing compliance and decreasing diastolic filling volume of the left ventricle. This may be associated with a variable degree of endocardial fibroelastosis. **B.** Long-axis view of fetal heart with aortic stenosis. Velocity across the aortic valve is 300 cm/s (angle correction prevents accurate estimation of aortic velocity).

on the severity of the obstruction. With critical valvular stenosis and a thick-walled left ventricle, it may not be possible to fill the ventricle adequately during diastole to maintain a sufficient systemic output.[17] This results in rapidly progressive congestive heart failure, metabolic acidosis, and a high neonatal mortality rate.[79] Early intervention in the neonate with either surgical valvotomy or catheter balloon valvuloplasty has improved the survival statistics for these children somewhat.

To date only isolated case reports are available to provide information about the evolution of the left ventricular outflow obstructive lesions, particularly critical aortic stenosis.[80] Doppler evaluation of flow in the stenosed artery may show an increased velocity; however, this is not a consistent finding.[13] A progressive gradient has been detected by Doppler evaluation in at least two fetuses with postnatally diagnosed critical aortic stenosis.[79,80] The diagnosis in utero is more likely to be suspected by the differential growth of the ventricles or great arteries. When there is valvular obstruction prenatally the affected great artery is often disproportionately small compared with the other great artery.[13] The specific etiology of the differential growth

remains speculative and is considered to be the effect of several hemodynamic alterations that result in reduced blood flow through the mitral valve, left ventricle, and aorta.[80] The presence of a poorly contractile left ventricle, left ventricular hypertrophy, a thickened and dome-shaped aortic valve, and, on serial studies, increasing disparity of right-to-left ventricular growth should strongly suggest severe left ventricular outflow obstruction from severe aortic stenosis. Doppler studies may show decreased flow antigrade across the mitral valve, reversed or bidirectional flow across the foramen ovale, or reversed flow in the distal aortic arch. Hornberger et al.[80] have described progression of the severity of obstruction in a fetus with critical aortic stenosis, as evidenced by an increase in the Doppler gradient and concomitant change in the morphology of the left ventricle on serial studies. The ability to recognize the fetus at risk for the progression of left heart obstruction in utero could facilitate the development of effective intrauterine therapy. To date, this is the only cardiac defect in which intrauterine intervention has been attempted. Balloon dilatation of the aortic valve has been successfully done in two fetuses with failing left ventricles during late gestation[81]; unfortunately neither of the two infants survived following delivery. That this defect can often be accurately identified in the fetus, particularly in the severest form; that it is frequently progressive with resultant severe and most often irreversible compromise of left ventricular function by the time of birth; that in the infant the restrictive aortic valve can be enlarged by the use of a transvenous dilating balloon catheter; and that this defect has a poor prognosis when there is critical aortic stenosis present brings this defect to the forefront for early interventional procedures in the fetus. Whether intervention can be undertaken before the damage to the left ventricle becomes irreversible remains yet to be determined.

Ebstein's Anomaly and Tricuspid Valve Dysplasia

Congenital tricuspid valve disease associated with tricuspid regurgitation is usually well tolerated in older infants and children.[82,83] Infants with anticipated higher levels of pulmonary vascular resistance often present with cardiomegaly, cyanosis, and congestive heart failure, and there is a greater incidence of death.[83] If the infant survives, the clinical symptoms generally improve as the pulmonary vascular resistance falls through the neonatal period. The congenital malformations of the tricuspid valve seen constitute a spectrum of changes from Ebstein's anomaly with isolated downward displacement of the valvular leaflets (Figure 14–15), through combinations of displacement and dysplasia, to exclusive dysplasia of normally attached leaflets.[84] The cardinal distinguishing feature of Ebstein's malformation is the downward displacement of the septal and mural leaflets and atrialization of the proximal right ventricle,[86] which should be identifiable on two-dimensional imaging. The difference between Ebstein's malformation and tricuspid dysplasia is generally academic in terms of functional effects, the incidence of associated lesions, and outcome.[85] Whether the defect is Ebstein's malformation or tricuspid dysplasia, the primary functional aberration of cardiac function is related to the degree of associated tricuspid regurgitation. Hornberger et al.[86] described three criteria, with at least two present, for suspecting significant tricuspid insufficiency: (1) marked right atrial enlargement; (2) half of the right atrium filled with the tricuspid regurgitant jet with color flow mapping; and (3) de-

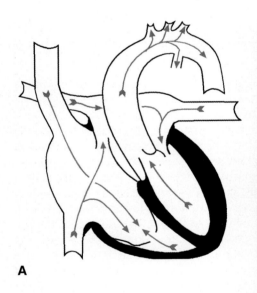

A

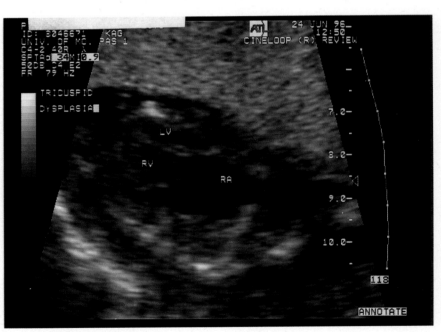

B

Figure 14–15. Ebstein's anomaly of the tricuspid valve. **A.** The downward displacement of the tricuspid valve orifice reduces the volume capacity of the right ventricle and increases the effective size of the right atrium. There is usually associated severe tricuspid insufficiency. (The pulmonary artery is not shown in this figure to show the tricuspid valve more clearly.) **B.** Tricuspid dysplasia. LV = left ventricle; RV = right ventricle; RA = right atrium. Note large right atrium due to "atrialization of the right ventricle."

tecting the regurgitant jet of tricuspid insufficiency at least halfway into the right atrium by pulsed Doppler. Serial evaluations frequently identified progressive right-sided cardiomegaly,[85-87] which was associated with poor outcome. Tricuspid insufficiency has been reported with otherwise normal cardiac anatomy, which was associated with maternal diabetes or the maternal use of indomethacin.[88] This was usually associated with a normal delivery.

The outcome of in utero detected tricuspid valve disease is generally poor, with reported mortality of 80% to 90%.[85,86] There are a number of indicators described for poor outcome; however, as Sharland et al.[85] have noted, the cases detected in fetal life are generally the most severe and therefore associated with poor outcome; therefore, fetal presentation itself should be regarded as an indicator of poor outcome.

TO SCAN OR NOT TO SCAN

The fetus with a cardiac defect, developing as it does in its cloistered environment within the uterus, does not present the typical clinical signs and symptoms of cardiac defects that are anticipated in the infant and child with similar defects. No murmurs are to be heard, no cyanosis is to be seen, and no early congestive heart failure is to be identified by direct examination. The fetus that should have a directed and detailed echocardiographic examination of the fetal heart must be identified by other criteria. Some of the factors that can identify the fetus at risk include the fetus with other somatic anomalies identified on ultrasound, fetal aneuploidy, or the fetus with growth retardation. Fetal cardiac defects should also be considered when the mother has been exposed to known teratogens (see Table 14–6) such as alcohol, anticonvulsants, lithium, or amphetamines or has underlying diseases that increase the incidence of cardiac defects such as rubella or diabetes mellitus. The presence of identified familial factors such as other family members with congenital cardiac defects (see Table 14–7) or a known genetic syndrome should alert the physician to the potential of a cardiac defect with this pregnancy. The presence of nonimmune hydrops indicates severe cardiac dysfunction (fetal equivalent of congestive heart failure). When this condition is identified, a complete cardiac evaluation by echocardiography should be done as immediately as is possible or the mother referred to a center where this evaluation is possible.

CONCLUSIONS

It may be anticipated that all of the structural cardiac defects defined in the newborn should also be identifiable

TABLE 14–6. CARDIAC MALFORMATIONS ASSOCIATED WITH KNOWN TERATOGENS

Potential Teratogen	Frequency of Cardiac Defect (%)	Malformation[a]
Alcohol	30	VSD, PDA, ASD
Amphetamines	5	VSD, PDA, ASD, TGA
Hydantoin	3	PS, AS, CA, PDA
Trimethadone	30	TGA, TOF, HLHS
Lithium	10	Ebstein's, TA, ASD
Thalidomide	10	TOF, VSD, ASD, Truncus
Retinoic acid	10	VSD
Rubella	35	PPS, PDA, VSD, ASD
Diabetes mellitus	5	TGA, VSD, CA
Lupus	40	Heart block
Phenylketonuria	10	TOF, VSD, ASD

[a]VSD, ventricular septal defect; PDA, patent ductus arteriosus; ASD, atrial septal defect; TGA, transposition of the great arteries; PS, pulmonary stenosis; AS, aortic stenosis; CA, coarctation of the aorta; TOF, Tetralogy of Fallot; HLHS, hypoplastic left heart syndrome; TA, tricuspid atresia; Truncus = truncus arteriosus.
Adapted, with permission, from Hess LW, Hess DB, McCaul JF, Perry KG: Fetal echocardiography. Obstet Gynecol Clin N Am: 1990; 17:41–79.

TABLE 14–7. RECURRENCE RISKS OF CONGENITAL CARDIAC DEFECTS WHERE THERE IS ONE AFFECTED FAMILY MEMBER (FIRST-DEGREE RELATIVE) WITH PERCENTAGE OF OFFSPRING AFFECTED

Cardiac Anomaly	Mother Affected	Father Affected	Prior Sibling Affected
Ventricular septal defect	6.0	1.0	3.0
Patent ductus arteriosus	4.0	2.5	3.0
Atrial septal defect	4.0	1.5	2.5
Tetralogy of Fallot	7.5	1.5	2.5
Pulmonary valvular stenosis	6.0	2.0	2.0
Coarctation of the aorta	4.0	2.0	2.0
Aortic valvular stenosis	15.0	3.0	2.0
Transposition of the great vessels	5.0	2.0	1.5
Atrioventricular canal	14.0	1.0	2.0
Truncus arteriosus	5.0	2.0	1.0
Tricuspid atresia	—	—	1.0
Ebstein's anomaly	—	—	1.0
Hypoplastic left heart syndrome	—	—	9.9

Adapted, with permission, from Hess LW, Hess DB, McCaul JF, Perry KG. Fetal echocardiography. Obstet Gynecol Clin N Am: 1990; 17:41–79.

on fetal echocardiography. Some of the identified defects in the postnatal period, such as persistence of the ductus arteriosus and patency of the foramen ovale, however, are a normal component of fetal circulation and become abnormal only in their persistence in the postnatal environment. The spectrum of cardiac defects identified by fetal ultrasound is also affected by the selection of pregnancies to be screened as well as the resolution and limitations of the equipment currently available. For example, fewer mothers who had a previous child with a mild heart defect were referred for elective screening than those who had a previous child who died of major congenital cardiac disease.[90] Similarly, with the resolution limitations of current ultrasound equipment, the detection rate is lower with milder cardiac anomalies[7,8,12,14,90–92] that produce minimal or no significant changes in the fetal circulation. In reported series where larger numbers of pregnancies were scanned and compared with the postnatal presence of cardiac defects, very few or no fetuses were identified with isolated simple lesions such as atrial septal defects or ventricular septal defects.[12,93,94] Milder forms of defects and defects that might be progressive, such as valvular pulmonary or aortic stenosis and coarctation of the aorta, would not affect fetal hemodynamics and should also be expected to have a lower fetal detection rate. The cardiac defects described here represent those that produce more identifiable changes in cardiac structure or more profoundly alter fetal cardiac hemodynamics and so are more readily identifiable in the fetus. As a consequence these also are frequently more devastating to the developing fetus and have a poorer anticipated outcome. Fortunately, the currently undetected cardiac anomalies are more minor and their contribution to perinatal mortality and morbidity is negligible.[94]

Fetal echocardiography is different from that in the newborn infant. Although in some respects it may be easier, with the visualization of the fetal heart not as obscured by the lungs as in the neonate,[93] the fetal heart being small (less than 1 cm overall length)[18] in earlier pregnancy, and being imaged from a distance that varies by maternal factors such as obesity or obscured by previous maternal abdominal surgery,[95] all of which can affect the ability to resolve essential details of the fetal cardiac structure. There are also some normal structures that can simulate abnormalities in the fetal heart,[96,97] affording pitfalls that should be avoided. Over the last decade the knowledge base of both normal and abnormal fetal cardiac structure and function has increased dramatically and may be expected to continue to increase over the next decade. Additionally, newer equipment and techniques, such as three-dimensional scans,[98] can improve the ability and accuracy of imaging the fetal heart in increasing detail and improving diagnostic capabilities.

As the capabilities of the ultrasonographer continue to increase, so do the questions regarding the role and application of these capabilities. Should all expectant mothers be screened? Although many of the lethal cardiac lesions such as hypoplastic left or right heart syndromes may be identifiable by the midtrimester, pediatric cardiovascular techniques also continue to progress, making these defects less lethal to the neonate. The four-chamber view, however, does not detect even all of the serious defects, and even with multiple views those defects that do not significantly alter in utero hemodynamics, such as atrial or ventricular septal defects, cannot currently be identified with any confidence. The general application of multiple views requires significant additional training of the technician and expertise of the physician reading the examination. Additionally, since there is evidence that there is progression of some forms of congenital cardiac defects in utero, such as aortic or pulmonary valvular stenosis, not all defects are appreciable in the midtrimester or the functional significance may not be identified until later pregnancy. The ethical implications arising from this technology are addressed in Chapter 24 of this book. Currently, mothers who have a congenital cardiac defect, or who have had a previous child with a serious congenital heart defect, or in whom there are indications of other fetal abnormalities or chromosomal defects or signs of fetal distress such as hydrops, should have a complete echocardiographic evaluation.

The real benefits of prenatal diagnosis of congenital cardiac defects (see Figures 14–16 to 14–27 for common fetal cardiac pathology) have been best summarized by Mellick et al.,[93] who described three advantages: first, that the parents could be appropriately counseled before delivery, and more realistic informed consent for any anticipated procedures could be obtained; second, that delivery could be planned for a center that would be able to manage the anticipated cardiac defect effectively; and third, that the anxiety of the family with a previously affected child can be eliminated if an unaffected fetus is defined. The developing potential for intrauterine intervention for the fetus with cardiac defects using attempts at balloon angioplasty of aortic stenosis in the fetus[81] suggest an additional advantage of prenatal screening. Mellick also noted that the outcome of the fetus was affected little by early diagnosis: With the severity of the malformations that are more likely to be seen in early pregnancy, the mortality rate among affected fetuses is very high both in utero and in the neonatal period. Accurate antenatal diagnosis, however, offers the greatest chance for a successful outcome of the pregnancy where a severe cardiac defect exists.

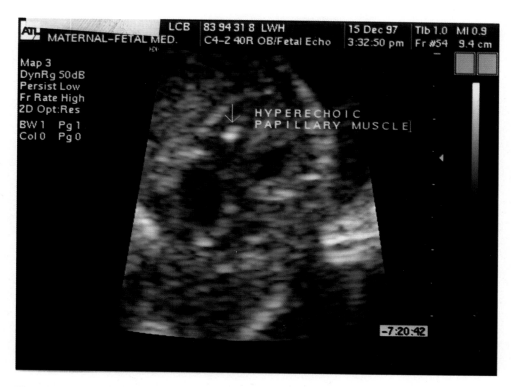

Figure 14–16. Hyperechoic papillary muscle. Usually a normal variant although may be associated with Down syndrome.

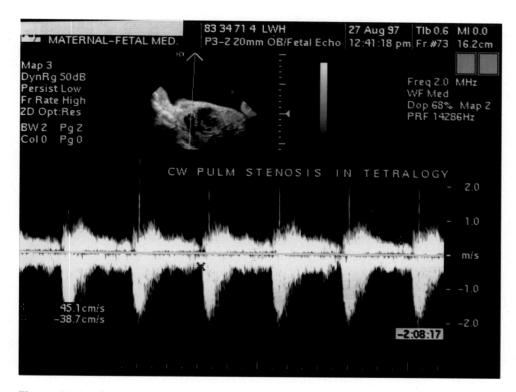

Figure 14–17. Continuous wave (CW) Doppler evaluation of the pulmonary valve revealing pulmonic stenosis with velocity of 200 cm/s across the valve.

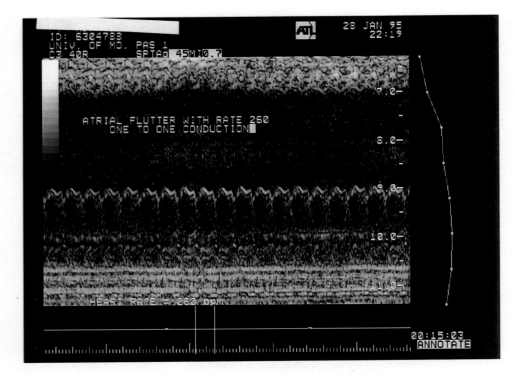

Figure 14–18. M-mode evaluation revealing atrial flutter with one-to-one conduction at a heart rate of 260 beats per minute.

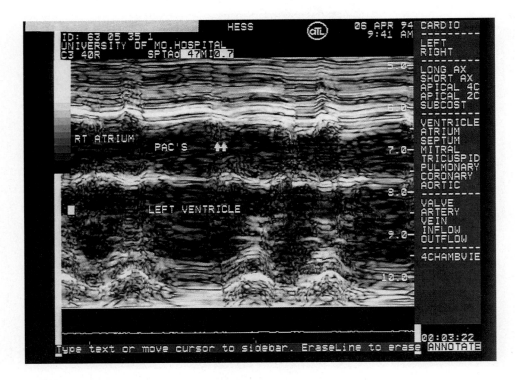

Figure 14–19. M-mode evaluation revealing premature atrial contractions (PACs) marked with a double arrow.

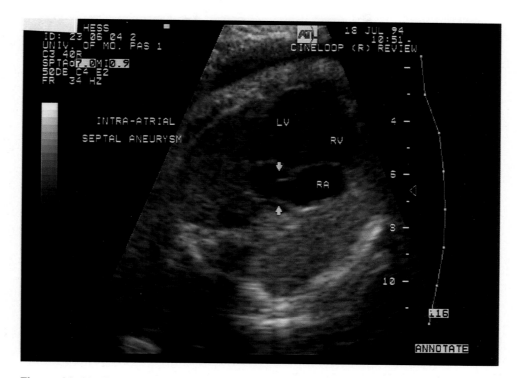

Figure 14–20. Four-chamber fetal heart revealing an atrial septal aneurysm which may be associated with atrial arrhythmias. LV = left ventricle; RV = right ventricle; RA = right atrium.

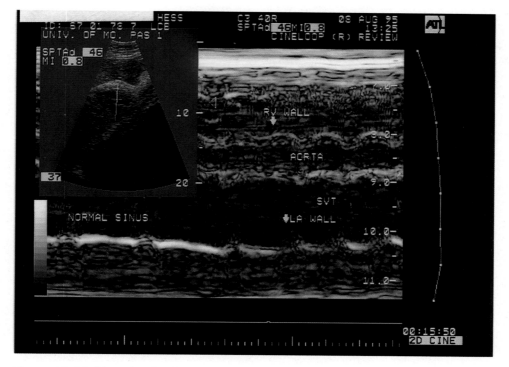

Figure 14–21. M-mode of a fetus in normal sinus rhythm that develops supraventricular tachycardia (SVT). RV = right ventricle; LA = left atrium.

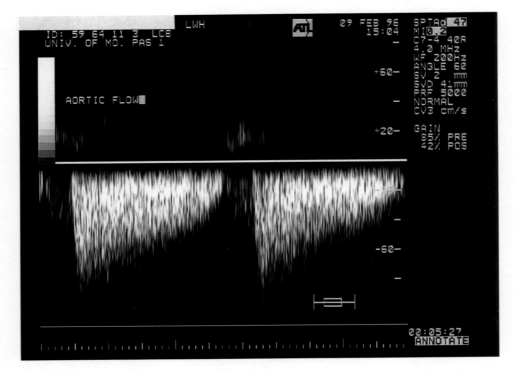

Figure 14–22. Severe aortic regurgitation in a fetus undergoing pulse Doppler evaluation.

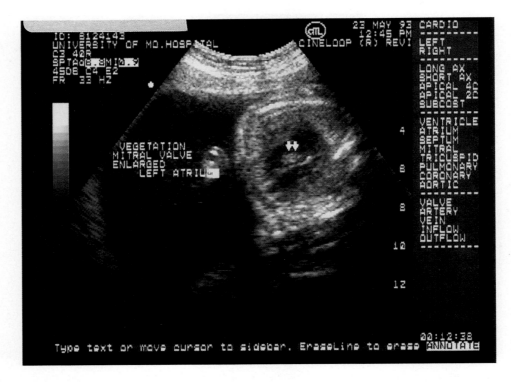

Figure 14–23. A vegetation on the mitral valve of a fetus with in utero toxoplasmosis.

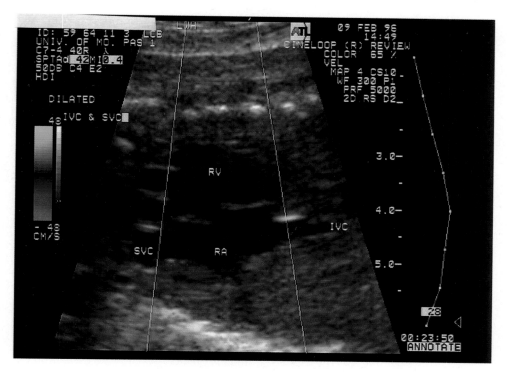

Figure 14–24. Long-axis view of the great veins demonstrating a dilated inferior vena cava (IVC) and superior vena cava (SVC). RV = right ventricle; RA = right atrium.

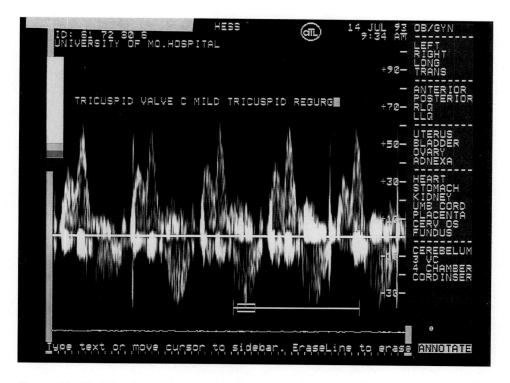

Figure 14–25. Pulse Doppler evaluation of the tricuspid valve demonstrating the E and A waves during diastole and mild tricuspid regurgitation during systole.

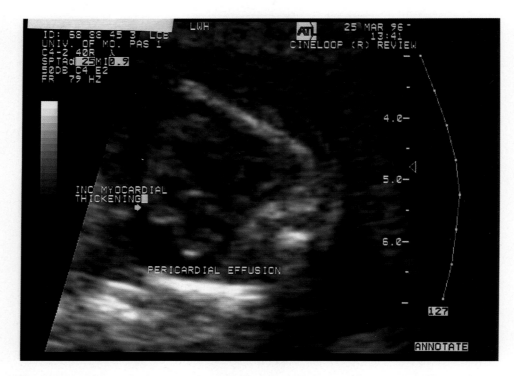

Figure 14–26. Four-chamber views of the fetal heart showing global myocardial wall thickening and severe pericardial effusion.

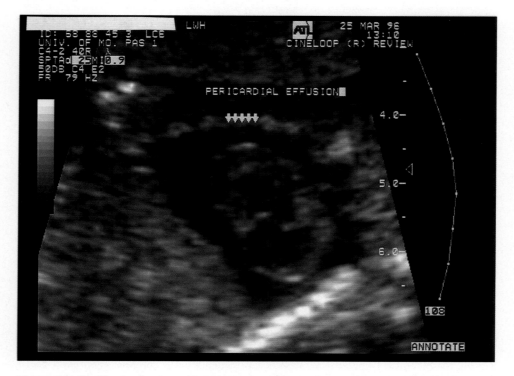

Figure 14–27. Short-axis view of fetal heart from Figure 14–26 showing pericardial effusion.

REFERENCES

1. Hofman JI, Christian R: Congenital heart disease in a cohort of 19,502 births with longterm follow up. *Am J Cardiol.* 42:641–7, 1987.

2. Lian ZH, Zack MM, Erickson JD: Paternal age and the occurance of birth defects. *Am J Hum Genet.* 39:648–60, 1986.

3. Rudolph AM: In *Congenital Diseases of the Heart.* Chicago: Year Book Medical Publishers, Inc.; 1974: pp. 1–16.

4. Keith JD, Rowe RD, Vlad P: In *Heart Disease in Infancy and Childhood.* New York: Macmillan; 1978: pp. 4–6.

5. Mitchell SC, Korones SB, Berendes HW: Congenital heart disease in 56,109 births. *Circulation.* 43:323–32, 1971.

6. Gasul BM, Arcilla RA, Lev M: In *Heart Disease in Children.* Philadelphia: JB Lippincott; 1966: p. 2.

7. Smythe JF, Copel JA, Kleinman CS: Outcome of prenatally detected cardiac malformations. *Am J Cardiol.* 69:1471–4, 1992.

8. Allan LD, Sharland GK, Milburn A, et al.: Prospective diagnosis of 1,006 consecutive cases of congenital heart disease in the fetus. *J Am Coll Cardiol.* 23: 1452–8, 1994.

9. Bound JP, Logan WFWE: Incidence of congenital heart disease in Blackpool, 1957–1971. *Br Heart J.* 39:445–50, 1977.

10. Feldt RH, Avasthey P, Yoshimasu F, et al.: Incidence of congenital heart disease in children born to residents of Olmstead County, Minnesota, 1950–1969. *Mayo Clin Proc.* 46:794–9, 1971.

11. Richards MR, Merritt KK, Samuels MH, et al.: Congenital malformations of the cardiovascular system in a series of 60,503 infants. *Pediatrics.* 15:12–32, 1955.

12. Stoll C, Alembik Y, Dott B, et al.: Evaluation of prenatal diagnosis of congenital heart disease. *Prenat Diagn.* 13:453–61, 1993.

13. Lindsey A, Baker EJ: Prenatal diagnosis and correction of congenital heart defects. *Br J Hosp Med.* 9:513–22, 1993.

14. Lindsey DA: Echocardiographic detection of congenital heart disease in the fetus: Present and future. *Br Heart J.* 74:103–5, 1995.

15. Brook MM, Silverman NH, Villegas M: Cardiac ultrasonography in structural abnormalities and arrhythmias. *West J Med.* 159:286–300, 1993.

16. Patton BM: In *Human Embryology.* New York: McGraw-Hill; 1968: pp. 500–83.

17. Dawes GS: In *Foetal and Neonatal Physiology.* Chicago: Year Book Medical Publishers; 1968: pp. 91–105.

18. Santulli TV: Fetal echocardiography: Assessment of cardiovascular anatomy and function. *Clin Perinatol.* 17:911–41, 1990.

19. Schmidt KG, Silverman NH, Hoffman JIE: Determination of ventricular volumes in human fetal hearts by two-dimensional echocardiography. *Am J Cardiol.* 76:1313–6, 1995.

20. Shiraishi H, Silverman NH, Rudolph AM: Accuracy of right ventricular output estimated by Dopplar echocardiography in the sheep fetus. *Am J Obstet Gynecol.* 168:949–53, 1993.

21. Sahn DJ, Lange LW, Allen HD, et al.: Quantitative real-time cross-sectional echocardiography in the developing normal human fetus and newborn. *Circulation.* 62:588–97, 1980.

22. Tan J, Silverman NH, Hoffman JIE, et al.: Cardiac dimensions determined by cross-sectional echocardiography in the normal human fetus from 18 weeks to term. *Am J Cardiol.* 70:1459–67, 1992.

23. Ursell PC, Byrne JB, Fears TR, et al.: Growth of the great vessels in the normal human fetus and in the fetus with cardiac defects. *Circulation.* 84:2028–33, 1991.

24. Pegg W, Michalak M: Differentiation of sarcoplasmic reticulum during cardiac myogenisis. *Am J Physiol.* 21: H22–31, 1987.

25. Marsh JD, Allen PD: Developmental regulation of cardiac calcium channels and contractile sensitivity to [Ca]$_0$. *Am J Physiol.* 256:H179–85, 1989.

26. Anversa P, Ricci R, Olivetti G: Quantitative structural analysis of the myocardium during physiologic growth and induced cardiac hypertrophy: A review. *J Am Coll Cardiol.* 7:1140–9, 1986.

27. Weil SR, Russo AP, Heckman JL, et al.: Pressure-volume relationship of the fetal lamb heart. *Ann Thorac Surg.* 55:470–5, 1993.

28. Gilbert RD: Control of fetal cardiac output during changes in blood volume. *Am J Physiol.* 238:H80–6, 1980.

29. Thornberg KL, Morton MJ: Filling and arterial pressures as determinants of RV stroke volume in the sheep fetus. *Am J Physiol.* 244:H565–3, 1983.

30. Thornberg KL, Morton MJ: Filling and arterial pressures as determinates of left ventricular stroke volume in fetal lambs. *Am J Physiol.* 251:H961–8, 1986.

31. Morton MJ, Thornberg KL: The pericardium and cardiac transmural filling pressure in the fetal sheep. *J Dev Physiol.* 9:159–68, 1987.

32. Reller MD, Morton MJ, Reid DL, et al.: Fetal lamb ventricles respond differently to filling and arterial pressures and to in utero ventilation. *Pediatr Res.* 24:621–6, 1987.

33. Shaddy RE, Tyndall MR, Teitel DF, et al.: Regulation of cardiac output with controlled heart rate in newborn lambs. *Pediatr Res.* 24:577–82, 1988.

34. Grant DA, Kondo CS, Maloney JE, et al.: Changes in pericardial pressure during the prenatal period. *Circulation.* 86:1615–21, 1992.

35. Hecher K, Campbell S, Harrington K, et al.: Assessment of fetal compromise by Doppler ultrasound investigation of the fetal circulation. *Circulation.* 91:129–38, 1995.

36. Tulzer G, Khowsathit P, Gudmundsson S, et al.: Diastolic function of the fetal heart during second and third trimester: A prospective longitudinal Doppler-echocardiographic study. *Eur J Pediatr.* 153:151–4, 1994.

37. Wladimiroff JW, Stewart PA, Burghouwt MT, et al.: Normal fetal cardiac flow velocity waveforms between 11 and 16 weeks of gestation. *Am J Obstet Gynecol.* 167: 736–9, 1992.

38. Weber HS, Botti JJ, Baylen BG: Sequential longitudinal evaluation of cardiac growth and ventricular diastolic filling in fetuses of well controlled diabetic mothers. *Pediatr Cardiol.* 15:184–9, 1994.

39. Bartelds B, van Bel F, Teitel DF, et al.: Carotid, not aortic, chemoreceptors mediate the fetal cardiovascular re-

sponse to acute hypoxemia in lambs. *Pediatr Res.* 34: 51–5, 1993.

40. Berning RA, Silverman NH, Villegas M, et al.: Reversed shunting across the ductus arteriosus or atrial septum in utero heralds severe congenital heart disease. *J Am Coll Cardiol.* 27:481–6, 1996.

41. Sharland GK, Sunder SK, Allan LD: The use of colour Doppler in fetal echocardiography. *Int J Cardiol.* 28: 229–36, 1990.

42. Gembruch U, Hansmann M, Redel DA, et al.: Fetal two-dimensional Doppler echocardiography (colour flow mapping) and its place in prenatal diagnosis. *Prenat Diag.* 9: 535–47, 1989.

43. Shultz SM, Pretorius DH, Budorick NE: Four-chamber view of the fetal heart: Demonstration related to menstrual age. *J Ultrasound Med.* 13:285–9, 1994.

44. American College of Obstetricians and Gynecologists: *Ultrasound in Pregnancy*. ACOG Technical Bulletin No. 187. Washington, DC: American College of Obstetricians and Gynecologists; 1993.

45. Davis GK, Farquar CM, Allan LD, et al.: Structural cardiac abnormalities in the fetus: Reliability of prenatal diagnosis and outcome. *Br J Obstet Gynecol.* 97:27–31, 1990.

46. Simpson LL, Marx GR: Diagnosis and treatment of structural fetal cardiac abnormality and dysrhythmia. *Semin Perinatol.* 18:215–27, 1994.

47. Allan LD: Diagnosis of fetal cardiac abnormalities. *Arch Dis Child.* 64:964–8, 1989.

48. Sharland GK, Lockhart SM, Chia SK, et al.: Factors influencing the outcome of congenital heart disease detected prenatally. *Arch Dis Child.* 66:284–7, 1991.

49. Gembruch U, Knöpfle G, Chatterjee M, et al.: Prenatal diagnosis of atrioventricular canal malformations with up-to-date echocardiographic technology: Report of 14 cases. *Am Heart J.* 121:1489–97, 1991.

50. Machado AVL, Crawford D, Anderson RH, et al.: Atrioventricular septal defect in prenatal life. *Br Heart J.* 58: 352–5, 1988.

51. McGahan JP, Choy MC, Parrish MD, et al.: Sonographic spectrum of fetal cardiac hypoplasia. *J Ultrasound Med.* 10:539–46, 1991.

52. Blake DM, Copel JA, Kleinman CS: Hypoplastic left heart syndrome: Prenatal diagnosis, clinical profile, and management. *Am J Obstet Gynecol.* 165:529–34, 1991.

53. Allan LD, Sharland G, Tynan MJ: The natural history of the hypoplastic left heart syndrome. *Int J Cardiol.* 25: 343–6, 1989.

54. Rosenthal A, Dick M: Tricuspid atresia. In: Adams FH, Emmanouilides GC, Reimenschneider TA, eds. *Heart Disease in Infants, Children, and Adolescents*, 4th ed. New York: Macmillan; 1989: p. 348.

55. Allan LD, Crawford DC, Tynan MJ: Pulmonary atresia in prenatal life. *J Am Coll Cardiol.* 8:1131–6, 1986.

56. Fyfe DA, Kline CH: Fetal echocardiographic diagnosis of congenital heart disease. *Pediatr Clin N Am.* 37:45–67, 1990.

57. Norwood WI, Lang P, Hansen D: Physiologic repair of aortic atresia-hypoplastic left heart syndrome. *N Engl J Med.* 308:23–6, 1983.

58. Guntheroth WG, Cyr DR, Winter T, et al.: Fetal Doppler echocardiography in pulmonary atresia. *J Ultrasound Med.* 5:281–4, 1993.

59. Moller JH, Neal WA: In *Heart Disease in Infancy*. New York: Appleton-Century-Crofts; 1981.

60. Lee WL, Smith RS, Comstock CH, et al.: Tetralogy of Fallot: Prenatal diagnosis and postnatal survival. *Obstet Gynecol.* 86:583–8, 1995.

61. Hornberger LK, Benacerraf BR, Bromley BS, et al.: Prenatal detection of severe right ventricular outflow tract obstruction: Pulmonary stenosis and pulmonary atresia. *J Ultrasound Med.* 13:743–50, 1994.

62. Benacerraf BR: Sonographic detection of fetal anomalies of the aortic and pulmonary arteries: Value of four-chamber view vs direct images. *Am J Radiol.* 163:1483–9, 1994.

63. Kirk JS, Riggs TW, Comstock CH, et al.: Prenatal screening for cardiac anomalies: The value of routine addition of the aortic root to the four-chamber view. *Obstet Gynecol.* 84:427–31, 1994.

64. Gembruch U, Weinraub Z, Bald R, et al.: Flow analysis in the pulmonary trunk in fetuses with tetralogy of Fallot by colour Doppler flow mapping: Two case reports. *Eur J Obstet Gynecol Reprod Biol.* 35:259–65, 1990.

65. Rudolph AM, Heymann MA, Spitznas U: Hemodynamic considerations in the development of narrowing of the aorta. *Am J Cardiol.* 30:514–25, 1972.

66. Gersony WM: Coarctation of the aorta. In: Adams FH, Emmanouilides GC, Reimenschneider TA, eds. *Heart Disease in Infants, Children, and Adolescents*, 4th ed. New York: Macmillan; 1989: pp. 188–98.

67. Allen LD, Crawford DC, Tynan M: Evolution of coarctation of the aorta in intrauterine life. *Br Heart J.* 52:471–3, 1984.

68. Wielenga G, Dankmaeijer J: Coarctation of the aorta. *J Pathol Bacteriol.* 95:265–74, 1968.

69. Allen LD, Chita SK, Anderson RH, et al.: Coarctation of the aorta in prenatal life: An echocardiographic, anatomical, and functional study. *Br Heart J.* 59:356–60, 1988.

70. Hornberger LK, Weintraub RG, Pesonen E, et al.: Echocardiographic study of the morphology and growth of the aortic arch in the human fetus. *Circulation.* 86: 741–7, 1992.

71. Sharland GK, Chan KY, Allan LD: Coarctation of the aorta: Difficulties in prenatal diagnosis. *Br Heart J.* 71:70–5, 1994.

72. Hornberger LK, Sahn DJ, Kleinman CS, et al.: Antenatal diagnosis of coarctation of the aorta: A multicenter experience. *J Am Coll Cardiol.* 23:417–23, 1994.

73. Feit LR, Copel JA, Kleinman CS: Foramen ovale size in the normal and abnormal human fetal heart: An indication of transatrial flow physiology. *Ultrasound Obstet Gynecol.* 1:313–9, 1991.

74. Jatene AD, Fontes VF, Paulista PP, et al.: Anatomic correction of transposition of the great vessels. *J Thorac Cardiovasc Surg.* 72:364–70, 1976.

75. Kirklin JW, Colvin EV, McConnell ME, et al.: Complete transposition of the great arteries: Treatment in the current era. *Pediatr Clin N Am.* 37:171–7, 1990.

76. Brown DL, DiSalvo DN, Frates MC, et al.: Sonography of the fetal heart: Normal variants and pitfalls. *Am J Radiol.* 160:1251–5, 1993.

77. Hutha JC, Carpenter RJ, Moise KJ, et al.: Prenatal diagnosis and postnatal management of critical aortic stenosis. *Circulation.* 75:573–6, 1987.

78. Jouk PS, Rambaud P: Prediction of outcome by prenatal Doppler analysis in a patient with aortic stenosis. *Br Heart J.* 65:53–4, 1991.

79. Robertson MA, Byrne PJ, Penkoske PA: Perinatal management of critical aortic valve stenosis diagnosed by fetal echocardiography. *Br Heart J.* 61:365–7, 1989.

80. Hornberger LK, Sanders SP, Rein AJJT, et al.: Left heart obstructive lesions and left ventricular growth in the midtrimester fetus. *Circulation.* 92:1531–8, 1995.

81. Maxwell D, Allan L, Tynan MJ: Balloon dilitation of the aortic valve in the fetus: A report of two cases. *Br Heart J.* 65:256–8, 1991.

82. Genton E, Blount SG: The spectrum of Ebstein's anomaly. *Am Heart J.* 73:395–425, 1967.

83. Kumar AE, Fyler DC, Miettinen OS, et al.: Ebstein's anomaly: Clinical profile and natural history. *Am J Cardiol.* 28:84–95, 1971.

84. Palladini D, Chita SK, Allan LD: Prenatal measurement of the cardiothoracic ratio in the evaluation of heart disease. *Arch Dis Child.* 65:20–3, 1990.

85. Sharland GK, Chita SK, Allan LD: Tricuspid valve dysplasia or displacement in intrauterine life. *J Am Coll Cardiol.* 17:944–9, 1991.

86. Hornberger LK, Sahn DJ, Kleinman CS, et al.: Tricuspid valve disease with significant tricuspid insufficiency in the fetus: Diagnosis and outcome. *J Am Coll Cardiol.* 17:167–73, 1991.

87. Oberhoffer R, Cook AC, Lang D, et al.: Correlation between echocardiographic and morphological investigations of lesions of the tricuspid valve diagnosed during fetal life. *Br Heart J.* 68:580–5, 1992.

88. Respondek ML, Kammermeier M, Ludomirsky A, et al.: The prevalence and clinical significance of fetal tricuspid valve regurgitation with normal heart anatomy. *Am J Obstet Gynecol.* 171:1265–70, 1994.

90. Allan LD, Crawford DC, Handerson RH, et al.: Spectrum of congenital heart disease detected echocardiographically in prenatal life. *Br Heart J.* 54:523–6, 1985.

91. Marasini M, Cordone M, Pongiglione G, et al.: In utero ultrasound diagnosis of congenital heart disease. *J Clin Ultrasound.* 16:103–7, 1988.

92. Ott WJ: The accuracy of antenatal fetal echocardiography screening in high- and low-risk patients. *Am J Obstet Gynecol.* 172:1741–9, 1995.

93. Mellick JD, Radford DJ, Galbraith AJ: Fetal echocardiography in the diagnosis of congenital heart disease. *Aust Paediatr J.* 25:356–60, 1989.

94. Achiron R, Glaser J, Gelernter I, et al.: Extended fetal echocardiographic examination for detecting cardiac malformations in low risk pregnancies. *Br Med J.* 304:671–4, 1992.

95. DeVore GR, Medearis AL, Bear MB, et al.: Fetal echocardiography: Factors that influence imaging of the fetal heart during the second trimester of pregnancy. *J Ultrasound Med.* 12:659–63, 1993.

96. Brown DL, Roberts DJ, Miller WA: Left ventricular echogenic focus in the heart: Pathologic correlation. *J Ultrasound Med.* 13:613–6, 1994.

97. Brown DL, DiSalvo DN, Frates MC, et al.: Sonography of the fetal heart: Normal variants and pitfalls. *Am J Radiol.* 160:1251–5, 1993.

98. Zosmer N, Jurovic D, Jauniaux E, et al.: Selection and identification of standard cardiac views from three-dimensional volume scans of the fetal thorax. *J Ultrasound Med.* 15:25–32, 1996.

99. Hess LW, Hess DB, McCaul JF, et al.: Fetal echocardiography. *Obstet Gynecol Clin N Am.* 17:41–79, 1990.

CHAPTER FIFTEEN

Management of Fetal Cardiac Arrhythmias

Joshua A. Copel, Alan H. Friedman, and Charles S. Kleinman

Fetal arrhythmias are common even in normal fetuses but can be the source of much parental and physician anxiety. In this chapter we review the more common fetal arrhythmias, including their detection, electrophysiology, medical and intrapartum management, and postnatal prognosis. Fetal arrhythmias should be assessed beginning with a general fetal evaluation, as part of a full fetal echocardiogram. This evaluation is necessary because it is not uncommon for certain arrhythmias, such as complete heart block or atrial flutter, to be associated with structural heart disease.

It is difficult for obstetricians and radiologists to become familiar with all aspects of the diagnosis and management of fetal arrhythmias. In general, decisions regarding interventions, including medications, should only be undertaken in conjunction with a pediatric cardiologist with a special interest in electrophysiology and with Maternal–Fetal Medicine subspecialists.

Fetal antiarrhythmic therapy requires an understanding of the underlying electrophysiology of the arrhythmia and knowledge of fetomaternal pharmacology and the pharmacokinetics of the drugs being administered. All antiarrhythmic drugs can cause significant toxicity to both mother and fetus, so the risks and benefits of fetal treatment must be carefully considered before any treatment is begun. Although space constraints preclude detailed discussion of all options and all drugs, an extensive review of the electrophysiology of fetal tachyarrhythmias and the drugs in common use for their treatment can be found in a number of reviews.[1,2]

INITIAL IDENTIFICATION

The most common presentation of fetal arrhythmias is by auscultation at a routine prenatal visit. Initially one may hear an apparent skipped beat, or an extra beat. At other times a sustained or paroxysmal rapid or slow fetal heart rate may be heard. If a tachycardia is heard, the referring practitioner should attempt to determine the rate and whether it begins and ends abruptly, because normal fetal heart accelerations begin and end gradually and usually have maximal rates below 200 to 210 beats per minute (BPM). Abrupt changes, on the other hand, especially if the rate is over 200 BPM, are more often associated with pathologic tachycardias. A mild tachycardia (200 to 220 BPM), in the setting of ruptured membranes or labor, should be evaluated by standard obstetric testing for reassurance about fetal status, particularly looking for evidence of fetal infection or other forms of potential fetal compromise.

Fetal bradycardias also need to be distinguished from physiologic events. Brief slowing of the fetal heart rate is common when patients lie supine, perhaps because of the supine-hypotension syndrome.[3] Transient slowing of the fetal heart rate with an immediate return to normal does not require fetal echocardiography. These episodes are caused by variable-type fetal heart rate decelerations, which occur as isolated physiologic events in the midtrimester. Once fetal viability is reached, recurrent slowing with return to the baseline rate suggests the need for standard assessment of fetal well-being (e.g., nonstress test, amniotic fluid volume assessment, biophysical profile).

Fetuses with persistent rates over 200 BPM or below 100 BPM require expedited evaluation, whereas those with irregular heart rates require less urgent assessment. There is still benefit in fetal echocardiography for fetuses with irregular heart rates. For example, 51 fetuses were referred to the Yale Fetal Cardiovascular Center in 1995 for evaluation of irregular heart rates, 49 of which were either in a normal rhythm when evaluated or had benign extrasystoles. However, one fetus had atrial flutter with variable block, and another had a malignant form of supraventricular tachycardia, eventually dying after extended intensive fetal treatment. Both presented to their referring obstetricians simply with irregular fetal heart rates.

EVALUATION TECHNIQUES

Optimally, fetal cardiac rhythm would be evaluated with an electrocardiogram. There is currently no reliable means to obtain a fetal electrocardiogram demonstrating p waves externally. Since most fetal arrhythmias require diagnosis before the onset of labor, we must rely on noninvasive approaches.

Fetal cardiac motion results from electrical activity. M-mode ultrasound, which depicts motion as a function of time, can be used to evaluate cardiac rhythm.[4–6] The M-mode sampling cursor should be placed through both the fetal atrium and the ventricle, which allows the relative timing of atrial and ventricular contractions to be determined (Figure 15–1). Electrical activity can then be inferred based on the timing of the mechanical events. The desired alignment is not always easy to obtain and is heavily dependent on fetal position, fetal movement, and fetal breathing.

Pulsed Doppler can similarly be used to identify the fetal rhythm by visualizing intracardiac flow.[6–8] Placement of the cursor in the left ventricle at the junction of the mitral inflow tract and the left ventricular outflow tract, using an apical four-chamber view, provides a view of flow both into and out of the ventricle (Figure 15–2). Flow velocity waveforms from the pulmonary arterial and venous circulations have also been advocated for this purpose,[9] although in our experience this approach is considerably more difficult.

Color Doppler M-mode combines the temporal information of M-mode with flow information from the color Doppler. It can be used to determine timing of atrial and ventricular systole with cursor placement similar to that for standard M-mode evaluation.

ELECTROPHYSIOLOGY OF FETAL ARRHYTHMIAS

Although the numbers may vary, it is not unusual for fetal cardiovascular centers to receive approximately 15% of their referrals for abnormalities of cardiac rhythm.[10] Fetal arrhythmias can be defined as any irregularity of rhythm or any sustained regular rhythm outside the range of 100 to 160 BPM.[11]

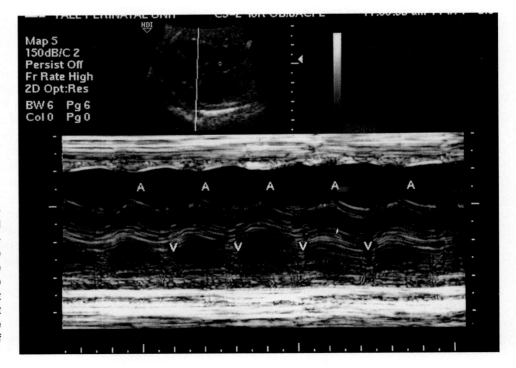

Figure 15–1. M-mode echocardiogram showing normal atrial (A) and ventricular (V) contraction relationship. Orienting image at the top of the figure shows the M-mode cursor passing, from top to bottom, through the right atrium, tricuspid valve, and right ventricle, which contains the moderator band near the apex of the heart.

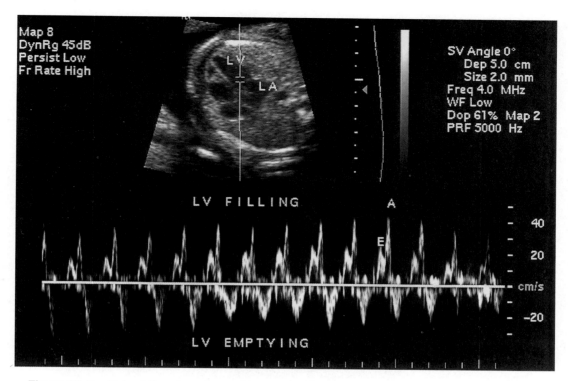

Figure 15–2. Pulsed Doppler echocardiogram showing normal left ventricular filling and emptying. The sample volume is placed in the left ventricle (LV) just below the mitral valve at the junction of ventricular inflow and outflow. Flow into the ventricle is seen above the baseline, and out of the ventricle below the baseline. Biphasic ventricular filling is demonstrated with less flow during the early, passive phase (E) of diastole than during the active atrial contraction phase (A). LA, left atrium.

Specific Fetal Arrhythmias

Isolated Extrasystoles

Extrasystoles, most often a result of premature atrial contractions, are the most common fetal arrhythmia and usually present as an irregular fetal heart rate. These benign and self-limited irregularities can cause a great deal of anxiety for the parents. Depending on the timing of the extrasystole in the cardiac cycle, there may be apparent pauses in the fetal heart rate lasting up to ¾ of a second, a frightening interval for the parents. Based on our experience, these arrhythmias are almost always supraventricular extrasystoles in origin, rather than true pauses in fetal cardiac rhythm, and comprise approximately 85% of the fetal arrhythmias that we encounter. Occasionally, however, these extrasystoles may be junctional or ventricular in origin.[12] Several studies have shown that isolated ectopy is usually a self-limited process, and just as in the newborn, it almost always carries a benign prognosis.[13–16] Interestingly, these arrhythmias usually resolve before labor or, alternatively, shortly after delivery.[4]

The diagnosis is established by the demonstration of premature movement of the posterior atrial wall on M-mode echocardiography (Figure 15–3). Alternatively, Doppler flow analysis can be used to demonstrate passive E wave filling of the ventricle during ventricular diastole, with the premature A wave (representing active atrial contraction corresponding to the electrocardiographic p wave) appearing close to, or even superimposed upon, the E wave. If the premature A wave is not obscured in the passive filling phase, the time to the next A wave can be seen to be the same as that between normal beats, a result of resetting of the atrial pacemaker.

The origin of isolated extrasystoles in the heart (i.e., atrial versus junctional versus ventricular) can be determined, but doing so is time consuming and difficult and occasionally impossible. It also has little practical significance, since isolated extrasystoles are important only as clues to the risk of future sustained tachyarrhythmias.[17] When these occur the underlying mechanism is secondary to reentry circuits, usually via accessory conduction pathways at the atrioventricular junction.[1] We have seen sustained fetal or neonatal

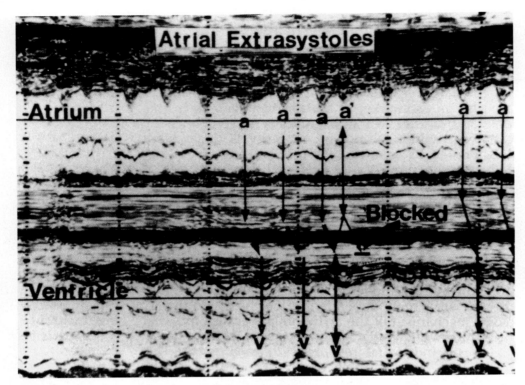

Figure 15–3. Ladder diagram analysis of fetal cardiac rhythm using dual M-mode recording of atrial and ventricular activity. Upper portion is atrial wall motion (a), which is interrupted by an extrasystole (a'). Simultaneous recording of ventricular wall motion below shows regular contractions (v) following normal conduction delay. The atrial extrasystole has encountered the AV node during its refractory period, so the beat is blocked and there is no ventricular response. (*Reprinted, with permission, from Kleinman CS, Copel JA. Fetal cardiac arrhythmias: Diagnosis and therapy. In Creasy RK, Resnick R, eds.* Maternal–Fetal Medicine, Principles and Practice, *3rd ed. Philadelphia: WB Saunders; 1994.*)

supraventricular tachycardia in only a few fetuses with isolated extrasystoles, with an approximate incidence of under 0.5% of fetuses with extrasystoles. Most of these occur prenatally, but we have seen one case manifest 3 days after birth in a neonate who had blocked atrial bigeminy in utero but was found to have Wolff-Parkinson-White syndrome on the neonatal electrocardiogram (ECG).

In 1985, we reported that 1% of fetuses with premature atrial contractions had concomitant structural heart disease.[18] In light of this, a full fetal echocardiographic evaluation should be undertaken in all patients demonstrating such ectopy. Furthermore, ~0.4% of such patients will develop a reentrant tachycardia later in pregnancy,[13,18,19] which is the basis for our recommendation that any fetus with premature extrasystoles be auscultated weekly throughout pregnancy to rule out the possible development of a sustained tachycardia.

Supraventricular Tachycardia

Fetal supraventricular tachycardia is most frequently found with a ventricular rate of 240 to 260 BPM, despite the fact that several differing mechanisms have been implicated as possible causes of the arrhythmia. Among these are (1) an automatic focus above the bundle of His but below the sinus node, which is separate from and faster than the sinus nodal pacemaker (Figure 15–4); (2) a reentrant or reciprocating mechanism, related to a circular movement of electrical energy, arising at or dependent on the atrioventricular junction with a monotonous, 1:1 ratio of atrial to ventricular rate (Figure 15–5); (3) atrial flutter or fibrillation with typically high atrial rates of 300 to 500 BPM and a variable degree of atrioventricular nodal block, yielding lower, and often irregularly irregular, ventricular rates (Figure 15–6).[1,11]

An automatic atrial focus is a mechanism of atrial tachycardia wherein the tachycardia originates in atrial muscle, at a site remote from the sinoatrial or atrioven-

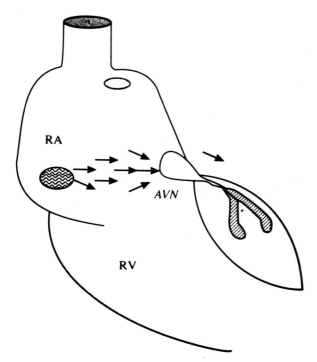

Figure 15–4. Schematic diagram of the cardiac conducting system in a patient with an automatic atrial tachycardia. An ectopic focus within the atrial muscle has taken over pacemaker activity from the sinus node. RA, right atrium; RV, right ventride; AVN, atrioventricular node. (*Reprinted, with permission, from Kleinman CS, Copel JA. Fetal cardiac arrhythmias: Diagnosis and therapy. In Creasy RK, Resnick R, eds. Maternal–Fetal Medicine, Principles and Practice, 3rd ed. Philadelphia: WB Saunders; 1994.*)

tricular node. Atrial flutter and fibrillation can be considered to be such rhythms; however, their mechanism is unique and is considered separately. In automatic atrial focus, sometimes also referred to as ectopic atrial tachycardia, the atrial activity continues in the presence of block of the atrioventricular (AV) node.[20] This block at the AV node may be spontaneously induced in the fetus or may be the result of antiarrhythmic medication. The atrial tachycardia results from abnormal automaticity of a section of atrial muscle, or rarely from triggered activity within the atrial tissue. In the former mechanism, the tachycardia is not induced or terminated by atrial extrasystoles, whereas in the latter mechanism, the tachycardia may be induced by atrial extrasystoles.

Reentrant tachycardias usually utilize the atrioventricular node as part of the pathway that conducts electrical energy.[1] These reciprocating tachycardias may occur within the AV node itself, or may use accessory AV pathways. The former are referred to as AV node reen-

try tachycardias (AVNRT) and the latter are referred to as AV reentry tachycardias (AVRT).

In AVNRT, there are dual pathways in the AV junctional region that serve as the substrate for the tachycardia. In this mechanism, the dual pathways have differing electrophysiologic conduction properties, one being a fast pathway with a shorter conduction time and a longer refractory period, and the other being a slow pathway with a longer conduction time and a shorter refractory period. Reentrant tachycardia occurs when there is unidirectional block in one of the pathways and an early extrasystole occurs. This allows conduction over the alternate pathway, with ensuing retrograde conduction over the previously blocked pathway, allowing for reentry into the AV node and thereby setting up a tachycardia circuit. In typical AVNRT, the slow pathway conducts in the anterograde direction, with the fast pathway being used for the retrograde conduction.

AVRT requires the presence of a discrete accessory pathway outside the atrioventricular node that conducts an impulse from the atrium to the ventricle. There are several different types of bypass tracts: those that connect the atrium to the His bundle, those that connect the AV node to the ventricle, and those that connect the His bundle to the ventricle. The most common, however, is the connection between the atrium and the ventricle. When this bypass tract conducts anterograde to the ventricle, there is ventricular preexcitation on the ECG, and the patient is said to have Wolff-Parkinson-White (WPW) syndrome. This diagnosis is generally made postnatally by examination of the electrocardiogram. However, we have noted that when the left atrium contracts before the right atrium, as may occur with a left-sided accessory pathway, there may be reversal of flow across the foramen ovale.[21] Preexcitation syndromes may be diagnosed prenatally, even in the absence of an electrocardiogram, in certain patients. The presence of the accessory pathway is necessary but not sufficient for reentrant tachycardia to occur, and not all patients (fetal and postnatal) necessarily develop arrhythmia. When there is tachycardia in these patients, it is referred to as either orthodromic or antidromic.

Orthodromic AVRT is said to occur when conduction from the atrium to the ventricle occurs along the normal conduction tissue and then travels back up from the ventricle to the atrium over the accessory pathway. Antidromic AVRT occurs when the atrium excites the ventricle through the accessory pathway and the ventricle in turn sends a retrograde impulse to the atrium up the AV node tissue. AVRT can also occur in a heart with a concealed pathway, which refers to an accessory pathway that is incapable of anterograde conduction but can conduct in the retrograde direction. Usually, AVRT or AVNRT is initiated by a premature atrial or ventricu-

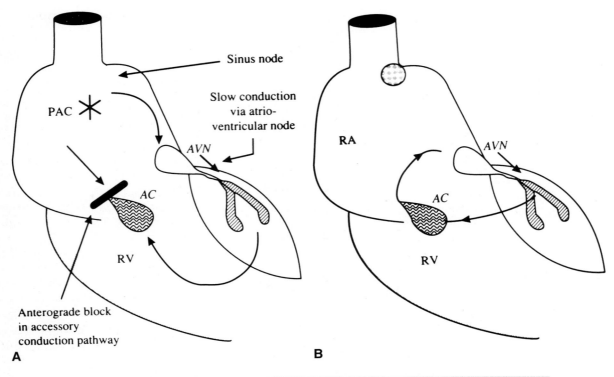

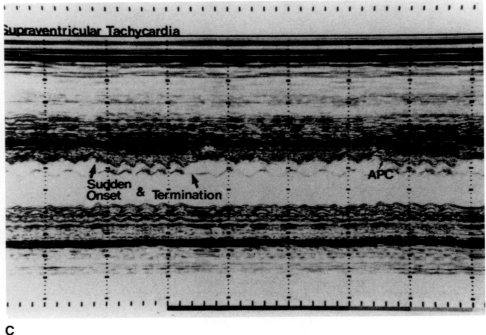

Figure 15–5. A. Schematic diagram of the cardiac conducting system in a patient with an accessory conducting pathway (AC). To establish orthodromic reciprocating supraventricular tachycardia, a premature atrial contraction (PAC) has occurred with a critical coupling interval that is shorter than the effective refractory period in the accessory conduction pathway. The impulse encounters the atrioventricular node (AVN) after its shorter refractory period and conducts slowly through the AVN node and the ventricular muscle and then encounters the AC in a retrograde fashion. RV, right venticle. (*Reproduced with permission, from Kleinman CS, Copel JA. Electrophysiologic principles and fetal antiarrhythmic therapy. Ultrasound Obstet Gynecol: 1991; 1:286.*) **B.** After retrograde reentry of the electrical impulse into the atrial muscle through the accessory pathway a circular movement of electrical energy is established. RA, right atrium. Other definitions as in part **A.** (*Reproduced, with permission, from Kleinman CS, Copel JA: Electrophysiologic principles and fetal anatiarrhythmic therapy. Ultrasound Obstet Gynecol: 1991; 1:286.*) **C.** M-mode echocardiogram of ventricular wall motion in a fetus having short runs of supraventricular tachycardia. The ventricular wall movements at a rate of 240 to 260 BPM occur in short paroxysms that are of sudden onset and termination. The onset of these episodes follows an extrasystole, further evidence that this dysrhythmia is a reentrant tachycardia. (*Reprinted, with permission, from Kleinman CS, Copel JA. Fetal cardiac arrhythmias: Diagnosis and therapy. In Creasy RK, Resnick R, eds.* Maternal–Fetal Medicine, Principles and Practice, *3rd ed. Philadelphia: WB Saunders; 1994: pp. 84–104.*)

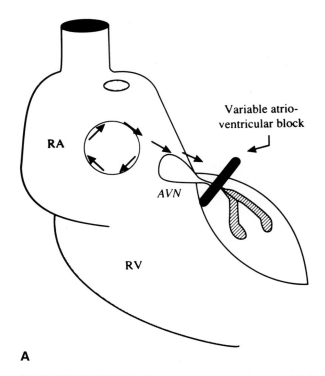

A

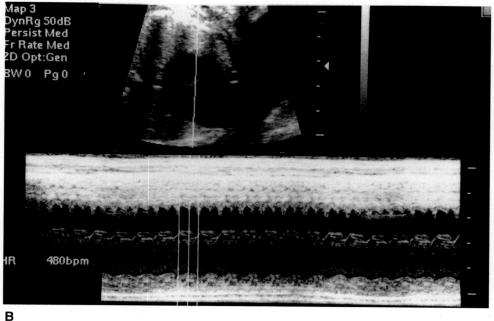

B

Figure 15–6. A. Schematic diagram of the cardiac conducting system in a patient with atrial (RA) flutter. In this situation the atrium (RA) flutters at a regular rate, governed by a circular movement of electrical energy. The wavefront of this movement is completely contained within the atrial muscle. The usual atrial rate in atrial flutter in the fetus is between 400 and 500 BPM. The ventricular rate is usually less than the atrial rate because of a variable degree of atrioventricular block at the level of the atrioventricular node (AVN). RV, right ventricle. (*Reprinted, with permission, from Kleinman CS, Copel JA. Electrophysiologic principles and fetal antiarrhythmic therapy.* Ultrasound Obstet Gynecol: *1991; 1:286.*) **B.** M-mode echocardiogram of a fetus with atrial flutter and 2:1 atrioventricular block. The atrial rate is measured at 580 BPM, and is represented by the upper portion of the M-mode tracing. The lower, ventricular portion shows contractions only in response to every other atrial contraction.

lar complex with block in one of the pathways while there is conduction over the other, with subsequent retrograde excitation over the previously blocked pathway, thereby setting up a reentrant circuit.

Atrial Flutter and Fibrillation

Atrial flutter typically occurs at extremely fast and regular atrial rates, with variable block through the AV node, yielding lower ventricular rates (Figure 15–6 B). It is not uncommon for the ventricular response rate to be half of the atrial rate (2:1 block), but higher degrees of AV block can also occur. When the degree of block varies, the ventricular response may become irregular. The mechanism of atrial flutter is generally thought to be a macroreentrant one, usually within the atrial muscle itself. Like the automatic or ectopic atrial tachycardias, atrial flutter does not resolve with block at the AV node. When the atrial depolarization is completely disorganized, without any effective contraction, atrial fibrillation exists. This is typically associated with variable AV node block, yielding an irregularly irregular ventricular response. Atrial fibrillation is relatively rare in the fetus.

Ventricular Tachycardia

Unlike fetal supraventricular tachycardia, fetal heart rates are highly variable in ventricular tachycardia and may be as fast as 400 BPM or as slow as 170 BPM. There are a number of different mechanisms that have been proposed to explain the electrophysiology of ventricular tachycardia. Ventricular tachycardia may occur through a reentrant mechanism. In the fetus who has had myocardial ischemia and/or infarction, the mechanism may be enhanced automaticity and triggered activity. The diagnosis can be made using M-mode echocardiography with the beam of interrogation transecting the atrium and the ventricle. This may reveal atrioventricular dissociation with the ventricular chamber contracting at a faster pace than the atrial chamber. Our experience has shown that ventricular tachycardia is a rare arrhythmia in the fetus, and it is our belief that not all of these fetuses require antiarrhythmic therapy.

It is extremely important to differentiate fetal ventricular tachycardia from fetal supraventricular tachycardia, since a misdiagnosis of supraventricular tachycardia and the administration of digoxin via the mother to a fetus with ventricular tachycardia may elicit life-threatening ventricular fibrillation.[1] The critical issue for the fetus with a tachycardia is a thorough analysis of the cardiac rhythm to define whether it is supraventricular or ventricular in origin. A meticulous, accurate analysis of the electrophysiology and the functional consequences of any arrhythmia is essential to the formulation of a rational management strategy for these fetuses.

Bradyarrhythmias

The most common etiology for fetal bradyarrhythmias, with ventricular rates less than 60 BPM, is fetal complete heart block.[22,23] According to Michaelsson and Engle,[24] complete heart block is a rare prenatal condition with an incidence of about 1 in 20,000 live births.

Approximately half of these fetuses have structurally normal hearts.[25] The mothers of these fetuses almost invariably produce one or both of two anti-RNA antibodies, designated anti-Ro and anti-La, which cross the placenta and damage the His-Purkinje fibers of the conducting system, causing fetal heart block, typically after 18 to 20 weeks.[25–29] These antibodies are also often found in patients with Sjögren syndrome, so they have also been designated SS-A and SS-B, respectively.

Patients may present with complete (third-degree) block, or second-degree block, which in our experience progresses to third-degree block. This observation implies that there are intermediate stages of fetal first- and second-degree block before the onset of complete heart block. Diffuse fetal myocarditis has also been described in these fetuses, resulting from damage to cardiac myocytes from the same antibodies.[30]

The sinoatrial node, located at the junction of the superior vena cava and the right atrium, functions as the intrinsic pacemaker of the atrium, maintaining a higher baseline rate than the intrinsic rate for the atrioventricular junction and the ventricles. In the fetus the atrial rate is usually 110 to 160 BPM, whereas intrinsic idioventricular rates range from 40 to 80 BPM. It is important to compare the atrial and ventricular contraction patterns over time to ensure that a fetus is actually in complete heart block rather than in atrial bigeminy, in which atrial activity is irregular.

Another group of fetuses with complete heart block have underlying structural cardiac abnormalities, usually involving complex lesions with abnormal development of the central portion of the heart, where the atrioventricular node is located. An example of this group is left atrial isomerism with an atrioventricular septal defect.[8,25] The defect interrupts the electrical connection between the atria and ventricles, resulting in independent electrical function of the upper and lower heart. These fetuses often also have the situs abnormalities that are seen in atrial isomerism (e.g., asplenia, polysplenia). The prognosis is quite poor for these fetuses, especially if hydrops develops.

Another complex type of congenital heart disease associated with complete heart block is atrioventricular–ventriculoarterial discordance, also known as physiologically corrected transposition, or levotransposition, of the great arteries. In this disease, the left atrium empties into the right ventricle (atrioventricular discordance), which then ejects the oxygenated blood received from the left atrium into the aorta (ventriculoarterial discordance). The conduction system is abnormally placed in these hearts and the incidence of heart block developing during pre- and postnatal life is in excess of 50% for these patients.

The experience at the Yale Fetal Cardiovascular Center has demonstrated that all mothers of fetuses with normal cardiac structure and complete atrioventricular block can be shown to have circulating autoantibodies with the use of sensitive assays.[2,8] A ventricular rate of 55 BPM or greater has been correlated with a favorable outcome. In general, approximately 85% of the fetuses found to have complete AV block with a structurally normal heart will survive the neonatal period.[25] Once a fetus has been found to have complete atrioventricular block, close echocardiographic follow-up is necessary to evaluate the patient for the development of hydrops fetalis. Nonimmune hydrops can be thought of as end-stage congestive heart failure in the fetus.[31] Hydrops fetalis can result from structural heart disease, arrhythmias, or a combination of the two. The presence of hydrops fetalis is a poor prognostic sign and when it is found in the patient with structural heart disease (with or without complete heart block), it is almost always fatal.[25,31]

TREATMENT OF FETAL ARRHYTHMIAS

When isolated extrasystoles are found, we reassure the parents and suggest avoidance of possible stimulating drugs (e.g., caffeine, cocaine, pseudoephedrine, and most importantly, β-mimetic tocolytics). Should preterm labor develop, alternative agents, such as intravenous magnesium or oral nifedipine, may be preferable to β-mimetics if the extrasystoles are still present.

There is an approximately 0.4% risk of developing supraventricular tachycardia among fetuses with premature atrial extrasystoles. To address this risk we recommend weekly auscultation of the fetal heart, with the plan to evaluate the heart again if tachycardia is suspected. The 1-week interval between fetal heart rate checks minimizes the risk of developing nonimmune hydrops from sustained fetal supraventricular tachycardia between visits. The fetus with frequent premature beats, or atrial bigeminy, can be managed in the same way. Surveillance can be discontinued after several visits without any ectopy. There may be an advantage in terms of convenience to prolonged fetal monitoring by nonstress testing, but we believe that several minutes of auscultation with any fetoscope or Doppler auscultation device should be sufficient to detect a fetus having recurrent episodes of supraventricular tachycardia, at substantially lower cost than weekly nonstress testing.

A variety of different pharmacologic therapies have been used to treat the fetus with arrhythmias, including digoxin, flecainide, procainamide, and amiodarone, to name just a few (Figure 15–7).[32–41] It is imperative that the physician bear in mind that each of these therapies carries with it inherent risks both for the fetus and for the mother. We recommend that whenever pharmacologic therapy of a fetal arrhythmia is undertaken, informed consent be obtained. For a particular drug to be effective in treating fetal arrhythmias it must be able to undergo uniform maternal absorption and reliable transplacental transfer and achieve therapeutic levels in the fetus without causing toxicity or severe maternal or fetal side effects. Maternal side effects and complicated clinical problems can be minimized with direct delivery of the medication into the fetus via cordocentesis,[42,43] a process that carries a small risk, especially for the fetus who may require multiple drug administrations.

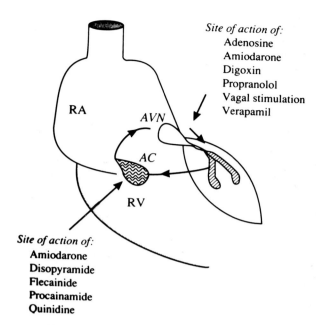

Figure 15–7. Schematic diagram of the cardiac conducting system in a patient with an accessory conducting pathway and reciprocating orthodromic supraventricular tachycardia. This diagram demonstrates the site of action of various drugs that have been used to treat this arrhythmia. RA, right atrium; RV, right ventricle; AVN, atrioventricular node; AC, accessory conducting pathway. (*Reprinted, with permission, from Kleinman CS, Copel JA. Electrophysiologic principles and fetal antiarrythmic therapy.* Ultrasound Obstet Gynecol: *1991; 1:286.*)

In general, we avoid the use of rigid algorithms for the pharmacologic therapy of fetal arrhythmias; instead, we use a team approach including a maternal–fetal medicine specialist and a pediatric cardiologist to determine the appropriate individualized therapy. The salient factor in treating a fetal arrhythmia is the accurate diagnosis of the fetal rhythm. With this in mind, the following discussion briefly reviews some of the medical therapies that may be utilized in the fetus with an arrhythmia.

When a reentrant supraventricular tachycardia is found in a very preterm fetus without evidence of hydrops, we first observe with a fetal monitor for an extended period of time (i.e., several hours). In contrast, if the fetus is at term, we generally recommend delivery for postnatal diagnosis and management of the tachycardia. The extended fetal monitoring demonstrates the proportion of time that the fetus experiences the tachycardia, which can further influence the management strategy. When the amount of time spent in supraventricular tachycardia is relatively short, the team may determine that intervention is unnecessary, whereas a more aggressive approach may be undertaken if the tachycardia is incessant. In the latter case, a reasonable first-line therapy is the maternal intravenous administration of digoxin.[1,32] Digoxin leads to slowing of conduction through the AV node, thereby blocking the circus pathway of the reentrant tachycardia.

When fetal hydrops exists, fetal blood sampling for drug levels as well as for direct introduction of medications may be performed. Adenosine, with its extremely short half-life and few side effects, blocks conduction through the AV node and is an effective therapy for direct administration into the fetus with supraventricular tachycardia.[44] If successful control of the tachycardia is achieved with adenosine, the fetus can then be loaded with digoxin at the dose of 20 μg/kg (estimated fetal dry body weight), followed by maintenance therapy through maternal dosing. It is important to remember that the maternal requirements to maintain therapeutic digoxin levels are often increased during pregnancy and dosing should be adjusted accordingly. It is important to remember that maternally administered adenosine is *not* useful, because its short half-life and rapid protein binding render it ineffective to the fetus. In addition, adenosine is also not an effective therapy for other supraventricular tachycardias (automatic, ectopic, atrial fibrillation). Adenosine, then, can be expected to result in only a brief conversion to sinus rhythm. Although lacking prophylactic properties against recurrent tachycardia, even a brief episode of sinus rhythm represents a therapeutic trial that ascertains that the underlying electrophysiologic mechanism is reentrant. Further therapy can be guided by this knowledge.

Other therapies that may be required if digoxin is unsuccessful in controlling fetal supraventricular tachycardia include the direct fetal administration of procainamide followed by oral maternal therapy,[34,35] or the oral administration of flecainide to the mother,[41,45,46] although the use of such antiarrhythmics may carry risk to both the mother and the fetus.

Digoxin is our first-line therapy for fetal atrial flutter. We begin with an intravenous maternal load of 1 mg over 12 h (e.g., 0.5 mg to start followed by two doses of 0.25 mg 6 and 12 h later). If cardioversion does not occur with this single therapy, we next administer flecainide orally to the mother, bearing in mind that flecainide alters the metabolism of digoxin, leading to increased serum digoxin levels.[47] It is appropriate, therefore, to decrease the digoxin dose by approximately half when it is given in conjunction with flecainide and to monitor both the mother and the fetus closely for any detrimental effects. When atrial flutter does not respond to therapy with digoxin and flecainide, amiodarone may be considered, which can be administered orally to the mother only after withholding flecainide for 48 h. Amiodarone has been used in Europe as a direct fetal infusion.[48] Amiodarone has a half-life of several weeks, which makes it an attractive option for the treatment of fetal arrhythmias since it can be given much less often than other drugs. On the other hand, any side effects will persist because of this prolonged half-life. However, the complications of this drug must not be ignored, including fetal hypothyroidism, which can be significant.[49–51]

Whereas the experience with fetal ventricular tachycardia is limited, it appears that the primary indication for therapy is the presence of hydrops fetalis and a ventricular rate in excess of 200 BPM. In this case, lidocaine may be given directly to the fetus by umbilical vessel injection. If this therapy is successful, the mother can be given the type-1B agent, mexiletine, or a type-1A agent, such as quinidine or procainamide, or a type-1C agent, such as flecainide.[1] It is imperative that the diagnosis of ventricular tachycardia be accurate and not be confused with supraventricular tachycardia, because therapy for the latter, which includes digoxin, can be potentially dangerous if administered as treatment of the former.

It is important to bear in mind that any of the antiarrhythmic agents listed in this chapter can have serious side effects for the mother, in addition to the increases in serum digoxin levels mentioned previously.[47] Proarrhythmic effects are seen in up to 8% of patients on flecainide[52] and can also be seen with any of the type-1C agents, and with quinidine.[53] Although the loss of a fetus with a presumably treatable fetal arrhythmia is a tragedy, the iatrogenic loss of a previously healthy mother, who is taking medications solely on behalf of her fetus, would be an even greater catastrophe.

The only effective treatment for fetuses with bradycardia caused by structural heart disease is postnatal surgery and pacemaker placement. The picture may be different for the structurally normal group, for we have recently reported that high-dose maternal steroids may be beneficial in some cases of immunologic fetal complete heart block.[54] We used dexamethasone, because it is not inactivated by the placenta, maximizing fetal exposure. We have never seen reversion of second-degree heart block spontaneously, but this did occur with steroid treatment in one fetus in our series, and transient reversion of complete heart block to second-degree block occurred in one other, as did permanent reversion from mixed second- and third-degree block to second-degree block. In contrast, we have never observed spontaneous resolution of AV block.

Plasmapheresis has also been suggested to treat fetal heart block in the past, to reduce maternal antibody loads.[55,56] There have also been a few reports of attempted fetal pacemaker placement; however, there have been no fetal survivors.[57,58]

INTRAPARTUM MANAGEMENT

Patients with extrasystoles can be managed with standard fetal monitoring approaches in labor. Antenatal fetal heart rate testing is not necessary for these fetuses. Occasionally, the frequency of the premature beats may seem to obscure the baseline rate, but looking at an overview of the tracing usually permits appreciation of the true baseline rate and any accelerations or decelerations that may be present.

Fetal complete heart block may be amenable to external fetal heart rate monitoring,[8] although in our experience this is successful only about a third of the time. For external monitoring to succeed, atrial contractions must be followed by directing the fetal monitor to the AV valves. Internal monitoring will only demonstrate the ventricular rate, as internal monitoring uses the R–R interval of the ECG to calculate heart rate. When external monitoring is not feasible, our approach is to perform elective cesarean delivery at term because we are not able to maintain assurance of fetal well-being in labor. If fetal transcutaneous oxygen saturation monitoring becomes accepted as an alternative to heart rate monitoring in labor, vaginal delivery may become a more attractive option.[59,60]

POSTNATAL OUTLOOK OF FETAL ARRHYTHMIAS

The postnatal outlook of the infant who had a fetal arrhythmia depends on the severity and duration of the fetal arrhythmia. For most infants, a precise diagnosis can be quickly established in the immediate newborn period with a 12-lead electrocardiogram. With this simple test, one can determine whether there is preexcitation of the ventricle, as in the Wolff-Parkinson-White syndrome, and whether the accessory pathway is right or left sided. Automatic atrial arrhythmias can be accurately diagnosed with the electrocardiogram. Intravenous administration of adenosine may be used as a diagnostic tool in such patients, since AV block occurs with continuing electrocardiographic evidence of atrial tachycardia, whereas atrioventricular block results in sudden cessation of AVRT or AVNRT. When necessary, a newborn infant can undergo a transesophageal electrophysiologic study with pacing to further delineate the mechanism of arrhythmia and to provide treatment.

When fetal arrhythmias persist into the newborn period, treatment can be quickly administered. This may be by the intravenous route through an umbilical or percutaneous catheter. Transesophageal pacing can be performed to convert certain arrhythmias. In the unstable newborn with a reentrant arrhythmia, synchronized electrical cardioversion can be delivered in the controlled setting of the neonatal intensive care unit.

With advances in pharmacotherapy in combination with new radiofrequency catheter ablation techniques performed at the time of electrophysiologic testing, the long-term outlook for the fetus and infant with arrhythmias continues to improve.

CONCLUSIONS

We have reviewed common fetal arrhythmias and their pathogenesis and treatment. Before any intrauterine antiarrhythmic therapy is initiated certain underlying concepts should be remembered:

- The arrhythmia must be accurately diagnosed.
- Any underlying structural heart disease must be identified.
- The value of intrauterine therapy versus delivery must be considered.
- The risks and benefits of intrauterine therapy per se should be explored.
- Treatment requires appropriate maternal and fetal monitoring, including inpatient initiation of maternal medications.
- Treatment must be preceded by full informed consent.

These decisions require extensive discussions with our patients and cannot be undertaken unilaterally by physicians. Furthermore, close collaboration between pediatric cardiologists and obstetricians is required for optimal results. We firmly believe that such interventions should be reserved for tertiary centers, to concentrate the experience and skills that are needed to provide the best outcomes, and because these are the locations best able to develop the necessary multidisciplinary teams. The institution providing care should also be prepared to care for any maternal or fetal complications that may ensue. The field of fetal antiarrhythmic therapy has been one of the earliest examples of fetal treatment, and its successes can be a model for other areas of fetal therapy if we bear these principles in mind.

REFERENCES

1. Kleinman CS, Copel JA: Electrophysiologic principles and fetal antiarrhythmic therapy. *Ultrasound Obstet Gynecol.* 1:286, 1991.
2. Martinez E, Tan ASA, Kleinman CS, et al.: Fetal cardiac implications of maternal system diseases. *Prog Pediatr Cardiol.* 5:91, 1996.
3. Mendoza GJ, Almeida O, Steinfeld L: Intermittent fetal bradycardia induced by midpregnancy fetal ultrasonographic study. *Am J Obstet Gynecol.* 160:1038, 1989.
4. Kleinman CS, Donnerstein RL, Jaffe CC, et al.: Fetal echocardiography: A tool for evaluation of in utero car-

diac arrhythmias and monitoring of in utero therapy: Analysis of 71 patients. *Am J Cardiol.* 51:237, 1983.

5. Silverman NH, Enderlein MA, Stanger P, et al.: Recognition of fetal arrhythmias by echocardiography. *J Clin Ultrasound.* 13:255, 1985.

6. Cameron A, Nicholson S, Nimrod C, et al.: Evaluation of fetal cardiac dysrhythmias with two-dimensional, M-mode, and pulsed Doppler ultrasonography. *Am J Obstet Gynecol.* 158:286, 1988.

7. Strasburger JF, Huhta JC, Carpenter RJ, et al.: Doppler echocardiography in the diagnosis and management of persistent fetal arrhythmias. *J Am Coll Cardiol.* 7:1386, 1986.

8. Kleinman CS, Copel JA, Hobbins JC: Combined echocardiographic and Doppler assessment of fetal congenital atrioventricular block. *Br J Obstet Gynaecol.* 94:967, 1987.

9. DeVore GR, Horenstein J: Simultaneous Doppler recording of the pulmonary artery and vein: A new technique for the evaluation of a fetal arrhythmia. *J Ultrasound Med.* 12:669, 1993.

10. Smythe JF, Copel JA, Kleinman CS: Outcome of prenatally detected cardiac malformations. *Am J Cardiol.* 69:1471, 1992.

11. Baumann P, Copel JA, Kleinman CS: Management of the fetus with cardiac disease. *Ultrasound Quart.* 10:57, 1992.

12. Kleinman CS: Prenatal diagnosis and management of intrauterine arrhythmias. *Fetal Ther.* 1:92, 1986.

13. Kallfelz HC: Cardiac arrhythmias in the fetus—Diagnosis, significance and prognosis. In Godman MJ, Marquis RM, eds. *Heart Disease in the Newborn.* Edinburgh: Churchill Livingstone; 1979: p. 401.

14. Southall DP, Richards J, Hardwick RA, et al.: Prospective study of fetal heart rate and rhythm pattern. *Arch Dis Child.* 55:506, 1980.

15. Bernstine RL, Winler JE, Callagan, DA: Fetal bigeminy and tachycardia. *Am J Obstet Gynecol.* 101: 856, 1968.

16. Kendall B: Abnormal fetal heart rates and rhythms prior to labor. *Am J Obstet Gynecol.* 99:71, 1967.

17. Kleinman CS, Copel JA: Fetal cardiac arrhythmias: Diagnosis and therapy. In Creasy RK, Resnick R, eds. *Maternal-Fetal Medicine, Principles and Practice,* 3rd ed. Philadelphia: WB Saunders; 1994.

18. Kleinman CS, Copel JA, Weinstein EM, et al.: In utero diagnosis and treatment of fetal supraventricular tachycardia. *Semin Perinatol.* 9:113, 1985.

19. Gillette PC: The mechanism of supraventricular tachycardia in children. *Circulation.* 54:133, 1976.

20. Knudson JM, Kleinman CS, Copel JA, et al.: Ectopic atrial tachycardia in utero. *Obstet Gynecol.* 84:686, 1994.

21. Kleinman CS, Dubin AM, Nehgme RA, et al.: Left atrial tachycardia in the human fetus: Identifying the fetus at greatest risk for developing nonimmune hydrops fetalis. (Manuscript submitted for publication.)

22. Crawford D, Chapman M, Allan L: The assessment of persistent bradycardia in prenatal life. *Br J Obstet Gynaecol.* 92:941, 1985.

23. Shenker L, Reed KL, Anderson CF, et al.: Congenital heart block and cardiac anomalies in the absence of maternal connective tissue disease. *Am J Obstet Gynecol.* 157:248, 1987.

24. Michaelsson M, Engle MA: Congenital complete heart block: An international study of the natural history. *Cardiovasc Clin.* 4:85, 1972.

25. Schmidt KG, Ulmer HE, Silverman NH, et al.: Perinatal outcome of fetal complete atrioventricular block: A multicenter experience. *J Am Coll Cardiol.* 91:1360, 1991.

26. Scott JS, Maddison PJ, Taylor PV, et al.: Connective-tissue disease, antibodies to ribonucleoprotein, and congenital heart block. *N Engl J Med.* 309:209, 1983.

27. Taylor PV, Scott JS, Gerlis LM, et al.: Maternal antibodies against fetal cardiac antigens in congenital complete heart block. *N Engl J Med.* 315:667, 1986.

28. Litsey SE, Noonan JA, O'Connor WN, et al.: Maternal connective tissue disease and congenital heart block: Demonstration of immunoglobulin in cardiac tissue. *N Engl J Med.* 312:98, 1985.

29. Taylor PV, Scott JS, Gerlis LM, et al.: Maternal antibodies against fetal cardiac antigens in congenital complete heart block. *N Engl J Med.* 315:667, 1986.

30. Horsfall AC, Venables PJW, Taylor PV, et al.: Ro and La antigens and maternal autoantibody idiotype in the surface of myocardial fibres in congenital heart block. *J Autoimmun.* 4:165, 1991.

31. Kleinman CS, Donnerstein RL, DeVore GR, et al.: Fetal echocardiography for evaluation of in utero congestive heart failure: A technique for study of nonimmune fetal hydrops. *N Engl J Med.* 306:568, 1982.

32. Kerenyi TD, Gleicher N, Meller J, et al.: Transplacental cardioversion of intrauterine supraventricular tachycardia with digitalis. *Lancet.* 2:393, 1980.

33. Lingman G, Ohrlander S, Ohlin P: Intrauterine digoxin treatment of fetal paroxysmal tachycardia. *Br J Obstet Gynaecol.* 87:340, 1980.

34. Dumesic DA, Silverman NH, Tobias S, et al.: Transplacental cardioversion of fetal supraventricular tachycardia with procainamide. *N Engl J Med.* 307:1128, 1982.

35. Given BD, Phillippe M, Sanders SP, et al.: Procainamide cardioversion of fetal supraventricular tachyarrhythmia. *Am J Cardiol.* 53:1460, 1984.

36. Spinnato JA, Shaver DC, Flinn GS, et al.: Fetal supraventricular tachycardia: In utero therapy with digoxin and quinidine. *Obstet Gynecol.* 64:730, 1984.

37. Golichowski AM, Caldwell R, Hartsough A, et al.: Pharmacologic cardioversion of intrauterine supraventricular tachycardia. A case report. *J Reprod Med.* 30:139, 1985.

38. Lasson JR, Beytout M, Jacquetin B, et al.: Traitement d'une tachycardie supraventriculaire foetale: Association digoxine-amiodarone. *Coeur.* 15:315, 1985.

39. Arnoux P, Seyral P, Llurens M, et al.: Amiodarone and digoxin for refractory fetal tachycardia. *Am J Cardiol.* 59:166, 1987.

40. Hansmann M, Gembruch U, Bald R, et al.: Fetal tachyarrhythmias: Transplacental and direct treatment of the fetus—A report of 60 cases. *Ultrasound Obstet Gynecol.* 1: 162, 1991.

41. Allan LD, Chita SK, Sharland GK, et al.: Flecainide in the treatment of fetal tachycardias. *Br Heart J.* 65:46, 1991.

42. Younis JS, Granat M: Insufficient transplacental digoxin transfer in severe hydrops fetalis. *Am J Obstet Gynecol.* 157:1268, 1987.

43. Weiner CP, Thompson MIB: Direct treatment of fetal supraventricular tachycardia after failed transplacental therapy. *Am J Obstet Gynecol.* 158:570, 1988.

44. Camm AJ, Garratt CJ: Adenosine and supraventricular tachycardia. *N Engl J Med.* 325:1621, 1991.

45. Kofinas AD, Simon NV, Sagel H, et al.: Treatment of fetal supraventricular tachycardia with flecainide acetate after digoxin failure. *Am J Obstet Gynecol.* 165:630, 1991.

46. Perry JC, Ayres NA, Carpenter RJ: Fetal supraventricular tachycardia treated with flecainide acetate. *J Pediatr.* 118:303, 1991.

47. Smith TW: Digitalis: Mechanisms of action and clinical use. *N Engl J Med.* 318:358, 1988.

48. Gembruch U, Manz M, Bald R, et al.: Repeated intravascular treatment with amiodarone in a fetus with refractory supraventricular tachycardia and hydrops fetalis. *Am Heart J.* 118:1335, 1989.

49. Laurent M, Betremieux P, Biron P, et al.: Neonatal hypothyroidism after treatment by amiodarone during pregnancy. *Am J Cardiol.* 60:942, 1987.

50. Rovet J, Ehrlich R, Sorbara D: Intellectual outcome in children with fetal hypothyroidism. *J Pediatr.* 110:700, 1987.

51. Bowers PN, Fields J, Schwartz D, et al.: Amiodarone-induced pulmonary fibrosis in infancy. *PACE* (in press).

52. Morganroth J, Anderson JL, Gentzkow GD: Classification by type of ventricular arrhythmia predicts frequency of adverse cardiac events from flecainide. *J Am Coll Cardiol.* 8:607, 1986.

53. Opie LH: Calcium channel antagonists. Part IV: Side effects and contraindications, drug interactions and combinations. *Cardiovasc Drugs Ther.* 2:177, 1988.

54. Copel JA, Buyon JP, Kleinman CS. Successful in utero therapy of fetal heart block. *Am J Obstet Gynecol.* 173:1384, 1995.

55. Barcaly CS, French MA, Ross LD, et al.: Successful pregnancy following steroid therapy and plasma exchange in a woman with anti-ro (SS-A) antibodies. *Br J Obstet Gynaecol.* 94:369, 1987.

56. Bierman FZ, Baxi L, Jaffe I, et al.: Fetal hydrops and congenital complete heart block: Response to maternal steroid therapy. *J Pediatr.* 112:646, 1988.

57. Carpenter RJ, Strasburger JF, Garson A, Jr, et al.: Fetal ventricular pacing for hydrops secondary to complete atrioventricular block. *J Am Coll Cardiol.* 8:1434, 1986.

58. Walkinshaw SA, Welch CR, McCormack J, et al.: In utero pacing for fetal congenital heart block. *Fetal Diagn Ther.* 9:183, 1994.

59. Dildy GA, Clark SL, Loucks CA: Preliminary experience with intrapartum fetal pulse oximetry in humans. *Obstet Gynecol.* 81:630, 1993.

60. Dildy GA, Clark SL, Loucks CA: Intrapartum fetal pulse oximetry: Past, present, and future. *Am J Obstet Gynecol.* 175:1, 1996.

CHAPTER Sixteen

Early Stabilization and Medical Management for Congenital Cardiac Disease

Elizabeth J. P. James

The immediate care of the newborn with congenital heart disease (CHD) has changed remarkably over the past 10 years in large part because of advances in intrauterine diagnosis of the fetus with heart disease.[1] Not only does early diagnosis permit fetal treatment (pharmacologic therapy of the fetus,[2,3] for example), but it also gives those responsible for the care of these newborns the ability to plan for early management beginning at the time of birth.

The newborn with CHD previously was most often a surprise to the obstetrician, pediatrician, or neonatologist caring for these infants. Current ultrasonographic and fetal echocardiographic techniques have given those caring for these newborns detailed advance knowledge about the infant's cardiac structure and function. This attendant information is essential to facilitating the infant's successful stabilization and early treatment.

In addition, intrauterine diagnosis gives the parents information about their infant's likely course at birth. At this point they have time to consider various options of treatment without being under the pressure to decide quickly (as when a newborn with an unexpected cardiac defect demands immediate attention). They then have the ability to speak with the pediatric cardiologist and pediatric cardiothoracic surgeon at length and explore treatment options thoroughly. Under such circumstances, true informed consent for treatment can be obtained.

In the event that the fetus has a defect that is ex-

pected to require immediate surgical intervention, the mother's delivery should be planned to take place in the hospital, where all the baby's cardiac and neonatal care can be given. It must be remembered that the fetus with stable in utero heart disease frequently changes at the point of birth to an unstable newborn because of the physiologic changes that take place in fetal circulation at delivery.[4] Planned early intervention can make the difference between a successful and an unsuccessful outcome. It is essential that the pediatric cardiologist or neonatologist be aware of the impending delivery of an affected fetus, preferably many days in advance, and that arrangements be made for a competent team to attend the delivery.

COEXISTING CONDITIONS

It is frequently pointed out that newborns do not usually have more than one disorder. However, this rule is broken more frequently in the case of CHD than with many other problems.[5] The following problems require immediate attention in the newborn with CHD, even though they may not be etiologically related to the cardiac defect.

Asphyxia

The infant with CHD may suffer from the effects of placental insufficiency and present with low Apgar scores, respiratory depression, and metabolic acidosis. The treatment should duplicate that of similar infants without heart disease and includes the standard neonatal resuscitative measures of physical stimulation, positive-pressure breathing, and establishment of an adequate heart rate, along with correction of the acid–base derangement. Hypovolemia[6] should be judiciously corrected, however, with care being taken not to administer a fluid overload inadvertently. It is helpful to establish venous and arterial access in such infants in the resuscitation room, since arterial and venous lines are most likely to be required later, and at the time of resuscitation it is usually not clear whether the infant's condition may be partially or totally a result of the cardiac disease.

Prematurity and Pulmonary Pathology

Preterm delivery and its attendant pulmonary immaturity can significantly adversely affect the infant with cardiac disease. The use of surfactant[7,8] in the resuscitation room can improve the course of the pulmonary disease in those infants with known lung immaturity. Group B streptococcal pneumonia and lung malformations can likewise exist in infants with heart disease and should be sought in those babies who demonstrate significant respiratory distress. An early chest x-ray examination frequently helps to clarify the role of lung disease in the clinical picture.

Hypoglycemia

It is important to remember that a low blood glucose level can have long-term sequels if not detected and promptly treated.[9] Routine screening for hypoglycemia must be done and appropriate dextrose infusions must be given, using 10% or 15% glucose solutions through appropriate lines.[10]

Other Anomalies

Cardiac disease is frequently associated with a constellation of other anomalies involving many organ systems.[11] A careful search should be made for chromosomal abnormalities (if not already diagnosed prenatally) and for syndromes that include heart disease (e.g., VATER syndrome, gastrointestinal, genitourinary, and central nervous system anomalies).[12,13]

RELATED CONDITIONS REQUIRING IMMEDIATE MANAGEMENT

Congenital heart disease is frequently associated with life-threatening problems, present at birth or appearing shortly thereafter, that require immediate management in order to stabilize the condition of the infant and permit definitive treatment. Because of the expected occurrence of such complications, it is essential to monitor the infant with pulse oximetry, transcutaneous oxygen and carbon dioxide monitors, and arterial blood pressures, as well as with standard cardiorespiratory monitoring. Central arterial and venous catheter placement (using the umbilical artery and umbilical vein) frequently proves helpful.

Decreased Cardiac Output

Decreased cardiac output, from whatever cause, results in poor perfusion of vital organs and progressive deterioration of their functioning.[14] When cardiac output is only mildly or moderately decreased, the infant exhibits tachycardia and peripheral vasoconstriction in an attempt to maintain blood pressure. Examination of the infant shows delayed capillary refill and cool extremities, along with poor peripheral pulses. As cardiac output decreases further, metabolic acidosis progresses (which, in turn, decreases myocardial function), and the infant shows tachypnea and agitation. Peripheral pulses disappear, and cyanosis of the extremities may become marked. Hypotension and a narrowed pulse pressure are present.[15]

In infants with a high probability of poor tolerance of a fluid load, volume expansion should be undertaken with caution.[6] In the absence of evidence of an already existing fluid overload, it is usually safe to administer a 10- to 20-mL/kg bolus of normal saline intravenously in an attempt to improve perfusion. If, however, evidence of venous congestion or pulmonary vascular distension appears, such a bolus should not be repeated.

The use of inotropic agents can be helpful in improving systemic circulation.[15] Dobutamine[16] stimulates myocardial β-1 receptors and should be used when there is significant left ventricular dysfunction. A beginning infusion rate of 5 µg/kg/min is appropriate and can be increased to 15 µg/kg/min to achieve the desired response.

Supplemental oxygen is helpful in improving tissue oxygenation but should be used cautiously in those infants whose systemic circulation is ductal dependent.[15]

Infusion of prostaglandin E1 should be started in those infants with ductal-dependent defects to maintain patency of the ductus arteriosus.[17] An initial intravenous infusion of 0.1 µg/kg of body weight per minute should be given. Once a therapeutic response is noted, it may be possible to decrease the dosage to 0.05 µg/kg/min. Infants with restriction of pulmonary blood flow should show an increase in P_{O_2}, and infants with restriction of systemic flow should show improvement in blood pressure and pH.

The most significant side effect of prostaglandin infusion is apnea,[18] occurring in 10% to 12% of treated infants. Apnea is seen most frequently in preterm infants and generally occurs during the first hour of treatment. Close monitoring of respiratory function must be done, with rapid intubation if apnea occurs. If the neonate must be transported while prostaglandins are being administered, intubation and mechanical ventilation should be initiated before transport.

It may be desirable to sedate and initiate mechanical ventilation in all infants with decreased cardiac output as a means of decreasing energy expenditure and therefore decreasing oxygen need.[19] Anemia should also be corrected in order to maximize oxygen delivery to tissues.[20] Irradiated cytomegalovirus (CMV)-negative washed packed red blood cells should be used when transfusion[20] is needed, since cardiac transplantation[20] may eventually be indicated for management of the heart disease. Cold stress must be avoided, because the resultant increase in oxygen consumption can be most detrimental to the infant.

Arrhythmias

With the widespread use of obstetrical ultrasound, it has become common for intrauterine arrhythmias to be detected before delivery.[3] The presence of fetal bradycardia (heart rate under 60 BPM) invariably raises the question of whether or not the fetus is hypoxic and demands immediate delivery. Such rates, if associated with continued normal fetal movements, are likely not immediately life threatening and are most frequently a result of complete heart block rather than acute asphyxia.[21,22] If fetal movements decrease, delivery is recommended.[22]

As many as half of the cases of congenital complete heart block may be caused by maternal collagen vascular disease.[22] Others are associated with structural heart defects such as single ventricle and truncus arteriosus.[22]

Management of complete heart block usually consists of placement of a pacemaker, preferably before the development of cardiac failure.

Fetal tachycardia, or fetal heart rate of greater than 220 BPM, is most commonly due to supraventricular tachycardia[22] (paroxysmal atrial tachycardia). Atrial flutter (associated with Ebstein's anomaly, coarctation of the aorta, endocardial fibroelastosis, and pulmonary atresia) and atrial fibrillation (associated with those structural defects with left atrial enlargement)[22] are also known to result in fetal heart rates in excess of 200 BPM. Such rates constitute an obstetrical emergency, and intrauterine conversion to a sinus rhythm (via maternal medication) or delivery followed by extrauterine conversion must occur promptly to avoid life-threatening

cardiac failure. Supraventricular tachycardia is associated with l-transposition[22] and with Ebstein's anomaly, where there is an increased incidence of Wolff-Parkinson-White syndrome.[22] Whatever the etiology, it is important to remember that coexisting acidosis, hypoxia, and electrolyte abnormalities must also be corrected.

Cardioversion may be accomplished by electric, physical (vagal stimulation), or pharmacologic means. The most effective vagal means of conversion is the sudden application of a cold stimulus to the infant's face. A large plastic bag filled with finely crushed ice is quickly applied to the entire face (including the forehead, ears, and chin) and held in place for approximately 10 s. It is important to have established intravenous access and resuscitation equipment immediately available before conversion attempts, because these maneuvers may result in a more ominous ventricular arrhythmia.[23] Carotid massage and eyeball pressure are ineffective, can be dangerous, and should not be used for vagal stimulation.

Rapid intravenous digitalization[23] may be used for pharmacologic conversion when the baby is not decompensated and time permits such an approach. One half of the calculated digitalizing dose (the digitalizing dose for a term infant is 0.04 mg/kg iv) is given intravenously, followed after 1 h by one fourth of the digitalizing dose (0.01 mg/kg, or 10 μg/kg). The final one fourth (another 0.01 mg/kg) is given 1 h later, so that complete digitalization may be accomplished in 2 h. It is wise to measure blood digoxin concentrations after the second dose to ensure that appropriate levels are being achieved.

Intravenous adenosine[24] has also been used for successful pharmacologic conversion. Propranolol[23] is useful in maintenance of a normal sinus rhythm when digoxin alone has been unsuccessful in the prevention of recurrent problems.

Electrical cardioversion[22] is used when the baby is in a compromised state and rapid treatment is necessary. Cardioversion using 0.25 to 1.0 W-s/kg is usually successful. The lower dose should be used initially. Successful cardioversion should be followed by digitalization.

When supraventricular tachycardia is accompanied by significant hypotension, the choice of a sympathomimetic agent becomes important.[23] Isoproterenol, levarterenol, and epinephrine should not be used, since they are associated with the production of ventricular fibrillation in such infants.[23] Phenylephrine[23] is the better choice, since it produces no cardiac stimulation.

SPECIFIC CARDIAC DEFECTS

The newborn with CHD presents clinically with cyanosis, congestive heart failure and respiratory distress,

TABLE 16–1. HYPOPERFUSION SYNDROMES

Obstruction of Left Ventricular Outflow
    Coarctation of the aorta
    Interrupted aortic arch
    Aortic stenosis
    Hypoplastic left heart
Obstruction of Left Ventricular Inflow
    Supravalvular mitral ring
    Mitral stenosis
    Cor triatriatum
    Total anomalous pulmonary venous return
Myocardial Disease
    Myocarditis and/or cardiomyopathy
    Endocardial fibroelastosis
    Glycogen storage disease
    Coronary artery anomalies
Arrhythmia
    Supraventricular tachycardia
    Complete heart block

signs of decreased cardiac output, or a combination of these. It is helpful to distinguish these presentations because this facilitates identification of the specific cardiac defect.

For the neonate who presents with cyanosis, the most important diagnostic possibilities include those defects characterized by decreased pulmonary blood flow (caused either by right ventricular inflow or outflow obstruction) and those defects with noncommunication of the pulmonary venous return with the systemic arterial outflow (e.g., transposition of the great vessels and Taussig-Bing anomaly).[23]

Defects with obstruction to right ventricular inflow include tricuspid atresia, hypoplastic right heart syndrome, and Ebstein's anomaly. Right ventricular outflow obstructions include pulmonary atresia and/or stenosis without ventricular septal defect, single ventricle with pulmonary stenosis or atresia, and tetralogy

TABLE 16–2. IMMEDIATE STABILIZATION FOR FREQUENTLY ENCOUNTERED DEFECTS[a]

Defect	Presentation	Immediate stabilization
ASD	Asymptomatic	None needed
VSD	Asymptomatic until pulmonary vascular resistance falls; CHF	Digitalis; diuretics for CHF
TGA, no VSD	Cyanosis, ↑ RR	PGE1 infusion
Tricuspid atresia	Cyanosis	PGE1 infusion
Pulmonary valve atresia, no VSD	Cyanosis	PGE1 infusion
Tetralogy of Fallot with severe PS	Cyanosis ± SGA Frequent associated anomalies	PGE1 infusion
Ebstein's anomaly of tricuspid valve	Cyanosis	PGE1 infusion
TAPVR:		
Cardiac or supracardiac	Asymptomatic until CHF develops with ↑ pulmonary flow	Usually not needed; treat CHF if present
Infradiaphragmatic	RDS symptoms with pulmonary venous obstruction	Mechanical ventilation with ↑ PEEP
Truncus arteriosus	Mild cyanosis, ↑ RR with left-sided failure	Digitalis; diuretics for increased pulmonary flow
Lesions with low systemic output:	Respiratory distress with ductal closure ↓ pulses	PGE1 infusion Mechanical ventilation with ↑ PEEP
HLHS	Ashen color	↓ supplemental O$_2$
Critical AS	Metabolic acidosis	Diuretics
Coarctation	Associated DiGeorge syndrome frequent[b]	Inotropes[c]
Interrupted aortic arch type B[b]	Hypoglycemia	

[a]ASD, atrial septal defect; VSD, ventricular septal defect; CHF, congestive heart failure; TGA, transposition of the great arteries; PS, pulmonary valve stenosis; SGA, small for gestational age; TAPVR, total anomalous pulmonary venous return; RDS, respiratory distress syndrome; RR, respiratory rate; HLH, hypoplastic left heart syndrome; AS, aortic stenosis; PGE1, prostaglandin E1; PEEP, positive end expiratory pressure.

[b]Interrupted aortic arch, type B, indicates interruption of the arch between the left common carotid artery and the left subclavian artery, representing left fourth aortic arch atresia and not simply a total coarctation (referred to as "type A"). Type B is frequently associated with DiGeorge syndrome, whereas type A is not.[26]

[c]Dopamine infused at a dose of 2 to 5 μg/kg/min increases renal blood flow and can therefore improve renal output in those infants with severe cardiac failure and poor urine production. Dobutamine (5–10 mg/kg/min) stimulates myocardial β–1 receptors[16] and is useful when there is significant impairment of left ventricular function.[27] The intravenous infusion (for both dopamine and dobutamine) can be calculated rapidly by the formula[28]: 6 3 weight (kg) 5 mg to be added to iv solution to make 100 mL. Infusion of the resulting solution at 1 mL/h delivers 1 μg/kg/min.

of Fallot. Lesions that may present with significant cyanosis, depending on the amount of obstruction or shunting, include truncus arteriosus and total anomalous pulmonary venous return. The latter can present with more or less severe signs of congestive heart failure, depending on the amount of obstruction to pulmonary venous return.

Ventricular septal defects[25] are rarely symptomatic initially but show congestive failure as pulmonary vascular resistance progressively falls. A similar mechanism for the development of congestive failure exists when there is an endocardial cushion defect or atrioventricular canal. The presence of an atrial septal defect[25] alone is usually suspected by the auscultation of a murmur and is not generally symptomatic in the immediate neonatal period.

The presence of a patent ductus arteriosus[25] is so common, occurring almost universally in the small preterm infant, that we have come to regard it as an expected problem, most often easily corrected pharmacologically with indomethacin.

Defects characterized by presentation with hypoperfusion may be divided into those with obstruction of left ventricular outflow, those with obstruction of left ventricular inflow, myocardial disease, and arrhythmias (Table 16–1).

In the event of delivery of an infant with unanticipated cardiac disease, the physician can take productive steps toward stabilization while simultaneously arranging for expeditious transport (Table 16–2). It is appropriate to begin an infusion of prostaglandin E1 whenever cyanotic CHD appears likely and whenever there is impaired pulmonary or systemic blood flow. Such treatment can be lifesaving, permitting transport of the infant to the care of a competent pediatric cardiothoracic surgeon.

SUMMARY

This chapter summarizes the information needed to manage newborns initially with congenital heart disease. It covers associated problems both related and unrelated etiologically to the primary cardiac defect and outlines the appropriate initial approach to frequently encountered cardiac problems in the neonate. Emphasis is placed on the importance of prenatal diagnosis and delivery in an appropriate care setting in order to maximize the likelihood of a good outcome.

REFERENCES

1. Copel JA, Pilu G, Green J, et al.: Fetal echocardiographic screening for congenital heart disease: The importance of the four-chamber view. *Am J Obstet Gynecol.* 157: 648–55, 1987.
2. Meijboom E, van Engelen AO, van de Beck EW, et al.: Fetal arrhythmias. *Curr Opin Cardiol.* 9:97–102, 1994.
3. Gow R, Hamilton R: Diagnosis and therapy for fetal tachycardia and other fetal rhythm abnormalities. *Curr Opin Pediatr.* 3:838, 1991.
4. Friedman AH, Fahey JT: The transition from fetal to neonatal circulation: Normal responses and implications for infants with heart disease. *Semin Perinatol.* 17: 106–21, 1993.
5. Fanaroff AA, Martin RJ (Eds.): *Neonatal-Perinatal Medicine, Diseases of the Fetus and Infant,* 6th ed.: St. Louis: CV Mosby; 1997: p. 1112.
6. Jaimovich DG, Vidyasagar D (Eds.): *Handbook of Pediatric and Neonatal Transport Medicine.* Philadelphia: Hanley & Belfus; 1996: pp. 131, 151.
7. Kattwinkel J, Bloom BT, Delmore P, et al.: Prophylactic administration of calf lung surfactant extract is more effective than early treatment of respiratory distress syndrome in neonates of 29 through 32 weeks' gestation. *Pediatrics.* 92:90–8, 1993.
8. OSIRIS Collaborative Group: Early versus delayed neonatal administration of a synthetic surfactant—The judgment of OSIRIS. *Lancet.* 340:1363-9, 1992.
9. Koivisto M, Blanco-Sequeiros M, Krause U: Neonatal symptomatic and asymptomatic hypoglycemia: A follow-up study of 151 children. *Dev Med Child Neurol.* 14: 603–14, 1972.
10. Fanaroff AA, Martin RJ (Eds.): *Neonatal-Perinatal Medicine, Diseases of the Fetus and Infant.* St. Louis: CV Mosby; 6th ed. 1997: p. 1458.
11. Kirby ML, Waldo KL: Role of neural crest in congenital heart disease. *Circulation.* 82:332-40, 1990.
12. Weaver DD, Mapstone CL, Yu P: The VATER association: Analysis of 46 patients. *Am J Dis Child.* 140:225–9, 1986.
13. Wyse RKH, Al-Mahdawi S, Burn J, et al.: Congenital heart disease in CHARGE association. *Pediatr Cardiol.* 14: 75–81, 1993.
14. Jaimovich DG, Vidyasagar D (Eds.): *Handbook of Pediatric and Neonatal Transport Medicine.* Philadelphia: Hanley & Belfus; 1996: p. 99.
15. Jaimovich DG, Vidyasagar D (Eds.): *Handbook of Pediatric and Neonatal Transport Medicine.* Philadelphia: Hanley & Belfus; 1996: p. 100.
16. Jaimovich DG, Vidyasagar D (Eds.): *Handbook of Pediatric and Neonatal Transport Medicine.* Philadelphia: Hanley & Belfus; 1996: p. 153.
17. Freed MD, Heymann MA, Lewis AB, et al.: Prostaglandin E1 in infants with ductus arteriosus–dependent congenital heart disease. *Circulation.* 64:899–905, 1981.
18. Lewis AB, Freed MD, Heymann MA, et al.: Side effects of therapy with prostaglandin E1 in infants with critical congenital heart disease. *Circulation.* 64:893–8, 1981.
19. Jaimovich DG, Vidyasagar D (Eds.): *Handbook of Pediatric and Neonatal Transport Medicine.* Philadelphia: Hanley & Belfus; 1996: p. 97.
20. Jaimovich DG, Vidyasagar D (Eds.): *Handbook of Pediatric and Neonatal Transport Medicine.* Philadelphia: Hanley & Belfus; 1996: p. 98.

21. Friedman AH, Copel JA, Kleinman CS: Fetal echocardiography and fetal cardiology: Indications, diagnosis and management. *Semin Perinatol.* 17:76–88, 1993.

22. Lees MH, King DH: The cardiovascular system. In Fanaroff A, Martin RJ (Eds.): *Neonatal-Perinatal Medicine, Diseases of the Fetus and Infant,* 4th ed. St. Louis: CV Mosby; 1987: pp. 679–84.

23. Heymann MA, Teitel DF, Liebman J: The heart. In Klaus MH, Fanaroff AA (Eds): *Care of the High-Risk Neonate,* 4th ed. Philadelphia, WB Saunders; 1993: pp. 357–70.

24. Van Hare GF: Neonatal arrhythmias. In Fanaroff AA, Martin RJ (Eds.): *Neonatal-Perinatal Medicine, Diseases of the Fetus and Infant,* 6th ed., St. Louis: CV Mosby; 1997: pp. 1167–81.

25. Zahka KG, Patel CR: Congenital defects. In Fanaroff AA, Martin RJ (Eds.): *Neonatal-Perinatal Medicine, Diseases of the Fetus and Infant,* 6th ed. St. Louis: CV Mosby; 1997: pp. 1154–5.

26. Gessner IH, Victorica BE: *Pediatric Cardiology, A Problem Oriented Approach.* Philadelphia: WB Saunders; 1993: p. 112.

27. Stopfkuchen H, Schranz D, Huth R, et al.: Effects of dobutamine on left ventricular performance in newborns as determined by systolic time intervals. *Eur J Pediatr.* 146:135–9, 1987.

28. American Academy of Pediatrics, Committee on Drugs: Emergency drug doses for infants and children. *Pediatrics.* 81:462–5, 1988.

CHAPTER SEVENTEEN

Interventional Cardiology in the Fetus

Guy A. Carter

Balloon valvuloplasty is becoming the treatment of choice for severe obstructive cardiac defects in the neonate, including critical aortic[1-4] and pulmonary stenosis,[5-8] coarctation of the aorta,[9,10] and palliative intervention for some cyanotic defects such as tetralogy of Fallot.[11-13] This technique, as are the corresponding surgical approaches, is associated with an increasing number and severity of complications as the size of the patient decreases.[14,15] However, it is less invasive or traumatic to the infant or potentially the fetus than a surgical procedure and offers conceivably more promise than intrauterine surgery to alter the outcome of the compromised fetus with obstructive cardiac defects.

A technique to dilate stenotic pulmonary valves was described by Rubio and Lason[16] in 1954. Pragmatically, the effective utilization of the techniques and availability of the special balloon catheters for dilating the congenitally stenotic valves of the aortic and pulmonary outflow tracts have been described only since 1982.[17] Over the decade and a half since that time, this technique has become the de facto procedure of choice for the initial treatment of congenital, acquired, and postoperative recurrent stenotic lesions not only of the pulmonary and aortic valves, but also of a multitude of other stenotic lesions. Concordantly, as miniaturization of the catheters has continued to progress, the technique has been continually extended to smaller and younger infants.

TECHNIQUE

Rao,[18] among others, has described the procedure for valvuloplasty or angioplasty in infants and children. Balloon valvuloplasty in the neonate or infant is typically done transvenously, either through a percutaneous entry into the femoral artery or vein or via the umbilical ves-

sels. Under fluoroscopic control in the cardiac catheterization laboratory, a diagnostic catheter is advanced across the stenotic area, using a flexible guide wire as necessary to assist the catheter course through the stenotic lumen. A valvuloplasty guide wire (which typically is a stiffer wire) is then advanced through the catheter and into the more distal vessel or is coiled into the cardiac chamber as appropriate, and the delivery catheter is withdrawn. The preselected valvuloplasty catheter is then advanced over the wire and positioned with the balloon centered over the stenotic lesion. The guide wire provides additional support for the catheter during the dilating procedure and remains in position. The balloon is then inflated until the "waist" in the balloon created by the stenotic valve disappears. Usually one to three inflations are done to assure that the stenotic lesion is appropriately enlarged. After the balloon catheter is withdrawn, the guide wire, which has remained in position, can be used to direct a diagnostic catheter for postprocedure pressure determinations to evaluate the effectiveness of the valvuloplasty. A surgical modification has been described[4] for the unstable neonate with critical aortic stenosis wherein, after cardiopulmonary bypass is initiated, the balloon catheter is inserted through the left ventricular wall at the apex and then directed antegrade across the aortic valve for the dilating procedure.

The observed complications of this procedure in the neonate include those associated with the process of dilating the lesion and of insult to the entry vessel. The process of valve dilatation is typically tearing of the valve raphe, or tearing of the valve leaflets, or occasionally avulsion of the valve leaflets.[19] The stiffer guide wire used to direct and stabilize the balloon catheter, and the stiffer balloon catheter itself, may perforate the wall of the ventricle or the vessel with resultant bleeding. During the inflation period the balloon occupies the total luminal area and occludes blood flow. During this time ventricular slowing is observed, but normal rate and rhythm are usually recovered after deflation of the balloon. This slowing is minimized by using brief inflation–deflation cycles. If the catheter is not positioned within the lumen (i.e., through a perforated valve leaflet), more severe structural damage to the valve is created, with resultant severe insufficiency. Complications involving the iliac and femoral arteries occur frequently[14] and are related to the larger size of the balloon catheters compared to the usual diagnostic catheters and the changes in the balloon configuration following the inflation–deflation cycle. These include thrombosis and resultant loss of pulse, or tearing and disruption of the arterial continuity with persistent blood loss at the entry site. The use of a sheath for entry can minimize the vessel damage, but it is not always possible to introduce or remove the balloon catheter through a sheath. The incidence of vessel injury is increased with larger balloon catheters and smaller infants and neonates.

Maxwell and colleagues[20,21] have reported the utilization of the balloon procedure to dilate a stenotic aortic valve in three fetuses at 28 to 33 weeks' gestation. Their procedure involved the insertion of a transabdominal chorionic villus sampling needle through the apex of the left ventricle into the ventricular chamber using echocardiographic imaging. A guide wire was inserted through the needle and directed across the aortic valve into the aorta and used to guide a balloon catheter to the aortic valve. One child so treated has been reported as living at 4 years of age,[21] and in the other two they reported little associated tissue damage to the fetus noted on autopsy after delivery.

With the application of the balloon catheter dilatation procedures to the fetus, the unique circumstances of approaching one patient through another individual must be considered. This requires that the risks to both the fetus and the mother be weighed against the potential benefits to the fetus from the procedure. The access utilizes established procedures for the intrauterine cardiac or umbilical vessel puncture for blood sampling. Premature labor may be induced in the mother, and hemorrhage from the puncture site is possible both in the mother and the fetus. If the needle crosses the lung fields or other tissue in the fetus, associated tissue damage may ensue.

CRITICAL AORTIC STENOSIS

The diagnosis of severe or critical aortic stenosis in the neonate encompasses a spectrum of infants with aortic annular hypoplasia, valvular dysplasia, hypoplasia of the left ventricle, mitral valve anomalies, and endocardial fibroelastosis.[4] With the severe obstruction to blood flow across the aortic valve, the infant is frequently unstable with progressive, and often intractable, congestive heart failure and metabolic acidosis shortly following birth,[2–4] resulting in death without aggressive early intervention. Even with intervention, the left ventricle frequently fails to maintain an adequate output, related to the degree of ventricular dysfunction and associated endocardial fibroelastosis, which equates to a high mortality rate. The infant with a small left ventricle at birth has the poorest prognosis, with reported mortality rates approaching 100%.[3] Endocardial fibroelastosis or other malformations are also associated with increased mortality rates.[1–4] The degree of left ventricular dysfunction appears to reflect the severity of the obstruction, and the developmental age at which the obstruction becomes significant. Progressive changes in the degree of obstruction from the aortic stenosis have been noted on serial echocardiographic studies in utero.[22] Typically, the more severe the degree of obstruction, the earlier the defect presents clinically. When aortic stenosis is identified prior to birth by fetal echocardiography the prognosis for the infant is particularly poor. Maxwell et al[20] noted that of 12 instances in which severe aortic stenosis was diagnosed in the fetus and the mother elected to continue the pregnancy, 2 fetuses died before delivery and, following birth, none of the other 10 survived. Only 4 survived long enough to undergo treatment with balloon valvuloplasty.

The application of balloon valvuloplasty to critical aortic valve stenosis in the fetus is becoming the primary focus for the intrauterine utilization of this technique. The rationales for this course are that aortic valve disease can be accurately diagnosed before birth by fetal echocardiography; that when prenatally diagnosed the prognosis of severe aortic stenosis is very poor; and that there is a progressive deterioration of left ventricular size, anatomy, and hemodynamics as the fetus develops with severe aortic stenosis. This leads to the hypothesis that with intrauterine relief of the outflow obstruction at an early stage of this disease, the adverse and irreversible left ventricular changes may be diminished or averted, and the outcome potentially improved. The initial reports by Allan's group at Guy's Hospital[20,21] demonstrate the feasibility of this adaptation of balloon valvuloplasty procedures in the fetus. Modifications of the transventricular procedure described as a surgical procedure at C. S. Mott Children's Hospital[4] to an intrauterine percutaneous procedure have been shown to be effective, with little or no collateral tissue damage. It remains to be shown that the defect can be identified and intervention undertaken at a fetal age sufficiently early to alter the course of hemodynamic changes, and before the development of irreversible left ventricular damage, resulting in left ventricular hypoplasia, or endocardial fibroelastosis, with resultant left ventricular dysfunction and eventual death. Additional experience with this technique and the development of smaller and more specially designed catheters will clarify the applicability of this technique and the potential to alter the previously reported course of this defect.

CRITICAL PULMONARY VALVULAR STENOSIS

Similar to the underdevelopment of the left ventricle with severe aortic valvular stenosis, critical pulmonary valvular stenosis is commonly associated with underdevelopment of the right ventricle, tricuspid valve, right ventricular outflow tract, and pulmonary artery.[23] At birth, critical pulmonary stenosis or atresia restricts or prevents the flow of blood directly from the right ventricle into the lungs; the neonate therefore presents dependent on the ductus arteriosus for pulmonary perfusion and clinically with severe cyanosis and frequently death as the ductus arteriosus closes. Early intervention with transluminal balloon valvuloplasty has been shown to improve the survival rate significantly for these infants.[5–8] Similar to cases of critical aortic stenosis, the presence of a significantly hypoplastic right ventricle at birth adversely affects the results obtained by valvuloplasty. The prenatal diagnosis of severe right ventricular outflow tract obstructions (critical pulmonary stenosis or pulmonary atresia) can be made accurately by Doppler evaluation when there is right atrial enlargement (most likely from tricuspid insufficiency or decreased right ventricular compromise), right ventricular hypoplasia, and retrograde flow in the pulmonary artery.[24] Unlike severe aortic stenosis, serial fetal evaluations of severe pulmonary stenosis have not been reported. In the neonate, pulmonary balloon valvuloplasty has been an effective initial therapy and has been utilized successfully even with membranous pulmonary atresia.[8] The techniques that were used at Guy's Hospital[20] for intrauterine balloon valvuloplasty of the aortic valve should be equally applicable for critical pulmonary stenosis or atresia. In their text, Maxwell et al.[20] reported recognizably entering the right ventricle during one attempt, indicating that this entry should be equally as feasible as access to the left ventricle. At present this continues to exist only as a potential therapeutic modality.

OTHER CARDIAC DEFECTS

In addition to aortic or pulmonary stenosis, balloon valvuloplasty and angioplasty are also frequently used in the neonate with coarctation of the aorta. The process of balloon angioplasty for coarctation of the aorta produces enlargement of the vessel by disrupting the intima and media at the coarctation site.[25] Recent studies have shown that balloon dilatation of unoperated coarctation is a safe and effective modality of treatment [9,10] and can be employed in the neonate through either a femoral arterial or an umbilical arterial approach. At the Children's Hospital at the University of Missouri, Dr. Lababidi has recently successfully dilated a coarctation in a 500-g premature infant (unpublished data, 1997). Although this suggests that successful dilatation should be feasible in the fetus, the application of this technique before birth is limited by the greater difficulty in diagnosis of coarctation in the fetus and the more frequent presence of significant tubular hypoplasia of the aortic arch with coarctation when diagnosed in the fetus. The presence of tubular hypoplasia has been associated with decreased effectiveness of balloon angioplasty for coarctation.[9,10] Also, since in the absence of other severe malformations as hypoplastic left heart syndrome, coarctation of the aorta does not as consistently as critical aortic or pulmonary stenosis produce as severe or as rapidly progressive deterioration of the infant, the urgency for intrauterine intervention is more likely to be attenuated for this defect.

There has been an increasing indication that balloon valvuloplasty may be an effective palliative procedure for tetralogy of Fallot, and it does result in reduced cyanosis.[11–13] Whether this procedure will result in increased size of the right ventricular outflow tract or the pulmonary arteries at the time of eventual total repair is yet to be documented. In that the fetus with tetralogy of Fallot is not typically compromised before birth, and the neonate can be effectively palliated or repaired shortly after birth by surgical intervention or balloon valvuloplasty, fetal intervention in this defect is more likely to await the further development and refinement of the techniques directed toward severe aortic or pulmonary stenosis.

CONCLUSIONS

The use of transvenous balloon angioplasty catheters to relieve obstructive lesions in infants and children has rapidly become the primary treatment of choice in the older infant and child. Although the risks are increased in the neonate, this procedure compares favorably with the more extensive surgical repair in this age group. Extending the application to the fetus adds the potential for favorably altering the course of the more severe ventricular outlet obstructive defects but also adds the risks of maternal complications to the procedural risks to the fetus, a factor that must also be taken into consideration. The field of interventional transcatheter repair or palliation of obstructive cardiac defects, however, appears to have a significant potential for favorably altering the adverse hemodynamics during the development of the fetus through later pregnancy. In theory, this could provide a significant improvement in outcome for the more severe obstructive cardiac defects by preventing the development of the secondary changes of ventricular or arterial hypoplasia considered to result from the decreased or altered blood flow patterns. The challenges for the future with this technique are to ensure that an accurate diagnosis can be made at an appropriately early stage of development before irreversible changes have occurred and to demonstrate that effective intervention initiated at an appropriate time can favorably alter the course of the cardiac defect. Further experience with this technique to better define the results and development of the special catheters needed are necessary for this potential to attain any reasonable degree of reality.

REFERENCES

1. Wren C, Sullivan I, Bull C, et al.: Percutaneous balloon dilitation of aortic valve stenosis in neonates and infants. *Br Heart J.* 58:608–12, 1987.
2. Kasten-Sportes CH, Piechaud JF, Sisi D, et al.: Percutaneous balloon valvuloplasty in neonates with critical aortic stenosis. *J Am Coll Cardiol.* 13:1101–5, 1989.
3. Bu'Lock F, Joffe HS, Jordan S, et al.: Balloon dilitation (valvuloplasty) as first line treatment for severe stenosis of the aortic valve in early infancy: Medium term results and determinates of survival. *Br Heart J.* 70:546–53, 1993.
4. Mosca RS, Iannettoni MD, Schwartz SM, et al.: Critical aortic stenosis in the neonate. *J Thorac Cardiovasc Surg.* 109:147–54, 1995.
5. Rey C, Marache P, Francart C, et al.: Percutaneous transluminal balloon valvuloplasty of congenital pulmonary valve stenosis, with a special report on infants and neonates. *J Am Coll Cardiol.* 11:815–20, 1988.
6. Khan MA, Al-Yousef S, Huta JC, et al.: Critical pulmonary valve stenosis in patients less than 1 year of age: Treatment with percutaneous gradational balloon pulmonary valvuloplasty. *Am Heart J.* 117:1008–14, 1989.
7. Caspi J, Coles JG, Benson LN, et al.: Management of neonatal critical pulmonic stenosis in the balloon valvotomy era. *Ann Thorac Surg.* 49:273–8, 1990.
8. Fedderly RT, Lloyd TR, Mendelsohn AM, et al.: Determinants of successful balloon valvotomy in infants with critical pulmonary stenosis or membranous pulmonary atresia with intact ventricular septum. *J Am Coll Cardiol.* 25:460–5, 1990.
9. Wren C, Peart I, Bain H, et al.: Balloon dilitation of unoperated aortic coarctation: Immediate results and one year follow up. *Br Heart J.* 58:369–73, 1987.
10. Huggon IC, Qureshi SA, Baker EJ, et al.: Effect of introducing balloon dilatation of native aortic coarctation on overall outcome in infants and children. *Am J Cardiol.* 73:799–807, 1994.
11. Sreeram N, Saleem M, Jackson M, et al.: Results of balloon pulmonary valvuloplasty as a palliative procedure in tetralogy of Fallot. *J Am Coll Cardiol.* 18:159–65, 1991.
12. Rao PS, Wilson AD, Thapar MK, et al.: Balloon pulmonary valvuloplasty in the management of cyanotic congenital heart defects. *Cath Cardiovasc Diagn.* 25:16–24, 1992.
13. Sluysmans T, Neven B, Lintermans J, et al.: Early balloon dilatation of the pulmonary valve in infants with tetralogy of Fallot. *Circulation.* 91:1506–11, 1995.
14. Burrows PE, Benson LN, Williams WG, et al.: Ileofemoral arterial complications of balloon angioplasty for systemic obstructions in infants and children. *Circulation.* 82:1697–704, 1990.
15. Stanger P, Cassidy SC, Girod DA, et al.: Balloon pulmonary valvuloplasty: Results of the valvuloplasty and angioplasty of congenital anomalies registry. *Am J Cardiol.* 65:775–83, 1990.
16. Rubio V, Lason L: *Treatment of Pulmonary Valvular Stenosis and Tricuspid Stenosis Using a Modified Catheter.* Washington, DC: Second World Congress on Cardiology, Program Abstracts II: p. 205, 1954.
17. Kan JS, White RI Jr, Mitchell SE, et al.: Percutaneous balloon valvuloplasty: A new method for treating congenital pulmonary valve stenosis. *N Engl J Med.* 307:540–2, 1982.
18. Rao PS: Balloon valvuloplasty and angioplasty in infants and children. *J Pediatr.* 6:907–14, 1989.
19. Walls JT, Lababidi Z, Curtis JJ, et al.: Assessment of percutaneous balloon pulmonary and aortic valvuloplasty. *J Thorac Cardiovasc Surg.* 88:352–6, 1983.
20. Maxwell D, Allan L, Tynan MJ: Balloon dilitation of the aortic valve in the fetus: A report of two cases. *Br Heart J.* 65:256–8, 1991.
21. Allan LD, Maxwell DJ, Carminati M, et al.: Survival after fetal aortic balloon valvuloplasty. *Ultrasound Obstet Gynecol.* 5:90–1, 1995.
22. Hornberger LK, Sanders SP, Rein AJJT, et al.: Left heart obstructive lesions and left ventricular growth in the midtrimester fetus. *Circulation.* 92:1531–8, 1995.
23. Freed MD, Rosenthal A, Bernhard WF, et al.: Critical pulmonary stenosis with a diminutive right ventricle in neonates. *Circulation.* 48:875–81, 1973.
24. Hornberger LK, Benacerraf BR, Bromley BS, et al.: Prenatal detection of severe right ventricular outflow tract obstruction: Pulmonary stenosis and pulmonary atresia. *J Ultrasound Med.* 13:743–50, 1994.
25. Lock JE, Niemi T, Burke BA, et al.: Transcutaneous angioplasty of experimental coarctation. *Circulation.* 66:1280–6, 1982.

CHAPTER EIGHTEEN

Surgical Interventions and Corrections for Congenital Heart Disease

Donald C. Watson, Jr.

Congenital heart disease (CHD) in a newborn can be devastating to a family. Fortunately, the occurrence of these abnormalities is under 1% of all live births (Table 18–1). Also fortunately, a great many of these abnormalities can be effectively cured and a large portion can be treated to allow survival in the short term. The length and quality of life is highly dependent on the severity of the abnormality. Since cardiac surgery is relatively new, the first closed heart procedure having been done in 1945[1] and the first open heart procedure having been performed in 1953,[2] we are steadily improving the outcome of infants and children with severe congenital heart abnormalities. This chapter begins with a fundamental approach to viewing the anatomy and physiologic consequences of CHD. Specific common congenital heart abnormalities are then reviewed using these principles to establish the current surgical options. Results in the treatment of these abnormalities are described. For a more detailed review of these topics, the reader is referred to standard cardiologic and cardiac surgical texts.[3–6] For the convenience of the reader, a glossary and a list of abbreviations appear at the end of this chapter.

GENERAL PRINCIPLES

Anatomic Realities

All of the known forms of CHD can be broken down into three fundamental anatomic realities, or a combination of these realities. By placing these abnormalities in various locations in the heart or great vessels and varying their severity, all forms of CHD can be constructed. This approach is highly functional and allows us to explain the natural subsequent physiologic consequences and develop a surgical strategy for treating these patients.

Obstruction

Obstruction to the flow of blood through a natural pathway is the first anatomic reality. The simplest example is coarctation of the aorta (CoA), in which a narrowing exists in the vicinity of a ligamentum arteriosum and blood flow to the lower body is impeded.

Extra Pathway

An extra pathway, allowing blood to flow to an abnormal location, is another anatomic reality. The simplest example is an atrial septal defect (ASD). The extra pathway, a hole in a normally intact atrial septum, allows blood to flow abnormally from the higher pressure left atrium (LA) into the right atrium (RA). Blood flow through the right heart is thus increased.

Abnormal Connection

An abnormal connection, facilitating abnormal blood flow patterns, is the third reality. For example, in transposition of the great arteries (TGA), the aorta arises from the right ventricle (RV) and the pulmonary artery (PA) arises from the left ventricle. Systemic venous blood returning to the RA proceeds to the RV and then proceeds to the aorta abnormally. Likewise, oxygenated pulmonary venous blood comes from the pulmonary veins to the left ventricle and then to the PA. Blood flow patterns with this abnormality are obvious.

TABLE 18–1. PERCENTAGE OF LESIONS IN INFANTS AND CHILDREN WITH CONGENITAL HEART DISEASE

Lesion	Canada (%)	New England (%)
Ventricular septal defect	28	16
Pulmonary stenosis	10	3
Patent ductus arteriosus	10	6
Tetralogy of Fallot	10	9
Aortic stenosis	7	
Atrial septal defect	7	3
Coarctation of the aorta	5	8
Transposition of the great arteries	5	10
Atrioventricular septal defect	3	5
Total anomalous pulmonary venous return	1	3
Tricuspid and pulmonary atresia (intact septum)	2	6
Hypoplastic left heart syndrome		7
Single ventricle		2

Data from Keith JD, Rowe RD, Vlad P. Heart Disease in Infancy and Childhood. New York: Macmillan Publishing Co., Inc.; 1978; and Fyler DC, Buckley LP, Hillenband WE, et al. Report of the New England Regional Infant Cardiac Program. Pediatrics: 1980; 65:375.

Physiologic Consequences

As a result of these anatomic realities, physiologic consequences in the amount and/or distribution of blood flow arise. Three fundamental consequences arise that can be used to construct the total physiologic consequence for a complex problem.

Reduced Flow

The first physiologic impact is reduced amount of blood flow to a region of the body. CoA provides a simple example. Blood flow to the lower body is impeded by the narrowing in the aorta in the vicinity of the ductus arteriosus.

Excessive Flow

The second fundamental physiologic consequence is abnormally increased blood flow to a region in the body. ASD provides a simple example, in which right-sided cardiac output is abnormally high because of a left-to-right shunt across the ASD.

Admixture

The third fundamental physiologic consequence is an admixture lesion. That is, the distribution of blood flow to various parts of the body is abnormal. TGA provides an example. Systemic blood is passed through the right heart and then ejected through the aorta to return to the systemic circulation; this situation is clearly abnormal and, unless other compensating lesions are present, life limiting.

All of these adverse physiologic consequences shorten a patient's life expectancy. The degree of shortening is directly related to the magnitude of the physiologic impact and the complexity of the heart disease. Operative and treatment modalities can be developed recognizing these physiologic consequences and taking into account the anatomic realities.

Surgical Principles

The strategy for developing operations to correct congenital heart disease begins with recognition of physiologic consequences.

Flow Augmentation

Specifically, lesions that have decreased flow to a region are treated by increasing flow. Two basic operative principles may be utilized: A direct repair of the anatomic obstruction or bypassing the region that is obstructed. In either case, every effort is made to use autologous material. Frequently grafts (polytetraflouroethylene, Dacron, bovine pericardium, for example) are used. A third principle is to augment the obstructed area using a prosthetic material. The specific principles used depend on the location of the obstruction and the available tissue.

Flow Restriction

When increased flow is the physiologic consequence, the surgical principle used is either to correct the anatomic abnormality directly or to add an obstruction in the region of increased flow. As an example, the patient with a ventricular septal defect (VSD) has increased pulmonary flow as a result of left-to-right shunting across an extra pathway in the ventricles. Currently, the strategy to reduce pulmonary overcirculation is a direct approach on the VSD, closing that defect, usually with a patch. Before the advent of safe cardiopulmonary bypass (CPB) in the neonate and infant, the surgical strategy was to reduce pulmonary overcirculation by placement of a PA band, narrowing the PA so that the excess of blood flow to the lungs was restricted. This strategy is used today for certain complex lesions.

Redistribution

The third physiologic consequence, admixture of blood flow, is treated surgically by a redistribution of blood flow using either a primary repair of the anatomic abnormality or creating an additional maldistribution that compensates for the native disease. A primary example of these principles is surgical treatment for TGA. Currently, surgical techniques have been so refined and the perioperative course is sufficiently well developed that the arterial switch operation (ASO) (Jatene procedure[7]) with coronary artery translocation can be achieved with a high degree of success. Before development of this technique, surgeons treated transposition by creating intraatrial baffles (Mustard[8] and Senning[9] procedures) that directed systemic venous blood into the morphologic left ventricle and then perfused the lungs for oxygenation. The baffle was positioned so that pulmonary venous blood, oxygenated blood, was directed into the morphologic RV and then to the systemic circulation. Thus, creating a compensating admixture lesion helps solve the original congenital admixture lesion. Unfortunately, the morphologic RV is performing systemic work and the tricuspid valve is the systemic AV valve.

Categories of Surgical Repair

Open versus Closed

Operations to correct congenital heart abnormalities can be categorized in several ways. A simple way to think about cardiac operations is whether or not CPB, the heart–lung machine, is used to facilitate the repair. Procedures using CPB are characterized as open procedures. Procedures that do not involve CPB are closed procedures.

Anatomic versus Physiologic versus Palliative

A second way to describe cardiac procedures is to characterize the type of repair generated by the procedure. Anatomic repairs are those in which the sequence of blood flow through the body is correct and the proper chambers are performing their normal tasks. Specifically, systemic desaturated blood is passed through the RA, the RV, the PA, and then to the lungs. Oxygenated pulmonary venous blood passes through the LA, through the LV, out the aorta, and to the systemic circulation. Physiologic corrections involve operations in which the sequence of blood flow is proper, but the chambers used to generate flow are abnormal. As an example, in atrial baffling for TGA, systemic venous blood passes into the LA, the LV, and then into the PA and lungs. Pulmonary venous blood passes into the RA, the RV, and then to the aorta and body. Obviously, the LV is generating pulmonary output and the RV is generating systemic output. This arrangement is physiologically correct but anatomically abnormal. A third type of repair is the palliative repair that includes all operations which are not anatomic or physiologic and are aimed to improve the patient's physiologic status. An example is placement of a systemic artery to PA shunt to increase the paucity of PA blood flow associated with tetralogy of Fallot (TOF). The details are described below.

Unique Methods of Cardiac Surgery

Cardiopulmonary Bypass

To facilitate the process of intracardiac repairs, the CPB machine, first used in 1954,[10] must be used to allow a quiet, bloodless operative field. This device intercepts systemic venous blood in the RA or venae cavae and delivers arterial blood to the ascending aorta. The heart–lung machine provides three principle functions that act in parallel to the patient's native heart and lung. Carbon dioxide is removed, oxygen is added, and pressure is generated. Additionally, the temperature can be regulated and many other secondary functions can be implemented. It can be seen that with placement of the heart–lung machine in parallel with the native heart and lung, the surgeon has the option of using either the machine or the native structures to perform cardiac and pulmonary functions. When CPB is established, systemic venous blood is diverted from the heart, pulmonary venous flow is absent except for bronchial collaterals, and the operative field can be made blood-free. Additionally, the heart can be stopped so that the operative field can be made still to facilitate the precision of an operation.

Aortic Cross-Clamping

To further facilitate a bloodless and quiet operative field, frequently the ascending aorta is cross-clamped proximal to the aortic infusion cannula. This allows the heart to become flaccid and eliminates coronary venous return. The proximal ascending aorta is usually infused with a cardioplegic solution to optimize preservation of the myocardium during this period of anoxia. A great deal of work has gone into developing the optimum cardioplegic solution, the details of which are beyond the scope of this chapter. Hypothermia and hyperkalemia are primary modalities of protection. An aortic cross-clamp time of an hour or less is well tolerated whereas a few hours can be used with good results if the repair requires a lengthy time of aortic cross-clamping.

Circulatory Arrest

There are certain circumstances, for example, hypoplastic left heart syndrome (HLHS), in which the existence of the heart–lung machine with flow to the patient is not possible during the operative repair. Perfusion of the aorta is impossible at the time that the surgeon is augmenting the aorta. During this time, circulatory arrest is induced and the cannulae are removed. This strategy, considered by some to be the ultimate in bench surgery, necessitates cooling the patient to below 18° C before the induction of circulatory arrest and minimizing the circulatory arrest time to under 45 min to optimize long-range outcome. Some surgeons use this technique to facilitate even simple procedures. Results to date, however, suggest that the avoidance of circulatory arrest is beneficial to a patient's long-range outcome.[11]

OBSTRUCTIVE LESIONS

Coarctation of the Aorta

CoA is a narrowing in the distal aortic arch. This narrowing in the aortic wall in the vicinity of the ductus arteriosus impedes blood flow to the lower body. In its extreme form, interruption of the aortic arch and severe aortic hypoplasia develop.

Embryology

The exact cause for CoA is not certain. Many theories hypothesize extension of ductal contractile tissue onto the aorta, alteration of blood flow patterns, or migration of neural crest tissue. It is highly likely that one or all of these mechanisms plays a role.

Types of Coarctation of the Aorta

Historically, CoA has been described as proximal, directly opposite, or distal to a ligamentum arteriosum or patent ductus arteriosus (PDA). The location of the CoA is not as critical as the size of the transverse aortic arch. If the CoA is too small to allow life-sustaining lower body perfusion after repair, the patient is a candidate for a much more extensive procedure, transverse aortic augmentation. The most severe form of CoA is interrupted aortic arch, in which no communication exists between the ascending and descending aorta. In *type A interruption*, the obstruction is between the left subclavian artery and the descending aorta. In *type B interruption*, the most common type, the obstruction is between the left carotid and the left subclavian artery. In the most severe form of interrupted aortic arch, the obstruction is proximal to the left carotid artery. Additional extracardiac abnormalities are likely, e.g., DiGeorge syndrome.

Natural History

In its mildest form, CoA may not be recognized until later in life, when arm hypertension is diagnosed in a routine physical. Excessive pressure work and systemic hypertension in the upper body can lead to congestive heart failure (CHF), stroke, and arterial sclerosis, among other things. Untreated, in the most severe form (interrupted aortic arch), about 90% of patients can be expected to die in the neonatal period. A similarly grave prognosis is present for patients with hypoplastic transverse arch syndrome.

Indications for Operation

In the mild form, operation may be avoided unless severe upper body hypertension or LV failure develop. The presence of an interrupted aortic arch, commonly associated with a VSD, or severe transverse aortic arch hypoplasia mandate a prompt operation. The patient's hemodynamic burden can be ameliorated with prostaglandin E1 (PGE1). Patient outcomes are optimized if this ductal vasodilator is instituted before the development of a deteriorating course, particularly metabolic acidosis. A principal consequence of high-dose PGE1 therapy is apnea, treated easily by endotracheal intubation.

Operative Procedures and Outcomes

The principal objective of a simple repair is to relieve the aortic obstruction in a way that reduces the likelihood of future stenosis. Three fundamental approaches can be used: resection of the CoA ridge with end-to-end anastomosis (simple or extended), patch augmentation, or subclavian flap angioplasty. All procedures are done through a left thoracotomy. The exact type of procedure to be done often requires direct examination of the structures by the operating surgeon. Often the transverse arch is small but large enough to allow sufficient lower body flow to maintain organ function while the transverse arch grows. Operative mortality is in the 5% range for infants.

Operative repair of transverse aortic arch hypoplasia cannot be achieved simply by clamping vessels and approximating opened segments. CPB with deep hypothermia and circulatory arrest is required. The techniques are similar to those used with interrupted aortic arch repair. A patch is placed (usually homograft material but other prosthetic substitutes have been used) in the transverse arch, which has been opened longitudinally from the adequate size ascending aorta around the transverse arch into the descending aorta, well through the region of the CoA. A median sternotomy approach is used.

Interrupted aortic arch repair also requires CPB and deep hypothermia with circulatory arrest via a median sternotomy. The ascending aorta and PDA are cannulated to provide arterial perfusion to the whole body while a single venous cannula is placed in the RA. With extensive mobilization of all structures, a single primary anastomosis of the ascending and descending aorta can be achieved. Concomitant lesions, VSD, and interatrial communication can be closed simultaneously. Single-stage repair carries about a 20% mortality rate. Attempts at two-stage procedures, a primary procedure to connect the ascending and descending aorta and a secondary procedure to close the VSD, carry a higher mortality and morbidity rate and are to be avoided.

Re-CoA is the most common late complication of CoA repair and has the highest rate, 20%, in patients who are repaired during neonatal life. Restenosis can easily be treated by balloon dilatation with a high degree of success, about 80%.

Pulmonary Stenosis

In the simplest form, obstruction at the valve level with fused commissures or a dysplastic valve is present. In the more complex form, diffuse hypoplasia of the entire right ventricular outflow tract (RVOT) is present. In the extreme form, pulmonary atresia, other compensating abnormalities must be present.

Embryology

In simple pulmonary stenosis, the pulmonary valve, a triradiant structure, has fused commissures. Other pulmonary valve abnormalities, a bicuspid orifice or narrowing of the sinotubular junction (junction of the sinus and tubular portion of an artery), may also be present. Subvalvular and infundibular obstruction may also be observed but are usually a consequence of RV hypertension and muscle hypertrophy.

Types of Pulmonary Stenosis

Pulmonary stenoses are characterized by the level of the obstruction and are valvular, subvalvular (infundibular), or supravalvular (at the sinotubular junction).

Natural History

For simple right ventricular outflow tract obstruction (RVOTO), the likelihood of sudden death, the most feared complication, is related to the RV pressure and RVOT gradient. Patients with initial gradients of under 40 mm Hg are likely to require no therapy. Debate exists and data are conflicting concerning the need for treatment of patients with moderate pulmonary valve stenosis. Some have advocated treatment because of the likelihood of significant gradient increase over the years or a decrement in systolic and diastolic function of the RV. Newer data and exercise-inducible high gradients or ischemia seem to support more aggressive therapy. Severe RVOTO, greater than 80 mm Hg gradient or a RV pressure that is greater than LV pressure, requires therapy. Worsening of the RVOTO and RV function can be expected. Sudden death and cyanosis or hypoxemia with their attendant consequences are well recognized.

Indications for Treatment

The severity of the RVOTO guides the treatment. Mild abnormalities can be observed. A moderate gradient would at a minimum require close follow-up and, under certain circumstances, therapeutic intervention. An increase in gradient, a decrease in ventricular function, or an extreme concern about the possible devastating sequelae would argue for treatment. Patients with a severe RVOT gradient, greater than 80 mm Hg, or equalization of the ventricular pressures should be treated with relief of RVOTO.

Procedures and Outcomes

In recent years, placement of a percutaneous transvenous balloon catheter has been used in the treatment of pulmonary stenosis with a high degree of success, particularly when the gradient is at the valvular level. In the more common and typical thin, doming valve, balloon pulmonary valvuloplasty relieves obstruction by splitting a commissure. Balloon techniques are less successful when the pulmonary valve is dysplastic or an important component of the RVOTO is at the subvalvular level. For these more severe abnormalities, surgical valvotomy, valvectomy, patch augmentation, and/or infundibulectomy are required with CPB. Concomitant lesions such as an ASD can be repaired simultaneously.

In properly selected patients, a high degree of success can be achieved with balloon pulmonary valvuloplasty. Remote long-term follow-up is still limited but persistent relief of RV hypertension is well recognized. Acutely, the RVOT gradient can be reduced by about 50 mm Hg. When necessary, operative correction is associated with a very low mortality and long-term follow-up demonstrates no strong evidence of restenosis. New onset or residual pulmonary valve regurgitation are common with both balloon and operative techniques. Only in severe pulmonary valvular regurgitation is there a likelihood of long-term RV dysfunction secondary to the regurgitant fraction.

Aortic Stenosis

In the simplest form, obstruction at the valve level, fused commissures or a dysplastic valve are present. In the more complex form, diffuse hypoplasia of the entire left ventricular outflow tract (LVOT) is present. In the extreme form, aortic atresia, other compensating abnormalities must be present.

Embryology

In simple aortic stenosis, the triradiant aortic valve has fused commissures. Other aortic valve abnormalities, a bicuspid orifice, or narrowing of the sinotubular junction may also be present. Subvalvular and supravalvular obstruction may also be observed.

Types of Aortic Stenosis

Aortic stenoses are characterized by the level of the obstruction and are valvular, subvalvular (fibromuscular), or supravalvular (at the sinotubular junction).

Natural History

For simple left ventricular outflow tract obstruction (LVOTO), the likelihood of sudden death or CHF is related to the LV pressure and LVOT gradient. Patients with initial gradients of under 40 mm Hg are likely to require no therapy. Severe LVOTO, greater than 50 mm Hg gradient, requires therapy. With severe obstruction, worsening of the LVOTO and LV function can be expected. Sudden death and CHF with their attendant consequences are well recognized.

Indications for Treatment

The severity of the LVOTO guides the treatment. Mild abnormalities can be observed. A moderate gradient requires close follow-up and, under certain circumstances, therapeutic intervention. An increase in gradient, a decrease in ventricular function, or a concern about the possible devastating sequelae indicate treatment. Patients with a severe LVOT gradient, greater than 50 mm Hg, should be treated with relief of the LVOTO.

Procedures and Outcomes

In recent years, placement of a percutaneous transluminal balloon angioplasty catheter has been used with a high degree of success for the treatment of aortic stenosis in the infant. This is particularly useful when the gradient is at the aortic valvular level. Balloon aortic valvuloplasty relieves obstruction by splitting a commissure in the more common and typical thin, doming valve. Balloon techniques are less successful when the aortic valve is dysplastic or an important component of the LVOTO is at the subvalvular level. Surgical valvotomy and/or fibromuscular ridge excision are required with CPB. Concomitant lesions can be repaired simultaneously.

In properly selected patients, a high degree of success can be achieved with balloon aortic valvuloplasty. Remote long-term follow-up is still limited but persistent relief of LV hypertension is well recognized. Acutely, the LVOT gradient can be reduced by about 50 mm Hg. Need for operative correction is associated with a 20% mortality risk. Long-term follow-up demonstrates some evidence for restenosis. New onset or residual aortic valve regurgitation are seen with both balloon and operative techniques. In severe aortic valvular regurgitation, there is a likelihood of long-term LV dysfunction secondary to the regurgitant fraction.

Pulmonary Atresia

With extreme RVOTO, patients have pulmonary atresia. The physiologic state of the patient depends on other concomitant lesions, specifically, extra pathways through a PDA, atrial septum, and ventricular septum. Extrauterine life is not possible without an ASD or a VSD and a PDA. The usual circumstance is an intact ventricular septum, but a VSD may be present. The size of the RV depends on flow through it. A normally sized RV can be present if severe tricuspid regurgitation or a VSD is present. With no flow through the right heart, the RV is likely to be quite small and nonfunctional ("peach pit") and represents a variant of hypoplastic right heart syndrome (HRHS).

Embryology

Pulmonary atresia with intact ventricular septum may be secondary to an inflammatory process leading to RVOTO, but it probably occurs after completion of cardiac septation. The normal RV consists of the inlet (sinus), trabecular, and infundibular (conus) regions. In pulmonary atresia with intact ventricular septum, the ventricle is diminutive. Rarely is it normal or large (10% of patients). The RV may be more normal in size when there is tricuspid regurgitation or a VSD.

Types of Pulmonary Atresia

The most common type is pulmonary atresia with intact ventricular septum. Concomitant ASD or VSD and PDA or MAPCAs (much less likely) are required for neonatal survival. The degree of hypoplasia of the RV often dictates the clinical course. Simple discoid pulmonary valve atresia is much more easily handled than severe HRHS with a tiny RV and coronary artery sinuses or fistulae. These fistulae are quite problematic when the ventricular myocardium depends on fistulous flow for coronary perfusion (about 10% of patients). With pulmonary atresia, RV pressure increases from isovolumic contraction contribute to maintenance of sinusoids present early in embryonic myocardium. Coronary fistulae create coronary steal and result in ischemia of the distal myocardium. Proximal stenoses occur in the native coronary arteries and result in ventricular-dependent myocardial perfusion.

A second type of pulmonary atresia is associated with a VSD. Physiologically, this represents an extreme form of TOF.

Natural History

If untreated, about half of patients with pulmonary atresia with intact septum die within 2 weeks. Hypoxemia and metabolic acidosis are related to closure of the PDA. At 6 months after birth, approximately 90% of patients will have died. The acute intervention to prevent early death is the administration of PGE1 to ensure a PDA. Saturations should be maintained in the 80% range.

Indications for Operation

The mere presence of pulmonary atresia with intact ventricular septum mandates surgical intervention to augment an underperfused pulmonary vascular bed secondary to obstruction of the RVOT. Assuming a PDA and a nonrestrictive ASD, the type of operation depends on the size of the RV, which is closely related to the size of the tricuspid valve. The presence of coronary artery sinusoid/fistulae also alters the decision about type of operation, but not necessarily the need for an operation. In extreme cases of RV-dependent coronary artery blood flow, cardiac transplantation should be considered. Patients with large tricuspid valves and RV chambers should receive procedures that allow the right heart to be maintained and grow. Extremely small RV chambers and tricuspid valves are not likely to develop into viable pumping chambers and should be staged with the idea of a single ventricle repair long term.

Procedures and Outcomes

In the simplest form of pulmonary atresia with intact ventricular septum (the RV is of normal size and discoid pulmonary atresia is present), the pulmonary valve can simply be opened to allow antegrade flow. In a rare circumstances, this is all that is required to provide life-sustaining pulmonary flow. A new communication between the RV and the PA can be established in one of three ways. A balloon catheter can be placed across the RVOT after wire perforation of a thin pulmonary valve. The balloon catheter can be dilated to sufficient size to allow adequate pulmonary blood flow. In a second alternative, through a median sternotomy, the pulmonary valve can be forcefully and bluntly dilated to a normal caliber, allowing sufficient blood flow. This can be achieved via the transventricular or transatrial route. In a third option, through a median sternotomy, with the distal main PA clamped to preserve ductal flow to the branch pulmonary arteries, the proximal PA is opened and the pulmonary valve is incised. Blind dilatation may be required if visibility cannot be established by infundibular pressure after initial opening of the pulmonary valve. Trial occlusion of the PDA, either operatively or by weaning of the prostaglandin, will test the adequacy of pulmonary blood flow created in this way.

In more extreme cases of RV outflow hypoplasia, a more radical approach may be required to establish RV to PA continuity. A transannular patch can be placed, most commonly with CPB. Some have argued that patch placement and expected ventricular growth, even in extreme cases, lead to an improved likelihood for a long-term biventricular repair. In severe cases where RV outflow is insufficient to sustain life in the absence of a PDA, a shunt can be placed to augment pulmonary flow. The shunt replaces the PDA physiologically and can be placed from the ascending aorta to the main PA, from the innominate artery to the right branch PA, or from the subclavian artery to the PA. The choice of which shunt to use depends on the surgical approach and the preference of the surgeon. Studies suggest that the placement of a modified Blalock-Taussig shunt, a polytetraflouroethylene interposition graft between the left subclavian artery and the left PA, provides optimum short-term survival.

A second-stage palliation is often required at the end of the first year of life after the PVR has become normal. Patients with a previously placed fixed diameter shunt outgrow this shunt and require additional procedures to treat hypoxemia. A bidirectional Glenn shunt[12,13] from the distal end of the superior vena cava (SVC) to the side of the right main-branch PA, with oversewing of the proximal SVC and takedown of previous shunts, has proved to be quite useful. In patients with no functional RV, a hemi-Fontan-type procedure can be performed. In this procedure, a bidirectional Glenn is performed as above. The proximal SVC is anastomosed to the PA confluence and a dam is placed at the SVC entrance into the RA, thus preventing a PA to RA short circuit. The total pulmonary flow is identical to that of a Glenn procedure, only SVC flow. This prevents systemic venous hypertension caused by copious pulmonary flow and avoids the adverse consequences of systemic venous hypertension.

A third-stage physiologic repair is performed in patients without a functioning RV. This procedure, a completion Fontan, creates or opens an anastomosis between the RA and the PA confluence, depending on whether a bidirectional Glenn or a hemi-Fontan has been performed. The ASD is closed, preventing desaturated blood from entering the systemic circulation. Early mortality is attributable directly to high PVR, LV dysfunction, or distortion of the caval PA pathways. If the patient is in the high-risk Fontan group, specifically if pulmonary arteriolar resistance is high or LV dysfunction is present, a fenestrated Fontan can be placed. This strategy places a hole in the partition, creating the pathway between the IVC and the pulmonary arteries. This allows a small amount of right-to-left shunting and prevents systemic venous hypertension. After Fontan physiologic correction, patients with a PA pressure in excess of 20 mm Hg or a transpulmonary gradient in excess of 6 mm Hg have a high risk of succumbing.

In extreme cases of pulmonary atresia with an intact ventricular septum, patient survival after 1 year is approximately 70%. Patients who have an RV that can be used and subsequently develop a biventricular repair have more favorable results. Patients whose anatomy is more favorable, receiving a valvotomy or transannular patch, have a better outcome than those whose anatomy precludes any procedure other than a shunt alone. Valvotomy plus a patch has approximately an 80% 1-year survival rate. The risk of a bidirectional Glenn and hemi-Fontan is relatively small and is under 5% operative mortality. The risk of Fontan physiologic correction with the advent of fenestration has been reduced to under 10% operative mortality. Obviously, patients who have an RV that responds to therapeutic efforts for growth and ultimately have a biventricular repair have better survival rates. The long-term outcome of patients with RVOTO is importantly related to the adequacy of the RV and its potential for growth.

Tricuspid Atresia

Complete obstruction of the pathway from the RA to the RV occurs in approximately 2% of infants born with CHD and is present in approximately 5% of the patients born prematurely. In the absence of other lesions, pulmonary flow is restricted to PDA flow.

Embryology

The cause of tricuspid atresia is not certain but has been hypothesized to be a malalignment of the ventricular septum in relationship to the atria, with absence of the RV sinus.

Types of Tricuspid Atresia

The details defining the types of tricuspid atresia depend on great vessel relationships and the presence or absence of a VSD and pulmonary stenosis. Approximately half of patients have normal great vessels and a small restrictive VSD with pulmonary stenosis. About 10% of patients have normal great vessel relationships without a VSD and, hence, pulmonary atresia.

Physiologic Consequences

The physiologic consequences relate to obligatory right-to-left shunting across a required ASD and insufficient pulmonary blood flow requiring that life be sustained by a PDA, facilitated by PGE1 after birth. If a large VSD is present and there is no RVOTO, markedly increased pulmonary flow develops as the pulmonary vascular resistance (PVR) falls after birth. The presence or absence of an extra pathway and the degree of an additional obstruction at the pulmonary valve level determine the patient's clinical course.

If the great vessels are transposed, namely, if the aorta comes off the RV, the physiologic consequences are similar to those in HLHS except that the RV is hypoplastic in tricuspid atresia with TGA. The physiologic aspects are similar to those of HLHS.

Natural History

Without an adequate interatrial communication or source of pulmonary blood flow, patients with tricuspid atresia and RV hypoplasia succumb. A patent foramen ovale is present in two thirds of patients with tricuspid atresia, and about one third have a true ASD. A PDA is required to sustain life shortly after birth. If a VSD is present, the magnitude of additional pulmonary blood flow depends on the size of the VSD and the degree of RVOTO. The need to augment pulmonary blood flow can be determined by the degree of systemic saturation and the events associated with weaning of PGE1. If hypoxemia ensues with prostaglandin weaning, an alternative source of pulmonary blood flow is required and placement of a systemic to PA shunt facilitates recovery.

In tricuspid atresia associated with an unrestrictive VSD and no RVOTO, the problem associated with the normally decreasing PVR is massive pulmonary overcirculation. CHF ensues. If this anatomic and physiologic setup persists, elevated PVR and eventually Eisenmenger's syndrome (fixed pulmonary arteriolar vascular disease) develop and the surgical therapeutic options are limited.

Indications for Operation

Typically patients with tricuspid atresia, normally related great vessels, restrictive VSD, or critical RVOTO present with hypoxemia. PGE1 therapy facilitates a PDA, reduces PVR, and provides beneficial pulmonary flow while arrangements can be made for surgical intervention. The physiologic problem is insufficient pulmonary blood flow and is easily treated by placement of a systemic to PA shunt.

If the patient presents with tricuspid atresia, normally related great vessels, a large VSD, and unrestrictive pulmonary blood flow, the physiologic consequence, pulmonary overcirculation, does not usually demand treatment until later in life, perhaps at a few weeks or months of age, when the PVR falls. Since this represents a physiologic increase in pulmonary blood flow, the primary strategy is to add an obstruction to the RVOT.

Procedures and Outcomes

For patients with restricted pulmonary blood flow, the most common source for systemic blood is the subclavian artery. Flow can be directed to the PA either by a direct connection, by ligating the distal vessels, or by placement of a polytetrafluoroethylene graft between the subclavian artery and the ipsilateral PA. Efforts are made to establish as large a shunt as possible, because the flow-restricting orifice is the native proximal subclavian artery. Larger grafts have a lower thrombosis rate. If a small graft (3- to 4-mm prosthesis) is placed, long-term aspirin is administered to inhibit platelet adhesiveness, intimal growth, and eventual thrombosis.

In patients with excessive pulmonary blood flow, obstruction is added by placement of a PA band. Many techniques are used to establish the tightness of the band, but establishing a systemic saturation in the 75% to 80% range with the patient in his or her normal physiologic state is the objective. A left thoracotomy is performed and an umbilical tape is passed around the PA. This tape can be secured to a fixed diameter or made adjustable, at the surgeon's preference, to the degree necessary to restrict pulmonary flow.

Eventually, with the placement of a systemic to PA shunt or a PA band, depending on the physiologic situation, the patient outgrows the shunt or band. Hypoxemia, cyanosis and polycythemia are the usual consequences. At a point when the systemic saturation is under 70% or the hemoglobin is above 17 gm%, an additional procedure should be performed. If saturations fall below

60% and hemoglobin is above 20 gm%, an urgent procedure should be considered. By this time, the patient is usually old enough, with a sufficiently low PVR, to allow placement of a systemic venous to PA shunt, a Glenn-type procedure.

In the classic Glenn procedure,[14] the distal SVC is anastomosed to the distal right PA, and the proximal aspects of both the SVC and the PA are oversewn. The advantages of a Glenn procedure over the addition of another systemic to PA shunt include a reduction of volume of flow across the patent foramen ovale, a reduction in LV volume work, and a lower risk of pulmonary vascular obstructive disease. Recently, the classic Glenn shunt has been replaced by the bidirectional Glenn shunt, namely connection of the distal SVC to the side of the right branch PA, allowing blood flow to the right and left lungs. The proximal SVC is oversewn. If, ultimately, a total caval to pulmonary anastomosis is considered, the proximal SVC can be anastomosed to the underside of the main PA and a dam placed between the proximal SVC and the RA. This, in combination with a bidirectional Glenn, is considered a hemi-Fontan type procedure. All additional sources of pulmonary flow are usually taken down; specifically, shunts are ligated or the main PA is detached from the heart and the PA stumps are oversewn. This latter circumstance prevails when there is a residual RV to PA pathway either related to the original anatomy or associated with placement of a PA band. The bidirectional caval pulmonary anastomosis (bidirectional Glenn) and the hemi-Fontan are preformed via median sternotomy with CPB. Rarely, a bidirectional Glenn can be placed off CPB by using a shunt between the SVC and the RA during the placement of the anastomosis. A hemi-Fontan, however, is not possible without CPB.

The physiologic result is that total pulmonary flow is supplied by the SVC only. Inferior vena cava (IVC) blood flow passes into the RA and subsequently through the ASD to mix with the pulmonary venous return. Patient systemic saturations after this procedure are in the 85% range. Relative hypoxemia is compensated for by an increase in hemoglobin. Patients tolerate this physiology quite well. In the long term, however, optimal treatment is provided by directing all of the systemic venous blood flow to the pulmonary circulation. At approximately 2 years of age, when the pulmonary arteriolar resistance has fallen to a satisfactory level, total caval PA connection[15] or Fontan procedure[16] can be established.

Historically, the first approaches that were widely used to direct systemic venous blood into the pulmonary circulation used a direct RA to PA connection. Fontan and Baudit[16] initially described this principle and outlined 10 commandments that were not to be violated in using this strategy. Recently,[15] direct connection between the vena cavae and the PA has lowered or eliminated many risks associated with the Fontan direct RA to PA connection. The same physiologic result is achieved; all systemic venous blood is directed to the pulmonary circulation. Coronary sinus blood may or may not be directed to the pulmonary circulation (see below). Ideally, diversion of all systemic venous blood to the pulmonary circuit is appropriate if the PVR is under 4 Wood units, the pulmonary arteries are of sufficient size and anatomy to allow an unobstructed connection, and LV function is sufficiently compliant to allow a low postoperative mean PA pressure. Confounding issues, systemic AV valve regurgitation, LVOTO, and operative age under 2 years should be considered on an individual basis. Important considerations for a total systemic venous to PA–type operation are the pulmonary arteriolar resistance index, the LV end-diastolic pressure, and the respective systemic and pulmonary flows.

A source of confusion exists here concerning terminology. "Fontan procedure" has become a generic term for any operation that directs systemic venous blood to the pulmonary circuit. Hence, the distinction between total caval PA anastomoses and RA to PA anastomoses (classic Fontan) has been lost. These days, most surgeons are performing total caval PA anastomosis and including it in the subset labeled Fontan procedure. In the total caval pulmonary anastomosis, the distal SVC is anastomosed into the side of the undivided right PA and the proximal SVC orifice is opened widely and connected to the underside of a confluent PA. Then a tunnel inside the atrium is placed directing IVC blood through the proximal SVC entrance into the PA. The anastomosis of the baffle in the vicinity of the IVC may or may not include the coronary sinus. If the coronary sinus is included in the IVC pathway, the risk of heart block increases. If the coronary sinus is left on the pulmonary venous side of the baffle, mild systemic desaturation, in the 94% range, ensues and is well tolerated. In high-risk Fontan procedures, specifically ones in which the total pulmonary resistance may be elevated, the baffle within the atrium may be fenestrated, decompressing the systemic venous hypertension. A right-to-left shunt ensues that allows a small amount of systemic venous flow into the LA. This increases systemic cardiac output and reduces systemic saturation. The fenestration may be a fixed hole placed in the baffle or an adjustable hole using special techniques. In either circumstance, the objective is to reduce the deleterious effects of systemic venous hypertension and augment cardiac output. The systemic desaturation associated with this is usually well tolerated, particularly when oxygen carrying capacity is enhanced by red blood cell transfusion.

Systemic venous hypertension can be quite problematic in the post-Fontan patient, particularly when the PA pressure exceeds 20 mm Hg. Hydrostatic pressure gradients exist favoring the transudation of fluid into the interstitial space and serous cavities. Edema, pleural effusion, ascites, protein-losing enteropathy, and hepatic and renal dysfunction may develop. These problems have been partially ameliorated by utilization of the total caval PA connection rather than RA to PA connection. Hormonal responses associated with RA hypertension and atrial natriuretic hormone have been implicated. An intraatrial baffle excludes the RA from the higher pressure systemic venous circuit. Morbidity and mortality have been improved by use of the total caval PA connection technique for implementing the Fontan principle.

Hypoplastic Left Heart Syndrome

HLHS is a spectrum of abnormalities characterized by severe obstruction at one or more levels of LV inflow or outflow. In the most common form, aortic valve atresia leads to hypoplasia of the ascending aorta and the aortic arch. The left ventricle (LV) and mitral valve are severely hypoplastic or atretic. In contrast to the RV side, HLHS represents a single syndrome; isolated mitral or aortic atresia are not commonly seen.

The physiologic consequences are similar in HRHS with TGA, in which a hypoplastic ascending and transverse aorta arises from a small RV. In this situation, the presence of a VSD, more commonly seen in HLHS with TGA, may have salutary effects on the size of the RV and the ascending aorta. The larger the defect, the larger the RV and the ascending aorta are likely to be. In the extreme, however, when there is no VSD with HRHS and TGA, the physiologic consequences are similar to HLHS which is discussed in detail here. The reader can perform the proper translations when the treatment modalities are used for hypoplastic right heart with TGA.

Embryology

The embryologic cause of HLHS is not understood. Multiple developmental abnormalities related to limited LV inflow or outflow are likely causal. This abnormality is the fourth most common defect presenting in infancy, but the likelihood of death is diminishing with current modalities of treatment.

Types of Hypoplastic Left Heart

HLHS is a collection of lesions with global left-sided hypoplasia. Approximately one quarter of these patients have either a double-outlet RV or a common AV septal defect malaligned to the RV. Although considerable variations exist in the anatomy, the physiologic consequences are similar.

Physiologic Consequences

Because HLHS is resentative of an obstructive lesion, the LV and hence LA outflow are nonexistent. Therefore, an additional pathway, an ASD or a stretched foramen ovale, permits pulmonary venous drainage. Additionally, since there is no LV output, systemic blood flow must be provided by the RV through a PDA. The RV supplies both the systemic and the pulmonary circulations in parallel. Mixture of oxygenated and unoxygenated blood occurs in the RA. The relative amounts of pulmonary and systemic flow determine saturation. Since RV cardiac output is relatively fixed, an increase in saturation indicates increased pulmonary flow and may represent reduced systemic flow, producing an unmet perfusion need in the systemic circulation and consequent systemic shock with metabolic acidosis. A satisfactory physiologic state for these patients requires a delicate balance between the pulmonary and systemic flows, which primarily depends on the balance of pulmonary and systemic vascular resistances. The absence of a patent unrestrictive ductus arteriosus or an improperly restrictive interatrial communication are also quite important. If a PDA is not present, there is no systemic flow; a widely patent interatrial communication facilitates unrestricted pulmonary flow and consequent low systemic outflow.

Natural History

Untreated, these patients ultimately die and represent 25% of neonatal cardiac deaths within the first week of life. Patients with HLHS present with either systemic shock and severe metabolic acidosis related to closure of the PDA or a severe imbalance of pulmonary and systemic flows resulting in CHF or hypoxemia. Treatment of a closing PDA requires PGE1. An imbalance in pulmonary and systemic flow ratios may be more difficult to treat and is counterintuitive. The HLHS patient often presents with relative hypoxemia, that is, saturations in the 80% range. The instinctive treatment for this abnormality of the neonate is often oxygen. Oxygen has two deleterious effects in patients with HLHS: It facilitates PDA closure with its consequent systemic shock or it facilitates preferential blood flow to the lungs because of pulmonary arteriolar vasodilatation while sacrificing systemic blood flow. Systemic shock with pulmonary overcirculation is therefore created. The saturation will likely increase but at great detriment to perfusion of other vital organs. The ideal saturation for a patient with HLHS is in the 70% to 75% range, with a hematocrit in the 50% range. Oxygen carrying capacity is preserved and discrepant pulmonary and systemic flows are not created.

The adequacy of the interatrial communication is an important determinant of patient outcome. If no ASD is present, neonatal mortality is almost assured. An ideal circumstance is one in which the LA pressure is about 10 mm Hg higher than the RA pressure. The elevation in pulmonary venous pressure limits pulmonary blood flow and hence reduces the risk of systemic shock caused by stealing through the pulmonary circulation. In patients with essentially balanced pulmonary and systemic circulation, little additional therapy is likely to be required. In patients who have systemic hypoperfusion, in which the pulmonary to systemic flow ratio (Q_p/Q_s) is much greater than 1, a deliberate hypoventilation or inspired CO_2 without supplemental oxygen is likely to be beneficial. Occasionally, the inspirated O_2 fraction can be reduced to under 21% to avoid pulmonary arteriolar vasodilatation. Patients who have remarkably reduced pulmonary flow and hypoxemia should be treated with increased inspirated O_2, hyperventilation, and efforts to increase systemic vascular resistance. Hypothermia may be helpful in reducing oxygen demand.

Indications for Operation

Because of the near certainty of death soon after birth in patients with HLHS, operation should be considered. The three strategies used are: (1) cardiac transplantation; (2) staged palliative repair consisting of a Norwood procedure,[17] a bidirectional Glenn, and an eventual Fontan-type procedure; and (3) supportive care. The last of these options is nonsurgical and must be arrived at only after the family has a thorough understanding of the other two options, which have become increasingly successful with additional experience. The long-term results of cardiac transplantation and staged correction are similar. A primary disadvantage to cardiac transplantation is that it requires a donor organ, an increasingly scarce resource. Staged repair has improving long-term results, presents an option that can be applied shortly after birth, and allows caretakers and parents to be active rather than passive in the neonate's recovery.

Operative Procedures and Outcomes

Cardiac Transplantation

Since the anatomic abnormalities in HLHS are so severe, some have felt the best option to be total replacement of the heart. Coordination of donors and recipients is performed by the United Network for Organ Sharing (UNOS), a federally mandated program to ensure equitable distribution of organs. The donor heart must be of an appropriate size to the recipient and have a compatible ABO blood group. Donor organ availability remains a limiting factor. A large fraction of neonates with HLHS are lost because of the consequences of the intensity of medical management required while waiting for a donor organ.

Once a donor heart is identified, the surgical steps required for transplantation are not dissimilar from those in the adult. Median sternotomy and CPB are required. The surgical technique is relatively standard. The one exception is that because of the small size of the patient and the inadequacy of the aortic arch, circulatory arrest is used while the operation is performed. The donor organ is retrieved with enough distal aorta to augment the patient's hypoplastic arch. Once the LA, RA, and ascending aortic anastomoses are performed, CPB can be resumed and the final anastomosis, PA, can be performed. Anastomotic growth has been confirmed and is usually not a problem long term, whether absorbable or nonabsorbable suture is used. The donor heart is preserved in a usual manner. Ischemia of greater than 5 h is tolerated but requires additional postoperative cardiotonic support. Long term, these patients are at a consistent risk of rejection. Long-term therapy may include cyclosporin A, FK506, azathioprine, prednisone, rabbit anti-thymocyte globulin, or monoclonal OKT3. Baseline antirejection therapy consists of cyclosporin and azathioprine, with or without prednisone. Rejection episodes are treated with anti-thymocyte globulin and OKT3. Rejection avoidance and treatment protocols vary from center to center. Data collected by the International Society for Heart and Lung Transplantation suggest that infants with cardiac transplantation have about a 70% 1-year survival and a better than 65% 3-year survival. Some centers have reported an 82% 5-year survival in newborns.

Staged Repair for HLHS

This multiple operation strategy requires careful planning and knowledge of the changing physiology in maturing neonates and infants. An initial palliative procedure must be performed that allows survival shortly after birth until the PVR decreases. This initial palliation, described and refined by Norwood et al.,[17] results in construction of a neoaorta and creation of a pulmonary circulation supplied by a modified Blalock-Taussig shunt. The ventricular volume work of the single RV is equal to both the systemic and the pulmonary blood flow, quite demanding of a morphologic RV. Successful outcomes depend on balancing these two circulations. After the neonate matures, the PVR diminishes and the patient outgrows the systemic to PA shunt. Hypoxemia and polycythemia ensue. At this point, the second stage, a bidirectional Glenn is placed. The pulmonary and cephalad systemic circulations are therefore placed in series and RV volume work is reduced. Ultimately, the third-stage palliation, a Fontan-type correction (see above), is implemented and all of the systemic venous return is directed to the pulmonary circulation. Volume load on the RV is further minimized by this series connection of the pulmonary and all the systemic circuits.

Stage I palliation, the Norwood procedure, has two fundamental anatomic objectives: creation of an unobstructed pathway (replacing the previous PDA) from the RV to the systemic circulation and to provide a systemic source of blood flow to the PA. The single morphologic RV has its function preserved by avoiding excess pressure and volume work. Additionally, PVR changes are allowed to progress normally. The technical aspects of this procedure require use of CPB and circulatory arrest. After the induction of circulatory arrest, the PA is transsected above the sinotubular junction and the PDA is divided. The PA side of the ductus arteriosus is oversewn and the distal PA is usually patch closed, isolating the PA confluence. The ascending, transverse, and descending aortas are opened longitudinally to allow placement of a vascular graft, usually a hemi-PA homograft, to be sutured to augment the distal aortic arch around to the proximal ascending aorta. The homograft is fashioned in such a way that the proximal PA is incorporated into the anastomosis so that RV outflow is directed solely to the neoaorta. Pulmonary blood flow is established by placing a polytetraflouroethylene shunt from the innominate artery to the top of the right PA. The size of the shunt is critically important in that it is a determining factor in the balance of pulmonary and systemic flow ratios. Since pulmonary flow is now restricted in part by the size of the shunt, the intraatrial septum is excised. At an appropriate time, CPB is resumed and the patient resuscitated and treated per protocol.

It is noteworthy that the physiologic state of a patient's post–stage I repair, Norwood procedure, is identical to the physiologic status preoperatively. Fine tuning of the Q_p/Q_s by proper sizing of the polytetraflouroethylene shunt can take place, but the patient is physiologically essentially the same as preoperatively. Since no corrective maneuver was performed at stage I palliation, these patients require intensive management postoperatively with assiduous attention to detail. Injudicious use of ventilation, oxygenation, volume administration, inotropic agents, and after-load–reducing agents can have deleterious effects on the precariously balanced pulmonary and systemic flow ratios since RV output is relatively fixed in amount. The pulmonary vascular bed is notoriously unstable in the neonate. After stage I palliation, 70% of deaths in these patients occur during their initial hospitalization. Although survival rates after a stage I palliation, Norwood procedure, are in the 60% range across the country, some centers have reported survival rates in the high 80% and low 90% range. After a successful stage I palliation and maturation so that the patient outgrows his or her pulmonary to sys-

temic shunt, the surgical operations utilized are similar to those used in the treatment of tricuspid atresia. This series of operations, bidirectional Glenn or hemi-Fontan followed by a completion Fontan, are a final common pathway for patients who receive treatment for a functional single ventricle. In tricuspid atresia with TGA and without a VSD, the functioning ventricle is the morphologic LV. In hypoplastic left heart, the functioning ventricle is the morphologic RV.

EXTRA PATHWAY LESIONS

Patent Ductus Arteriosus

A persistent extra pathway between the aortic arch in the vicinity of the left subclavian artery and the PA is typically a PDA. As the PVR falls, flow increases through this extra pathway and pulmonary overcirculation ensues. A PDA may be life sustaining if concomitant congenital heart disease is present that limits pulmonary flow.

Embryology

If one of the six paired aortic arches remains patent, a communication between the aorta in the vicinity of the left subclavian artery and the PA persists. The PDA is usually on the left but can be on the right. Factors associated with persistent patency include prematurity, hypoxemia, rubella, and possible genetic and environmental factors.

Types of Patent Ductus Arteriosus

A PDA may exist in an infant in a variety of shapes and sizes. These differences help explain the varying forms of presentation. The typical PDA has a large aortic end that tapers toward the PA and becomes narrowest at the PA end. In neonates, problematic PDAs are usually tubular and straight, although they can be very tortuous.

Physiologic Consequences

Shortly after birth, pulmonary vascular and systemic vascular resistances are similar. With advancing age, the PVR falls. A left-to-right, aortic to PA shunt develops. The degree of excess pulmonary overcirculation varies with the amount of closure of the ductus arteriosus and the degree of pulmonary vascular resistance decrease. If there is no narrowing of the PDA and the PVR falls to normal, high-flow, hyperkinetic, pulmonary hypertension is the rule. Neonates with compromised pulmonary function may become worse as pulmonary flow increases. This abnormal flow increases volume load on the LA and LV. CHF often ensues, which complicates treatment of ventilator-bound neonates.

An aorticopulmonary window (APW), an extra pathway between the ascending aorta and the main- or right-branch PA can be confused for a large PDA. The physiologic consequences, natural history, and indications for operation are the same as for a large PDA.

Natural History

Shortly after birth, with the first few breaths of extra-uterine life, lungs expand and the PVR falls. Simultaneously, the PDA begins to constrict. Normally this constriction continues and the ductus is functionally closed by 24 h of age. Structural closure is usually complete by 2 to 3 weeks of life. If a ductus arteriosus remains open after 3 months of life, an abnormal response is certain.

Indications for Operation

Typically a patient with a PDA is asymptomatic and presents to the cardiologist with an incidental murmur. However, neonates, particularly premature neonates, may present with signs of CHF in the presence of concomitant pulmonary disease. Indomethacin, an inhibitor of cyclooxygenase and a potent constrictor of a ductus arteriosus, may facilitate closure. Factors that contribute to failure of ductal closure include insufficient smooth muscle within the ductus arteriosus, oxygen sensor insufficiency, prostaglandin excess, furosemide, excess fluids, surfactant replacement therapy, hypocalcemia, and theophylline, among others. The patient who is unresponsive to medical management should be considered for operative closure.

Procedures and Outcomes

A myriad of techniques have been used for mechanical closure of a PDA. In the neonate, the most common technique uses a left thoracotomy. The PDA is either suture ligated or clip occluded. CPB is not required. Historically, a chest tube was usually placed, but recent experience has suggested this is not always necessary. The neonate who is ventilator bound requires continued management in an intensive care setting. Typically, this is a safe and relatively easy procedure, but mortality and morbidity may occur.

In older patients, on an elective basis, this same surgical approach may be used. Other techniques have been developed that seem attractive. Some have used the thoracoscope with three or four incisions, dissection of the PDA, and placement of an occluding clip. As patients become older, they become candidates for transvascular catheter closure, using either two opposing umbrellas or an intraductal coil. These transvascular techniques, particularly the former, have been in the development stage for over two decades. The transcatheter coil placement technique, a relatively new strategy, is gaining acceptance and may ultimately be applied to younger patients. Persistent patency of the ductus arteriosus is more likely with the transcatheter technique. Injuries to the recurrent nerve, thoracic

duct, possible ligation of the left PA, descending aorta or carotid artery, all rare but potentially morbid if not catastrophic consequences of thoracotomy techniques, are avoided.

With closure of the PDA, all physiologic sequels associated with the left-to-right shunt are ameliorated. If a persistent ductus arteriosus is present, the physiologic consequences are in direct proportion to the magnitude of the left-to-right shunt. The possibility of bacterial endocarditis in association with a PDA is eliminated by closure of the extra pathway.

The presence of an APW demands repair with CPB, aortic cross-clamping, and placement of a patch in the extra pathway. Operation is curative in the absence of other anomalies.

Atrial Septal Defect

A persistent extra pathway, a result of either deficiency in the atrial septum or failure of closure of the fossa ovale between the atria, causes an ASD. Since LA pressure is higher than RA pressure, this extra pathway allows left-to-right shunting and volume loading of the right heart.

Embryology

Normally, a septum primum, extending from the atrial roof, connects with fused endocardial cushions on the floor of the atrium. A septum secundum, also arising from the atrial roof, resides on the right side of the primum septum. An interatrial opening, the foramen ovale, is formed. In utero, RA blood passes through this one-way valve into the LA. Postnatally, the one-way valve is closed by relatively higher LA pressure. Absence of a portion of the atrial septum allows persistent interatrial communication.

Types of Atrial Septal Defect

These defects are categorized by the portion of the atrial septum that is absent or deficient: patent foramen ovale, secundum, primum, and sinus venosus. Failure of fusion of the septum primum and septum secundum causes a patent foramen ovale. Deficiency of the primum septum in the region of the foramen ovale causes a secundum ASD. Failure of the septum primum to fuse with the endocardial cushions causes a primum ASD. Failure of development of the atrial septum in the vicinity of the SVC and the RA is associated with partial anomalous pulmonary venous return and forms a sinus venosus ASD. A wide variety of atrial defects with respect to size, shape, and location can be seen and, in the extreme, a common atrium develops.

Physiologic Consequences

Since LA pressure is higher than RA pressure, an extra pathway between the atria allows left-to-right shunting proportionate to the size of the defect and ventricular diastolic function. The larger the defect and the more compliant the RV, the greater the left-to-right shunt. Increased shunting produces additional volume work for the RA and RV. High pulmonary flows can develop without a concomitant rise in right-sided pressures because of the ability of the pulmonary vascular bed to vasodilate and the RV to be compliant.

Natural History

The likelihood of ASD closure depends directly on the size and location of the defect. Rarely does an isolated ASD become problematic in the neonatal period. Concomitant disease, either cardiac or noncardiac, may adversely affect the consequences of an interatrial communication. Death from an isolated ASD is unusual in the first two decades. Long term, death is usually associated with progressive right heart failure, atrial arrhythmias, and, rarely, irreversible pulmonary vascular disease.

Indications for Operation

Typically, ASD closure is recommended with a persistent left-to-right shunt and a Q_p/Q_s of greater than 1.5 to 1. Operation is seldom indicated in neonates or infants. Closure in association with surgical treatment of other severe CHD is common. In the current era of deciding about cardiac operations without catheterization, echocardiographic evidence of RV volume overload argues for closure. Paradoxical embolus is a risk in even the smallest ASDs. Because of this risk, particularly in association with pregnancy, some have argued that all ASDs should be closed. In the adult patient, cerebrovascular accidents of unknown etiology in association with an ASD have led some to close these hemodynamically insignificant alternative pathways.

Procedures and Outcomes

Most commonly, the ASD is closed using CPB through a median sternotomy. The exact technique for closure depends on the size and shape of the defect as well as on the nature of the border of the defect. Primary closure can be achieved when the defect is small and there is firm ASD tissue in the rim. If the defect is large or there is friable ASD tissue, a patch can be used. The patch material may be Dacron, polytetraflouroethylene, pericardium, or any other commercially available endovascular substitute. In older patients, a right anterolateral thoracotomy or transverse bilateral submammary incisions have been used. A ministernotomy, the lower one half of the sternum with limited skin incision, has recently been used with considerable success and small external scar. Other variations on the technical scheme have been used and are limited basically by the imagi-

nation of the surgeon. In all cases, CPB has been required to put the heart at rest while the defect is closed.

A second alternative closure technique is a percutaneous, transvenous route using two opposing umbrellas of wire and Dacron. These techniques have been developed for over a decade. They are limited to patients who have relatively small central defects with excellent surrounding septal tissue. Additional transcatheter techniques have been introduced but none has received approval as a standard procedure at this time.

ASD closure is associated with nearly zero mortality. Mortality is usually associated with other complicating and confounding issues. Surgical closure rate is close to 100%. Hospital stay postoperatively in the routine situation is 2 to 3 days. Patients, if appropriately managed postoperatively, can resume normal activity, with the exception of strenuous upper body activities, within 1 week.

Ventricular Septal Defect

An extra pathway between the LV and the RV results in a VSD. Since LV pressure is much higher than RV pressure, the physiologic consequence is increased flow through the right heart.

Embryology

The interventricular septum is a fusion of the primary folds at the apex, the inlet septum from posterior inferior tissue, and the conal ridge superiorly. Absence or underdevelopment of one of these regions permits an interventricular communication.

Types of Ventricular Septal Defect

The most common type, membranous VSD, results from failure of merger of the conal ridge with the fused endocardial cushions from the inlet septum. This accounts for about 75% of defects requiring operative correction. The defect lies immediately beneath and superior to the septal leaflet of the tricuspid valve. The second most common type, inlet, also known as an AV-type defect, is found beneath the septal leaflet of the tricuspid valve and represents a failure of development of the posterior inferior ventricular septum. Infundibular defects, also described as conal, intracristal, or supracristal, result as an incomplete development of the conal ridge. Muscular VSDs are present in the trabecular septum, may be multiple, and result from failure of the apical primary fold to develop. In the extreme, absence of the entire ventricular septum is called a common ventricle. Since operative repair is more challenging in common ventricle than the above-mentioned types of VSD, a functional single-ventricle repair strategy has been developed for this disease.

Physiologic Consequences

Flow into the pulmonary circuit as a result of a left-to-right shunt across the VSD is related to the size of the defect and the level of the PVR. Small and medium-sized VSDs usually have a pressure gradient between the LV and RV and hence are termed restrictive. Large defects, usually equal to or greater than the aortic valve annulus, are nonrestrictive and in the absence of other anomalies permit massive pulmonary flow and RV and PA hypertension. In this situation, the Q_p/Q_s is determined by the ratio of pulmonary and systemic vascular resistance.

In the newborn period, the PVR is high. As the newborn matures, the PVR falls and shunting from left to right develops. Between 4 and 6 weeks of life, in patients with unrestrictive VSDs, increasing left-to-right shunting causes CHF. Patients with small and moderate VSDs present with less severe symptoms or, if the VSD is tiny, may only have a heart murmur. With large VSDs, there is high pulmonary flow and hyperkinetic (high-flow) RV and PA hypertension. Relatively decreased systemic perfusion and increased work of breathing leads to activation of the renin-angiotensin system, salt and water retention, systemic vasoconstriction, increased left-to-right shunting, and worsening CHF.

With persistent pulmonary overcirculation, the pulmonary vascular bed vasoconstricts at the arteriolar level and the PVR increases. Progressive pulmonary arteriopathy leads to the development of irreversible pulmonary vascular disease. As the PVR increases, the left-to-right shunting decreases, the PA and RV pressures remain systemic, and the PA hypertension is related more to PVR changes rather than to increased amounts of pulmonary flow (hyperkinetic hypertension). Pulmonary vascular disease may develop within 2 years of life and culminates with the development of Eisenmenger's complex when the PVR is greater than the systemic vascular resistance. A right-to-left shunt then ensues. Every effort should be made to prevent this devastating consequence.

Indications for Operation

Perimembranous and muscular VSDs, particularly when small, have a greater than 80% spontaneous closure rate. CHF in an infant requires medical management; oral cardiotonics, systemic after-load–reducing drugs, and diuretic agents are helpful. Infants with large perimembranous defects who have continued CHF and failure to thrive or recurrent pulmonary infections should have surgical VSD closure. About one third of patients with a small defect will develop VSD-related complications. Many factors should be considered in the decision about VSD closure, but data tend to support surgical closure.

The presence of an intracristal, supracristal, or subarterial VSD is an indication for closure. Because of a venturi effect and velocity across the adjacent aortic valve leaflet—and probable injury to that leaflet—repair should be performed even for small defects. Inlet, AV canal–type defects do not close spontaneously. Arguments for closure are similar to those described above for perimembranous defects.

Muscular VSDs present a spectrum of anomalies. With few small defects, spontaneous closure is the rule and no operative intervention is required. Infants having multiple large muscular defects may require an operation shortly after birth. Surgical closure in this group can be difficult.

A method for ameliorating the physiologic consequences of pulmonary overcirculation is PA banding, in which the PA is narrowed to restrict blood flow to the pulmonary circuit. This technique is used only for extreme cases of multiple muscular VSDs, for common ventricle, or for those who have absolute contraindications for CPB. However, closure of large VSDs is the current desired technique, almost regardless of the patient's size in the absence of other confounding problems.

Procedures and Outcomes

Typically for perimembranous, inlet, supracristal, and solitary muscular VSDs, CPB is instituted and the aorta cross-clamped to facilitate exposure. Perimembranous and inlet VSDs are approached through the RA. A patch is sutured in place. Suture techniques are variable, depending on the surgeon, but all produce reliable closure rates. Intra- or supracristal VSDs may also be approached through the PA and across the pulmonary valve. Alternatively, a RVOT ventriculotomy provides an unencumbered view of the outlet VSD. Muscular defects require a sequence of approaches through the RA, the RV, and, if all else fails, the LV. Every effort is made to avoid a left ventriculotomy because of the adverse long-term consequences.

The 30-day mortality, in ideal cases, is under 1%. Mortality increases with repair of multiple VSDs, preoperative myocardial dysfunction related to CHF, persistent postoperative pulmonary hypertension, sepsis, or a technically suboptimal procedure. Long-term results are excellent and justify the practice of closing large defects early in life.

Transvascular closure of VSD is possible but isolated to very special circumstances and remains investigational. These techniques may be useful for muscular defects or residual postoperative VSDs that are remote from surrounding vital structures. This technique is currently investigational but may become useful in our treatment armamentarium.

Atrioventricular Canal

Atrioventricular (AV) defects are the coexistence of two extra pathways. The atrial and ventricular septa are absent immediately above and below the tricuspid and mitral valves. The tricuspid and mitral valves are malformed such that there is a single-inlet AV valve. The physiologic consequence, assuming no AV valve dysfunction, is a large left-to-right shunt and pulmonary overflow. Partial AV canal defects exist. AV valve dysfunction can complicate the clinical course.

Embryology

In AV-canal defect, the septum primum, after its growth toward the AV valves, is not met by endocardial tissue growing upward from the dorsal and ventral walls in the region of the AV valve. These endocardial cushions also fail to form the inlet ventricular septum and join the upward growing trabecular ventricular septum. These cushions also form the septal leaflets of both the mitral and the tricuspid valves. Failure of maturation of this tissue prevents development of the juxtaposed mitral and tricuspid annuli. A single ventricular valve is formed supplying both the RV and the LV. A defect is thus created in the center of the heart where the lowermost portion of the atrial septum and the superiormost portion of the ventricular septum are absent; a single AV valve to both ventricles is formed secondary to failure of development of the septal leaflet of the tricuspid and mitral valves.

Types of AV Canal

Variations in anatomy for AV-canal (endocardial cushion) defects are quite numerous. The size and shape of AV valve components, the number and types of attachments of the leaflets to the underlying structures, and the degree of override can be quite variable. A simple classification allows initial description of these abnormalities. The failure to form of the separate septal leaflets of the tricuspid and mitral valves allows the persistence of a superior bridging leaflet, which in fact is composed of the superior component of the mitral septal leaflet and the superior component of the tricuspid septal leaflet. A Rastelli classification is based on the nature of this superior leaflet. In the type A defect, the superior bridging leaflet has a cleft over the interventricular septum, with numerous chordal attachments to the septum. The depth of this cleft can be complete, dividing the superior bridging leaflet into its two components, the superior component of the tricuspid septal leaflet and the superior component of the mitral septal leaflet. In type C AV-canal defect, the superior bridging leaflet has no cleft and no attachments to the interventricular septum. In a type B defect, the superior bridging leaflet has a variable cleft and a variable amount of attachment to the ventricular septal crest.

Partial AV-canal defects, ostium primum ASDs, have an intact ventricular septum, absent lower atrial septum, and usually a cleft in the septal leaflet of the mitral valve. Two separate orifices for the AV valves are present. A detailed morphologic analysis shows abnormalities in the location of the common tricuspid–mitral annulus onto the crest of the ventricular septum, specifically displaced toward the apex, which is usually of no physiologic consequence. AV-canal defects can be associated with other forms of complex and severe congenital heart disease. Approximately 30% of children with Down syndrome have some form of AV defect.

Physiologic Consequences

As with ASDs and VSDs, a relatively high pulmonary flow compared to systemic flow can be well tolerated. As PVR falls, the Q_p/Q_s becomes even higher and CHF develops. If the PVR fails to fall, CHF and failure to thrive may not ensue. Symptoms are worsened by the occurrence of AV valve regurgitation, an extra pathway for ventricular flow during systole.

Natural History

The development of severe CHF may lead to an 80% mortality in the first 2 years of life. If an infant survives his or her first year of life, a 50% chance of living to 5 years can be expected. Respiratory distress, failure to thrive, pulmonary infections, and arrhythmias contribute to these adverse outcomes. Infants who do survive convert hyperkinetic pulmonary hypertension to high-resistance pulmonary hypertension, thus reducing the intracardiac shunt. These infants tend to develop irreversible pulmonary vascular disease at a young age. Infants with Down syndrome seem particularly prone to this unwelcome sequel. Irreversible pulmonary vascular disease may develop within the first 2 months of life in a child with Down syndrome and AV defect.

Indications for Operation

The presence of an AV defect, complete or partial, is an indication for repair. Mitral valve insufficiency may hasten the development of symptoms. The optimal timing for repair depends on the severity of the lesion and the associated symptoms. The simplest form, partial AV defect, primum ASD, and the absence of symptoms, may be fixed after infancy but before schooling begins. More severe forms, complete AV defect, particularly when associated with AV valve regurgitation, may require operation in the first few months of life. In general, it is best to wait for the PVR to fall so that a more favorable pulmonary vascular bed reactivity is present at the time of CPB and in the postoperative state. Once irreversible PVR changes occur, however, the operative risk is increased. If the PVR level is high, usually greater than 10 Wood units/m^2, most surgeons would consider

VSD closure contraindicated. In patients with an initial pure left-to-right shunt, the development of elevated PVR can be suspected with the onset of right-to-left shunting and cyanosis. Commonly, however, shunting at the atrial and ventricular levels is bidirectional and early onset of low systemic saturations, in the high 80% range, may not be an ominous sign for PVR changes. Any child under 4 months of age should be considered for AV-canal repair and the status of pulmonary arteriolar resistance changes tested. Without repair, pulmonary arteriolar resistance changes that are progressive, make dismal outcomes certain. Operative repair seems to ameliorate the development of pulmonary arteriolar vascular changes in most patients.

Procedures and Outcomes

AV defects, whether partial or complete, are repaired via median sternotomy with CPB. The defect is exposed through the RA. The most critical step is analysis of the defect so that repair can be designed to optimize mitral valve function and minimize the chances for remote complications. Several surgical strategies have evolved, emphasizing the number of patches and type of material used to close the septal defects. Whether the newly constructed septal leaflet of the mitral valve receives closure of the cleft between the superior and inferior components depends on the function of the newly constructed valve. Stages required for successful repair are VSD patch closure, ASD patch closure, repair of the mitral valve so that it is competent, and repair of the tricuspid valve so that its function is optimized.

In repair of partial AV canal, no VSD is present. The cleft in the septal leaflet of the mitral valve may or may not be suture repaired, depending on the valve function. An ASD patch is placed to avoid injury to the AV node. Commonly, the ASD patch is placed such that the coronary sinus drainage returns to the LA. This has the consequence of mild systemic desaturation, in the 94% range. A favorable surgical outcome is expected. Long-term results are quite favorable, although these patients do have a real risk of the development of subaortic stenosis.

Occasionally, a patient has contraindications, absolute or relative, to CPB. Since the physiologic consequence of AV canal is increased pulmonary flow, these patients can be palliated by placement of a PA band to control CHF. Most centers prefer, in suitable patients, to perform total correction.

Postoperative recovery can be difficult in these patients. Pulmonary vascular hypertensive crises are common. Dysrhythmias are more common after repair of complete AV canal defects than in other CHD. The severity of residual mitral insufficiency adds to complicating factors. Rarely, if a patient has extreme difficulty in recovering, the mitral valve is re-repaired

or replaced at a subsequent time. In general, patients with a hemodynamically satisfactory repair have an operative mortality rate of under 2%. Remote follow-up is required for the development of subaortic stenosis and progression of mitral valve regurgitation.

Single Ventricle

Single ventricle, also known as double-inlet ventricle or univentricular heart, represents, in its simplest form, complete absence of the ventricular septum. This extra pathway produces the physiologic consequence, in the absence of other abnormalities, of markedly increased pulmonary flow as in a VSD. In single ventricle, one morphologic ventricular type, left or right, dominates. The AV and ventriculoarterial connections may be variable. Obstructions along any part of one of the pathways may be present.

Embryology

Single ventricle is an arrest of early cardiac development. Anatomic variations associated with this abnormality are numerous. Although not certain, an abnormal transfer of the inlet parts of the primary heart tubes probably causes a single ventricle. The primitive atria are connected to the inlet aspect of the primary heart tube, which develops into the LV. Blood passes from this inlet tube into the bulbus cordis, which becomes an RV. Defective intraventricular septation probably causes double-inlet LV. Transference of the primitive AV junction to the outlet component probably causes double-inlet RV. Great vessel development depends on the timing of arrest. Every conceivable permutation is possible.

Types of Single Ventricle

The initial nomenclature describes the morphologic type of ventricle, left or right. Approximately 75% of single ventricles are double-inlet LVs. Secondary descriptions include whether the nondominant ventricle is to the left or the right side and whether there is ventricular arterial concordance or discordance. About 60% of double-inlet LVs have a left-sided RV and ventricular arterial discordance. About 70% of double-inlet RVs have a leftward LV and ventricular arterial concordance. In about 10% of single ventricles, the morphologic type of the ventricle is undetermined. It is noteworthy that AV conduction tissue in patients with single ventricle has no resemblance to a normal heart. When patients are considered with this diagnosis, each individual case is unique.

Physiologic Consequences

Without other CHD, three scenarios develop depending on the location and degree of ventricular outlet obstruction. If the pulmonary outflow tract is obstructed, hypoxemia, cyanosis, and acidosis develop as the PDA closes spontaneously. PGE1 ameliorates this difficulty by allowing the ductus to stay open and provide adequate pulmonary perfusion. If the aortic outflow tract is obstructed, systemic blood flow is PDA dependent. As the PDA closes, systemic shock and acidosis develop. PGE1 with opening of the ductus arteriosus ameliorates this consequence. A third scenario occurs when neither the systemic nor pulmonary outflow tract is obstructed. In this situation, PDA closure does not threaten perfusion of either the lungs or the body. As the PVR falls, pulmonary flow increases and CHF develops. In severe forms, with high Q_p/Q_s, systemic flow may be quite marginal. Aggressive medical management may be required in the early resuscitative phase.

Natural History

Although natural history studies are fraught with difficulties, primarily because they represent data of referral centers seeing patients who had survived infancy, most believe that single ventricle has a terrible prognosis. Early studies have difficulties in diagnosis of morphology because of the absence of modern cardiac imaging techniques. Referral center studies describe patients who have received a surgical intervention.

Indications for Operation

The anatomy of the patient dictates the physiologic status of the single ventricle variant and determines when to proceed with operation. In extreme cases, severe or expectedly severe hypoxemia resulting from decreased pulmonary flow, severe or expectedly severe reduction in systemic perfusion caused by aortic inflow (ductal-dependent) obstruction, or severe or expectedly severe CHF caused by unobstructed aortic and pulmonary outflow tracts determines the need for operation. Rarely, a patient will have an unobstructed aortic outflow and an obstructed pulmonary outflow tract that is just the right amount to prevent CHF. In this circumstance, waiting for ominous signs or symptoms is warranted. As a rule, patients with single ventricle should be expected to require one or more operations, depending on the anatomy and consequent physiology.

Procedures and Outcomes

Because of the wide variation in physiologic consequences, a single best surgical intervention for patients with double-inlet ventricle cannot be determined. All initial procedures are palliative and subsequent procedures for the most part provide physiologic repair. Often a decision has to be made concerning multiple relatively low-risk palliative operations and compared to a more risky radical procedure, which may provide better long-term results if successful. Currently, the surgical treatment pendulum leans toward the more radical approach, with the idea of optimizing long-term results once the perioperative risks have passed. The surgical approach depends on the exact anatomy and physiology of the single-ventricle variant.

Neonates who have diminished pulmonary flow are best served by placement of a systemic to PA shunt. In the long term, subsequent systemic to PA shunts will cause volume overload of the dominant ventricle, which has long-term adverse sequels. These shunts have been replaced by a bidirectional Glenn or hemi-Fontan at about 1 year of age. Subsequently, if the patient is a suitable candidate, a completion Fontan or cavopulmonary connection can be performed. Fontan physiologic correction for double-inlet LV has about an 85% in-hospital survival. Five-year survival is about 70%.

Patients with an obstructed LVOT in the extreme are handled similarly to HLHS patients. An initial stage I Norwood is performed. This is followed by a bidirectional Glenn or hemi-Fontan and, finally, by a completion Fontan.

In patients without obstructed systemic or PA outflow tracts, CHF develops as PVR falls. Two strategies have developed: PA banding followed by bidirectional Glenn- and Fontan-type correction, or ventricular septation. In the former approach, a PA band is placed to restrict pulmonary overcirculation and relieve symptoms of CHF while reducing the chance of pulmonary vascular disease. This can be performed at relatively low perioperative risk. Subsequently, at about 1 year of age, a bidirectional Glenn can be placed and finally a completion Fontan can be achieved. This leads to a long-term physiologic repair.

Ventricular septation, a second alternative, has been attempted and carries a quite high operative mortality rate and a high likelihood of complete heart block. In the 1970s, an operative mortality of about 50% and a late mortality of about 20% could be expected. Of the 35% of survivors, only 75% have had a fair to good result. A substantial incidence of persistent septal defects or AV valve dysfunction has discouraged more recent attempts. A wide variety of morphologic variants mitigates against successful ventricular septation. For that reason, most centers prefer the multiple staged physiologic repair route.

A subset of patients who receive a PA band develop subaortic stenosis which can be solved by subaortic septal resection or a Norwood-type procedure. Historically, a modified Damus-Kaye-Stansel procedure, similar in physiologic consequences but varied in the detail of anastomoses when compared to the Norwood procedure, also provides an option for physiologic improvement. Long term, both the Norwood and Damus-Kaye-Stansel palliated patients receive a bidirectional Glenn and proceed to completion with a cavopulmonary repair at about 2 years of age. Because of the complex anatomy, these Fontan patients are not as well off as those treated for tricuspid atresia, but they do have about an 85% 1-year survival.

Unique situations develop in patients with single ventricle that allow the surgeon to exercise creativity in designing an operation. Given the proper circumstances, an ASO with atrial septectomy and aortic arch repair may be required. In extreme circumstances, when patients have failed therapeutic alternatives or no satisfactory alternative exists, cardiac transplantation may be of benefit. Patients who receive transplantation after multiple operations for complex congenital heart disease have about a 70% perioperative survival. Once these patients get through this high-risk interval, their long-term results track the results of patients receiving transplantation for other less risk-prone etiologies.

OBSTRUCTION WITH EXTRA PATHWAY LESIONS

Tetralogy of Fallot

This condition, TOF, first described in 1672, is one of the most common forms of cyanotic congenital heart disease. The two anatomic features most important are RVOTO at one or several levels of varying degrees and an extra pathway between the ventricles. The aorta is also deviated to the right and the RV is hypertrophied, hence the term "tetralogy." The physiologic consequence depends highly on the degree of RVOTO. In mild forms of obstruction, pulmonary overcirculation may develop. In severe forms of RVOTO, insufficient pulmonary blood flow with consequent cyanosis and polycythemia may develop. In absolute RVOTO, pulmonary atresia with VSD, alternative pathways for pulmonary flow are required to sustain life. Patients with concomitant ASD are said to have pentalogy TOF.

Embryology

Incomplete rotation of the bulbotruncal region causes failure of the infundibular ventricular septum to align with the trabecular ventricular septum and explains the VSD associated with TOF. Abnormal separation of the distal bulbus caused by anterior placement of the bulbotruncal ridges results in unequal separation of the outflow tracts and leads to RVOTO. Other theories have been hypothesized but cannot be verified by all observers.

Types of Tetralogy of Fallot

The degree of RVOTO, in the absence of other important abnormalities, determines the clinical presentation. The VSD is usually large, subaortic, perimembranous, and associated with malalignment of the conal septum. The RVOTO may be mild or absolute (pulmonary atresia) and may occur at one or several positions in the RVOT (infundibular, valvular, main PA, branch PA). Patients with TOF are characterized by degree and posi-

tion of RVOTO. Additionally, if there is severe aortic overriding such that the aorta is more than 50% off the RV, double-outlet right ventricle (DORV) is present. With a subaortic VSD, treatment of DORV is similar to TOF. Patients with pulmonary atresia and VSD are separated diagnostically from other forms of TOF but have physiologic consequences and require similar operative strategies as TOF.

Physiologic Consequences

In mild forms of RVOTO, patients act similarly to those with VSD and mild pulmonary stenosis (PS). Left-to-right shunting persists, as in patients with VSD and no RVOTO. Patients with this abnormality are considered pink TOF. As RVOTO becomes more severe, bidirectional shunting may occur. Changes in systemic vascular resistance and degree of RVOTO, e.g., infundibular "spasm," can produce changes in the pulmonary to systemic flow ratio. A severe episode of right-to-left shunting causes a hypercyanotic (tet) spell. These spells are reversed by squatting, which increases systemic vascular resistance, systemic vascular resistance–increasing drugs, reduction of infundibular muscle tone (beta blockade), and intravascular volume loading. Patients with absolute RVOTO, pulmonary atresia, usually have alternative sources of pulmonary blood flow, either natural (main aorta to PA collateral arteries, MAPCAs), or surgically created shunts. These alternative sources are more stable than RV infundibular muscle and do not allow the hypercyanotic spell. These patients often are cyanotic and polycythemic, but stable. The aortic overriding and RV hypertrophy have little physiologic consequence. These factors are important to the surgeon, however, when achieving anatomic repair.

Natural History

As can be predicted, the long-range outlook without repair depends on the severity of the RVOTO and alternative sources of pulmonary blood flow. Approximately 30% of patients do not survive to 6 months of age. At 2 years, approximately 50% will have died. Although, rarely, patients have been diagnosed as adults, only 20% reach 10 years of age. When pulmonary atresia is associated with TOF, only one half reach their first birthday. Operative intervention, palliative or reparative depending on the circumstances, offers these children a much improved quantity and quality of life.

Indications for Operation

The degree of systemic desaturation and cyanosis is the prime variable used in deciding about when an operation should be undertaken. In the absence of hypoxemia or cyanosis, reparative operations are usually performed at the end of infancy to ameliorate the long-term adverse consequence of RV hypertension and the resultant development of long-term arrhythmias. The specific type of operation, palliative versus corrective, depends on numerous variables. Current trends in centers routinely treating complex heart disease show favorable results with properly selected patients who have early correction. Patients with systemic saturations under 75%, polycythemia with hematocrits over 55%, or significant or persistent hypercyanotic spells should receive operation.

Procedures and Outcomes

Two strategies have been used in treatment of TOF: palliation with subsequent correction versus immediate correction. Since the primary physiologic consequence is reduced pulmonary blood flow, palliation uses various methods of shunting blood from a systemic artery to the PA circulation. The first blue baby operation, performed in 1944 by Blalock at Taussig's suggestion,[1] joined the innominate artery to the right PA, thus making a systemic artery to PA shunt. Today, the operative technique has been refined and any operation designed to direct subclavian artery blood flow to the PA has been termed the Blalock-Taussig (B-T) shunt. When a piece of prosthetic material, typically polytetraflouroethylene, is interposed between the subclavian artery and the PA, a modified B-T shunt has been performed. Classically, standard B-T shunts are performed on the side opposite the arch, usually the right side, to prevent kinking of the proximal subclavian artery. Modified B-T shunts are performed on the side of the arch because of the ease of exposure of the subclavian artery. Other types of shunts are used today, specifically from the ascending aorta to the main PA. Additionally, palliation may be achieved by placement of a RVOT patch. Although most institutions prefer early one-stage repair for TOF, palliation may be indicated in specific circumstances: extremely small PAs, an anomalous left anterior descending coronary artery crossing the RVOT, severe concomitant lesions that preclude total repair, or the presence of a contraindication to CPB, e.g., severe, long, unrelenting, hypercyanotic spell or sepsis. Patients who present with symptoms as neonates usually have one or more of these circumstances and may require an early palliative shunt.

The second strategy for operation is total correction, which consists of median sternotomy, CPB, closure of the VSD, relief of the RVOTO, and if present, closure of the ASD. If there are no contraindications, a general trend toward open correction in early infancy exists. Debate persists concerning the best strategy for complex patients with TOF, particularly when risk factors for death (multiple VSDs, Down syndrome, large aortopulmonary collaterals, AV-canal defect, or early age) are present.

The main consideration, surgically, when planning a total correction, is the strategy used to relieve RVOTO. In the simplest form, mild infundibular obstruction, simple resection of infundibular bands provides satisfactory relief of obstruction. In more extreme forms, an augmentation patch may be required from the RV across the PV annulus and even into one or more branches of the PA. This renders the PV insufficient, which is usually well tolerated in 90% of patients provided no other residual abnormalities are present. Patients with pulmonary atresia and VSD require replacement of a conduit, usually a pulmonary homograft valved conduit from the RV to the branch PAs. Placement of a conduit early in life and at a small patient size requires a future operation when the patient outgrows the size of the initial conduit.

Outcomes are quite favorable when compared to the natural history. Although debate exists about treatment of complicated patients with TOF early in life, single-stage total correction is reasonable for simple disease. Properly selected patients have an operative mortality with total correction of less than 7%. Risk factors predictive for operative mortality include the need for a transannular patch, residual postrepair RVOTO (RV to LV pressure ratios of greater than 0.65), and persistent uncontrolled hypercyanotic spells at the time of repair. Late outcomes are quite favorable, with over 85% of patients living into their third decade of life. About 80% of patients have a normal life without intellectual or exercise impairment. A persistent concern is the incidence of sudden death, particularly in patients with right bundle branch block (a common consequence of infundibular resection) and premature ventricular contractions. Pulmonary valve (PV) regurgitation may present a risk factor for RV dysfunction and dysrhythmias, while the use of the transatrial approach may improve the long-term results. Data supporting these hypotheses are currently being developed.

ABNORMAL CONNECTION LESIONS

Transposition of the Great Arteries

TGA exists in its simplest form when the aorta arises from the RV and the PA arises from the LV. The AV connections are normal. In the absence of other abnormalities, the physiologic consequence is an admixture lesion in which blue systemic blood is pumped again to the systemic circulation and red pulmonary venous blood is pumped back to the pulmonary circuit. Thus, a blue and a separate red circuit exit in parallel. Without some communication between these two circuits, patient survival is unexpected. In the neonate, a PDA and patent foramen ovale provide extra pathways that allow a life-sustaining shunt of oxygenated blood to the systemic side and desaturated blood to the pulmonary side. In simple TGA, the ventricular septum is intact and no additional alternative pathway is available to mitigate adverse consequences of these parallel circuits.

Embryology

Although complex and still speculative, TGA development appears to involve abnormal rotation and septation of the truncus artery in the primitive heart. Abnormal truncal septation can be associated with a myriad of other abnormalities. Coronary artery anatomy is quite variable. The main coronary ostia, however, do arise from the aortic sinuses adjacent to the PA. Surgical techniques devised to transplant coronary arteries, developed late in the history of treatment for TGA, have allowed anatomic correction early in life.

Types of Transposition of the Great Arteries

Most commonly, TGA refers to a heart with atrial situs solitus, concordant AV connection, and discordant ventriculoarterial connection with intact ventricular septum and is the main subject of this section. Malrotation abnormalities of the great vessels also involve discordant AV and discordant ventriculoarterial connections, congenitally corrected TGA. In congenitally corrected TGA, the LA enters a morphologic RV that gives off the ascending aorta and coronaries. The RA enters the morphologic LV, which supplies the PA. In congenitally corrected TGA, without other abnormalities, e.g., VSD, the physiologic consequence is nil. In the absence of other abnormalities, these patients can be expected to lead normal lives, although an increased incidence of heart block is present.

Physiologic Consequences

The separate parallel pulmonary and systemic circulations in TGA in the absence of other abnormalities cause life-threatening systemic desaturation. Mixing of these two circulations via a PDA, an ASD, a patent foramen ovale (PFO), or a VSD is required to maintain life. This allows some oxygenated blood from the pulmonary circuit to enter the systemic circuit and an equal amount of desaturated blood from the systemic circuit to enter the pulmonary circuit. Patients with restrictive intercirculation communications present with severe systemic hypoxemia, acidosis, and eventual cardiovascular collapse. Patients with large intercirculation communications do not suffer from systemic hypoxemia but may develop CHF related to ineffective ventricular volume work, particularly on the pulmonary side. The surgical options for TGA parallel improving techniques in cardiac surgery.

Natural History

Without intervention, survival beyond 6 months is unlikely. Approximately 90% of patients do not reach their first birthday. Patients with severe hypoxemia do not survive the newborn period. Patients who have adequate mixing and hence large intercirculation communications develop pulmonary vascular disease even with an intact ventricular septum and limit long-range treatment options. Importantly, early in life, as pulmonary vascular resistance falls, LV mass diminishes. This is particularly important to patients who are to receive anatomic repair because the LV becomes the systemic, high-pressure pumping chamber. Operations designed to use the LV as the systemic ventricle must be performed before significant LV mass involution. A large VSD allows maintenance of LV mass and provides an opportunity for several surgical strategies for correction.

Indications for Operation

Most infants with TGA are diagnosed early in life. Patients with limited intercirculation communication may progress to cardiovascular collapse. Other patients who are recognized early and treated before intercirculation limitation, e.g., PGE1, allow a more deliberate evaluation and consideration of options. If intercirculation communication is limited, an emergency balloon atrial septostomy (BAS), facilitating interatrial shunting, can convert an emergency situation into a more elective circumstance. Occasionally the atrial communication must be created surgically, a Blalock-Hanlon procedure.[18] Improvement in oxygenation allows resolution of metabolic acidosis and an improved patient preoperative status that facilitates better perioperative results. After BAS and patient stabilization, a more deliberate weighing of the options is possible. Historically, before the ASO, patients received BAS, were weaned from support, and ultimately discharged. Cardiologic follow-up focused on the degree of hypoxemia, cyanosis, and polycythemia. Some months after birth, usually before the first birthday, systemic hypoxemia (saturations under 70%) or polycythemia (hematocrit over 55%) prompted surgical intervention. Operations early in the treatment of TGA consisted of an atrial switch procedure (Mustard[8] or Senning[9]).

The current surgical strategy for TGA is early repair before LV mass involution, usually before discharge after birth. PGE1 and BAS allow for sufficient stabilization of neonates so that a relatively elective ASO can be performed. Currently, operation within the first 14 days of age permits satisfactory results with ASO. If a patient cannot maintain adequate systemic oxygenation after BAS and remains PGE1 dependent, an operation may be required earlier. Some infants, because of complicating factors, are not able to have ASO within the first 2 weeks of life. Primary ASO has been performed up to 8 weeks of life, whereas others prefer a two-stage procedure where a PA band is placed to allow training of the LV mass over a 2-week interval. These patients can be quite challenging during the interval between operations. When the LV appears adequately prepared to maintain systemic cardiac output, ASO is performed.

Procedures and Outcomes

Early surgical treatment, before the mid-1980s, centered on the concept that two admixture lesions can cause physiologic correction. Both the Mustard and the Senning operations, atrial switch procedures, provide a physiologic repair. In these procedures, systemic venous blood is baffled through the atrium into the morphologic LV and, hence, to the pulmonary circulation. Concomitantly, the pulmonary venous blood is directed into the morphologic RV and, hence, to the aorta. Serial pulmonary and systemic circulations were thus created and established a physiologic repair. However, the morphologic RV was dedicated to performing systemic work and the tricuspid valve was designated the systemic AV valve. Early results were quite favorable. Over 90% of patients could be expected to reach their first birthday. Long-term follow-up, however, has shown a disturbing incidence of dysrhythmias, tricuspid insufficiency, and failure of the systemic RV. These sequels precipitated an alarming death rate of patients in their teenage years. Other surgical alternatives were explored.

In the mid-1980s, surgical techniques allowed development of the ASO procedure. In this procedure, the great vessels are transsected and the proximal PA is anastomosed to the distal aorta and the proximal aorta is anastomosed to the distal PA. Surgical techniques allow satisfactory translocation of the coronary arteries, an early era limitation of this operation, to the neoaortic sinuses, the proximal PA. Concomitant repair of other abnormalities is performed. This provides an anatomic correction for TGA, since the pulmonary and systemic circulations are in series and the LV does systemic work. In properly selected patients, operative mortality is under 10%. Improving techniques, both surgical and in postoperative management, have further improved these results. Early mortality is now similar to the atrial switch procedure, whereas long-term results seem improved. Since this procedure was popularized in the mid-1980s, an analysis of patients in their late teens and early 20s is not possible. Preliminary evidence suggests that the PV functions well as the systemic semilunar valve. Refinements in operative techniques will further improve the long-term outcomes. ASO appears to be the best surgical option for treatment of TGA with intact ventricular septum (IVS).

If a large VSD is present the physiologic consequences are similar to a large VSD except that systemic desaturation is present. The degree of systemic desaturation depends on the mixing at the VSD level. Operative repair of TGA with large VSD (Rastelli procedure) consists of VSD patch closure so that the LV pumps into the aorta. The PA is divided and the proximal end oversewn. A conduit is placed from the RV to the distal PA.

Truncus Arteriosus

In truncus arteriosus, a single great artery, attached to the heart by a single semilunar valve, gives rise to the aorta, PA, and coronary arteries. The PAs are functionally attached to an ascending aorta and a large VSD allows RV and LV output through this single truncal artery.

Embryology

A failure of proper septation of the truncus arteriosus and the conal ventricular septum causes truncus arteriosus. Failure of neural crest cell migration causes two opposing spiral ridges to fail to divide the truncal artery and join a conal septum that has failed to separate the ventricles. The single truncal valve usually has three leaflets (70%) but may have four (25%), increasing the chance of truncal valve regurgitation. About 30% of these patients have DiGeorge syndrome.

Types of Truncus Arteriosus

Four basic types, depending on the nature of the PA attachment to the truncal artery, exist. The most common types, I and II, are of similar consequence for the surgeon. As more has become known about this lesion, the classification system has been amplified.

Physiologic Consequences

The patient's physiology depends on the degree of proximal PA obstruction at aortic attachment. If no obstruction is present, pulmonary flow increases as PVR decreases and CHF develops. If obstruction is present, CHF may not develop until later in life. Obstruction to one PA branch can facilitate preferential flow to the opposite side.

Natural History

Without operative repair, these neonates die in infancy. If other lesions are present, such as interrupted aortic arch or truncal valve insufficiency, death may occur during the neonatal period. If a patient survives early life, irreversible pulmonary vascular disease is the rule. Branch PA stenosis can favorably influence outcome.

Indications for Operation

As with many pulmonary overcirculation scenarios, such as CHF or failure to thrive, recurrent pulmonary infections argue for operative correction. Some correctly believe that a neonate with truncus arteriosus should have an operation early in life, just after neonatal PVR falls. With improved perioperative management, infants receiving repair early, before development of ominous signs, have a better operative prognosis.

Procedures and Outcomes

Repair consists of VSD closure, detachment of the main and branch PAs from the truncal artery, and establishment of RV to distal PA continuity, usually with a valved homograft conduit. CPB with aortic cross-clamping is necessary. Some use circulatory arrest, although this is not required. Operative survival is > 80%. Risk is increased in patients with arch interruption, truncal valve insufficiency, coronary anomalies, and neonatal age > 100 days.

Total Anomalous Pulmonary Venous Connection

The absence of a direct connection between the pulmonary vein and the LA requires that an abnormal connection be present from the pulmonary veins to the systemic circulation for newborn viability. Total anomalous pulmonary venous return (TAPVR) can also be considered an obstructive lesion with absolute obstruction (atresia) between the pulmonary veins and the LA. An abnormal connection between the pulmonary venous and the systemic venous circulation allows viability. This admixture lesion requires that an ASD be present so that the body can be perfused. A PDA also allows systemic circulation by right-to-left shunting.

Embryology

Through a complex sequence of septation, invagination, and incorporation, the common pulmonary vein becomes attached and communicates with the LA. Failure of common pulmonary vein incorporation into the LA and persistence of one of the alternative connections to the pulmonary venous system causes TAPVR. If only a part of the pulmonary vein and alternative connection development is aberrant, partial anomalous pulmonary venous return (PAPVR) develops. An ASD or PDA is required to allow neonatal survival.

Types of TAPVR

An alternative route must be present to allow pulmonary venous flow. This route characterizes TAPVR and is supracardiac, intracardiac, infracardiac, or mixed. In the most common, supracardiac, the pulmonary veins drain superiorly through a left SVC into the left innominate vein. In the intracardiac type, a direct connection exits between the pulmonary veins and the coronary sinus, which then drains into the RA. In approximately 20%, the pulmonary vein confluence drains inferiorly through the diaphragm into the portal venous system. Connections to the ductus venosus, hepatic veins, and IVC are possible. Infracardiac TAPVR is usually associated with obstruction, a medical and surgical emergency. The mixed type involves more than one of the sites of anomalous pulmonary venous connection.

Physiologic Consequences

In all forms of TAPVR, all systemic and pulmonary venous blood returns to the RA, where complete mixing is assumed. Blood then either can pass through an ASD or the tricuspid valve. Because the pulmonary arteriolar resistance usually decreases after birth, most of the blood enters the RV. RV volume overload and CHF develop. The amount of right-to-left shunt at the atrial level is in part dependent on the size of the ASD. If the ASD is unrestrictive, the magnitude of shunting depends on the systemic and pulmonary resistance ratios. If the pulmonary veins are obstructed, a high Q_p/Q_s can be expected. If allowed to persist, pulmonary arteriolar vascular obstructive disease develops. Since mixed pulmonary and systemic venous blood enter the LA and then the LV, systemic desaturation and cyanosis can be anticipated. The degree of desaturation depends on the restrictedness of the ASD and degree of obstruction of the alternative pathway draining the pulmonary vein confluence.

If the alternative pathway draining the pulmonary vein confluence is obstructive, pulmonary venous and consequent pulmonary arterial hypertension develop. This decreases pulmonary flow and amplifies right-to-left shunting. Additionally, there are fewer oxygenated red cells mixing with the systemic venous return, causing a more severe systemic hypoxemia. Cardiac output may be limited by the anatomic venous obstruction combined with a restrictive ASD or ductus arteriosus. Often these neonates are hemodynamically unstable and require urgent treatment. Because some of the problems are anatomic and cannot be controlled physiologically, prompt operation or institution of extracorporeal membrane oxygenation (ECMO) may be necessary. ECMO allows optimization of the preoperative patient, providing hemodynamic stability and multiple organ system resuscitation before an additional insult of cardiac repair associated with circulatory arrest.

Natural History

A patient's presentation depends on the magnitude of pulmonary venous obstruction, the size of the ASD, and associated cardiac abnormalities. Patients without pulmonary venous obstruction and an unobstructive ASD may be asymptomatic in the neonatal period and have only mild tachypnea. As pulmonary blood flow increases with decreasing PVR, CHF and failure to thrive may develop. In the long term, irreversible pulmonary arteriolar resistance changes can be expected.

Pulmonary venous obstruction causes patients to present with tachypnea, cyanosis, and often hemodynamic instability as a newborn. TAPVR can be mistaken for persistent fetal circulation or respiratory distress in the newborn. A restrictive ASD causes hemodynamic instability with acidosis as the PDA closes and PVR diminishes. Patients with a restrictive interatrial communication have about a 20% chance of living to their first birthday. Most of these patients die before their first 6 months of life. In general, the prognosis also depends on the degree of obstruction in the extracardiac pulmonary venous channels. The greater the degree of obstruction, the more urgent the need for operative correction. No medical treatment or palliation is useful in determining ultimate outcome. BAS may temporarily benefit patients with a restrictive ASD.

Indications for Operation

Most surgeons and pediatric cardiologists believe the primary indication for surgical intervention is the presence of TAPVR. Debate exists about the timing of procedures. Patients with pulmonary venous outflow obstruction and low cardiac output require prompt, even emergency, correction. Similarly, patients with a restrictive ASD and a closing PDA also require urgent operative treatment. Other patients without pulmonary venous obstruction and a sufficient ASD may present later in life with pulmonary congestion and tachypnea and without ominous signs of cardiovascular collapse. These operations can be performed semielectively but should not be delayed for nonspecific reasons.

Procedures and Outcomes

Operation requires median sternotomy and CPB with circulatory arrest. The surgical objective is the creation of a pulmonary venous confluence to LA connection, ASD closure, ligation of the PDA, and possibly ligation of the pulmonary venous alternative pathway (supracardiac or infracardiac). In supra- and infracardiac types, the pulmonary venous confluence, a structure distinct from the LA, is incised longitudinally and anastomosed to the longitudinally incised LA. In the intracardiac type, the coronary sinus septum is removed, allowing direct pulmonary venous drainage into the LA. The ASD is closed. Techniques vary among centers on the exact methodology of repair. Techniques may also vary depending on the anatomic status of the patient.

With operative correction and improved intra- and postoperative management, operative mortality has decreased from the 50% range in the 1960s to the 10% range in the current era. Risk factors for perioperative mortality include infracardiac connection, small interatrial pathway, pulmonary venous obstruction, pulmonary hypertension, low systemic saturation, and small LV dimensions. Patients without these factors have an excellent perioperative risk and are considered anatomically corrected after operation. Correction of TAPVR in the newborn period is associated with a relatively low initial mortality and good long-term outcome.

CONCLUSION

Although the spectrum of congenital heart disease is broad and complex, the use of three anatomic realities (obstruction, extra pathway, and abnormal connection) applied at various locations and to varying degrees, permits a functional knowledge of these abnormal hearts. These realities translate into physiologic impairments (increased flow, decreased flow, admixture) which, when viewed by the surgeon, translate into strategies for treatment. Using tools specific to the congenital cardiac surgeon, anatomic, physiologic, or palliative procedures can be achieved. A major thrust, with improved perioperative care of these critically ill neonates, infants, and children, has been total correction as the initial procedure. When this is not possible, many therapeutic options exist that allow improved quality and quantity of life for patients with these devastating lesions.

ABBREVIATIONS

APW	Aorticopulmonary window
ASD	Atrial septal defect
ASO	Arterial switch operation
AV	Atrioventricular
B-T	Blalock-Taussig
BAS	Balloon atrial septostomy
CHD	Congenital heart disease
CHF	Congestive heart failure
CoA	Coartctation of the aorta
CPB	Cardiopulmonary bypass
DORV	Double-outlet right ventricle
ECMO	Extracorporeal membrane oxygenation
HLHS	Hypoplastic left heart syndrome
HRHS	Hypoplastic right heart syndrome
IVC	Inferior vena cava
IVS	Intact ventricular septum
LA	Left atrium, atrial
LV	Left ventricle, ventricular
LVOT	Left ventricular outflow tract
LVOTO	Left ventricular outflow tract obstruction
MAPCAS	Main aortopulmonary collateral arteries
PA	Pulmonary artery
PAPVR	Partial anomalous pulmonary venous return
PDA	Patent ductus arteriosus
PFO	Patent foramen ovale
PS	Pulmonary stenosis
PV	Pulmonary valve
PVR	Pulmonary vascular resistance
Q_p/Q_s	Pulmonary to systemic flow ratio
RA	Right atrium, atrial
RV	Right ventricle, ventricular
RVOT	Right ventricular outflow tract
RVOTO	Right ventricular outflow tract obstruction

SVC	Superior vena cava
TAPVR	Total anomalous pulmonary venous return
TGA	Tranposition of the great arteries
TOF	Tetralogy of Fallot
VSD	Ventricular septal defect

GLOSSARY

Aortic stenosis   Narrowing of the aortic outflow, subvalvular, valvular, or supravalvular

Atrial septal defect   Abnormal extra pathway in the atrial septum between the atria

Atrioventricular canal   Defects that involve atrial septum, ventricular septum, tricuspid, and/or mitral valve; endocardial cushion defect, atrioventricular septal defect

Atrioventricular septal defect   Defects that involve atrial septum, ventricular septum, tricuspid, and/or mitral valve; atrioventricular canal, endocardial cushion defect

Bidirectional Glenn   Connects distal SVC to top to right PA; proximal SVC is oversewn

Blalock-Taussig shunt   Subclavian artery to PA shunt; is modified when a tube graft is used between vessels

Coarctation of the aorta   Localized narrowing of the aortic lumen, usually at the ligamentum arteriosus

Eisenmenger's reaction (disease)   Pulmonary vascular obstructive changes; irreversible

Endocardial cushion defect   Defects that involve atrial septum, ventricular septum, tricuspid, and/or mitral valve; atrioventricular canal, atrioventricular septal defect

Fontan procedure   Systemic venous return is directed to the PA using prosthetic conducts or direct vascular connection; primarily used for tricuspid or pulmonary atresia

Glenn procedure   Distal SVC to distal right PA anastomosis, end-to-end; proximal ends are oversewn

Mustard procedure   Used in transposition of the great arteries to redirect systemic venous blood to the anatomic left atrium, left ventricle, and hence to the pulmonary artery; pulmonary venous blood is directed to the anatomic right atrium, the right ventricle, and out the aorta; uses either pericardium or prosthetic material within the atrium

Patent ductus arteriosus   Persistent communication between the aorta and the PA distal to the left subclavian artery

Patent foramen ovale   Opening in the atrial septum at the site of the fossa ovalis

Pulmonary atresia with intact ventricular septum   Absence of the pulmonary valve orifice, separation of the right ventricle from the pulmonary artery by tissue; no interventricular communication is present

Pulmonic stenosis   Narrowing of the pulmonary outflow tract; may involve muscular infundibulum, valve, or peripheral pulmonary artery

Rashkind procedure   Balloon atrial septostomy performed at cardiac catheterization to improve intraatrial mixing of venous and oxygenated blood

Rastelli procedure   Left ventricular blood is directed out the aorta using a complex ventricular septal defect patch; the proximal PA is oversewn and a valved conduit is placed between the RV and distal PA; used primarily in TGA with a large ventricular septal defect and tetralogy of Fallot or double-outlet right ventricle with severe pulmonary stenosis

Senning procedure   Intra- and extraatrial baffling using atrial wall and a prosthesis to direct blood flow, as in a Mustard procedure

Tetralogy of Fallot   Ventricular septal defect, pulmonic stenosis, overriding aorta, and right ventricular hypertrophy

Total anomalous pulmonary venous return   Return of pulmonary venous blood through anomalous channels to the right atrium

Transposition of the great arteries   Abnormal great artery connection with the aorta arising from the anatomic right ventricle and the pulmonary artery arising from the anatomic left ventricle

Tricuspid atresia   Absent tricuspid orifice, with patent atrial septum, enlarged mitral orifice, and rudimentary right ventricle

Ventricular septal defect   Abnormal communication between the left and right ventricle through the ventricular septum

Waterston shunt   Ascending aorta to right pulmonary artery anastomosis; is modified by placement of a tube graft between these great arteries

REFERENCES

1. Blalock A, Taussig HB: The surgical treatment of malformations of the heart. *JAMA.* 128:189, 1945.
2. Gibbon JH: Application of a mechanical heart and lung apparatus to cardiac surgery. *Minn Med.* 37:171, 1954.
3. Garson A, Bricher JT, McNamara TW (Eds.): *The Science and Practice of Pediatric Cardiology.* Philadelphia: Lea & Febiger; 1990.
4. Nichols DG, Cameron DE, Greely WJ, et al. (Eds.): *Critical Heart Disease in Infants and Children.* St. Louis: CV Mosby; 1995.
5. Mullins CE, Mayer DC: *Congenital Heart Disease—A Diagrammatic Atlas.* New York: Alan R. Liss; 1988.
6. Keith JD, Rowe RD, Vlad P: *Heart Disease in Infancy and Childhood.* New York: MacMillan; 1978.
7. Jatene AD, Fontes VF, Paulista PP, et al.: Successful anatomic correction of transposition of the great vessels. A preliminary report. *Arq Bras Cardiol.* 28:461, 1975.

8. Mustard WT: Successful two-stage correction of transposition of the great vessels. *Surgery.* 55:469, 1964.

9. Senning A: Correction of the transposition of the great arteries. *Ann Surg.* 182:287, 1975.

10. Austin JW, Harner DL: *The Heart-Lung Machine and Related Technologies of Open Heart Surgery.* Phoenix: Arrowhead Press; 1990.

11. Newburger JW, Jonas RA, Wernovsy G, et al.: A comparison of the perioperative neurologic effects of hypothermic circulatory arrest versus low flow cardiopulmonary bypass in infant heart surgery. *N Engl J Med.* 329:1057, 1993.

12. Haller JA Jr, Adkins JC, Worthington M, et al.: Experimental studies on permanent bypass of the right heart. *Surgery.* 59:1128, 1966.

13. Lamberti JJ, Spicer RL, Waldman JD, et al.: The bidirectional cavopulmonary shunt. *J Thorac Cardiovasc Surg.* 100:22, 1990.

14. Glenn WWL, Patino JF: Circulatory bypass of the right heart, I. Preliminary observation on direct delivery of vena caval blood into pulmonary arterial circulation. Azygos vein—pulmonary artery shunt. *Yale J Biol Med.* 27:147, 1954.

15. de Leval MR, Kilner P, Geivillig M, et al.: Total cavopulmonary connection: A logical alternative to atriopulmonary connection for complex Fontan operations. Experimental studies and early clinical experience. *J Thorac Cardiovasc Surg.* 96:682, 1988.

16. Fontan F, Baudit E: Surgical repair of tricuspid atresia. *Thorax.* 26:240, 1971.

17. Norwood WI, Lang P, Hansen DD: Physiologic repair of aortic atresia—hypoplastic left heart syndrome. *N Engl J Med.* 308:23, 1983.

18. Blalock A, Hanlon CR: The surgical treatment of complete transposition of the aorta and the pulmonary artery. *Surg Gynecol Obstet.* 90:1, 1950.

CHAPTER NINETEEN

Late Cardiac Physiology Following Palliative and Surgical Repair of Congenital Cardiac Defects

Mark D. Reller

The purpose of this chapter is to introduce the reader to and familiarize him or her with the common surgical procedures utilized to both palliate and repair the common congenital cardiac defects seen by the pediatric cardiologist. This discussion includes a brief historical review of many of the surgical procedures, considers the usual indications for the surgical procedures, and reviews information about both short- and long-term sequelae. This review begins with the palliative procedures, followed by the corrective or reparative surgical procedures.

PALLIATIVE PROCEDURES

Systemic to Pulmonary Shunts

1. Classic and modified Blalock-Taussig shunts
2. Waterston shunt
3. Potts shunt

The primary indication for palliative shunts in children with congenital heart disease is hypoxemia (or cyanosis) that is secondary to restricted pulmonary blood flow when definitive corrective surgery is not possible or carries prohibitive risk to the patient. Currently, palliative shunts are used almost exclusively in infancy. Conditions for which palliative shunts are most frequently used include severe forms of tetralogy of Fallot (with hypoplastic pulmonary arteries), pulmonary atresia with or without ventricular septal defect (VSD), certain patients with tricuspid atresia (and severely restricted

pulmonary blood flow), and certain patients with single ventricle anatomy and restricted pulmonary blood flow.

Credit for the first systemic to pulmonary shunt goes to Drs. Blalock and Taussig for their pioneering work, which literally initiated the modern surgical era for congenital heart disease in 1945.[1] In physiologic terms, the "classic" Blalock-Taussig (B-T) shunt produces a "permanent ductus" by creating a direct anastomosis between the subclavian artery and the pulmonary artery, usually on the side opposite the aortic arch (Figure 19–1). In the early days of cardiac surgery, the most common condition treated was tetralogy of Fallot. The B-T shunts were placed surgically via either right or left thoracotomies. For historical purposes, two other systemic to pulmonary shunts were utilized and were known as the Waterston (an anastomosis between the ascending aorta and the right pulmonary artery) and the Potts (between the descending aorta and left pulmonary artery) shunts. Potential complications of any of the systemic to pulmonary shunts include the possibility of kinking or distorting the pulmonary arteries and the possibility of producing excessive pulmonary blood flow. This latter problem was particularly great for the Waterston and Potts shunts; many of these patients developed secondary pulmonary hypertension. For this reason, these shunts have been largely abandoned. However, adult survivors are still followed and frequently are seen in adult congenital heart disease clinics.

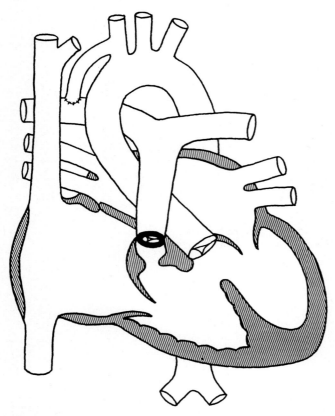

Figure 19-1. Diagram of classic Blalock-Taussig shunt with subclavian artery to pulmonary artery shunt for tetralogy of Fallot. *(Reprinted, with permission, from Mullins CE, Mayer DC.* Congenital Heart Disease—A Diagrammatic Atlas. *New York: John Wiley & Sons, Inc.)*

Currently, palliative shunts are utilized using synthetic Gortex tube grafts interposed between the subclavian artery (or centrally) and the pulmonary artery. These "modified B-T" shunts have allowed for better control of pulmonary blood flow, although some risk of distortion of the pulmonary artery still exists. In addition, similar to each of the systemic to pulmonary shunts, the modified B-T shunt flow has the potential to volume load the systemic ventricle. While this is less of a problem in the setting of tetralogy of Fallot, it can be a greater problem for patients with single-ventricle anatomy, in which the volume load can adversely impact diastolic function.[2] This may be a problem for patients who are potential Fontan candidates.

Cavopulmonary Anastomosis

1. Classic Glenn shunt
2. Bidirectional Glenn shunt

The classic Glenn shunt was first performed in the late 1950s. The Glenn shunt created an anastomosis be-

tween the end of the divided right pulmonary artery and the side of the superior vena cava, with ligation of the superior cava below the anastomosis. This cavopulmonary anastomosis produced flow to the right pulmonary artery only and was typically used as a palliative procedure in patients with tricuspid atresia (many went on to have an earlier version of the Fontan operation). The Glenn shunt generally provided good initial palliation. Unfortunately, many patients developed late problems associated with increasing cyanosis. The cyanosis was frequently a result of increasing pulmonary vascular resistance that resulted in secondary shunting of flow away from the lung via collateral vessels (azygous, etc.) to the inferior vena cava. In addition, many of these patients developed pulmonary arteriovenous malformations that also resulted in increasing cyanosis. It has recently been hypothesized that the pulmonary arteriovenous fistulae develop when hepatic flow is excluded from the pulmonary circulation (as was the case in the classic Glenn patients).[3] The exact etiology for this possible explanation is as yet lacking.

In the early 1980s, many centers began utilizing the so-called bidirectional Glenn, whereby an anastomosis is created between the superior vena caval and undivided pulmonary arteries (Figure 19–2). Currently, many centers view the bidirectional Glenn as the "first stage Fontan" (hemi-Fontan) in any patient with single-ventricle anatomy, and it is being increasingly performed at an earlier age (at under 6 months). The procedure is performed via a midline sternotomy approach. The predominant advantage of the cavopulmonary anastomosis is that it gives satisfactory oxygenation without producing a volume load to the systemic ventricle.[4] In some patients without significant hypoxemia in infancy (necessitating a modified B-T shunt), the bidirectional Glenn can be the first surgical procedure performed in the infant. However, careful patient selection is important, and the patient needs a cardiac catheterization preoperatively to evaluate the pulmonary artery anatomy and pressure.

Pulmonary Artery Banding

In the early 1950s, the first surgeries to band the pulmonary artery were reported. Unlike the palliative procedures already discussed, the purpose of pulmonary artery bands is to reduce pulmonary blood flow in patients who have increased pulmonary flow from their cardiac defects. These cardiac defects include large VSDs, AV septal (canal) defects, truncus arteriosus, certain tricuspid atresia situations (with unrestricted pulmonary blood flow), and similar single-ventricle anatomy situations. In most patients, the pulmonary

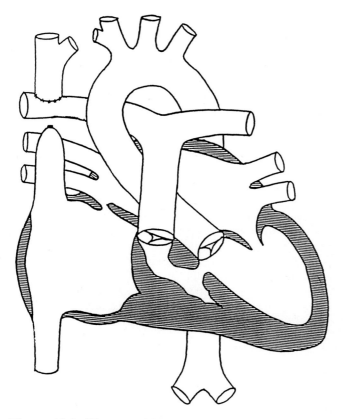

Figure 19-2. Diagram of bidirectional Glenn with superior vena cava to pulmonary artery shunt for tricuspid valve atresia and restrictive VSD. *(Reprinted, with permission, from Mullins CE, Mayer DC.* Congenital Heart Disease—A Diagrammatic Atlas. *New York: John Wiley & Sons, Inc.)*

bands are performed surgically via a left anterolateral thoracotomy. Common risks associated with banding include possible migration of the band and obstruction of (usually) the right pulmonary artery, the potential need for pulmonary artery reconstruction at the time of debanding, and the possibility of the banding's being too loose (and leaving the patient at risk for pulmonary hypertension). Other important risks include possible worsening of AV valve regurgitation in patients with AV septal defects and, importantly, the potential for producing significant cardiac hypertrophy. This latter problem is of particular concern for patients with single-ventricle anatomy, where hypertrophy can result in significant subaortic obstruction (from restriction of the bulbo-ventricular foramen or "outlet chamber"). In addition, cardiac hypertrophy can have an adverse impact on ventricular compliance (and hence diastolic filling) in potential Fontan patients with single-ventricle anatomy. In the current era, pulmonary artery banding plays a limited role in surgical management.[5]

Atrial Septectomy

In 1948, Drs. Blalock and Hanlon[6] performed the first successful atrial septectomy. The indication for performing an atrial septectomy is to achieve better intracardiac mixing at the atrial level. Historically, this was commonly performed as a palliative procedure in patients with d-transposition of the great vessels to improve mixing and hence arterial saturation. The surgery is generally performed via a right thoracotomy. Other cardiac lesions that continue to require atrial septectomies as part of their surgical repair are mitral and tricuspid valve atresias. In patients with single-ventricle and mitral atresia, it is particularly important that pulmonary venous return be unobstructed. An atrial septectomy is also a routine part of the Norwood repair in patients with hypoplastic left heart syndrome.

In 1966, Raskind and Miller[7] first reported their experience of performing balloon atrial septostomies via a cardiac catheterization. Many patients with d-transposition of the great vessels continue to have balloon atrial septostomies as their first palliative procedure before definitive surgical repairs. The Raskind procedure initiated the era of catheter intervention procedures.

CORRECTIVE SURGICAL PROCEDURES

Repair of Atrial Septal Defect

In 1953, Dr. John Gibbon[1] was the first to close an atrial septal defect (ASD) (utilizing a pump oxygenator) and so was the first to perform an open-heart surgical repair of a cardiac defect. The long-term risks of unoperated ASDs include pulmonary hypertension and atrial dysrhythmia (supraventricular tachycardia atrial fibrillation) secondary to right heart enlargement. Currently, it is recommended that all children with pulmonary to systemic shunt ratios greater than 1.5 and right ventricular enlargement have surgical closure electively in the first several years of life. The location of the ASD varies, with the secundum type (midatrial septum) being the most common. Other types include the ostium primum ASD (partial atrioventricular, or AV, septal defect), located in the inferior septum and frequently associated with mitral valve abnormalities (cleft), and the sinus venosus ASD, located in the superior–posterior aspect of the atrial septum and commonly associated with partial anomalous pulmonary venous return from the right lung. Secundum defects can be closed primarily or by patch closure. The primum and sinus venosus defects invariably require patch closure. Most atrial defects are closed via a midline sternotomy incision, although secundum defects are occasionally closed via a right thoracotomy approach. Currently, the major risk associated with surgical closure of the ASD is essentially that associated with extracorporeal perfusion and general anesthesia. The major long-term risk in operated patients is that of atrial dysrhythmia, and this risk appears to be greater in those patients operated on later in life. Last, catheterization devices are likely to play an increasingly greater role in closure of secundum ASDs and patent foramen ovale.

Repair of Ventricular Septal Defect

The first ventricular septal defect (VSD) was given surgical closure by Dr. Lillehei in 1955[1] using cross-circulation techniques. Because VSD is the most common congenital cardiac defect, experience rapidly accumulated in subsequent years. The usual indications for surgical closure of VSD include congestive failure (and failure to thrive), pulmonary hypertension resulting from the left-to-right shunt, and left ventricular volume overload. Most VSDs requiring surgery have a pulmonary to systemic shunt ratio greater than 2.0, although closure is generally recommended for shunts with ratios of greater than 1.5 when associated with left ventricular enlargement. Performed via a midline sternotomy, most VSDs are now closed through a transatrial approach to avoid a ventriculotomy. As with ASDs, VSDs can be closed either primarily or via patch closure. Although perimembranous defects are the most common, another common location is in the muscular (apical) septum. Muscular defects can be multiple and sometimes require a left ventriculotomy to better visualize the defects and to reduce the risk of residual shunt. Supracristal (subarterial) defects are relatively uncommon. However, their location requires an approach via either a high ventriculotomy in the right ventricular outflow tract or a transpulmonary approach. The major risk associated with supracristal defects is prolapse of the aortic valve; if present, this prolapse requires resuspension of the valve leaflets at the time of surgery.

Surgical risks associated with closure of VSDs include injury to conduction tissue. Right bundle branch block is not uncommon and does not appear to be associated with risk for serious arrhythmia. In the current era, the incidence of complete heart block is quite low (< 1%). Incomplete closure is another risk, although frequently the residual shunt is small. The major long-term risk associated with small residual shunts is infectious endocarditis. Pulmonary hypertension is another risk, especially in those patients operated later on in life (less common in the current era). Pulmonary hypertension in this setting can be progressive in spite of previous repair. The current mortality associated with surgical closure of VSD is ~ 1%.

Repair of Atrioventricular Canal (AV Septal) Defects

Many infants and children with AV septal defects have Down syndrome (trisomy 21). Because many of these infants are predisposed to accelerated pulmonary hypertension, the trend has clearly been toward earlier surgical repair (typically between 3 and 6 months) in essentially all infants with complete AV septal defects. Most are now closed via a right atriotomy, and many surgeons currently prefer a double-patch repair of the atrial and ventricular defects. A surgical risk associated with repair is the relatively greater one of complete heart block (caused by the altered orientation of the His bundle–conduction tissue in this lesion). An additional risk with AV septal defects is abnormality of the AV valves, particularly the mitral, or left, AV valve. Postoperatively, patients need to be evaluated for either mitral stenosis or regurgitation. Long-term risks include the need for reoperation for significant mitral regurgitation (possibly requiring a prosthetic valve). As discussed with VSDs, another long-term risk is pulmonary hypertension, especially in infants with Down syndrome operated on later in life. Last, patients with AV septal defect are at risk for developing subaortic stenosis, and may require reoperation for this.

Repair of Tetralogy of Fallot

As previously noted, the Blalock-Taussig shunt initiated the modern era of surgical procedures for congenital heart disease. The first intracardiac repair for tetralogy of Fallot (TOF) was performed by Lillehei in 1954.[1] Initially, most patients with TOF underwent palliative shunts before definitive repair. Currently, most patients go directly to a primary intracardiac repair regardless of age. Exceptions to this are those patients with extremely small (hypoplastic) pulmonary arteries and those patients with coronary anomalies precluding standard repair. An alternative to shunting patients with hypoplastic pulmonary arteries is patch enlargement of the right ventricular outflow tract without closure of the VSD to increase antegrade flow into the pulmonary arteries. Because the natural history of TOF is progression of the pulmonary and subpulmonary obstruction, most patients undergo surgical repair in the first 6 months of life. Most patients with TOF have the defect repaired via a high right ventriculotomy approach, although some surgeons do the repair via a right atriotomy (more difficult but avoids the ventriculotomy incision). Surgical repair involves resection of the infundibular (subpulmonary) stenosis, patch closure of the VSD, and—if the pulmonary annulus is small—a transannular patch insertion (Figure 19–3).

Currently, the surgical risks associated with surgical repair are quite low for patients with typical TOF anatomy. The long-term results (many out > 25 years) have been quite good, with most patients free of cardiovascular symptoms.[8] Ventricular dysrhythmia has been of some concern and appears to be of greatest risk in those patients with increased right ventricular

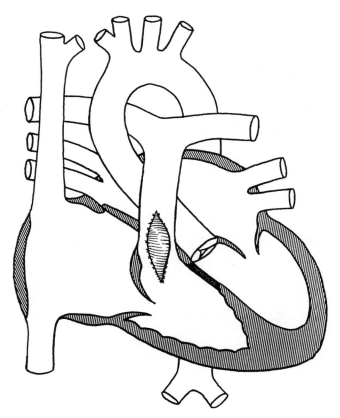

Figure 19-3. Diagram of postoperative tetralogy of Fallot with patch closure of VSD, infundibular resection, and transannular right ventricular outflow and/or main pulmonary artery patch. *(Reprinted, with permission, from Mullins CE, Mayer DC.* Congenital Heart Disease—A Diagrammatic Atlas. *New York: John Wiley & Sons, Inc.)*

pressure caused by residual stenosis (usually in the pulmonary arteries). These patients have been shown to be at risk for sudden death. Many postoperative patients have significant residual pulmonary insufficiency. In the absence of pulmonary arterial stenosis, this is usually well tolerated (at least for the short term). However, there is increasing evidence that right ventricular enlargement as a consequence of pulmonary insufficiency may cause late problems. Current management for patients with significant pulmonary insufficiency would be placement of a homograft conduit. Last, some TOF patients may develop aortic insufficiency, which is likely secondary to aortic annular dilatation commonly seen in TOF.

Rastelli Repair for Complex Heart Disease

The Rastelli repair[9] is reserved for patients with complex congenital heart disease, including patients with double-outlet right ventricle (DORV), transposition with VSD and pulmonary stenosis, and truncus arteriosus. It was first described in 1967. The Rastelli repair establishes

continuity between the left ventricle and the aorta by creating an intracardiac conduit via the VSD (Figure 19-4). Most patients require placement of a conduit (usually a homograft, currently) between the right ventricle and the pulmonary arteries. The major long-term risks associated with this surgical repair are developing conduit obstruction and need for replacement. These risks are greatest in the infant and the younger patient, where growth (and lack thereof of the conduit) may contribute to obstruction.

Truncus Arteriosus Repair

The first successful repair of a patient with truncus arteriosus was performed by McGoon in 1967.[10] Surgical repair includes detachment of the pulmonary arteries from the common truncus, closure of the VSD, and placement of a conduit (usually a homograft) from the right ventricle to the pulmonary arteries. Because most infants with truncus arteriosus develop cardiac symptoms at an early age, surgery is necessary in the first

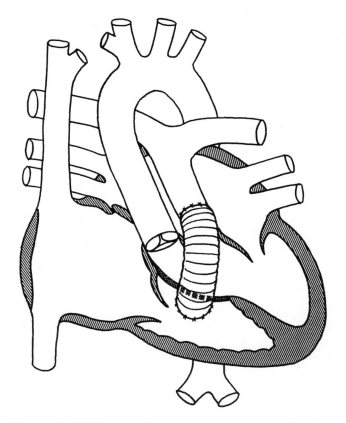

Figure 19-4. Diagram of postoperative Rastelli repair with intracardiac left ventricular to aortic tunnel and right ventricle to pulmonary artery conduit for d-transposition of the great arteries, VSD, and pulmonary stenosis. *(Reprinted, with permission, from Mullins CE, Mayer DC.* Congenital Heart Disease—A Diagrammatic Atlas. *New York: John Wiley & Sons, Inc.)*

months of life and carries a significant surgical mortality. Factors that increase the surgical risk include significant truncal valve insufficiency (usually requiring prosthetic valve replacement) and additional repair of aortic arch interruption, which can coexist, especially, in patients with DiGeorge syndrome. These patients are at risk for developing elevated pulmonary vascular resistance, especially in those patients where surgical repair is delayed. Long-term risks include the development of progressive truncal valve insufficiency (and/or occasional stenosis) that requires placement of a prosthetic valve and the long-term need for anticoagulation. Last, as already stated, the homograft conduits are at ongoing risk for developing obstruction either from degeneration of the valve or by development of diffuse calcification, both of which contribute to the need for conduit replacement.

Transposition of the Great Arteries

1. Atrial Repairs (Senning, Mustard)
2. Arterial Switch (Jatene)

Transposition of the great arteries (d-TGA) is the most common cyanotic congenital heart disease presenting in infancy. Before the modern era of surgical repair, the vast majority of these "blue babies" died of progressive cyanosis in the first months of life. The first palliative procedure available for d-TGA infants was an atrial septectomy (first performed by Blalock and Hanlon)[6] to enhance "mixing" of blood at the atrial level, thus improving the overall level of arterial oxygenation. In the early 1960s, Senning and Mustard[1] first performed successful intraatrial repair for children with d-TGA. In the Mustard repair, the atrial septum is excised and replaced with a large patch or baffle using either pericardium or synthetic patch material (i.e., Dacron). Alternatively, Senning created an intraatrial baffle using primarily flaps of atrial septum. Both repairs were similar in that the transposition was corrected by rerouting the venous inflows at atrial level but leaving the great vessels transposed (aorta from the right ventricle) (Figure 19–5). Early complications were not unusual and included superior vena caval obstruction (associated with pleural effusion and/or chylothorax) and pulmonary venous obstruction with the potential for pulmonary venous congestion and development of pulmonary hypertension. Long-term complications include not only baffle obstruction of systemic and pulmonary venous return, but also baffle leak (resulting in arterial desaturation) and dysrhythmia (including sinus node dysfunction, bradycardia, and atrial tachydysrhythmias). Patients with significant sinus node dysfunction often need pacemakers, and the development of atrial tachycardias are associated with the risk of sudden death. Some patients also develop significant subpulmonary obstruction of

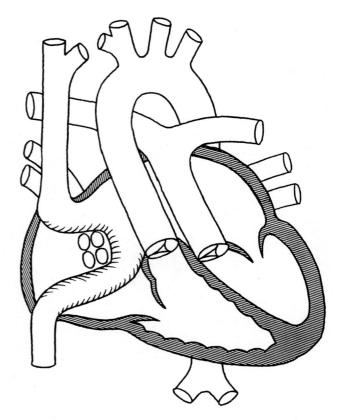

Figure 19-5. Diagram of postoperative Mustard (or Senning) atrial repair for d-transposition of the great arteries. *(Reprinted, with permission, from Mullins CE, Mayer DC.* Congenital Heart Disease—A Diagrammatic Atlas. *New York: John Wiley & Sons, Inc.)*

the left ventricular outflow tract. Last, some of these patients have—and many more will likely develop—significant right ventricular (systemic ventricle) dysfunction. In spite of these complications, a generation of d-TGA patients are alive today because of these surgical procedures.

The arterial switch repair of d-TGA was first successfully performed by Jatene in 1975.[11] Its major advantage is that it results in anatomic correction of transposition utilizing the left ventricle as the systemic ventricle. However, it was not until the 1980s that most centers in the United States began routinely performing the arterial switch. The surgery was initially found to have a significant "learning curve," with early attempts associated with increased mortality. The surgery involves division of both great vessels above the sinuses and then reanastomosis of each to the opposite vessel (i.e., aorta to the proximal native pulmonary artery and vice versa). In addition, and importantly, buttons of the coronary arteries have to removed from the native aorta and successfully reimplanted. For many centers, certain coronary anomalies (especially single coronary ostium) have been a relative contraindication for the arterial switch procedure. The major early risk associated with the arterial switch was the initial higher mortality in many centers. Long-term complications noted so far include the potential for developing neo-aortic valve incompetence as well as pulmonary arterial stenosis at the anastomotic suture line. Significant coronary problems and myocardial perfusion abnormalities have so far not been a major problem.[12] However, it is important to emphasize that the long-term results are significantly shorter for the arterial switch repair than for the atrial repairs previously discussed here.

Norwood Repair

Hypoplastic left heart syndrome (HLHS) is the most serious congenital cardiac defect with which an infant can be born, and unfortunately it is fairly common. Success with the Norwood repair for infants with HLHS was first reported in the late 1970s.[13] Unfortunately, many centers were unable to duplicate these early results (until recently), so this defect continues to be associated with a high mortality. The primary abnormality in HLHS is severe underdevelopment of the left ventricle, which is invariably associated with severe stenosis or atresia of both the mitral and the aortic valves. Because these patients have univentricular hearts (in this case the right ventricle), survivors of the Norwood procedure ultimately become candidates for a Fontan-type repair.

The Norwood procedure is usually performed in the first days to weeks of life (following stabilization of the infant on prostaglandin). The primary objective of the Norwood repair is to reconstruct a neoaorta that communicates with the right ventricle using the proximal portion of the main pulmonary artery and patch graft material (Figure 19–6). Flow to the pulmonary arteries is achieved using a modified B-T shunt either centrally from the neoaorta, or from the subclavian artery. Recent surgical results have suggested the B-T shunt should be somewhat restrictive in size.[14] Last, an atrial septectomy is performed so that pulmonary venous return can freely communicate from the left to the right atrium. The mortality for the Norwood procedure remains high in many centers relative to most other cardiac surgeries. However, increasing success has clearly been recognized in a growing number of centers. The long-term success, however, is still unclear, and survivors of the Norwood procedure still require staging to a Fontan repair (the first stage being the bidirectional Glenn).

Damus-Kaye-Stansel Operation

The Damus (or DKS) repair is utilized in the setting of complex cardiac lesions such as transposition with VSD, DORV with subpulmonary VSD, and certain univentric-

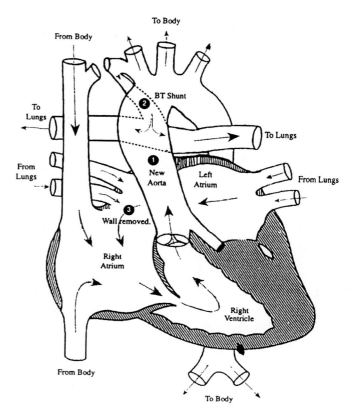

Figure 19-6. Diagram of the Norwood procedure with reconstructed neoaorta, transection of the pulmonary arteries, atrial septectomy, and placement of a modified Blalock-Taussig shunt for hypoplastic left heart syndrome. *(Reprinted, with permission, from, Hypoplastic left heart syndrome (HLHS): A guide for parents.* Prog Pediatr Cardiol*: 1996; 5:65–9, 1996.)*

ular hearts (particularly those with subaortic obstruction). The repair establishes flow from the left ventricle to the aorta by anastomosing the proximal end of the transected pulmonary artery to the side of the aorta (Figure 19–7). In addition, the VSD is closed, and flow from the right ventricle to the distal pulmonary artery is achieved with a conduit (usually homograft). In patients with single ventricle, the DKS repair can be done in conjunction with a Fontan-type repair.

Repair of Left-Sided Obstructive Lesions

1. Valvular Aortic Stenosis (AS)
2. Subvalvular AS
3. Supravalvular AS

Surgical commissurotomy for valvular AS has been the standard approach used since the earliest days of cardiac surgery. The major risk associated with commissurotomy is the development of significant aortic valve insufficiency. Unfortunately, the natural history of aortic valve disease is that of progressive restenosis and/or

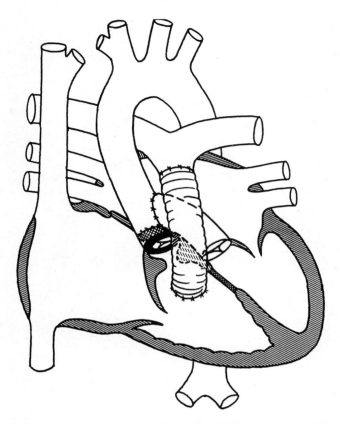

Figure 19-7. Diagram of Damus-Kaye-Stansel operation with pulmonary artery to ascending aorta (end-to-side) anastomosis, patch closure of VSD, and right ventricle to pulmonary artery conduit for d-transposition of the great arteries, VSD, and aortic obstruction. *(Reprinted, with permission, from Mullins CE, Mayer DC.* Congenital Heart Disease—A Diagrammatic Atlas. *New York: John Wiley & Sons, Inc.)*

insufficiency with potential need for prosthetic valve replacement. Within the last decade there has been an increasing role for catheter balloon valvuloplasty for aortic stenosis, and in many centers this has become the procedure of choice. Although it is not yet possible to call the results long term, the intermediate results indicate that balloon valvuloplasty produces similar relief of obstruction with comparable degrees of aortic insufficiency.[15]

Subaortic stenosis resulting from a discrete fribromuscular ridge or membrane is amenable to surgical excision, usually in conjunction with a septal myomectomy. The surgery is associated with a small but real risk for heart block as well as inadvertent creation of a ventricular septal defect. The long-term risk of subaortic stenosis is that of recurrence (in spite of septal myomectomy), with a risk as high as 15% to 20%.

Supravalvular AS is the least common type of obstruction and is associated with Williams (elfin facies) syndrome. Supravalvular AS is also sometimes seen as a familial type (with autosomal dominant inheritance and variable expression). The extent of obstruction is variable ranging from a discrete "hourglass" type at the sino-tubular junction to more diffuse hypoplasia of the ascending aorta. The usual repair involves removal of the obstructive ridge and patch enlargement of the involved portion of the aorta.

Konno-Rastan Procedure (Aortoventriculoplasty)

The Konno procedure is utilized when left-sided aortic obstruction is more extensive, with hypoplasia of the aortic annulus and/or tunnel subaortic obstruction of the left ventricular outflow tract. The surgical aortotomy incision creates enlargement of the anterior aortic root by extending the incision into the cephalad portion of the ventricular septum and excision of the aortic valve. A Dacron patch is sutured into the septal incision to enlarge the aortic valve annulus, with subsequent placement of a prosthetic aortic valve. The short-term risk associated with the procedure is that it is a major operation associated with increased mortality (relative to other cardiac surgeries). The long-term risks are primarily those associated with having a prosthetic valve and the need for anticoagulation.

Ross Procedure

The Ross procedure has enjoyed a recent resurgence of enthusiasm. Many centers currently are offering the Ross procedure as an alternative to prosthetic valve replacement in patients with severe aortic valve disease. The procedure involves excision of the aortic valve and placement of the pulmonary valve annulus and trunk into the aortic position with reimplantation of the coronary arteries. On the pulmonary side, a homograft conduit is placed between the right ventricle and the pulmonary artery. The Ross procedure can also be done in conjunction with an aortic root enlargement. The short- and long-term risks include the development of neoaortic valve insufficiency as well as the potential need to replace the homograft conduit.

Repair of Coarctation of the Aorta

The first surgical resection and end-to-end anastomosis repair of coarctation of the aorta was performed in 1945.[1] Subsequently, alternative repairs have been proposed, especially for more diffuse coarctation (with isthmic hypoplasia), such as prosthetic patch aortoplasty and the subclavian flap repair. Traditionally, elective surgical repair for the asymptomatic child was deferred until he or she was 4 years to 6 years of age, when the aorta has achieved more than 50% of its growth potential. Currently, most centers would repair coarctation regardless of age, and certainly if the obstruction were associated with any symptoms of congestive failure (seen mostly in infants), significant hypertension, or left ventricular hypertrophy.

The standard operation for discrete, localized (juxtaductal) coarctation is to perform resection of the posterior ledge with an end-to-end anastomosis performed via a left posterolateral thoracotomy. The major advantage of this approach is that it removes all abnormal tissue and involves no prosthetic material. The major disadvantage is that the end-to-end approach does not relieve the obstruction if a significant component of isthmic hypoplasia exists. There is also some risk of restenosis, particularly if the surgery is performed in infancy. However, at the current time, many centers would utilize balloon angioplasty procedures for recoarctation of the aorta. The role that balloon angioplasty should play in primary coarctation is still being debated, but it likely will increase in frequency.

An alternative approach to repair of coarctation is the patch aortoplasty, wherein the coarctation is resected and a prosthetic patch is sewn in to enlarge the coarcted segment. The predominant advantage of this approach is that it is well suited for enlargement of a long segment coarctation. The major long-term risk is that associated with the utilization of prosthetic material. In addition, there appears to be an important long-term risk associated with the development of aortic aneurysm formation. Another approach well suited to patients with longer segment coarctation is the subclavian flap aortoplasty. With this approach, the subclavian artery is transected, turned down, and sutured to the distal end of the aortic incision. The primary advantage of the subclavian flap repair is that it avoids prosthetic material and has growth potential. The major disadvantage is that it sacrifices the distal subclavian artery, although overt complications have been rare.

Early complications associated with any type of coarctation repair include the risk of hemorrhage, damage to adjacent structures (vagus and/or branches, phrenic nerve injury, chylothorax), and paraplegia from spinal cord ischemia (rare in the current era). In addition, significant rebound or paradoxical hypertension and postcoarctation syndrome (mesenteric arteritis and ischemia associated with severe abdominal pain and distention) are not uncommon complications in the immediate postoperative time frame. Late complications and risks include recurrence of the coarctation, development of hypertension despite satisfactory repair, endocarditis (endarteritis), cerebral aneurysm, and aortic aneurysm and dissection. Fortunately, many of these risks appear to be lessened when the coarctation is repaired earlier in life.

Fontan Procedure

The Fontan repair, initially described in 1971,[16] has been modified and revised repeatedly through the years. Used primarily in patients with tricuspid atresia initially, early Fontan repairs typically placed a valved conduit between the right atrium and the pulmonary artery, and were usually performed after a previous classic Glenn

shunt. These early Fontans invariably developed problems with obstruction at valve level. Later, modified Fontans involved a direct anastomosis between the right atrial appendage and the pulmonary artery. Currently, any patient with a univentricular heart with good ventricular function, low end-diastolic pressure, minimal AV valve regurgitation, and reasonably normal pulmonary artery anatomy (with low pressure) is considered a candidate for the Fontan operation.

As stated in the section Cavopulmonary Anastomosis, the current trend is to stage the Fontan by performing a bidirectional Glenn at an earlier age, before completion of the Fontan. The presumed advantage of staging the Fontan at an earlier age is to remove the volume load to the single ventricle (thus preserving diastolic function) and to "prepare" the pulmonary circulation before completion of the Fontan.[2,4] Many centers now complete the Fontan using the "lateral tunnel" technique, whereby inferior caval flow is baffled through the atrium into the lower portion of the divided superior vena cava and into the pulmonary artery (Figure 19–8). In addition, an increasing number of centers are

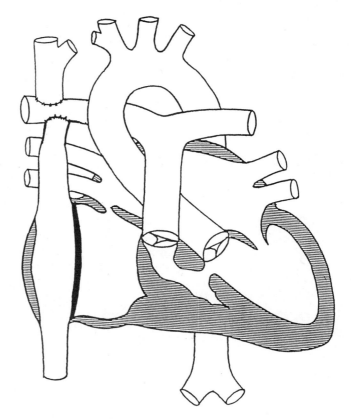

Figure 19-8. Diagram of lateral tunnel Fontan with cavolpulmonary anastomosis for tricuspid atresia. *(Modified, with permission, from Mullins CE, Mayer DC. Congenital Heart Disease—A Diagrammatic Atlas. New York: John Wiley & Sons, Inc.)*

fenestrating the Fontan; that is, a defect is created in the atrial baffle to allow "decompression" of central venous pressure. This may be particularly helpful in patients with mild elevations of pulmonary artery pressure, in whom fenestration is felt to reduce the incidence of postoperative complications.

Complications of the Fontan are unfortunately quite numerous. Short-term risks include problems with pleural effusion and chylothorax, often requiring lengthy hospitalization for chest tube drainage. Long-term complications include the risk for thrombus formation with the associated risk of paradoxical embolization and cerebrovascular accidents. Also, chronic increase in systemic venous pressure can result in hepatic dysfunction, venous distention, and protein-losing enteropathy from dilated lymphatics. Last, these patients are at risk for bradydysrhythmia (requiring pacemaker therapy) and atrial tachydysrhythmia. Ultimately, many Fontan patients develop progressive ventricular dysfunction with the potential need for transplant.

IN SUMMARY

The common surgeries for most of the congenital cardiac defects have been reviewed. Although the individual discussions for the various surgical procedures are necessarily brief, it is hoped that sufficient discussion exists to give the reader a good introductory concept of each. Certainly, more detailed information can be gained for any of the individual cardiac surgical procedures from either a pediatric cardiology textbook or from a cardiovascular surgery text.

ACKNOWLEDGMENT

Reprinted with permission by Chrestomathic Press, Inc. Originally published in *Pediatric Ultrasound Today* 1(9):121–36, 1996 and 1(10):137–52, 1996.

REFERENCES

1. Emmanouilides GC. Development of Pediatric Cardiology: Historical Milestones. In: Moss, Adams, eds. *Heart Disease in Infants, Children, and Adolescents including the Fetus and Young Adult*, 5th Edition. Baltimore: Williams & Wilkins; 1995.

2. Allgood NL, Alejos J, Drinkwater DC, et al.: Effectiveness of the bidirectional Glenn shunt procedure for volume unloading in the single ventricle patient. *Am J Cardiol.* 74:834-6, 1994.

3. Srivastava D, Preminger T, Lock JE, et al.: Hepatic venous blood and the development of pulmonary arteriovenous malformations in congenital heart disease. *Circulation.* 1217-22, 1995.

4. Pridjian AK, Mendelsohn AM, Lupinetti FM, et al.: Usefulness of the bidirectional Glenn procedure as staged reconstruction for the functional single ventricle. *Am J Cardiol.* 71:959-62, 1993.

5. Freedom RM.: The dinosaur and banding of the main pulmonary trunk in the heart with functionally one ventricle and transposition of the great arteries: A saga of evolution and caution. *J Am Coll Cardiol.* 10:427-8, 1987.

6. Blalock A, Hanlon CR. The surgical treatment of complete transposition of the aorta and the pulmonary artery. *Surg Gynecol Obstet.* 90:1–15, 1950.

7. Rashkind WJ, Miller WW. Creation of an atrial septal defect without thoracotomy: A palliative approach to complete transposition of the great arteries. *JAMA.* 196: 991–992, 1966.

8. Murphy JG, Gersh BJ, Mair DD, et al.: Long-term outcome in patients undergoing surgical repair of tetralogy of Fallot. *N Engl J Med.* 329:593-9, 1993.

9. Rastelli GC, McGoon DC, Wallace RB. Anatomic correction of transposition of the great arteries with ventricular septal defect and subpulmonary stenosis. *J Thorac Cardiovasc Surg.* 58:545–552, 1969.

10. McGoon DC, Rastelli GC, Ongley PA. An operation for the correction of truncus arteriosus. *JAMA.* 205:69–73, 1968.

11. Jatene AD, Fontes VF, Paulista PP. Anatomic correction of the great vessels. *J Thorac Cardiovasc Surg.* 72:364–370, 1976.

12. Hayes AM, Baker EJ, Kakadeker A, et al.: Influence of anatomic correction for transposition of the great arteries on myocardial perfusion: Radionuclide imaging with technetium-99m 2-methoxy isobutyl isonitrile. *J Am Coll Cardiol.* 24:769-77, 1994.

13. Norwood WI, Lang P, Castaneda AR, Campbell DN. Experience with operations for hypoplastic left heart syndrome. *J Thorac Cardiovasc Surg.* 82:511–519, 1981.

14. Chang AC, Farrell PE Jr, Murdison KA, et al.: Hypoplastic left heart syndrome: Hemodynamic and angiographic assessment after initial reconstructive surgery and relevance to modified Fontan procedure. *J Am Coll Cardiol.* 17:1143-9, 1991.

15. Justo RN, McCrindle BW, Benson LN, et al.: Aortic valve regurgitation after surgical versus percutaneous balloon valvotomy for congenital aortic valve stenosis. *Am J Cardiol.* 77:1332-8, 1996.

16. Fontan F, Bandet E. Surgical repair of tricuspid atresia. *Thorax.* 26:240–244, 1971.

CHAPTER TWENTY

Prenatal Diagnosis of Congenital Heart Disease

Robin D. Shaughnessy, Susan B. Olson, and Cheryl L. Maslen

Traditional teaching in pediatric cardiology has held that only a small proportion of congenital heart defects is directly due to genetic causes (both chromosomal anomalies and single-gene disorders). Such teaching argues that the majority of congenital heart disease (approximately 90%) is of "multifactorial" origin, resulting from vague genetic–environmental interactions. However, as scientific techniques become more sophisticated and we learn more about genetic regulation of cardiac development, it is becoming increasingly apparent that much of congenital heart disease (CHD), including seemingly sporadic cases, is caused by single-gene abnormalities rather than multifactorial events. It is also clear that different forms of CHD can arise from a common genetic defect, and that a single type of cardiac malformation can result from mutations at different loci in different individuals. Many of these observations have resulted because more patients with severe heart defects are surviving and having their own children.[1] Along with our expanded understanding of the etiology of many types of CHD has come the ability to perform prenatal genetic testing to diagnose many genetic defects associated with CHD. Such genetic testing is an ideal adjunct to prenatal echocardiography. However, current technology does not allow us simply to "rule out congenital heart disease," so it is helpful to have a particular diagnosis in mind (based on characteristic ultrasound findings) when submitting material for genetic testing. In addition, in those families in which a specific molecular diagnosis has been established, a high degree of certainty can be achieved for the presence or absence of a causative mutation.

INDICATIONS

Before proceeding with prenatal genetic testing, one must carefully consider the usefulness of the information to be obtained for a particular family. Whereas many parents desire as much information as possible before delivery of an infant, others would rather wait to obtain genetic information until after the baby is born when more clinical information is available. Genetic testing is therefore indicated if it will make a significant difference to the management of the pregnancy and delivery, or if the information may prepare or reassure the parents.

In conjunction with fetal echocardiography, there are several indications for genetic testing. The first would be the detection of a congenital heart defect on fetal echocardiography, especially if there is a positive family history for CHD. Some defects, such as atrioventricular canal, suggest a particular genetic diagnosis—in this case, trisomy 21. A second indication for testing would be a negative fetal echo in the presence of a strong family history, especially in the case of an echocardiographically "silent" diagnosis in the fetus, such as of Marfan's syndrome. Finally, prenatal genetic testing may also be considred when there has been previous fetal demise to rule out common genetic abnormalities. Knowing the cause of the previous infant's death can be helpful in directing the evaluation of the current pregnancy.

TISSUE TYPES

Amniotic Fluid

The first prenatal determination of a fetal karyotype by analysis of cultured amniotic fluid cells was reported in 1966.[2] It has since become the most common method for acquiring fetal tissue for analysis. *Amniocentesis* is the aspiration of amniocytes and amniotic fluid with a hypodermic needle under ultrasound guidance. The procedure is commonly performed at 15 weeks to 18 weeks gestation but may be done earlier or later if indicated. It is routinely offered for advanced maternal age, occurrence of a previous child or fetus with a chromosomal abnormality, known carrier status for a structural chromosomal abnormality, a family history of a biochemical or single-gene defect for which testing is available, or a family history of X-linked disease for which there is no direct diagnostic assay.[3]

Placenta

Chorionic villus sampling (CVS) is a placental biopsy, done either transvaginally or transabdominally, at 10 weeks to 12 weeks of gestation. The obvious advantage over amniocentesis is the ability to perform testing, and therefore have the results, earlier in the pregnancy. However, there are several complicating factors that must be acknowledged. One problem is the origin of the tissue being sampled. Maternal cell contamination and the presence of more than one cell line in a given sample (mosaicism) are both serious concerns. Maternal cell contamination, in which tissue from the maternal component of the placenta is inadvertently cultured either along with or instead of fetal tissue, occurs in approximately 1.8% of all CVS tests. True mosaicism, where both placental and fetal tissues are of mixed cell line origin, occurs in approximately 0.8% of all CVS cases and has been confirmed in the fetus by subsequent amniocentesis in approximately 25% of cases.[4] Confined placental mosaicism is associated with intrauterine growth retardation and fetal loss.[5] Another concern is the reported association of CVS with limb reduction defects.[6] For this reason, follow-up fetal ultrasound examination is recommended at 18 weeks' gestational age.

Cord Blood

Percutaneous umbilical blood sampling (PUBS), or cordocentesis, is useful in providing an independent fetal tissue sample for analysis when mosaicism has been identified by amniocentesis or when anomalies are detected by ultrasound late in gestation.[3]

Preimplantation Diagnosis

Although it is an experimental technique and not widely available, preimplantation screening for genetic disease is likely to become more common in the future. It is currently performed in conjunction with in vitro fertilization on single cells obtained by either polar body removal[7] or blastomere biopsy.[8] Such preimplantation diagnosis allows in vitro fertilization programs to avoid transferring genetically abnormal embryos to prospective mothers.

Noninvasive Methods

All of the techniques just given for obtaining fetal tissue for analysis involve risks to the mother, the fetus, or both. The normal presence of nucleated fetal cells in the maternal circulation, including cytotrophoblastic elements, fetal lymphocytes, and nucleated fetal erythroblastoid cells, permits low-risk and economically feasible access to fetal tissue for genetic analysis. The primary difficulty lies in the identification and separation of the fetal cells, although several techniques using immunologically specific markers are being developed.[4]

GENETIC TECHNIQUES

Traditional and Molecular Cytogenetics

Although human chromosomes were first observed in the late 1800s, it was not until 1956 that Tjio and Levan established that the complete karyotype consisted of 46 chromosomes. In 1959, Lejeune observed that patients with Down syndrome (i.e., trisomy 21) had an extra chromosome. By 1966, development of amniocyte culturing techniques allowed the prenatal diagnosis of certain chromosome abnormalities.[2] Chromosome analysis continues to play a fundamental role in prenatal genetic testing. The karyotype determines the number of chromosomes and their integrity. Since many types of chromosomal anomalies are associated with congenital heart defects (see Table 20–1), karyotyping should be considered for any fetus identified as having a congenital heart defect, especially if associated with other physical anomalies. Other important indications include a positive family history for genetic disorders and/or fetal loss.

To achieve analyzable chromosome preparations, dividing cells must be obtained. Cells are grown in culture and arrested for study at a time in the cell cycle (prometaphase to metaphase of mitosis) when the replicated chromosomes are condensed enough to allow individual identification. The chromosomes are stained to produce chromosome-specific banding patterns. The standard protocol used by most laboratories is treatment with trypsin followed by Wright stain. This produces a G banding pattern that gives the best definition of regions along the length of the chromosome. Other stains may be chosen to highlight specific regions of concern. Once the chromosomes have been photographed

TABLE 20–1. CONGENITAL HEART DEFECTS ASSOCIATED WITH SELECTED CHROMOSOMAL ABNORMALITIES

Diagnosis	Incidence of CHD (%)	Most Common Lesions
Trisomy 21	50	VSD or AVSD, PDA, ASD
Trisomy 18	>99	VSD, PDA, PS
Trisomy 13	90	VSD, PDA, dextroversion
Partial trisomy 22	40	TAPVC, VSD, ASD
del (4p)	40	ASD, VSD, PDA
del (5p) (*cri du chat*)	20	VSD, PDA, ASD
8 trisomy (mosaic)	50	VSD, ASD, PDA
9 trisomy (mosaic)	50	VSD, coarctation, DORV
del (13q)	25	VSD
del (19q)	50	VSD
del (22q)	70–95	IAA, TOF, TGA, truncus arteriosus
45,X	35	Coarctation, bicuspid aortic valve, AS, ASD

*a*ASD, atrial septal defect; AVSD, atrioventricular septal defect, DORV, double-outlet right ventricle; PDA, patent ductus arteriosus; PS, pulmonary stenosis; TAPVC, total anomalous pulmonary venous connection; VSD, ventricular septal defect; IAA, interrupted aortic arch; TOF, tetralogy of Fallot; TGA, transposition of the great arteries; del, deletion.

or captured by computer imaging, a karyotype is prepared for interpretation (Figure 20–1).

The ability to make an accurate diagnosis depends on the quality and band number of the karyotype. Each tissue type has its own optimum achievable level of quality and banding length. The routine band level for analysis in most laboratories ranges from less than 400 per haploid set (e.g., in bone marrow) to 850 (in peripheral blood). For thorough examination, 500 to 550 bands is the optimum. More subtle abnormalities require at least 650 bands. Microdeletions and some rearrangements may only be visualized at 850 bands or greater (high resolution) or may require more sophisticated molecular cytogenetic techniques.

The standard chromosome study requires the analysis of at least 20 cells. In addition, long-term tissue cultures, such as amniotic fluid cells, require analysis of cells from independent cultures and/or clones. These rules were created to address the possibility of mosaicism. If mosaicism is suspected, either by initial findings or by patient phenotype, additional cells may be analyzed.

Karyotyping detects abnormalities in both chromosome number and chromosome structure. The normal karyotype is diploid, with one haploid contribution from each parent. The term "aneuploidy" refers to an increase or decrease in the diploid number of one or several chromosomes. Trisomy is the most common form of aneuploidy and refers to the presence of three homologous chromosomes instead of the usual two (e.g., trisomy 21). Monosomy refers to the presence of only one chromosome of a homologous pair (e.g., 45,X, or Turner's syndrome). "Partial" monosomy or trisomy

indicates the loss or duplication of a portion of the chromosome. The term "polyploidy" is used when the abnormal number of chromosomes is a multiple of the haploid number (i.e., 23), such as triploidy (69 chromosomes) or tetraploidy (92 chromosomes). Aneuploidy is due to chromosome loss or nondisjunction. Polyploidy can most often be explained by multiple fertilization of the egg or cell cleavage errors.

Structural defects in chromosomes result from breaks and rearrangements and include such findings as deletions, translocations, and inversions. The nomenclature for describing a karyotype is standardized[9] and is expressed first by the total number of chromosomes, followed by the sex chromosome complement, and then any aberration detected. The short arm of a chromosome is referred to as *p* (for *petit*) and the long arm as *q*. Several examples of karyotype notations can be found in Table 20–2.

Fluorescent in Situ Hybridization

Whereas banding techniques represent the foundation for detecting chromosomal abnormalities, not all such chromosomal defects can be demonstrated using this technology. Therefore, a variety of other strategies have been developed to detect less obvious abnormalities. Fluorescent in situ hybridization (FISH) is a relatively new technique that greatly facilitates the chromosomal localization of cloned fragments of genomic DNA. It permits the identification of the chromosomal locus of a gene or sequence of DNA directly, not only on chromosomes but also within decondensed interphase nuclei.[10] Submicroscopic losses or rearrangements of genetic material can also be detected by FISH analysis. FISH is

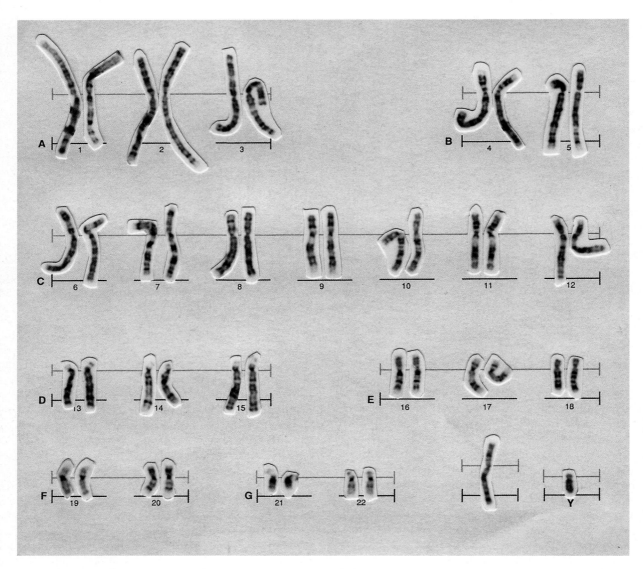

Figure 20-1. GTG-banded karyotype of normal male fetus at the 650-band level.

TABLE 20–2. EXAMPLES OF KARYOTYPE NOTATIONS THAT MAY BE ASSOCIATED WITH CONGENITAL HEART DISEASE

Karyotype	Definition
46,XY	Normal male
47,XX, +13	Female with trisomy 13
47,XY, +21	Male with trisomy 21 (Down syndrome)
46,XY, del (5p)	Male with *cri-du-chat* (caused by deletion of part of short arm of chromosome 5)
45,X	Female with Turner's syndrome

performed by preparing metaphase spreads or interphase nuclei on glass slides, which are then hybridized with fluorescence-labeled DNA pieces (probes). These probes are subsequently observed on the chromosome in question under a fluorescence microscope.[11]

One of the more exciting uses of FISH technology

in cardiology has been in the detection of chromosome 22q11 deletions, present in cases of velocardiofacial (VCFS) and the DiGeorge syndromes (DGS). These findings have been termed "CATCH-22" (for *c*ardiac anomalies, *a*bnormal facies, *t*hymic hypoplasia, *c*left palate, and *h*ypocalcemia—chromosome *22* deletion) and are associated with conotruncal and aortic arch anomalies. Using probes prepared from DNA clones shown to be deleted in many VCFS–DGS patients, it is a highly sensitive assay. Whereas cytogenetic studies detect deletions in approximately 25% of DGS and VCFS cases, molecular studies using probes for various locuses in the 22q11 region have detected submicroscopic deletions in more than 95% of the DGS cases and in 80% of VCFS who have not exhibited cytogenetic abnormalities.[12,13] The deletions are detected as absence of hybridized signal on one of the two chromosomes (Figure 20–2). Although the deletion can be readily detected, it

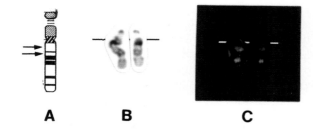

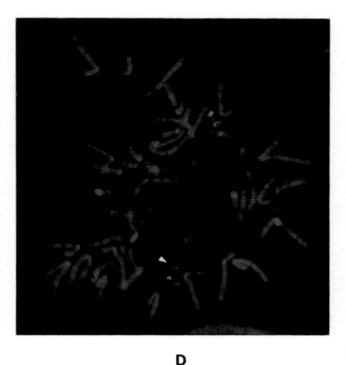

D

Figure 20-2. A. 850-band ideogram of chromosome 22 (ISCN, 1985) with arrows delineating breakpoints of the deleted region in velocardiofacial–diGeorge syndromes (VCFS–DGS). **B.** 850-band-level GTG-banded chromosomes 22 from a VCFS patient. The chromosome on the right is deleted. **C.** Chromosomes 22 from the deleted patient following fluorescent in situ hybridization (FISH) with the Vysis TUPLE1 probe (red) and terminal 22-specific identifier (green). The deleted chromosome (on the right) shows signal for the identifier region but is missing the signal for the VCFS–DGS region. **D.** Full metaphase spread of the TUPLE1 and identifier FISH. Chromosomes can be distinguished by the DAPI counterstain. The deleted chromosome 22 is indicated by the white arrowhead.

is not possible to predict the infant's phenotype. Therefore, if a deletion is detected prenatally the mother should be referred for fetal echocardiography to determine the presence or absence of associated heart defects. Conversely, if an aortic arch anomaly or conotruncal defect is detected on fetal echocardiography, one should consider prenatal testing for a 22q11 deletion. FISH has also been useful in the diagnosis of *cri-du-chat* syndrome [deleted chromosome 5 short

arm, associated with ventricular septal defect (VSD), atrial septal defect (ASD), and patent ductus arterioses (PDA)], Williams syndrome (associated with supravalvular aortic stenosis and peripheral pulmonary artery stenosis), and Wolf-Hirschhorn syndrome (deleted chromosome 4 short arm, associated with ASD, VSD, PDA, and tetralogy of Fallot).[14]

Linkage Analysis

Rapid progress over the last decade in the field of molecular genetics has enabled the mapping of a significant number of genes responsible for human disease. Linkage analysis maps the chromosomal locus of a gene responsible for a disease through the use of DNA markers that have known chromosomal locuses. It is based on the fact that coinheritance of two locuses on a particular chromosome depends on their distance from one another. During gametogenesis, recombination exchanges large blocks of genes between the homologous parent chromosomes. After meiotic reduction, the chromosomes transmitted to the offspring contain a new combination of alleles. The closer two genes are to each other on the chromosome, the less likely they are to undergo random exchange during recombination. Two locuses that are adjacent to each other (such as 1 cM [centimorgan], approximately 1 million bp, apart) almost always segregate together. In contrast, locuses far from one another on the same chromosome (greater than 50 cM) or on different chromosomes are inherited separately in a random fashion. The higher the likelihood of two alleles being coinherited, the tighter the linkage is said to be. Linkage analysis is performed to show whether a DNA marker with a known chromosomal locus cosegregates with inheritance of a disease in a particular family.[15,16]

The first step in linkage analysis is to identify a family with the disease of interest and establish a pedigree. Accurate diagnosis, and exclusion of that diagnosis, is of utmost importance because each member of the family must be classified as affected, unaffected, or unknown. A false positive or false negative diagnosis could cause an error in linkage determination. Once the pedigree is established, cosegregation of a DNA marker (with a known chromosomal locus) with the phenotype of the disease is analyzed. If a particular DNA marker is always observed when the disease is present in an individual, this indicates that the gene responsible for the disease is located near the marker gene (see Figure 20–3). Consequently, in addition to being a diagnostic technique, linkage analysis is a research tool, used to find the approximate locus for a gene of interest.

Two types of DNA markers are routinely used in linkage analysis. The first is restriction fragment length polymorphisms (RFLPs). An RFLP results when a silent variation in an individual's DNA sequence alters the

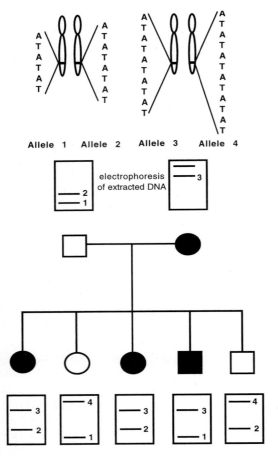

Figure 20-3. Linkage analysis. The polymorphic DNA marker (AT)n, where n is the number of repeats in a given allele, is present in each chromosome. Four variations in the number of DNA repeats are present in this family. Only allele 3 cosegregates with inheritance of the disease, indicated by full circles or squares. Allele 3 is not present in normal individuals, suggesting positive linkage of the DNA marker and the disease locus. Statistical analysis is performed to determine the actual odds of linkage.

recognition site of enzymes (restriction endonucleases) that cut DNA in a sequence-specific fashion. When human DNA from normal individuals is digested with a particular restriction enzyme, fragments of discrete lengths are obtained. Any change in a single base pair could abolish an existing restriction site or create a new one, altering the lengths of the fragments obtained. These fragments of varying length are known as polymorphisms. Polymorphic restriction sites occur throughout the human genome, and one or more is likely to be found in the region of the gene of interest. Each individual has two copies of each gene (one on each homologous chromosome), so a person could be homozygous or heterozygous for the presence or absence of a restriction site. Because linkage analysis studies the cosegregation of a DNA marker with inheritance of a disease, only heterozygous individuals provide useful

information with regard to inheritance of a particular allele in the family. Consequently, DNA markers based on RFLPs have a limited number of possible variations and limited informativity.[10,16]

A second type of DNA marker, which is now more commonly used in linkage analysis than RFLPs, is based on interindividual variations in the number of dinucleotide, trinucleotide, and tetranucleotide repeats in the human genome. Such markers are referred to as short tandem repeats (STRs) or satellite markers. STR markers occur very frequently in the human genome, approximately every 5000 bp. The advantage of STR markers lies in the great variability in the number of repeats among individuals. STR markers usually have 4 to 10 alleles in the population as compared with RFLP markers, which have 2 alleles. Consequently, STR markers are highly polymorphic and, therefore, more informative.[16]

Linkage analysis depends on accurate diagnosis of the disease, based on phenotypic expression, in affected family members. However, there may not be a clear-cut association between the presence of the genetic defect and development of the clinical manifestations of the disease. Some individuals, despite having the underlying genetic defect, may be phenotypically normal, i.e., *nonpenetrant*. When a disease is expressed in fewer than 100% of the persons who carry the gene defect, the disease is said to have *reduced penetrance*. For a particular disease with reduced penetrance, we refer to the proportion of persons carrying the disease allele and expressing the phenotype as a percentage of the total population carrying the disease gene (e.g., 80% penetrant). A potential source of error in linkage analysis is the incorrect assumption of percentage penetrance of the mutation. If the percentage penetrance of the disease is low, then the clinical manifestations are not present in many individuals with the mutation, leading to misdiagnosis as not carrying the mutant gene and reducing the chance of identifying positive linkage. Furthermore, in some diseases (such as hypertrophic cardiomyopathy), clinical manifestation is age dependent. That is, a young, phenotypically normal individual may have inherited the genetic defect and may develop the disease phenotype later in life. This young individual, too, could be misdiagnosed as unaffected. Finally, acquired disease may mimic the phenotype of a genetic disease, and those individuals may be misclassified as affected, leading to false positive linkage.[16]

Once the pedigree has been established and an appropriate DNA marker selected, actual linkage analysis is performed using computer-based statistical models to determine the odds of linkage of the marker and the disease. If the odds of cosegregation of a marker with the inheritance of the disease are 1000:1, the marker is considered to be linked to the locus for the disease.

This number correlates to a 95% probability of linkage and is considered to be significant. The likelihood ratio is expressed as the log of odds and referred to as an LOD score. An LOD score of 3, which correlates to a likelihood ratio of 1000:1, indicates positive linkage. An LOD score of −2 excludes the region as the locus of the candidate gene.[16] If tight linkage is established, the likelihood of an individual (or fetus) who has that marker also having the disease is determined. Linkage analysis has been used to establish the locuses for clinical syndromes such as Marfan's syndrome, the familial forms of total anomalous pulmonary venous return,[14] hypertrophic cardiomyopathy, and long Q-T syndrome.[10] Linkage analysis combined with FISH was instrumental in localizing the gene for Holt-Oram syndrome, an autosomal-dominant condition characterized by upper extremity deformities and cardiac septation defects (ASD, VSD, tetralogy of Fallot) to the gene *TBX5* on chromosome 12q2.[17,18]

DNA Diagnostics

There are several cardiac diseases that are not usually thought of as congenital diseases because they do not develop or present until later in life. However, they clearly have a genetic origin and are therefore congenital. Advances in molecular genetic techniques have allowed the localization of some of the genes responsible for these syndromes, thus making the option of presymptomatic diagnosis available for a limited number of diagnoses. Diagnosis of single-gene defects can be accomplished by directly analyzing the DNA of the patient, and peripheral blood is usually an adequate tissue source. Although not widely applicable (because of the limited number of diagnoses with known mutations) or widely available, presymptomatic diagnosis can be useful in planning surveillance and early therapy for affected individuals with the goal of preventing the more drastic sequels of some of these diseases. Since treatment may be beneficial early in infancy, prenatal diagnosis may be indicated for those families with positive family history for such genetic defects.

The long Q-T syndromes (LQTS) are characterized by prolongation of the Q-T interval on a 12-lead electrocardiogram, which indicates delayed cardiac repolarization and predisposes these patients to ventricular arrhythmias, syncope, seizures, and sudden death. With appropriate therapy the incidence of these symptoms can be decreased.[19] Unfortunately, sudden death may be the presenting symptom in a previously undiagnosed individual, and presymptomatic clinical diagnosis can be difficult because of the overlap in Q-T interval measurements between normal individuals and LQTS patients. Three inheritance patterns have been identified—the Romano-Ward syndrome (autosomal dominant), the Jervell and Lange-Nielsen syndrome (autosomal recessive, associated with sensorineural hearing loss), and sporadic (indeterminant inheritance). The most common is the Romano-Ward syndrome. Linkage analysis has demonstrated extensive genetic heterogeneity among affected families, with at least five different genes responsible for LQTS,[20,21] as summarized in Table 20–3. Approximately 50% to 60% of autosomal-dominant LQTS (LQT1) is due to defects in the *KVLQT1* gene, located at chromosome 11p15.5. The *KVLQT1* gene codes for a voltage-gated potassium channel in the myocardium, and mutant genes result in proteins with diminished function. Affected individuals are at risk for sudden death during periods of stress or excitement and may respond to medications that open these potassium channels. *KVLQT1* has recently been implicated in the development of the Jervell and Lange-Nielsen syndrome as well.[22] LQT2 (approximately 30% of autosomal-dominant LQTS) has been traced to defects in the *HERG* gene, located at chromosome 7q35–36, which codes for a different type of potassium channel. Affected individuals are particularly susceptible to hypokalemia, and therapy is directed at increasing serum potassium in order to activate the defective potassium channels. LQT3 (approximately 10% of autosomal-dominant LQTS) is due to defects in the gene *SCN5A*, found at chromosome 3p21–25, which codes for a voltage-gated sodium channel subunit. Patients having this gene are vulnerable to sudden death while

TABLE 20–3. MOLECULAR GENETICS OF THE LONG Q-T SYNDROMES

Subtype	Inheritance	LQTS (%)	Channel	Locus
LQT1	Autosomal dominant	~50	*KVLQT1*	11p11.5
LQT2	Autosomal dominant	~30	*HERG*	7q35–36
LQT3	Autosomal dominant	~10	*SCN*5A	3p21–25
LQT4	Autosomal dominant	<5	Unknown	4q25–27
LQT5	Autosomal dominant	~10	Unknown	Unknown
Jervel and Lange-Nielsen syndrome	Autosomal recessive	Rare	Unknown	Unknown

sleeping and may be treated with sodium channel blockers. Therefore, an accurate genetic diagnosis may be extremely important in determining which family members are at risk for sudden death and in choosing appropriate therapy for individuals with LQTS.[19] The gene for LQT4 (which is associated with severe sinus node bradycardia) has been located using linkage analysis to chromosome 4q25–27, but the gene has not yet been identified.[23]

Familial hypertrophic cardiomyopathy (FHC) is an autosomal-dominant disorder that can exhibit variable penetrance. It is characterized by ventricular (particularly septal) hypertrophy, with clinical manifestations ranging from a benign asymptomatic course to severe heart failure and sudden death. As in LQTS, sudden death may be the presenting symptom, especially in young athletes. Several genes on different chromosomes have been identified as responsible for the FHC phenotype (Table 20–4).[24–26] All code for sarcomeric proteins, the basic contractile units of the heart. Each genotype produces a slightly different phenotype, varying in such things as degree and distribution of hypertrophy, age at onset, and natural course of the disease. Once a mutation is detected in a particular family, all family members can be screened. Affected individuals require close medical follow-up and restriction from strenuous physical activity, with therapy based on the particular mutation and its natural course.[26]

Dilated cardiomyopathy (DCM) is estimated to be familial in at least 20% of cases.[25,27] It is characterized by left ventricular or biventricular dilation and impaired ventricular function, and is the leading indication for cardiac transplant. Without transplant, 5-year survival is <50%. The most common form of familial DCM is transmitted in an autosomal-dominant fashion, with age-related penetrance. It usually presents in the second or third decade. Less commonly, it is apparent in early childhood and is more severe. As with many other cardiac diseases, affected individuals may be asymptomatic and go undiagnosed until they are severely impaired. Linkage analysis has identified three genetic loci, 1q32, 9q13–22, and 3p22–25, but many families are not linked to these loci, indicating that there are other familial DCM genes. Although the mol-

ecular defects have not yet been characterized, presymptomatic diagnosis is sometimes possible using linkage analysis.

Marfan's syndrome is an autosomal-dominant disorder that affects an estimated 1 in 5000 live births. It has a complex constellation of clinical characteristics that include cardiovascular, skeletal, and ocular abnormalities. The wide range in both inter- and intrafamilial phenotypic variability can make clinical diagnosis difficult, particularly since there are phenotypic mimics.[28] In addition, some of the manifestations may not be apparent until later in life. A severe form of infantile Marfan's syndrome has been described, with serious cardiac pathology present in up to 94% of those patients.[29] Therefore, prenatal diagnosis may be indicated in cases of positive family history or characteristic findings on prenatal ultrasound or echocardiography. Marfan's syndrome is known to be due to mutations in the gene encoding the extracellular matrix protein, fibrillin-1.[28] To date, over 50 mutations have been reported and virtually every affected individual or family has a different mutation.[30] This makes direct mutation analysis impractical unless the mutation in a given family has already been characterized. However, linkage analysis is generally available and should be offered when there is a positive family history and a sufficient number of family members are available for analysis.

Coronary artery disease and arteriosclerotic peripheral vascular disease are the leading causes of morbidity and mortality in the United States. It has long been suspected that some families have a genetic predisposition to development of these conditions, thus putting them at increased risk for stroke, myocardial infarction, and venous thrombosis. It has been estimated that 10% of the population's risk for coronary artery disease is attributable to elevated levels of plasma homocysteine.[31] The remethylation of homocysteine to methionine requires the carbon donor 5-methyl tetrahydrofolate, formed by the action of the enzyme methylenetetrahydrofolate reductase (MTHFR). However, approximately 38% of the general population carries a defect in the gene coding for MTHFR.[32] Homozygosity for the mutation, present in approximately 10% of the population of the USA, results in clinically significant

TABLE 20–4. THE MOLECULAR GENETICS OF FAMILIAL HYPERTROPHIC CARDIOMYOPATHY (FHC)

Inheritance	FHC (%)	Protein	Locus
Dominant	30	β-cardiac myosin heavy chain	14q11
Dominant with reduced penetrance	15	Cardiac troponin T	1q3
Dominant	<5	α-tropomyosin	15q2
Dominant	Unknown	Cardiac myosin binding protein C	11p11.2
Dominant (single kindred)	Unknown	Unknown	7q3

hyperhomocysteinemia and may be the most common defect predisposing to vascular disease. The genetic defect can be screened for by digestion of a sample of the patient's DNA with a restriction enzyme, thus producing different size fragments for the mutant and wild-type alleles. Fortunately, homocysteine levels in patients with the MTHFR mutation can be decreased with the administration of folic acid, thus lowering the affected individual's risk of developing related disease.[31]

Thromboembolic diseases, most commonly manifested as deep venous thrombosis and resultant pulmonary emboli, are another major cause of morbidity and mortality in adults. Familial genetic predisposition is suspected to play a role in at least one third of cases.[33] A significant number of families have been found to have a genetic defect in the anticoagulant response to one particular anticoagulant protein, activated protein C.[34] The mutation alters the site where factor V is normally cleaved by activated protein C, causing persistence of the factor Va procoagulant that would normally be inactivated. Heterozygotes (2% to 7% of the general population) have a 3- to 10-fold increased risk for development of venous thrombosis; homozygotes are estimated to carry a 50- to 100-fold increased risk.[35] Presymptomatic diagnosis is useful in patients contemplating pregnancy or other situations that may further increase their risk for development of venous thrombosis. As with the MTHFR mutation, genetic screening is easily performed using a restriction enzyme that produces different sizes of DNA fragments depending on the presence or absence of the mutation.

GENETIC COUNSELING

The importance of genetic counseling cannot be overstated. It is imperative that parents have sufficient accurate information with which to make informed decisions about whether to conceive, avoid conception, undergo diagnostic testing, deliver a child or terminate a pregnancy.[36] To that end, genetic counseling should include information about the risks and benefits of testing, the diagnosis in question, its etiology (if known), the prognosis, and the recurrence risk, as well as issues related to psychology and reproductive options. Counseling should be nondirective, with information presented in a nonjudgmental and an unbiased manner. The parents can then make decisions based on medical information as well as their own religious, moral, cultural, social, and family backgrounds. Not all reproductive options are acceptable to all parents. Nevertheless, no assumptions should be made about a given couple's beliefs. All potential options should be presented in a sensitive manner. Parents should also understand that a decision to pursue prenatal diagnosis does not obligate them to

any further actions, such as terminating the pregnancy in the event of a positive diagnosis. It is very helpful to the couple and extended family members if a written summary of the counseling session is provided, allowing them to review the information at a later point.[37]

Parent support groups are available for a number of diagnoses (e.g., Marfan's, Noonan's, and Williams syndromes, and trisomies 13, 18, and 21), and parents should be given information about the appropriate group. Not only do they provide psychological support, but they can serve as educational resources as well. Many such groups are "online," making them available via a home computer to even the most isolated families.

SUMMARY

The last decade has seen major advances in traditional and molecular genetic techniques, as well as our understanding of the etiology of many cardiac diseases. There is no doubt that this body of knowledge is going to expand. With this knowledge has come the ability to make diagnoses at the earliest stages of life. Prenatal genetic diagnosis is a valuable adjunct to other diagnostic modalities, such as fetal echocardiography, and it behooves clinicians to become acquainted with the scope of genetic testing available in their own institutions and communities.

REFERENCES

1. Payne RM, Johnson MC, Grant JW, et al.: Toward a molecular understanding of congenital heart disease. *Circulation.* 91:494–504, 1995.
2. Steele MW, Breg WR: Chromosome analysis of human amniotic fluid cells. *Lancet.* 1:383–5, 1966.
3. Cohen MM, Rosenblum-Vos LS, Prabjakar G: Human cytogenetics: A current overview. *Am J Dis Child.* 147:1159–66, 1993.
4. Ledbetter DH, Zachary JM, Simpson JL, et al.: Cytogenetic results from the US collaborative study on CVS. *Prenat Diagn.* 12:317–45, 1992.
5. Kalousek DK, Howard-Peebles PN, Olson SB, et al.: Confirmation of CVS mosaicism in term placentae and high frequency of intrauterine growth retardation association with confined placental mosaicism. *Prenat Diag.* 11:743–50, 1991.
6. Firth HV, Boyd AP, Chamberlain P, et al.: Severe limb abnormalities after chorion villus sampling at 56–66 days' gestation. *Lancet.* 337:762–3, 1991.
7. Verlinsky Y, Ginsberg N, Lifchex A, et al.: Analysis of the first polar body: preconceptual genetic diagnosis. *Hum Reprod.* 5:943–6, 1990.
8. Handyside AH, Kontogianni EH, Hardy K, et al.: Pregnancies from biopsied human preimplantation embryos sexed by Y-specific DNA amplification. *Nature.* 344:768–70, 1990.

9. ISCN (1985): In Mitelman F, ed. *An International System for Human Cytogenetic Nomenclature.* Basel: S. Karger; 1995.

10. McQuinn T: Molecular biological approaches to genetic cardiac diseases. *Progr Pediatr Cardiol.* 6:1–18, 1996.

11. Ferguson-Smith MA, Andrews T: Cytogenetic Analysis. In Rimoin DL, Connor JM, Pyeritz RE, eds. *Emery and Rimoin's Principles and Practice of Medical Genetics,* 3rd ed. New York: Churchill Livingstone; 1996.

12. Lewin MB, Lindsay EA, Baldini A: 22q11 deletions and cardiac disease. *Progr Pediatr Cardiol.* 6:19–28, 1996.

13. Lindsay EA, Goldberg R, Jurecic V, et al.: Velo-cardio-facial syndrome: frequency and extent of 22q11 deletions. *Am J Med Genet.* 57:514–22, 1995.

14. Pierpont MEM: Genetic etiology of cardiac syndromes. *Progr Pediatr Cardiol.* 6:29-41, 1996.

15. Paulus-Thomas J, McCormack MK, Burlingham BT: Detection of genetic disorders by DNA analysis and applied molecular genetics. In: Filkins K, Russo JF, eds. *Human Prenatal Diagnosis,* 2nd ed. New York: Marcel Dekker; 1990.

16. Marian AJ: Molecular approaches for screening of genetic diseases. *Chest.* 108:255–65, 1995.

17. Li QY, Newbury-Ecob AR, Terrett JA, et al.: Holt-Oram syndrome is caused by mutations in TBX5, a member of the Brachyury (T) gene family. *Nature Genetics.* 15:21–9, 1997.

18. Basson CT, Bachinsky DR, Lin RC, et al.: Mutations in human TBX5 cause and limb and cardiac malformation in Holt-Oram syndrome. *Nature Genetics.* 15:30–4, 1997.

19. Garson A Jr, Dick M II, Fournier A, et al.: The long QT syndrome in children. *Circulation.* 87:1866–72, 1993.

20. Keating MT. Genetic approaches to cardiovascular disease. *Circulation.* 92:142–7, 1995.

21. Russell MW: The long QT syndromes. *Progr Pediatr Cardiol.* 6:43–51, 1996.

22. Neyroud N, Tesson F, Denjoy I, et al.: A novel mutation in the potassium channel gene KVLQT1 causes the Jervell and Lange-Nielsen cardioauditory syndrome. *Nature Genetics.* 15:186-9, 1997.

23. Schott J-J, Charpentier F, Peltier S, et al.: Mapping of a gene for long QT syndrome to chromosome 4q25–27. *Am J Hum Genet.* 57:1114–22, 1995.

24. Kelly DP, Strauss AW. Inherited cardiomyopathies. *N Engl J Med.* 330:913–9, 1994.

25. Durand J-B, Abchee AB, Roberts R: Molecular and clinical aspects of inherited cardiomyopathies. *Ann Med.* 27:311–7, 1995.

26. Abchee AB, Roberts R: Molecular genetics of familial hypertrophic cardiomyopathy. *Progr Pediatr Cardiol.* 6:63–70, 1996.

27. Ortiz-Lopez R, Schultz KR, Towbin JA: Genetic aspects of dilated cardiomyopathy. *Progr Pediatr Cardiol.* 6:71–82, 1996.

28. Ramirez F: Fibrillin mutations in Marfan syndrome and related phenotypes. *Curr Opin Genet Dev.* 6:309–15, 1996.

29. Morse RP, Rockenmacher S, Pyeritz RE, et al.: Diagnosis and management of infantile Marfan syndrome. *Pediatrics.* 86:888-95, 1990.

30. Dietz HC: Molecular etiology, pathogenesis and diagnosis of the Marfan syndrome. *Progr Pediatr Cardiol.* 5:159–66, 1996.

31. Boushey CJ, Beresford SAA, Omenn GS, et al.: A quantitative assessment of plasma homocysteine as a risk factor for vascular disease. *JAMA.* 274:1049–57, 1995.

32. Frosst P, Blom HJ, Milos R, et al.: A candidate genetic risk factor for vascular disease: a common mutation in methylenetetrahydrofolate reductase. *Nature Genetics.* 10:111–3, 1995.

33. Press RD, Goodnight SH: Predisposition to thrombosis by a factor V mutation causing hereditary resistance to activated protein C. *West J Med.* 162:450–2, 1995.

34. Svensson PJ, Dahlback B: Resistance to activated protein C as a basis for venous thrombosis. *N Engl J Med.* 330:517–22, 1994.

35. Ridker PM, Hennekens CH, Lindpainter K, et al.: Mutation in the gene coding for coagulation factor V and the risk of myocardial infarction, stroke, and venous thrombosis in apparently healthy men. *N Engl J Med.* 332:912–7, 1995.

36. Hollowell EE, Eldridge JE: The legal implications of current and future prenatal diagnostic and therapeutic techniques. In: Filkins K, Russo JF, eds. *Human Prenatal Diagnosis,* 2nd ed. New York: Marcel Dekker; 1990.

37. Greenberg F: Chromosomal abnormalities and heritable aspects of pediatric cardiology. In: Garson A, Bricker JT, McNamara DG, eds. *The Science and Practice of Pediatric Cardiology.* Philadelphia: Lea & Febiger; 1990.

CHAPTER TWENTY-ONE

Fetal Echocardiography in China

Shaoqing Wang

China is one of the countries that had an early start in the basic research and clinical application of fetal echocardiography. The ultrasound examination of the fetal heart was reported by X. Wang et al.[1] as early as 1964. Since the ultrasonic equipment in 1964 was quite limited, whether a fetus was alive or in distress could only be diagnosed on ultrasound evaluation of the fetal heart. Still, it was impossible with earlier technology to observe this detailed structure of the fetal heart and how it functioned. Later on, for reasons other than technological development, research in fetal cardiac ultrasound came to a standstill. It was not until 1989 that some Chinese scholars reorganized themselves and worked in cooperation on fetal echocardiography.[2] They used M-mode echocardiography, two-dimensional echocardiography, and Doppler echocardiography to observe the structure and hemodynamics of the fetal heart. Then there were other scholars who concentrated their research efforts into this field. Fan et al.,[3,4] Zhang et al.,[5] Liu et al.,[6] and Huang et al.[7] detected, respectively, the structure of the fetal heart, the flow spectrum of the atrioventricular valves and the semilunar valves, and used color Doppler flow imaging. To find out the best time for imaging the structure of different parts of the heart completely, Deng et al.[8] studied the various views and images of the fetal heart. To analyze the developmental evolution and systolic and diastolic function of the normal heart, Huang et al.[9,10] have concentrated their research in these areas.

EXAMINATION METHODS USED IN FETAL ECHOCARDIOGRAPHY

Equipment

Precise ultrasonic diagnosis relies on qualified ultrasonic images. The fetal heart is small in structure and it beats rapidly. Only equipment with high resolution, enough penetrating power, and real-time presentation can provide analytical images. At the present time, M-mode, two-dimensional, pulse wave, and color Doppler flow imaging are being used in China. The most frequently used equipment is the Acuson 128 XP. The Toshi SSH-65A is also in use. The transducer frequencies are 3.0 MHz to 3.5 MHz.

Echocardiography Practitioners

In China echocardiographic examinations are given directly to the patients by physicians with rich clinical experience so that an immediate diagnosis can be given. In case additional views of the heart are needed, they can be obtained at that time. The number of echocardiographic examinations performed by technicians is very limited.

The Examination Used in Fetal Echocardiography

In the study of fetal heart images, most scholars are more interested in finding some views that are similar to those after birth. The most frequently used views are the long axis of the left ventricle, the short axis of the great vessels, and the apical four-chamber view.[2-8,11,12] There are also scholars who agree with Allen et al.[13] in scanning the fetal chest along the vertical and horizontal axes to observe the various sections of the heart and its connections. It should be pointed out that basic views are obtained for the standard cardiac examinations, whereas in practice a complex malformation can only be diagnosed by a careful analysis of all the images, their movements and serial sectional views.

It is generally agreed that the fetal heart completes its formation at a gestational age (GA) of 12 weeks. Studies show that between 16 and 35 weeks' gesta-

TABLE 21–1. HEMODYNAMIC PARAMETERS OF THE MITRAL VALVE ORIFICE ($\bar{x} \pm$ SD)

GA (weeks)	PFV$_E$ (m/s)	PFV$_A$ (m/s)	$\bar{V}$ (m/s)	VTI (m)	mAV (m/s^2)	PPG (mm Hg)	MPG (mm Hg)	PHT (ms)	Slope (m/s^2)
Approximately 16–27	0.36 ± 0.06	0.51 ± 0.03	0.26 ± 0.01	0.046 ± 0.007	6.99 ± 1.70	1	0	23.0 ± 4.25	6.63 ± 1.22
Approximately 28–42	0.38 ± 0.02	0.54 ± 0.03	0.30 ± 0.01	0.061 ± 0.005	5.98 ± 0.81	1	1	26.61 ± 3.87	6.11 ± 0.99

Reprinted, with permission, from Huang XQ, et al. Detection of fetal cardiovascular anatomic and hemodynamic data by ultrasound. Chin J Physical Med: 1991; 13:133.

tional age, especially between 20 and 27 weeks, better images are obtained. At this GA, the heart is big enough; it is closer to the transducer, and there are no bony structures to prevent its view. At the same time the fetus is not in a fixed position and it is easier to make adjustments.[8] The fetal heart before 16 weeks is too small for the recognition of its detailed structures, whereas after 35 weeks the images are difficult to obtain because of the fetal fixed position and its shaped bony structures; the placental thickness, its calcification and position (between the transducer and the fetal heart); and the amnionic fluid, which is too much or too little. Some scholars in China have narrowed the favorable examination period down to 24 to 28 weeks' gestational age.

TWO-DIMENSIONAL ECHOCARDIOGRAPHY OF THE FETAL HEART

Cardiovascular anatomic structures detected by two-dimensional echocardiography in the heart of an adult can be seen in almost all fetal heart examinations. Examinations of fetal atrial and ventricular diameters, atrioventricular ring diameter, and large arteries have shown that fetal heart two-dimensional echo has the following features[2,7,14]: (1) right heart system > left heart system, pulmonary artery > aortic artery; (2) the diameters of large vessels, atria, and ventricles increase along with the gestational age; (3) the oval foramen (OF), ductus arteriosus (DA), and ductus venosus (DV) are in existence. After birth, pulmonary respiratory function begins and the oval foramen closes. Consequently the anatomic and physical function of the right heart system changes from an advantageous to a disadvantageous position and the left heart system becomes advantageous instead.

The circulation of a normal fetal heart has three physical short circuits: (1) Most of the right atrium flow goes to the left atrium through the oval foramen; (2) most of the pulmonary artery flow goes to the descending aorta through the ductus arteriosus shunt; and (3) placental flow returns to the inferior vena cava through the ductus venosus. The ultrasonic detections of oval foramen, ductus arteriosus, and ductus venosus are very important in the discovery of cardiovascular malformation and the detection of hemodynamics. Some scholars[15] use the main pulmonary artery branch view of the base of the heart and the rising aorta–aortic arch–descending aorta view to detect the ductus arteriosus of the normal fetuses in different positions. The results are: diameter, 0.364 ± 0.066 cm ($x \pm$ SD), and length, 0.856 ± 0.157 cm ($x \pm s$). The measurement result for the oval foramen, using an apical four-chamber view or an atrial two-chamber view, is as follows: diameter, 0.662 ± 0.101 cm ($x \pm s$).

Some scholars use the sagittal plane view near the center line or the oblique–horizontal view in the epigastrium to observe the ductus venosus. It is a narrow trumpetlike vessel between the left and right hepatic lobes. Starting from the umbilical sinus, it goes obliquely up and backwards and stops at the inferior vena cava. The diameter is smaller than 2 mm at its narrowest place.

FETAL PULSE WAVE ECHOCARDIOGRAPHY

Using pulse Doppler to detect the indexes of semilunar valve opening, the atrioventricular valve opening, and the vessel flow spectrum can help in understanding the fetal cardiovascular hemodynamic changes. The results (see Tables 21–1 through 21–4) indicate that fetal cardiovascular hemodynamics has the following features[7]: (1) right cardiac output is greater than left cardiac out-

TABLE 21–2. HEMODYNAMIC PARAMETERS OF THE TRICUSPID VALVE ORIFICE ($\bar{x} \pm$ SD)

GA (weeks)	PFV$_E$ (m/s)	PFV$_A$ (m/s)	$\bar{V}$ (m/s)	VTI (m)	mAV (m/s^2)	PPG (mm Hg)	MPG (mm Hg)	PHT (ms)	Slope (m/s^2)
Approximately 16–27	0.38 ± 0.05	0.52 ± 0.02	0.28 ± 0.01	0.046 ± 0.005	6.71 ± 1.76	1	0	23.78 ± 6.12	6.62 ± 0.99
Approximately 28–42	0.39 ± 0.03	0.56 ± 0.03	0.32 ± 0.02	0.062 ± 0.005	5.94 ± 0.62	1	1	28.39 ± 4.49	5.93 ± 0.96

Reprinted, with permission, from Huang XQ, et al. Detection of fetal cardiovascular anatomic and hemodynamic data by ultrasound. Chin J Physical Med: 1991; 13:133.

TABLE 21–3. HEMODYNAMIC PARAMETERS OF THE AORTIC VALVE ORIFICE ($\bar{x} \pm$ SD)

GA (weeks)	PFV (m/s)	$\bar{V}$ (m/s)	VTI (m)	AcT (ms)	DcT (ms)	mAV (m/s²)	mDV (m/s²)	ET (ms)	PPG (mm Hg)	MPG (mm HG)
Approximately 16–27	0.59 ± 0.07	0.34 ± 0.05	0.061 ± 0.009	41.74 ± 5.80	117.80 ± 7.36	15.12 ± 3.34	5.34 ± 0.73	159.70 ± 6.01	1.5	1
Approximately 28–42	0.68 ± 0.03	0.40 ± 0.01	0.075 ± 0.004	48.17 ± 6.53	116.58 ± 6.72	14.64 ± 3.25	5.76 ± 0.57	163.24 ± 7.07	2.5	1.5

Reprinted, with permission, from Huang XQ, et al. Detection of fetal cardiovascular anatomic and hemodynamic data by ultrasound. Chin J Physical Med: *1991; 13:133.*

put; (2) both the velocity and the volume of the late diastolic phase at atrioventricular valve opening (A) are greater than the early diastolic phase (E) (i.e., A/E > 1); (3) the peak velocity at tricuspid valve opening is greater than that at mitral valve opening; (4) the average flow acceleration at atrioventricular valve opening in the second trimester of pregnancy is greater than the acceleration at the third trimester; (5) the peak velocity at the aortic valve (A_0) is greater than the velocity at pulmonary valve opening (pA) (i.e., A_o/pA > 1.01 ± 0.07); (6) the pulmonary flow acceleration time is less than aortic flow; (7) the right-to-left shunt through the oval foramen and the pulmonary to aorta shunt through the ductus arteriosus both exist; (8) the peak velocity, velocity–time integral, and velocity average increase along with the gestational age at cardiac valves' opening.

Detailed evaluations have been done of the anatomic structure of the ductus arteriosus and the oval foramen and the indexes of hemodynamics (see Tables 21–5 and 21–6). Study results show the following features[15]: (1) The PFV, $\bar{V}$, PPG, and MPG of the DA during systole were obviously higher than other cardiac valve orifices. (2) The velocity of the DA was high during systole and low during diastole. This indicates that during the cardiac cycle the pulmonary artery pressure is higher than the descending aorta. (3) The ejection time of the DA was longer than that of the aorta (AO) and the pulmonary artery (PA). (4) The acceleration time of the DA was longer than that of the PA. This indicates that the descending aorta has less resistance than the pulmonary artery. (5) The valve of the foraman ovale

was opening twice during each cardiac period; therefore, the features of pulse wave echocardiography across the foramen ovale gives two peaks. This indicates that right atrial pressure is higher than the left atrial pressure whether in the systolic phase or in the diastolic phase. (6) There were good relationships about the velocity–time integral (VTI) between the DA and the OF ($r = 0.61$, $P < .001$).

The study of human fetal heart ductus venosus (DV) flow began in 1991.[16] The pulsatility of the DV blood flow had a characteristic pattern, reflecting a positive spectrum of ventricular systole, ventricular diastole, and atrial systole (see Table 21–7).[14] Probably one third of the umbilical vein (UV) blood is shunted through the DV in a normal human fetus.

FETAL HEART COLOR DOPPLER FLOW IMAGING

Fetal heart color Doppler flow imaging is very different from that of older children and adults. The following are the most important features[5,15]: (1) Different fetal positions and gestational ages may produce different color imaging for normal flows at cardiac valves even though the transducer is placed in the same area. This causes some difficulties in color Doppler examinations. For this reason, the flow colors cannot be taken as an indication of the different cardiac valve flows. On the other hand differences in anatomic structure, flow spectrum, phase, and area provide more reliable factors for judgement. (2) Different flow sources for mitral valves and tricuspid valves may be used to distinguish right

TABLE 21–4. HEMODYNAMIC PARAMETERS OF THE PULMONARY VALVE ORIFICE ($\bar{x} \pm$ SD)

GA (weeks)	PFV (m/s)	$\bar{V}$ (m/s)	VTI (m)	AcT (ms)	DcT (ms)	mAV (m/s²)	mDV (m/s²)	ET (ms)	PPG (mm Hg)	MPG (mm Hg)
Approximately 16–27	0.58 ± 0.04	0.34 ± 0.03	0.064 ± 0.008	40.14 ± 5.80	120.04 ± 6.74	15.42 ± 3.02	5.16 ± 0.80	160.17 ± 5.24	1.5	1
Approximately 28–42	0.67 ± 0.03	0.40 ± 0.02	0.078 ± 0.004	46.43 ± 5.91	117.98 ± 5.67	15.20 ± 3.06	5.74 ± 0.64	163.06 ± 6.42	2.5	1.5

Reprinted, with permission, from Huang XQ, et al. Detection of fetal cardiovascular anatomic and hemodynamic data by ultrasound. Chin J Physical Med: *1991; 13:133.*

TABLE 21–5. NORMAL PARAMETERS OF THE FETAL DUCTUS ARTERIOSUS

	PFVs (m/s)	PFVd (m/s)	$\overline{V}$ (m/s)	VTI (m)	mAV (m/s²)	mDV (m/s²)	AT (ms)	DT (ms)	ET (ms)	PPG (mm Hg)	MPG (mm Hg)	D (cm)	L (cm)
MV	1.080	0.303	0.503	0.133	15.121	9.509	72.139	110.613	175.871	4.859	1.362	0.364	0.856
SD	0.225	0.057	0.088	0.036	3.027	1.873	9.341	10.356	16.790	1.991	0.816	0.066	0.157
Max V	1.63	0.38	0.77	0.22	23.76	13.87	93.00	135.00	210.00	10.63	4.95	0.54	1.27
Min V	0.61	0.18	0.36	0.07	9.80	5.26	48.00	93.00	130.00	1.49	0.88	0.26	0.57

Reprinted, with permission, from Huang XQ, et al. The study of the anatomy and hemodynamics of the fetal ductus arteriosus and foramina ovale by echocardiography. Chin J Ultrasound Med: *1995; 11:673.*

atrium and left atrium. Since the inferior vena cava is easier to detect, the flow from it goes naturally to the right atrium. The flow at the oval foramen is always from right atrium to left atrium, and there should be no problem in distinguishing the right atrium and the left atrium by color flow. (3) The flow at normal valves is usually indicated by a single color and the velocity always below the color Doppler Nyquist limit. Therefore, an observation of mixed colors is a high indication of abnormal flow. (4) For the normal fetus, the color flow at the mitral valve is darker and narrower than that at the tricuspid valve. This indicates that the fetal right ventricle has a higher flow output than the left ventricle. An observation of a brighter and wider flow at the mitral valve than that at the tricuspid valve indicates a large amount of right-to-left shunt caused an atrial septal defect. (5) When the fetal heart rate is fast and the spectrum lacks a simultaneous electrocardiogram recording, it is difficult to distinguish systolic phase and diastolic phase. Doppler spectrum shape, sample position, anatomic structure, and flow distribution may help solve the difficulty. (6) No regurgitation has been found at fetal cardiac valves, whereas "physiologic regurgitation" is often found in color Doppler for normal

adults. Therefore, cardiac valve regurgitation is very important in the clinical examination of the fetal heart. (7) The right atrium–left atrium shunt at the oval foramen appears to be a slow and narrow flow beam passing horizontally through and vertical to the atrial septum. When the ejection beam appears oblique and more than 6 mm wide, it is a very good indication of a secundum atrial defect. Color Doppler flow imaging of the ductus arteriosus shows a mixed-color flow shunt from the pulmonary artery to the descending aorta. Therefore, color Doppler flow imaging is a highly recommended technology in the evaluation of fetal heart hemodynamics. The principles and features of fetal heart flow motion offered by color Doppler flow imaging are considered very important both in the study of fetal heart physiology and in the examination of fetal heart flow abnormality. But it should be pointed out that color Doppler flow imaging also has limitations in fetal heart detection since the fetal heart is small.[5] A high-spectrum transducer may produce an indication of a darker flow or no indication at all. The color flow signal is very weak when the fetal heart is far from the transducer. Using a low-frequency transducer may get better color indication, but the two-dimensional echo-

TABLE 21–6. NORMAL PARAMETERS OF THE FORAMINA OVALE

	PFVs (m/s)	PFVd (m/s)	$\overline{V}$ (m/s)	VTI (m)	D (cm)
MV	0.481	0.392	0.209	0.092	0.662
SD	0.888	0.065	0.049	0.021	0.101
Max V	0.65	0.52	0.31	0.15	0.87
Min V	0.30	0.21	0.11	0.06	0.46

Reprinted, with permission, from Huang XQ, et al. The study of the anatomy and hemodynamics of the fetal ductus arteriosus and foramina ovale by echocardiography. Chin J Ultrasound Med: *1995; 11:673.*

TABLE 21–7. BLOOD FLOW VELOCITY IN DV AND UV OF NORMAL FETUSES

	Mean	SD	Range	Number
DV PVVs (cm/s)	55.1	12.92	~90–~33	60
DV PVVd (cm/s)	47.45	13.87	~87–~21	60
DV PVAs (cm/s)	29.14	10.49	~55.08–~8.74	60
DV $\overline{V}$ (cm/s)	46.04	12.36	~77–~23.78	60
DV index	0.48	0.12	~0.75–~0.2	60
DV FV (mL/min)	27.53	12.17	~91.2–~11.4	60
UA velocity (cm/s)	17.9	4.71	~28–~8	50
UA/FV (mL/min)	86.2	37.8	~210.6–~36	50
DV/UV	0.32	0.16	~0.9–~0.14	50

Reprinted, with permission, from Ai H, Todros T. Blood flow velocity waveforms in the ductus venosus of normal fetuses. Chin J Ultrasound Med: *1996; 12:12.*

cardiography is obviously of lower quality. The fetal heart rate is fast, and the flow edge is unclear at real-time imaging, which may cause a greater error when the flow beam is being detected.

FETAL ECHOCARDIOGRAPHIC VALUE FOR CLINICAL USE

Fetal echocardiography is a new technology in diagnostic ultrasound. Its clinical use is popular in China and is mainly in the following four aspects.

1. Two-dimensional, pulse wave, and color Doppler flow imaging are used for normal fetal cardiology. The detection of fetal heart anatomic structure and hemodynamics have shown that the fetal right heart system is, as a rule, larger than the left heart system. Studies show that the anatomic structural features are [2,5,7,14,15] right heart > left heart, pulmonary artery > aortic artery; and the hemodynamic features that are the peak flow velocity at the tricuspid valve > that at the mitral valve, right heart flow output > that of left heart; and the systolic and diastolic flow at the foramen ovale are characteristic of right-to-left shunt. Moreover, normal fetal cardiovascular structure and flow index increase with GA. For all these reasons, echocardiography has become an important technique for the detection of fetal development.

2. Using echocardiography for early diagnosis of various cardiovascular malformations and tumors so as to stop the pregnancy in time is not only important but also practical in China's quality-birth project. Every year in China about 100,000 infants are born with congenital heart disease.[12] For this reason many Chinese scientists highly recommend that regular fetal echocardiographic examination be given to those who have a higher risk of malformation during pregnancy. There are many reports on such examinations of fetal echocardiography in China.[2,7,11,12,17,18] The fetal heart diseases reported are: atrial septal defect, ventricular

TABLE 21–8. NORMAL PARAMETERS OF LV SYSTOLIC FUNCTION IN THE EARLY PHASES OF HUMAN DEVELOPMENT

Group		Number	EF (%)	EDV (mL)	ESV (mL)	FS (%)	SV (mL)	CO (L)
Fetus	(A)	37	58.17 ± 7.21	4.63 ± 1.86	1.28 ± 0.77	33.05 ± 4.16	2.78 ± 1.16	0.406 ± 0.169
Neonates	(B)	32	60.62 ± 9.49	15.09 ± 4.22	6.43 ± 2.86	36.33 ± 5.01	8.72 ± 3.13	1.055 ± 0.379
Infants	(C)	30	63.96 ± 6.57	36.87 ± 6.23	9.55 ± 4.26	39.91 ± 3.87	21.19 ± 8.78	1.949 ± 0.808
Children	(D)	33	65.83 ± 6.13	43.92 ± 14.51	14.88 ± 8.14	40.19 ± 5.32	29.05 ± 9.16	2.556 ± 0.806
	P		<0.001	<0.001	<0.001	<0.001	<0.001	<0.001

Reprinted, with permission, from Huang XQ, et al. A study of the development and evolution of the left ventricular systolic function by complex echocardiography. Chin J Ultrasound Med: *1996; 12:41.*

TABLE 21–9. RELATIONSHIP OF EF OF LV AND FETAL AGE

Group	Number	r	p
A	37	0.71	<.01
B	32	0.92	<.001
C	30	0.94	<.001
D	33	0.82	<.001

Reprinted, with permission, from Huang XQ, et al. A study of the development and evolution of left ventricular systolic function by complex echocardiography. Chin J Ultrasound Med: 1996; 12:41.

septal defect, pulmonary atresia, single atrium, hypoplastic left heart syndrome, single ventricle, transposition of conducting arteries, intra-atrial septal aneurysm, duplex atrial myxoma, aortic coarctation, and pericardial effusion.

Using the ductus venosus flow indexes in the evaluation of central venous pressure change, by echocardiography, has provided the basis for the diagnosis of fetal heart diseases.[14]

3. The PHT, slope, PPG, and MPG detected by pulse wave at the atrioventricular valve have provided valuable data for the diagnosis of atrio-oventricular valve stenosis or incompetence.[17]

4. Multiple echocardiograph techniques (including the two-dimensional Simpson method, M-mode, and pulse wave) are used for normal fetal heart function detection. The detected EF, FS, SV, and CO are compared to those of neonates (24 h to 4 weeks), infants (1.5 months to 11 months) and children (1 year to 4 years). Study results show that for normal human heart the left ventricular systolic function is formed during the fetal phase, and there is a gradual increase after birth for a short period (see Tables 21–8 and 21–9). The increase may be an indication of the corresponding relativity of the neonate and infant in their ventricular EF and age. Normal systolic function is therefore an important and comparatively stable function that is formed in the fetal-phase circulation and continues to adult-phase circulation. This is quite different from the unstable fetal diastolic function.[10] These discoveries are important for studying the physiology and pathology of the fetal heart.

Pulse wave detection has been used for fetal cardiac flows at the left and right atrioventricular valves and at early and late diastolic stages. The indexes include: (1) PFV_E, PFV_A, PFV_E/PFV_A; (2) VTI_E, VTI_A, VTI_t, VTI_E/VTI_A; (3) PPG_E, PPG_A, PPG_E/PPG_A; (4) $\overline{V}$; (5) MPG; and (6) IVRT. The results are given in Tables 21–10 and 21–11. Comparisons have been made to

TABLE 21–10. HEMODYNAMIC PARAMETERS OF THE MITRAL VALVE ORIFICE ($\bar{x} \pm$ SD)

	Fetus	Neonates	Infants	Children	P
PFV_E (m/s)	0.38 ± 0.06	0.61 ± 0.09	0.72 ± 0.21	1.21 ± 0.48	<.001
PFV_A (m/s)	0.57 ± 0.08	0.63 ± 0.10	0.69 ± 0.14	0.41 ± 0.21	<.01
PFV_E/PFV_A	0.67	0.97	1.04	2.95	<.001
VTI_E (m)	0.30 ± 0.005	0.052 ± 0.014	0.096 ± 0.023	0.168 ± 0.031	<.001
VTI_A (m)	0.041 ± 0.004	0.062 ± 0.017	0.090 ± 0.025	0.058 ± 0.019	<.01
VTI_T (m)	0.071 ± 0.007	0.114 ± 0.028	0.186 ± 0.046	0.226 ± 0.047	<.001
VTI_E/VTI_A	0.73	0.84	1.07	2.90	<.001
PPG_E (kPa)	0.079 ± 0.023	0.169 ± 0.041	0.263 ± 0.052	0.877 ± 0.212	<.001
PPG_A (kPa)	0.165 ± 0.034	0.216 ± 0.065	0.214 ± 0.029	0.198 ± 0.059	<.01
PPG_E/PPG_A	0.48	0.78	1.23	4.43	<.001
$\overline{V}$ (m/s)	0.233 ± 0.12	0.36 ± 0.11	0.47 ± 0.17	0.78 ± 0.21	<.001
MPG (kPa)	0.077 ± 0.023	0.109 ± 0.033	0.204 ± 0.065	0.283 ± 0.069	<.001
IVRT (ms)	40.51 ± 6.92	46.11 ± 8.43	64.20 ± 13.14	80.58 ± 16.18	<.001

Reprinted, with permission, from Huang XQ, et al. Evaluation of the diastolic function of the fetus, newborn, infant, and young child by Doppler echocardiography. Chin J Ultrasonog: 1996; 5:125.

TABLE 21–11. HEMODYNAMIC PARAMETERS OF THE TRICUSPID VALVE ORIFICE ($\bar{x} \pm$ SD)

	Fetus	Neonates	Infants	Children	P
PFV$_E$ (m/s)	0.40 ± 0.18	0.56 ± 0.12	0.70 ± 0.26	1.82 ± 0.27	<.001
PFV$_A$ (m/s)	0.59 ± 0.10	0.46 ± 0.15	0.51 ± 0.19	0.35 ± 0.16	<.01
PFV$_E$/PFV$_A$	0.68	1.22	1.37	2.34	<.001
VTI$_E$ (m)	0.031 ± 0.004	0.079 ± 0.002	0.096 ± 0.037	0.120 ± 0.027	<.001
VTI$_A$ (m)	0.042 ± 0.003	0.066 ± 0.021	0.073 ± 0.022	0.055 ± 0.030	<.01
VTI$_T$ (m)	0.073 ± 0.006	0.145 ± 0.042	0.169 ± 0.056	0.180 ± 0.057	<.001
VTI$_E$/VTI$_A$	0.74	1.20	1.32	2.20	<.001
PPG$_E$ (kPa)	0.087 ± 0.024	0.162 ± 0.031	0.245 ± 0.041	0.302 ± 0.110	<.001
PPG$_A$ (kPa)	0.186 ± 0.049	0.120 ± 0.035	0.158 ± 0.036	0.096 ± 0.035	<.01
PPG$_E$/PPG$_A$	0.46	1.36	1.55	3.15	<.001
$\bar{V}$ (m/s)	0.26 ± 0.07	0.32 ± 0.11	0.43 ± 0.15	0.56 ± 0.11	<.001
MPG (kPa)	0.083 ± 0.021	0.130 ± 0.031	0.162 ± 0.041	0.185 ± 0.055	<.001
IVRT (ms)	39.66 ± 7.79	47.10 ± 9.35	69.48 ± 12.37	82.56 ± 15.28	<.001

Reprinted, with permission, from Huang XQ, et al. Evaluation of the diastolic function of the fetus, newborn, infant, and young child by Doppler echocardiography. Chin J Ultrasonog: 1996; 5:125.

those of neonates, infants, and children. Study results indicate that the right heart functions better than the left at fetal-phase blood circulation, so the PFV, VTI, and PPG at the left and right atrioventricular valves flows all appear to be E < A. This indicates that the fetal heart has a very good atrial compensation. It also indicates that fetal ventricular diastolic function is physically incomplete.[9] Comparative studies have observed the regular patterns of hemodynamics within the heart in the early development of human body, or fetal—neonate—infant—child. These patterns reveal that normal ventricular diastolic function undergoes a physical development: incompletion—transition—normal transition—normal.[9] Overall and detailed studies of ventricular diastolic function development features are very important and practical in the analysis and distinction of physical ventricular function and pathologic ventricular function.

SUMMARY

This chapter is a general review of the advancement of the basic research and clinical application of fetal echocardiography in China, with emphasis on and a detailed introduction to the examination methods of fetal echocardiography, two-dimensional echocardiography

detection of fetal heart, pulse wave, echocardiography, color Doppler flow imaging echocardiography, and their value for clinical use.

REFERENCES

1. Wang Xinfang, et al.: Diagnosis of pregnancy by ultrasound—Ultrasonic examination of the fetal heart. *Chin J Gynecol Obstet.* 10:267, 1964.
2. The Collaborated Group of Fetal Echocardiography: Clinical study of fetal echocardiography. *Chin J Gynecol Obstet.* 24:268, 1989.
3. Fan Dong-sheng, et al.: A real-time two-dimensional echocardiography study on 170 Chinese fetuses. *Chin J Ultrasound Med.* 6:100, 1990.
4. Fan Dong-sheng, et al.: Pulsed Doppler echocardiography study on 100 normal fetuses. *Nat Med J Chin.* 69:282, 1989.
5. Zhang Yun, et al.: Evaluation of fetal cardiac hemodynamics by the color Doppler flow imaging technique. *Chin J Phys Med.* 13:193, 1991.
6. Liu Ming-yu, et al.: Diagnosis and analysis of fetal heart with color Doppler flow imaging. *Chin J Phys Med.* 13:86, 1991.
7. Huang Xiao-qin, et al.: Detection of fetal cardiovascular anatomic and hemodynamic data by ultrasound. *Chin J Phys Med.* 13:133, 1991.
8. Deng Jing, et al.: Study on cross-sectional echocardiographic imaging in the fetus. *Chin J Phys Med.* 14:77, 1992.
9. Huang Xiaoqin, et al.: Evaluation of the diastolic function

of the fetus, newborn, infant and young child by Doppler echocardiography. *Chin J Ultrasonog.* 5:125, 1996.

10. Huang Xiaoqin, et al.: A study of the development and evolution of the left ventricular systolic function by complex echocardiography. *Chin J Ultrasonog.* 12:41, 1996.

11. Xi'an Medical University, et al.: Echocardiographic diagnosis of cardiovascular malformation in the fetus (Report of 7 cases). *Chin J Phys Med.* 12:79, 1990.

12. Duan Xueyun, et al.: Diagnosis of congenital heart disease in the fetus by echocardiography. *Chin J Ultrasound Med.* 11:43, 1995.

13. Allan LD, et al.: Echocardiographic and anatomical correlates in the fetus. *Br Heart J.* 44:444, 1980.

14. Ai Hong, Todros T: Blood flow velocity waveforms in the ductus venoses of normal fetuses. *Chin J Ultrasound Med.* 12:12, 1996.

15. Huang Xiaoqin, et al.: The study of the anatomy and hemodynamics of the fetal ductus arteriosus and foramina ovale by echocardiography. *Chin J Ultrasound Med.* 11:673, 1995.

16. Kiserud T, et al.: Ultrasonographic velocimetry of the fetal ductus venosus. *Lancet.* 338:1412, 1991.

17. Deng Jing, et al.: One case of fetal aortic coarctation by echocardiography. *Chin J Phys Med.* 12:128, 1990.

18. Zhao Li, et al.: One case of atrial myxoma. *Chin J Gynecol Obstet.* 30:630, 1995.

APPENDIX
ABBREVIATIONS

AcT (or AT)	Acceleration time
CO	Cardiac output
D	Diameter
DcT (or DT)	Deceleration time
DV	Ductus venosus
EDV	End-diastolic volume
EF	Ejection fraction
ESV	End-systolic volume
ET	Ejection time
FS	Fractional shortening
FV	Flow volume
IVRT	Isovolumetric relaxation time
L	Length
Max V	Maximum value
mAV	Mean accelerant velocity
mDV	Mean decelerant velocity
Min V	Minimum velocity
MPG	Mean pressure gradient
MV	Mean value
PFV	Peak flow velocity
PFV_A	A peak flow velocity
PFVd	Diastolic peak flow velocity
PFV_E	E peak flow velocity
PFV_S	Systolic peak flow velocity
PHT	Pressure half-time
PPG	Peak pressure gradient
PVAs	Peak velocity of atrium systole
PVVd	Peak velocity of ventricular diastole
PVVs	Peak velocity of ventricular systole
SD	Standard deviation
SV	Stroke volume
UV	Umbilical veins
$\overline{V}$	Mean velocity
VTI	Velocity–time integral

CHAPTER
TWENTY-TWO

Fetal Imaging in Developing Countries

Alfredo Jose Jijón-Letort and Alfredo González-Guayasamin

As in any developed country, in most of the third world obstetricians are constantly searching for ways to evaluate the unborn fetus. Numerous reports have been found in the literature concerning the use of ultrasound for prenatal diagnosis,[1-3] and also the use of nuclear magnetic resonance imaging,[4] Doppler flow,[5-7] color Doppler,[8] and fetoscopy.

The routine use of ultrasound during pregnancy, although not proven to be of real clinical benefit in prenatal care and probably not even cost effective, has become an integral part in the management of pregnancies. Where this technology is available, it is very infrequent that there is not at least one ultrasound examination done on every pregnant patient.

Ultrasound during pregnancy has proved to be safe for both the mother and her fetus, and no harmful effects have been documented,[9] with regard to malformations, growth retardation, and mental, neurologic, cognitive, visual, or auditive impairments; even fetal weight and height have been demonstrated not to change.[10]

With real-time ultrasound we could easily document the general conditions of the fetus, both anatomic and physiologic. An ultrasound examination, one that does not require very sophisticated equipment or an expert ultrasonographer, could identify the number of fetuses, fetal presentation, fetal cardiac activity, estimation of gestational age, placental location, and amount of amniotic fluid. This information could be useful for the obstetrician and would improve the management of that particular pregnancy. This is the rationale behind why many obstetricians or caretakers of pregnant women in third world countries usually have an inexpensive ultrasound machine in their offices, one that is portable and can be used for home visits.

Unfortunately, sometimes the ultrasound examination replaces an adequate history and physical exam,

and this could be a serious detriment to the pregnant woman's health.

TYPES OF MEDICAL CARE IN THIRD WORLD COUNTRIES

As in most of the world, third world countries have at least two different types of health care organizations that take care of patients: One is private, expensive, and not available for the general population, and the other is organized by the government for the local community, mostly indigent.

The first kind of health care is mostly organized in a pay per service arrangement, has its own hospitals and clinics, and is usually properly equipped with new, modern, and expensive tools. Within this group, there are also significant differences, most frequently related to the cost of the services provided. In most third world countries there are some institutions or hospitals with standards of care similar to the ones available in first world countries, such as the United States, and the physicians who work there are generally trained abroad.

The health care provided by the government in third world countries shows significant differences from one place to another. Some hospitals, usually located in the major cities, have adequate standards of care, equipment, personnel, and technology. Others, located generally in rural areas, have no equipment, insufficient personnel, extremely poor budgets, and little or no technology.

Table 22–1 shows the situations in which an ultrasound examination during pregnancy can be of benefit, according to the National Institutes of Health (NIH) Consensus Development Conference held in 1984 on the use of ultrasound during pregnancy.[11] The information gathered by ultrasound can be especially important in rural areas of third world countries, where ei-

TABLE 22–1. POTENTIAL BENEFITS OF AN ULTRASOUND EXAMINATION DURING PREGNANCY

1. Evaluation of the fetus: Gestational age, number, presentation, growth, malformations, fetal demise
2. Evaluation of the uterus: Malformations, vaginal bleeding of unknown etiology, fibroids
3. Adjunct to certain procedures: Amniocentesis, cordocentesis, fetoscopy, chorionic villi sampling, fetal transfusions, external versions, placement of a cerclage, etc.
4. Suspected abnormal pregnancies: Ectopic pregnancy, hydatidiform mole, abortions
5. Determination of placental location and placental pathology
6. Evaluation of the amniotic fluid

ther there is no medical care or it is so inadequate that a pregnant patient with a serious problem, such as placenta previa, would be sent to a major city where a cesarean section could be done.

There is a lot of controversy in the literature surrounding the establishment of ultrasound screening as a standard of practice. Several studies, including the RADIUS project,[12] have shown that there are no scientific data that support its routine use during pregnancy,[13] whereas others feel that its routine use is useful and affordable.[14]

ROUTINE ULTRASOUND EXAMINATION

Fetal Anatomy

Performing a routine ultrasound during pregnancy as a screening test for fetal malformations has been advocated by some authors.[15] A large multicentric study done in Belgium was able to identify a significant number of prenatal malformations.[16] In Hungary, another large study showed that a mid-second trimester screening program, checking maternal serum α-fetoprotein at 16 weeks along with a routine ultrasound screening at 18 weeks to 20 weeks, with the availability of termination of pregnancy, could significantly reduce the prevalence of severe major abnormalities at birth.[17]

In Perú, a routine level or basic ultrasound was done in 900 pregnant women. The authors found that this screening test had a detection rate of fetal malformations of 50%, with 99% specificity, 40% false positives, and 2% false negatives. They concluded that a level I ultrasound screening had an acceptable detection rate and excellent specificity for congenital anomalies, and should be a useful diagnostic procedure in low-prevalence populations.[18]

With regard to fetal cardiac malformations, a study done in Cuba demonstrated how useful an ultrasound examination could be for prenatal diagnosis.[19] For example, the finding of polyhydramnios is an indication

to perform a detailed ultrasound, since it has been shown that there is a 53% risk of fetal malformations related to this finding in pregnancies.[20]

Although many private obstetricians in third world countries do a routine ultrasound for this purpose, this could not, and most likely would not, become a general policy because of the tremendous costs that such generalized testing would involve. It will require ultrasound scanners and properly trained personnel. Furthermore, the difficulty in accessing some areas leads us to think that universal testing is not realistic. We also have to realize that a normal ultrasound examination does not completely rule out a fetal abnormality[21]; in fact, half of all anomalies are not detected by high-resolution ultrasonography in expert hands, as demonstrated by the RADIUS Study Group.

The ultrasonographic finding of a fetal malformation creates a new problem: what to do with the pregnant woman who has a malformed baby identified around the latter part of the second trimester. She would have to be sent to a tertiary care center where a new ultrasound done by an expert physician would confirm the finding. In third world countries access to tertiary care centers is not easy. There are few of these centers available; those that do exist are overwhelmed by the number of patients and the long waiting period for service. By the time the patient is seen, her pregnancy may be in the later second or third trimester when a termination is not possible. To diagnose malformations sooner, so that termination of pregnancy, if needed, becomes easier, the ultrasound must be performed earlier, which increases the error rate. A study in Israel demonstrated that an early transvaginal ultrasound examination between 13 and 16 weeks had to be followed by a transabdominal ultrasound between 18 and 20 weeks to be accurate.[22]

To complicate matters even more, some third world countries, especially in Latin America, are predominantly Catholic, and therefore abortion, even for fetal malformations, is not an acceptable option and may be illegal.

Table 22–2 enumerates the most important elements that, at the very least, an ultrasound examination should document. If the ultrasonographer is unable to identify all these structures he or she should refer the patient to somebody else.

Fetal Growth Curves

Because of racial, climatic, and altitude differences, using growth curves from developed countries may not be appropriate. Many reports have been found in the literature where doctors from different third world countries have developed their own fetal body measurements; these have allowed them to create local tables and growth curves.[23,24]

TABLE 22–2. FACTORS THAT AT THE VERY LEAST SHOULD BE RECOGNIZED ON A ROUTINE ULTRASOUND EXAMINATION DURING PREGNANCY

1. Fetal number, viability, and presentation
2. Placental location
3. Amniotic fluid volume
4. Estimation of the gestational age
5. The following fetal structures: Cerebral ventricles, spine, stomach, bladder, cord insertion and number of umbilical vessels, four-chamber heart, diaphragm, and fetal kidneys

Gestational Age Determination

Menstrual history may not be optimal in third world countries to properly determine the gestational age, and an ultrasound examination may help to determine it better. A study done in Chile showed a 24% discrepancy between ultrasonography and menstrual dating in all patients, and a 14% discrepancy in patients with optimal menstrual history. This suggests that an ultrasound examination during the first trimester is the gold standard to estimate the true gestational age.[25]

Determination of Fetal Well-Being

A modified biophysical profile, described in Perú, appears to be an important tool in fetal surveillance during pregnancy. The researchers evaluated seven parameters: fetal movements, respiratory movements, fetal tone, basal heart frequency, cardiac reactivity, amniotic fluid volume, and placental maturity.[26] Likewise, numerous reports try to correlate Doppler flows through different fetal vessels as indicators of well-being.[27,28]

An ultrasound may be very useful in determining when and where the delivery should take place and to help prepare both family and doctors to take care of the mother and newborn.

SURVEY FROM AROUND THE WORLD

We sent a letter to all obstetricians from third world countries who are affiliated fellows of the American College of Obstetrics and Gynecology, asking them to answer the following questions regarding the use of ultrasound during pregnancy.

1. Are there any governmental or institutional guidelines in your country with regard to the routine use of ultrasound during pregnancy? Has the society of OB-GYN of your country issued a special directive in this regard?
2. Who is responsible for performing the ultrasound examinations during pregnancies: obstetricians, midwives, radiologists, or medical technologists?
3. Are there any centers in your country where ob-

stetricians can refer their patients for a more detailed ultrasound?
4. Approximately what percentage of pregnancies in your country do not have an ultrasound done?
5. Do doctors in your country perform an ultrasound examination on each prenatal visit?

The responses to these questions are summarized in Table 22–3. Although the replies were fewer than expected, all of them have more or less the same problems.

1. There are no governmental or national society guidelines regarding routine ultrasound during pregnancy.
2. Most ultrasounds are done either by the obstetricians themselves or by radiologists, depending on where the equipment is located; in hospitals they are done by the radiologists. Except for one doctor from Saudi Arabia, there are no reports of medical technologist doing ultrasound examinations. Several of the respondents do state that many nonobstetricians are performing ultrasounds without any formal training.
3. In almost every country there are referral centers where the reputation of the obstetrician or the radiologist is the basis for a referral, but there is no organized system in place.
4. This question is very difficult to answer because

TABLE 22-3. ULTRASOUND SURVEY TO OBSTETRICIANS FROM THIRD WORLD COUNTRIES

Countries	Questions[a]				
	1	**2**	**3**	**4 (%)**	**5**
Argentina	No	Obst/Rad	Yes	?	No
Ecuador	No	Obst/Rad	Yes	60	No
Guatemala	No	Obst/Rad	Yes	?	No
Honduras	No	Obst/Rad	Yes	60	No
Iraq	No	Rad	No	90	Few
India	No	Obst/Rad	Yes	95	No
Perú	No	Obst/Rad	Yes	30–40	No
Saudi Arabia	No	Obst/Tec	Yes	50	No
Syria	No	Obst/Rad	Yes	30	No
Uruguay	No	Obst	Yes	?	No
Venezuela	No	Obst	Yes	30	30%

[a]Questions: (1) Are there any governmental or insitutional guidelines in your country with regard to the routine use of ultrasound during pregnancy? Has the society of OB-GYN of your country issued a special directive in this regard? (2) Who is responsible for performing the ultrasound examinations during pregnancies: obstetricians, midwives, radiologists, or medical technologists? (3) Are there any centers in your country where obstetricians could refer their patients for a more detailed ultrasound? (4) Approximately what percentage of pregnancies in your country does not have any ultrasound done? (5) Do doctors in your country perform an ultrasound examination on each prenatal visit?

there is little reliable information in this regard and most of the responses were rough estimates. In rural areas an ultrasound is very seldom available, so most of the pregnancies do not have any done. When the pregnancy is followed in large institutions or in private practice, however, almost 100% of the pregnancies have at least one ultrasound done.

5. Most pregnant women do not have an ultrasound examination done on each visit. In some places doctors use the ultrasound on every visit, but these are what we call a "social ultrasound," so that the mother and her family can see the baby, but there is no effort to do a routine screening of fetal parts, and most of the time there are no written reports.

CONCLUSIONS

Obstetricians all over the world share a common goal: to have patients with normal pregnancies and healthy babies.

With the new technology available, we can rule out most major fetal malformations, recognize the fetus that is in danger of dying in utero, identify several obstetrical complications, and perform a few invasive procedures for the purpose of diagnosis and treatment.

Unfortunately, this rapidly evolving technology is not always available in third world countries, since it is expensive and requires special training to be used properly.

The use of a routine ultrasound examination during pregnancy, although easy to suggest, is very difficult to implement. The benefits from such a screening test have not been proved cost effective even in developed countries. An ultrasound may be very beneficial for one particular patient, demonstrating an abnormal placenta, fetal growth retardation, or amniotic fluid abnormalities, but for the general population, such an examination may not be justified.

In third world countries we need to continue our efforts to be well informed about the current technology available, and its usefulness, limitations, and potential hazards, in order to provide the best care possible for the mother and her unborn baby.

ACKNOWLEDGMENTS

We acknowledge the letters received from the following doctors: Eduardo Castelnovo, Argentina; Roberto Robles, Guatemala; Roberto Figueroa Fuentes and Leonardo Pérez, Honduras; D. K. Tank, India; Khansa Al-Chalabi, Iraq; Manuel González del Riego, Luis Vega y Alfredo Salazar, Perú; Bernd D. Wittmann, Saudi Arabia; Ahmad M Dahman, Syria; Carlos Rodríguez, Uruguay; and Juan Rivero, Venezuela.

REFERENCES

1. Arista O, Pérez R, Pedraja D, et al.: Diagnóstico prenatal de las cardiopatías congénitas. *Rev Cuba Pediatr.* 60(4): 494–504, 1988.
2. Fernández M, Fuster F: Ultrasonido y monitoreo fetal electrónico en el embarazo múltiple. *Rev Med Costa Rica.* 60(524):113–6, 1993.
3. Ciapessoni NE, Sigura L, Pereyra AG: Diagnóstico ultrasonográfico de cefalotoracopagos (JANICEPS): A propósito de un caso. *Rev Argent Radiol.* 57(2):133–7, 1993.
4. Lacreta O: Emprego da imagem por ressonância magnetica nuclear (nucleografía) in obstetrics: Part 2. *J Bras Med.* 53(4):28–33, 1987.
5. Melo VH, Cabral ACV, Chaves NH: Doppler da arteria umbilical no diagnóstico do crescimento intra-uterino retardado. *Rev Med Minas Gerais.* 3(2):64–9, 1993.
6. Corral E, Ulloa A, Pérez N, et al.: Velocimetría Doppler: Resultados perinatales según valoración integral de resistencias. *Rev Chil Obstet Ginecol.* 58(3):179–89, 1993.
7. Cassis-Martínez R, Durán G, Bizueta C, et al.: Curvas de indices de resistencia y pulsatilidad en arteria umbilical de fetos normales entre las 20 a 40 semanas de gestación. *Rev Ecuatoriana Ginecol Obstet.* 4(3):28–9, 1995.
8. Raga F, Ballester MJ, Osborne NG, et al.: Role of color flow Doppler ultrasonography in diagnosing velamentous insertion of the umbilical cord and vasa previa. A report of two cases. *J Reprod Med.* 40(11):804–8, 1995.
9. American Institute of Ultrasound in Medicine Bioeffects Committee: Bioeffects considerations for the safety of diagnostic ultrasound. *J Ultrasound Med.* 7:S1–38, 1988.
10. Start CR, Orleans M, Haverkamp AD, et al.: Short- and long-term risks after exposure to diagnostic ultrasound in utero. *Obstet Gynecol.* 63:194–200, 1984.
11. National Institutes of Health Consensus Development Conference Consensus Statement: The use of diagnostic ultrasound imaging in pregnancy. NIH Publication No. 84-667. Bethesda, MD: NIH; 1984.
12. Ewigman BG, Crane JP, Frigoletto FD, et al.: Effect of prenatal ultrasound screening on perinatal outcome. *N Engl J Med.* 329:821–7, 1993.
13. Crane JP, LeFevre ML, Winborn RC, et al.: A randomized trial of prenatal ultrasonographic screening: Impact on the detection, management, and outcome of anomalous fetuses. *Am J Obstet Gynecol.* 171:392-9, 1994.
14. Routine ultrasound in pregnancy (Polzin) (Letter), (LeFevre et al.) (Reply). *N Engl J Med.* 172:242–3, 1995.
15. Goncalves LF, Jeanty P, Piper JM: The accuracy of prenatal ultrasonography in detecting congenital anomalies. *Am J Obstet Gynecol.* 171:1606–12, 1994.
16. Levi S, Hyjazi Y, Schaaps JP, et al.: Sensitivity and specificity of routine antenatal screening for congenital anomalies by ultrasound: The Belgian multicentric study. *Ultrasound Obstet Gynecol.* 1:102–10, 1991.
17. Papp Z, Toth-Pal E, Papp C, et al.: Impact of prenatal mid-

trimester screening on the prevalence of fetal structural anomalies: A prospective epidemiological study. *Ultrasound Obstet Gynecol.* 6(5):320–6, 1995.

18. Pinedo J, Espinoza M, Diaz J, et al.: Diagnóstico prenatal de anomalías congénitas por ultrasonido. *Ginecol Obstet Perú.* 40:45–8, 1994.

19. Arista O, Fernández I, Javech C, et al.: Diagnóstico prenatal ecocardiográfico en Cuba. *Rev Cub Obstet Gynecol.* 17:17–26, 1991.

20. San Martín J, Diaz J, Trelles J, et al.: Polihidramnios y su relación con anomalías congénitas. *Ginecol Obstet Perú.* 41(2):62–4, 1995.

21. Evans MI, Hume RF, Johnson MP, et al.: Integration of genetics and ultrasonography in prenatal diagnosis: Just looking is not enough. *Am J Obstet Gynecol.* 174:1925–33, 1996.

22. Yagel S, Achiron R, Ron M, et al.: Transvaginal ultrasonography at early pregnancy cannot be used alone for targeted organ ultrasonographic examination in a high risk population. *Am J Obstet Gynecol.* 172:971–5, 1995.

23. Faneite P, Salazar G, González X: Evaluación céfalo-abdominal fetal en embarazos normales. *Rev Obstet Ginecol Venezuela.* 53(3):143–8, 1993.

24. Batista JA, Batista JY, Batista HM: Cálculo aproximado de la edad gestacional mediante estudio ultrasonográfico. *Rev Cub Obstet Ginecol.* 19(2):91–103, 1993.

25. Galvez J: Ecografía sistemática en el primer trimestre del embarazo. *Rev Chil Obstet Gynecol.* 58(4)323–7, 1993.

26. Huamán M, Pacheco J, Rosales H, et al.: Perfil Biofísico Ecosonográfico. *Ginecol Obstet Perú.* 41:52–5, 1995.

27. Pereira AK, Cabral ACV: Estágio atual na propedéutica do retardo de crescimento intra-uterino. *Rev Med Minas Gerais.* 3:8–10, 1993.

28. Melo VH, Cabral ACV, Chavez NH: Doppler da arteria cerebral media fetal na predicao do crescimento intra-uterino retardado. *Rev Med Minas Gerais.* 4:11–4, 1994.

CHAPTER TWENTY-THREE

Legal Issues Associated with Fetal and Neonatal Cardiac Disease

Frank I. Clark

If physicians are asked to provide adjectives to describe a discussion of the law as it affects an area in which they practice medicine, words such as cold, sterile, inflexible, or detached are likely to be offered. Statutes may deserve such descriptions, but legal scholars are much more likely to view our common law system as being dynamic, flexible, and subject to change on a daily basis. John Locke viewed law as existing only for the public good.[1] For him, the purpose of law was not to restrain humankind but to preserve and enlarge its freedoms. Locke envisioned people who were free to exercise their individual liberties within the boundaries of a common law that possessed the flexibility to change as people's needs changed.

This describes the existing legal–ethical interface that is frequently projected as a template by law,[2] ethics,[3] and the medical profession[4] on various aspects of our current medical practices. The discrete legal doctrines that evolve in response to these varying medical issues are not always a perfect mirror of current social requirements. In recent years the pace of medical technological development in some areas has outstripped the ability of either legislatures or judges to respond in a timely manner to societal needs. Nonetheless, our legal system attempts to set the outer boundaries of behavior for both patient and physician; physicians and their patients are left to make ethically appropriate and medically intelligent choices within those legal boundaries. Whereas law has seemed slow to develop in a few instances, it has at other times either anticipated medical developments or actually driven changes in ethical medical practice.[5] Law will ultimately fashion a legal doctrine that can be relied on for initial direction. Knowledge of a particular legal doctrine and any potential deficiencies in that doctrine can provide crucial guidance and support to the clinician in solving current medical and ethical dilemmas.

Most of the current legal issues that can pose occasional medical and ethical predicaments in the field of fetal and neonatal cardiac disease involve the decision-making process between physician and the prospective parent(s). These include the issues of how the process should be shared between doctor and patient,[5] who will be allowed to make which decisions,[6] and, unique to the field of maternal–fetal medicine, will the decision be made in the best interests of the fetus or the mother.[7,8] It would therefore seem appropriate first to review the current status of the three legal doctrines that govern informed consent, parents as guardians of their children's interests, and real and perceived maternal autonomy be-fore discussing the impact of these respective doctrines on the specific legal issues raised by fetal and neonatal cardiac disease.

CURRENT LEGAL DOCTRINES

Informed Consent

The doctrine of informed consent has been in a process of development in the United States since 1914.[9] By 1983, a presidential commission composed of several eminent ethicists recognized that both the physician and patient had their own individual interests with respect to medical decisions.[10] The commission, in its report, attempted to strike a balance between the needs of medical paternalism and patient autonomy by proposing a model it named "shared decision-making."[10] In

1990, the Supreme Court recognized that certain aspects of this shared model were inconsistent with well-established law and held that the patient had the final right to refuse or consent to medical treatment.[11] As a result of over 90 years of development, it is worth noting that law and medical ethics have some mildly differing views as to both the function and application in principle of this doctrine. Legal scholars are inclined to discuss the doctrine of informed consent in terms of a few documentable objective facts[5,12]; physicians and ethicists (perhaps rightly so) tend to stress the adequacy of patient or surrogate comprehension as it relates to the patient's subjective needs in the consent process.[13–16] There is another factor in this dichotomy between law and ethics besides the perceived differences in objective and subjective reasoning: Unless a patient appears to be incompetent at the time consent is obtained, the law simply presumes adequate patient comprehension of properly transmitted information.[5] Because this is a chapter on legal issues, what follow follows is a lawyer's concise review of current doctrine.

As implied by the name itself, the doctrine of informed consent has two major elements: the delineation of specific medical information and consent to some action or inaction based on that information. The second element also involves the identification of who actually grants consent to a medical treatment plan or surgical procedure. As a general rule that grantor is statutorily defined by each state[17]; these statutes are relatively uniform and consistent. Assuming a competent patient 18 years of age or greater, it is the patient him- or herself who has the right to give consent (a federal right).[11] Most states grant similar status to the pregnant teenager.[18] If the mother-to-be is either incompetent or is otherwise incapacitated (drugs, coma, anesthesia, etc.), then states generally default first to a spouse and then the woman's parent(s) as surrogate grantors of medical consent.[17] It is also possible that an incapacitated woman has utilized some other legal instrument to control her decision making should she not be legally available to do so herself.[17] The prudent physician should know the specific consent requirements of his or her jurisdiction and should also timely inquire as to the existence of any surrogate decision-making instruments such as living wills, advanced health care directives, or durable powers of attorney for health care decisions.

Some physicians narrowly confuse a signed consent form with informed consent.[5] The piece of paper the patient signs bears witness to an exchange of information between the doctor and the patient. The nature and content of this encounter determines whether consent is truly informed. It is this first element of informed consent that has seen the most change and posed more

difficulty in recent years.[5,12] This should not be unexpected because the requirements regarding the scope and process of transmission of information between doctor and patient are with a few exceptions essentially derived from our common law. The American judiciary has fashioned a doctrine of informed consent that has driven medicine into making the transition from a model of medical paternalism to one of patient autonomy.[5] Although this change has made more than a few physicians feel disenfranchised, it will be demonstrated that a respect for patient autonomy is not synonymous with total patient control of the medical treatment plan.

How much information a physician must disclose to a patient (scope of disclosure) depends on the standard of disclosure utilized in the state in which the consent process is occurring. The majority of states have adopted the physician-based standard, which requires a doctor to divulge that information which a reasonable medical practitioner in the same or similar circumstances would disclose to a patient.[5] A significant minority of states have adopted the reasonable patient standard, which allows a jury to decide whether the average or reasonable patient would have wanted to be made aware of a particular fact.[5] The distinction between these two standards is primarily a technical one left to law: The former requires expert testimony to determine the need for a particular disclosure, whereas the latter does not. The following six common law requirements seem to be independent of which standard of disclosure a particular state may require.

First, the physician must discuss the actual or working diagnosis with the patient.[12] The doctor should include any laboratory results, diagnostic radiology, or other test results as a basis for making the diagnosis. The relevance of starting with the presumed diagnosis is the simple fact that all resulting treatment decisions will be based on the patient's knowledge and comprehension of her current condition. This is especially crucial for those situations where the patient may choose nonintervention and the natural outcome of the disease process in place of the physician's recommendations. Second, the physician is obligated to discuss the nature and purpose of the treatment he or she proposes.[19] The third requirement is the need to discuss the attendant risks and potential outcomes of the proposed treatment with the patient or surrogate decision maker.[19–21] This information must be current, objective, and discussed at a level of comprehension appropriate to the individual patient's abilities. Materiality of the risk is seen as the cornerstone in those states that follow the reasonable patient standard of disclosure.[19,21] In those states, remote nonmaterial risks or those commonly known to the patient can be omitted from disclosure; material risks such as death or paralysis, however infrequent, must be discussed. It is interesting to note that the actual probability of success for a particular procedure or treatment by the individual physician has rarely been discussed or weighed by the courts as a significant factor.[5] It can be speculated that this is a result of judicial reluctance to stand in the patient's shoes and make a subjective value decision. However, as managed care organizations develop larger comparative outcome databases, courts in the future may be more likely to require physicians to disclose and compare success in their own hospitals against other institutions or some published national standard.

The fourth factor to be discussed in the consent process is that of alternative choices. In addition to disclosing what the physician recommends as a primary choice, he or she should also disclose the risks, consequences, and probability of success for those alternative methods of diagnosis or treatment that the medical community acknowledges as being feasible.[20,22] The basis for this requirement is the judicial observation that failure to mention any alternative treatment choices puts the physician in the position of making the choice for the patient. A fifth and related factor is the obligation to inform the patient of the probable prognosis or outcome should the patient decline any tests or treatment choices the physician has offered or suggested.[23,24] This has been termed the *right to an informed refusal.*[5] Whereas to date this requirement is technically required by only a minority of states, it is strongly implied in dicta by the *Cruzan v. Director* decision.[11]

The sixth requirement pertains to the choice itself. Whether the patient or the surrogate decision maker agrees with the physician's recommendation, opts for the physician's second choice (feasible, but not really what the doctor wants to do), or decides to do nothing at all, courts have made it clear that the patient's "consent, to be efficacious, must be free from imposition upon the patient."[19] In *Meador v. Stahler and Gheridan*, the plaintiff requested and initially started a trial of labor for vaginal birth after prior section.[25] This child was ultimately delivered by a cesarean section after the mother signed the consent form. There was an unfortunate surgical complication. The plaintiff did not claim that the physicians performed the surgery in a negligent manner. Instead, she was able to convince a jury that the labor was progressing normally, that the physicians disregarded her expressed wishes, and that they gave an inaccurate representation of the risks and benefits of the approach she preferred. She also convinced the jury that she signed the consent form because of the allegedly emotionally coercive manner of the obstetricians.

In addition to juries, courts have recently begun to take notice of the unequal relationship between physi-

cian and patient.[5] As a result of the physician's dominant position, they have begun in certain circumstances to impose the obligation of a fiduciary duty on the doctor.[26] The application of this seemingly abstract legal doctrine to the informed consent process requires the physician to disclose any possible conflicts of interest or other information important to a patient in assessing physician motivations."[5] These conflicts may arise in something as intangible as the physician's desire to enroll patients in a promising research project[27] or as direct as the commercial value of a hairy-cell leukemia line.[26] This fiduciary requirement will probably see further application as courts are forced by unhappy patients to probe the myriad potential conflicts of interest inherent in modern managed care relationships.

The final obligation in this process of information transmission is suggested by common sense and is either required or inferred by judges in their decisions: The person granting consent must have the opportunity to ask questions of the physician during the process.[12] The prudent clinician should note in the medical record not only that the patient was afforded this opportunity to make enquiry, but also briefly the subject matter of any questions the patient may have asked. This simple step documents both the physician's efforts to be complete and the level of the patient's comprehension. It also minimizes the possibility that an angry patient can successfully argue that he or she did not understand the consequences of a prior choice.

The most contentious area of informed consent doctrine that continues to evolve at a relatively quick pace deals with the allocation of authority between physician and the grantor of consent. The issue more specifically asks what degree of latitude is to be afforded the patient who requests a form of treatment that the doctor objects to providing for reasons of efficacy, technical abilities, or moral beliefs.[28] It has long been taught that the physician could refuse to be coerced into providing treatment that the physician felt was medically futile or was in conflict with the physician's personally held moral beliefs.[4,17] It would also not seem wise from the patient's point of view to antagonize the treating physician by forcing him or her to provide this treatment. The case law seems ready to excuse physician performance when the physician lacks the requisite skills.[17] The balance of power, however, seems to shift toward the patient when the physician is either physically capable of providing the treatment requested by the grantor of consent or the treatment has already been employed. The physician who was treating Elizabeth Bouvia was ordered not to decrease her morphine dosing simply because the physician was of the opinion that it was no longer medically indicated.[29]

In another case physicians sought permission from her husband-guardian to discontinue medically futile life-sustaining treatment for an elderly woman in a persistent vegetative state.[30] He adamantly refused, so the physicians petitioned the court to replace the husband as guardian; the court determined the husband was the most appropriate guardian of his wife's interests and thus de facto allowed the treatment to continue for whatever subjective reasons were important to the husband. For some reason the anencephalic *Baby K* was intubated at birth; her mother successfully fought to maintain the right to have her infant reintubated as needed for respiratory failure.[31] Despite the apparent willingness of the physicians caring for *Baby L* to refuse to reintubate the child, the court signaled its intention to order the resumption of mechanical ventilation (the case is legally moot because another provider agreed to provide the care sought by the parents).[32] These cases have been discussed as examples of the failure of the futility argument employed by the treating physicians. The reality is that these cases are also powerful examples of a strong judicial prejudice against stopping prior or currently provided medical treatment that surrogate decision makers have requested to be continued on largely subjective grounds. Paris and Schreiber make a compelling argument that "it is now time for physicians to reassert the role of clinical judgment in treatment decisions."[28] To that argument should be added the caveat that there is a subtle inference in the case law that such a position stands a better chance of surviving a legal challenge if the treatment in question has never been employed for the particular patient.

In summary, the doctrine of informed consent appears to have asked American physicians to become educators of patients as well as healers. The physician is expected to offer a sufficient amount of current factual knowledge at a level of comprehension appropriate to the patient's ability to understand. In return, a competent person 18 years of age or greater is entitled to reflect on this objective information and consider any subjective values he or she may wish to attach to this information. The patient then has the right either to consent to a proposed medical or surgical treatment plan, to choose a medically feasible alternative treatment that may not be the physician's first choice, to choose not to treat his or her condition at all at this time, or finally, to decide that he or she lacks sufficient information to make a choice at that particular point in time and express a desire to delay the decision. It must be emphasized that the consent process is not a static event that is necessarily fixed in time. Instead, the transmission of medical information from physician to patient should be considered a fluid process that can be readily updated as new information is obtained.

Exercising the Best Interests of the Child

As it applies to medical issues, the doctrine of exercising the best interests of the child deals substantially with informed consent. There are only two legal differences from the preceding section. The first is a fairly straightforward concept. With the exception of the emancipated minor, children under the age of 18 are considered to lack the capacity to make medical decisions for themselves and the role of surrogate medical decision maker is almost always performed by the parents on behalf of their minor child.[6,17,18] The second difference is easy to articulate but may be extremely difficult to recognize in clinical practice: Once the surrogate has made a decision, the health care provider must determine that this decision is a reasonable one made in the child's best interests.[6,17,18,33] In essence, this added requirement asks the physician to preserve and possibly exercise the state's interest in protecting its minor citizens (*parens patriae*).[34,35] This societal, ethical, and legal expectation that the physician or other member of the health care team make what is essentially a value-laden subjective assessment of the parental decision has a long and tortured history that demands a brief review.

The constitutional law dealing with the allocation of authority between parents and the state to determine the societal expectations of the child's best interests began in 1923.[36] Medical decision making for critically ill infants did not become a national issue until 1982, when an Indiana trial court judge concluded that, after having been informed by their obstetrician, the parents of a newborn (Baby Doe) with trisomy 21 and tracheoesophageal fistula had the right to choose between surgical and medical treatment in the best interests of their child.[6]

The saga of Baby Doe generated an intense public debate in the lay press. The Bioethics Commission supported the legal and ethical reasoning of the judgment but criticized the decision because it felt an infant with trisomy 21 deserved the benefit of surgical intervention for a blocked intestinal tract.[37] The United States Office for Civil Rights viewed the situation as a denial of appropriate medical care to a disabled person[38] and The Department of Health and Human Services published a set of regulations collectively referred to as the Baby Doe rules.[39] A federal appellate court invalidated these rules for a lack of statutory authority.[40] In a related case, the Supreme Court noted that the agency failed to find a single case of discrimination in 49 reported cases that were reviewed prior to the rules being invalidated.[35] The Court also noted that these issues should be left to the discretion of the states.

Congress observed the public discussion and responded to the judicial invalidation of the Baby Doe rules by first holding public hearings and then passing the 1984 Federal Child Abuse Amendments.[6,41] These amendments provided the substantive basis for the Department of Health and Human Services to formulate new Baby Doe rules.[42] They are intended to establish guidelines for the medical treatment of seriously ill newborns. All "medically indicated treatment" was to be provided with three exceptions.[42] The first exception exempts treatment of the irreversibly comatose and the second exempts those treatments that would "merely prolong dying."[42] The third exception allows the physician to withhold treatment that would be "virtually futile in terms of the survival of the infant and [when] the treatment itself . . . would be inhumane."[42] The legislation attempts to shift the decision-making process from a subjective best interests test used by the parents to an objective reasonable medical judgment made by the physician in order to define "medically indicated treatment."[33] Finally, the amendments require that state law be utilized in all cases.[42]

The amendments and the current Baby Doe rules that are based on them envision that all newborns will receive medically indicated treatment at the direction of the treating physician unless the infant's condition qualifies for one of the three exceptions. Furthermore, the official interpretative guidelines appended to the Baby Doe rules state that these medical decisions must be devoid of all quality-of-life considerations.[42] Whereas purporting to require strict objectivity in their interpretation, the 1984 Federal Child Abuse Amendments have been legally dissected and shown by their very language to require intrinsically a subjective quality-of-life analysis in each of the three exceptions.[43] The second set of Baby Doe rules and the amendments that support them have never been tested in a courtroom[33] (search updated March 18, 1998). Unfortunately, their passage and publication did confuse and alter the clinical practice of many neonatologists.[44] Because the 1984 Federal Child Abuse Amendments do require the application of state law, it is instructive to review how state appellate courts have dealt with the issue of medical treatment of critically ill legal minors (the same legal principles apply to any child between birth and 17 years of age) since the Baby Doe rules were first promulgated.

Only decisions that are published in a prescribed manner can shape the common law; this process is almost exclusively the domain of appellate judges. A minimum of eight such cases dealing with medical treatment for critically ill children have been reported since 1984.[45–52] The first six cases all upheld the centuries old common law approach to the relationship of parent and child.[33] In every case parents or their surrogates were allowed to make medical treatment decisions in the best interests of their children. These decisions carefully balanced the child's right to care against the

child's right to refuse care that would not be of much benefit. Subjective values such as quality-of-life issues were clearly allowed to shape the parental determination of the child's best interests. None of these cases allowed the physician to decide what constituted the medically indicated treatment required by the second set of Baby Doe rules.[42] It is only after the parents have made their decision that the law asks the physician to make a determination that given the current clinical condition of the patient, the parental decision is a reasonable one which other similarly situated parents might make.[6,17,33] This secondary requirement has its origins in the common law[6] and, as mentioned earlier, has been constitutionally approved in principle by the Supreme Court. It must be noted that in recent years the requirement has found a statutory basis as well. The child abuse and neglect reporting statutes of all 50 states include failure to provide for the medical necessities of a child in their definitions of abuse or neglect.[6,33] The significance of this distinction is that these laws require providers other than just the physician to report suspected instances of medical abuse or neglect. One court noted the potential benefit of utilizing an ethics committee to resolve conflict between parents and doctors when there was a lack of consensus on the appropriate course of action, but pointedly noted also that an ethics committee consultation was not a legal requirement.[50] The judiciary somewhat reluctantly holds itself to be the final arbiter of the child's best interests when parent and medical providers cannot agree.[17,50]

The seventh case[51] is consistent with the legal reasoning of the first six but adds its own unique requirement to the common law. It deals with the elective withdrawal of either a terminally ill or a clinically dead newborn from life-sustaining medical treatment (LSMT). The family claimed a lack of informed consent to the withdrawal; the defendant physician sought summary judgment, arguing that the infant was "clinically dead" and that he had obtained parental consent to withdraw LSMT.[51] The trial court issued a directed verdict in favor of the doctor because the child was near death despite the doctor's actions and the parent appealed. The appellate court noted the presence of conflicting evidence with respect to the issue of informed consent and the time of death (nurse's notes recorded a heart rate 40 min after the physician declared the infant to be dead). The court wrote that the physician "had no right to decide, unilaterally, to discontinue medical treatment even if, as the record in this case reflects, the child was terminally ill and in the process of dying. That decision must be made with the consent of the parents."[51] The appeals court ordered the matter to a full trial so that a jury might hear the evidence and determine the facts. The appeals court essentially conceptualized the LSMT much like any other treatment modality and found that permission was required to terminate the treatment. The eighth and most recent case[52] upheld a hospital's right to remove a brain-dead infant from life support over the parent's objections. It is not clear upon what grounds the anesthesiologist father and attorney mother objected. The case can be read as judicial support for the argument of absolute physiologic futility; i.e., there is no requirement to continue treatment that has absolutely no objective physiologic chance of improving the patient's condition.

In summary, the current legal approach to determining both how and when to provide medical treatment for a critically ill newborn is governed by our common law as applied by state courts with a rare exception.[31,35,40] These outer boundaries of our medical and ethical behavior ask that we first provide parents or their surrogates with accurate medical information on which they may make what they consider to be a reasonable decision. The sufficiency of the amount of information required is determined initially by the parents.[53] They are allowed to consider subjective issues such as the infant's potential quality of life and how they will manage to care for this child in determining their child's best interest. Once they have made their decision, the health care provider has the obligation to represent societal interests by secondarily determining whether the parents have made a reasonable decision.[6,35] It appears that Judge Baker's original 1982 Baby Doe order is still valid law. Society is also likely still to be split on the reasonableness of a parental decision not to attempt surgical repair of a tracheoesophageal fistula in a child with trisomy 21.

Maternal Autonomy and Maternal–Fetal Conflict of Interests

The physician whose practice includes the management of pregnancy in most instances is in the unique position of shepherding the interest of two patients before the completion of the pregnancy. The clinician's concept of when the developing fetus has become an individual patient with its own medical treatment options may be influenced by the physician's level of training and experience.[54] The concept of fetus as patient is also rooted in ethical considerations that may influence the individual clinician's approach to pregnancy management as the gestation progresses.[8,54] A recent review discusses several potential and actual medical and surgical treatments for the developing fetus.[55] Intrauterine fetal aortic balloon valvuloplasty has also been reported.[56,57] There is, however, usually very little discussion or thought given to the fetus as patient in actual clinical practice for two reasons. First, the interests of mother and fetus are frequently identical and the appropriate medical treatment is therefore presumed.[7] The second reason is the observed tendency of many gravid women to assign the interests of their fetuses a higher priority than their own by accepting a higher degree of risk for themselves in order to benefit the interests of their fetuses.[58] Apparent maternal-fetal conflict therefore only arises when the best interests of mother and fetus become either objectively or subjectively not synonymous. This rare conflict generally occurs in only two clinical settings. The first situation develops when a pregnant woman has a complicating medical condition and articulates an informed autonomous treatment choice for her benefit that is felt by her physician to be inconsistent with the best interests of her fetus. The woman may be making her decision on the basis of objective information supplied by her physician or other sources, or she may be basing her decision on some subjective values that make her decision more difficult for the physician to accept and hence is perceived as conflict. The second situation occurs when the mother's health is fine, but the astute physician recognizes a fetal problem and proposes a treatment plan that would benefit the fetal patient (ethical beneficence)[8,54] but poses some degree of risk to the mother. The conflict arises when the woman has assessed these risks to her well-being and subsequently rejects the proposed treatment plan to benefit the fetal patient. These two situations can occur in any of the three discrete areas of maternal-fetal conflict currently recognized by the law[7]: employment choices, lifestyle choices, and health care choices made by pregnant women. The following discussion is limited to conflicts that arise in the course of making health care choices.

This is one of those areas mentioned earlier where legal and ethical reasoning can become divergent. Ethicists may pose the fundamental question as to when and under what circumstances should the gravid woman be allowed to make an autonomous choice that is not consistent with the best interests of her fetus.[8,54] Legal scholars are more likely to ask when—if ever—and under what circumstances is the gravid woman's physician allowed to become an advocate for the well-being of her fetus by subjugating maternal interests for those of the fetus.[7] As noted earlier, the law in this country has been slowly leading the discipline of ethics to accept autonomy as a guiding principle by granting it the legal status of an almost absolute personal right. In addition to formulating this overreaching principle, courts have been advised to avoid being pulled into "apparent but false conflicts between the interests of the pregnant woman and the interests of the fetus."[7] "False conflicts" are characterized as those that occur when a pregnant patient and her physician differ in their opinions of the fetal best interests.[7] Some alleged maternal-fetal conflicts have been viewed as "merely" an assertion of power by physicians over patients.[7] Most of the case law that has actually tried to balance the interests of mother and fetus is derived either from blood transfusion cases[59] (pregnant woman refuses a transfusion to save her life and the life of the fetus) or coerced cesarean sections[60] (pregnant woman refuses to consent for cesarean delivery arguably necessary to safeguard either her health or the life or health of her fetus). Although these earlier cases held for physician-recommended treatment over the mother's wishes, more recent cases have favored a requirement that the pregnant woman give a truly voluntary informed consent.[58] As a result, the legal scholarship in the United States is currently divided into majority and minority positions on this issue. Regardless of which position a legal scholar may choose, both positions agree that before a judge can order medical treatment on behalf of a fetus against the wishes of the mother, the judge absolutely must find that there is a legal reason on which to base the order.[7]

The prevailing majority position holds that the interests of the pregnant woman always prevail and therefore there is never any need to balance the competing interest of the woman and her fetus. A respected authority recently noted several legal theories supporting this position.[7] The first and most compelling argument is based on a theory of constitutional rights. It is noted that the pregnant woman does not give up any of her rights simply by becoming pregnant.[61] If truly voluntary informed consent is required from a nonpregnant woman before undergoing a medical treatment or surgery, then the pregnant woman should similarly be free to grant or refuse consent for the same treatment or procedure. Although the second reason given in support of strict maternal autonomy is stated in legal terms, ethicists should recognize a familiar theme. Simply stated, there is no legal (or ethical) theory that can (or should) force a person to undergo medical treatment with some degree of detriment solely for the benefit of another person.[62] For example, a tissue-compatible parent cannot be forced to donate a kidney to benefit his or her own child in renal failure. It is therefore reasoned that "there can be no greater legal obligations on pregnant women to serve the interest of their fetuses than there are on parents to serve the interests of their already-born children."[7] Third, there are cases in which the treating physicians testified that a cesarean section was required to safeguard the health of the fetus or mother and a subsequent vaginal delivery has proved them wrong.[63] Judges have noticed these results and are understandably skeptical of the objectivity of physician testimony. Fourth, the judiciary is aware that the medical circumstances of these cases often require an immediate hearing. Under these circumstances there will be legitimate concern that the pregnant woman will not have sufficient time to obtain and instruct counsel, the court will not have time to appoint a guardian ad litem for the fetus, and there will not be enough time

for expert witnesses other than the treating physician to become familiar with the case.[7,63] A fifth reason given to support judicial noninvolvement is really a matter of societal interest in public health. The American Public Health Association has pointed out that the threat of legal intervention adversely affects the physician-patient relationship and discourages some pregnant women from seeking care.[7] Finally, judges realize that there is no adequate method available to carry out court-ordered treatment against the mother's wishes.[7,58]

The minority position contends that the state's interest in preserving the health of children requires judges to balance the pregnant woman's interests against the interests of her fetus in being born as healthy as possible.[7] Bioethicists have attempted to articulate a source of ethical authority in support of fetal interests.[8,54,63] However, physicians who may in certain clinical settings feel strongly about intervening on behalf of the fetus are reminded that for a court to order such intervention on behalf of the fetus, it must find that the pregnant woman has a legal obligation to support the best interests of her fetus. Legal theory for finding this maternal obligation has begun to be found not in the doctrine governing maternal–fetal conflict in health care decisions, but in the somewhat parallel doctrine of maternal-fetal conflicts that arise because of maternal lifestyle choices. The South Carolina Supreme Court has upheld the conviction and sentencing of a mother for child abuse for exposing her fetus to cocaine during pregnancy.[64] The court found that South Carolina law would include a viable fetus in the category of children in need of protection (this case is not final pending appeal). A Wisconsin appellate court upheld a trial judge's decision to detain a fetus in a hospital to protect it from its cocaine-abusing mother, but the Wisconsin Supreme Court has recently overturned that decision[65] on the grounds that while *Roe v. Wade*[66] and *Casey*[67] do indeed establish the state's interest in the viable fetus, the state is still required to evidence that interest. The trial judge had initially established jurisdiction to hear the case on the grounds that the viable fetus was a child that could be protected under the child abuse and neglect laws of Wisconsin. The Wisconsin Supreme Court held that, since the state legislature had not specifically included the viable fetus in the statutory definition of a child in need of protection, the state had declined to express its interest in protecting the viable fetus.[65]

Other legal arguments for intervening include the fact that the viable fetus is treated as a person for other common law purposes[7] and so, it can be argued, should be treated as a person for purposes of medical decision making. It has also been observed that it is legally inconsistent to hold the physician accountable for damage to the fetal patient that results from maternal therapies and yet denies providers from doing what is necessary to preserve the health of the fetus.[7]

It may be shocking for some readers to consider that behavior which may be personally conceived as immoral and perhaps unethical is not necessarily also illegal.[7,62] Ethicists may be ahead of lawyers in finding justification for physician intervention on behalf of the fetal patient.[8,54,63] Failure of the current legal doctrine governing perceived maternal–fetal conflicts arising in the area of health care decision making to protect the fetus should not dissuade the physician from being an advocate for fetal interests. The doctrine of informed consent has taught us that the parental or maternal choice must be unfettered and that we as physicians cannot coerce our patient's decisions. There is a fine line between coercing what the physician perceives to be a morally or ethically correct decision and objectively telling a woman what the majority of other women in the same or similar circumstances have chosen to do in the past. This information frequently forms the basis of a physician recommendation and may take the form of the "directive counseling" proposed by Chervanak and McCullogh.[8,54] Presuming the physician has demonstrable knowledge of actual facts and the patient does not feel she has been directed to the point of being coerced, then there appears to be nothing that legally prohibits the physician from informing the patient of what the majority of other similarly situated women have chosen in the past. Finally, the physician must remember that *Roe v. Wade* established the state's interest in protecting the potential human life of the fetus.[66] The trimester analysis of *Roe* has been replaced by the *Casey* requirement that the fetus must only be viable for the state's interest to materialize.[67] This state interest seems to rebut the very logically crafted constitutional arguments presented earlier in this discussion. It is conceivable that the judiciary has yet to hear a case where the maternal intrusion is sufficiently slight to be outweighed by the fetal benefit.[63]

CURRENT LEGAL ISSUES

With the applicable legal doctrines discussed, it is now appropriate to apply them to the clinical practice of medicine. Four specific areas of conflict between physician and patient–fetal interests have been chosen for discussion. Hypothetical cases are utilized to illustrate the issues. Other areas of conflict can and do arise during pregnancy, but they do not relate directly to congenital heart disease.

Antenatal Assessment Issues

Several issues may arise when the physician is providing either preconceptual counseling or antenatal assessment for the gravid patient. Suppose the combination of history and screening tests indicate a risk of genetically related heart disease, but the patient refuses chromosomal evaluation. Does the physician incur any liability when the child is born with a defective heart? What steps should the physician undertake when there is a strong risk of congenital heart disease and he or she recommends fetal echocardiography but the patient declines the examination on the grounds that the knowledge gained will not change the outcome of the pregnancy? Finally, presume that the physician is a primary care provider in a capitated managed care system and determines that the gravid patient has become a high-risk pregnancy. Can this physician limit the scope of evaluation by ordering less expensive (and presumably less specific or sensitive) laboratory tests? Must this same physician feel bound by a clause in his or her contract which forbids mentioning to this high-risk patient that an out-of-network maternal–fetal specialist practices in the same local community? Truly informed consent is both the physician's guidepost and the defense for all of the above situations; the answers for the managed care scenario are aided by a recent federal decision.

The first scenario deals with the informed refusal of consent to a laboratory test or procedure to determine the risk of congenital disease.[23,24] As long as the physician documents in the medical record the facts that were given to the patient, the risks and benefits of the proposed testing, the opportunity of the patient to ask questions, and the reason given by the patient for the refusal, then the physician should have a more than adequate defense if he or she is later sued for failing to inform the parent(s) adequately. In the second scenario, the patient who refuses the fetal echocardiography on the grounds that the knowledge will not change the outcome of the pregnancy is probably not fully informed in making this refusal. It should be pointed out to the patient that despite the fact that she may have no immediate need for the information, it can be of tremendous help to the neonatologist in planning appropriate medical care in the infant's best interests. For example, if hypoplastic left heart syndrome is suspected, the neonatologist could begin to make antenatal plans to refer the patient to a transplant center once the diagnosis is confirmed postnatally.

The third scenario presents the difficult and complex relationship between managed care organizations and the doctrine of informed consent. Even if the physician in question has a gag clause in his or her contract, the impact on the practice of medicine still involves informed consent and not, strictly speaking, the tenets of contract law. A recent Eighth Circuit Court opinion dealt directly with these issues.[68] The patient was a gentlemen who presented to his health maintenance organization's (HMO) primary care physician with a positive family history and current signs and symptoms of cardiovascular disease. The primary care physician told the patient that referral to a cardiologist was not necessary. What the physician did not disclose was his financial incentive to make as few as possible covered specialty referrals and the potential penalty for making too many. The man died a few months later of heart failure and his widow sued the HMO for (among other causes of action) failing to disclose the financial arrangements between the physician provider and the HMO. The court agreed that this information should have been provided to the patient so that an informed decision about his health care could have been made. The court held that the HMO had a fiduciary duty to all its plan's participants to disclose any financial incentive that would discourage a physician from making a referral to a specialist. Although the results of this case are only binding in the eighth circuit, it is a federal appellate holding and would likely be viewed with respect in other circuits as well.

Termination as an Option

"During the last quarter of this century, no legal and political issue has so divided the United States as the issue of abortion."[69] Similarly, it is quite possible that the physician or the pregnant patient may have strong feelings about the subject as well. The control of patient access to pregnancy termination has been given to the individual states as long as it does not constitute an undue burden on the woman's right to seek termination.[67] The presumptive diagnosis of severe or life-threatening congenital heart disease may not occur until that portion of the pregnancy when the fetus may be presumed otherwise viable and a particular state may have regulated the patient's access to a termination procedure. Nonetheless, for the sake of discussion let us presume that a physician makes a probable diagnosis of severe or life-threatening congenital heart disease in a fetus and under appropriate state law time remains for the gravid patient to consider and seek termination of the pregnancy as an option. Does the physician have a legal obligation to mention this option? Although this situation is not likely to occur with great frequency, the prudent physician should be prepared both to recognize and to deal with the issues appropriately.

Despite all the recent social upheaval regarding abortion, a woman still has a constitutionally protected right to seek pregnancy termination under various state-based limiting terms and conditions.[67] There is a developing body of negligence tort law that has been termed either "wrongful life"[70] (child is the plaintiff) or "wrongful birth"[71–73] (parents are the plaintiffs). Although many states have taken statutory action to prohibit such cases,[74] the breach of duty in these cases is typically a physician failure to advise the prospective parents of a probable diagnosis and the available treatment options.

The parents argue that if they had been given this information, then they would have either chosen not to conceive or chosen to terminate the pregnancy. It is also clear that the previously discussed doctrine of informed consent requires the physician to discuss all reasonably feasible treatment choices. The answer to the question posed is therefore affirmative; termination is a legally available medical procedure and the physician has an obligation to discuss it as part of the consent process. The physician may inform the patient that he or she is personally opposed to the procedure and, if the patient chooses this treatment option, then the physician will fulfill his or her obligations to the patient by referral to an appropriate physician, institution, or state where the procedure may be performed. As a practical matter, even if the physician has reason to believe that the patient disfavors termination and will refuse this treatment option, the prudent physician will still discuss this option and note the patient's refusal in the medical record in order to protect against any subjective memory loss on the part of the patient with the passage of time.

Potential Maternal–Fetal Conflicts

Let us presume a hypothetical fetus that has by accurate dating reached 33 weeks' gestation and in whom a provisional diagnosis of complex congenital heart disease has been made. Let us presume also that the mother's medical course throughout the pregnancy has been totally unremarkable and that she herself has no current medical complications. The obstetrician has strongly recommended premature operative delivery because the infant is becoming hydropic and there is a chance of surgical intervention benefiting the infant. The prospective parents listen to the medical facts as well as the risk and benefit analysis on which the obstetrician makes this recommendation but choose instead to wait for a spontaneous vaginal delivery at some later time. They acknowledge their understanding that their infant is likely not to survive to be born alive if they wait for spontaneous onset of labor at term. Should the obstetrician consult the hospital ethics committee? Would it help if a neonatologist spoke with the parents?

Conversely, let us presume a 26-week fetus with complex but stable congenital heart disease. In this hypothetical case the mother has a complicating chronic medical condition that is now exacerbating to the point of seriously threatening the mother's life if the pregnancy is allowed to continue. The obstetrician has objectively informed the parent of the fetal condition and that, if delivered now, the infant's premature size virtually eliminates any possibility of surgical correction or palliation that can be of any benefit to the baby. The obstetrician tells the parents that there is a 96% chance of operative delivery of the fetus at this time will allow the mother's chronic condition to stabilize and of so being of substantial benefit to the mother. After she has answered the parent's questions, the obstetrician is shocked by the mother's request to continue medical management of her condition and indefinitely postpone operative delivery.

The first scenario presents a situation in which the obstetrician wishes to undertake a course of action based on what he or she feels is in the best interest of the fetus. The informed maternal patient has made a decision for herself regarding the risks of surgical delivery and the parents have jointly made a decision regarding their analysis of their child's best interests based on their values and beliefs. They have rejected the obstetrician's assessment of their infant's best interests and have reasonably determined instead that their child's best interests lie with opting to allow nature to take its course with the potential for a natural fetal demise. In the second case, the parents have also rejected the obstetrician's analysis of the fetal best interests and have determined at least for the time being to risk maternal health by making the fetal interest in survival the primary objective.

Both of these situations could be posed as examples of maternal-fetal conflict. In actuality, there is no real conflict of interest between mother and fetus; the maternal-fetal interests are synonymous. Both sets of parents balanced the maternal interests with the fetal interests and both sets presumably made what they considered to be a loving and reasonable decision to allow the fetal interests to control. It is the obstetrician who may be conflicted by presuming to make a subjective evaluation that is rightfully the mother's or parent's to make.[33] If the physician recommends treatment in the best interests of the mother, he or she is really making a value judgment that either the maternal interests outweigh the fetal interests or it is in the fetus's best interests to die. If the physician proposes intervention on behalf of the fetus, then he or she may be disregarding the subjective values the mother may place on the effects of such intervention on her person. Antenatal maternal consultation with the neonatologist can be of benefit in these high-risk obstetric cases.[53,75] The neonatologist may be better informed than the obstetrician to address specific parental concerns regarding any suffering or other burdens placed on the infant undergoing medical and surgical treatment for various cardiac anomalies. Hospital ethics committees can be a very useful resource for assisting the parties in resolving the issues underlying difficult cases of this nature. Nonetheless, whereas some courts have suggested in nonbinding dicta the usefulness of such ethics committees, there is no legal requirement for a physician to seek or a patient to accept a consultation with such an ethics committee.[50]

Withdrawal of Fetal and Neonatal Life Support

Let us presume that the obstetrician has made a reasonably firm diagnosis of congenital heart disease and other major anomalies in a fetus at 25 weeks' gestation and has so informed the mother. The mother has just presented with ruptured membranes and is in early labor. The infant is in the breech position. The mother has been fully informed of the objective medical facts. She has asked for a vaginal delivery with no intervention on behalf of the fetus in the delivery room. Should her request be honored? If it is honored, how should the labor be monitored? Should the obstetrician simply not notify his or her colleague (pediatrician or neonatologist) who would otherwise be caring for the infant? Is the health care provider who takes charge of this infant at birth obligated to assess the infant's potential viability by including an attempted resuscitation in his or her assessment? Can this infant be allowed to expire in the delivery area, or must it be taken to a neonatal intensive care unit first for a more complete assessment before any determination is made to discontinue LSMT? The answers to these questions depend primarily on the assessment and understanding of four critical factors: (1) To what degree of accuracy can the antenatal diagnoses be relied upon? (2) Presuming the antenatal information is correct, has the mother been given accurate information regarding her infant's mortality and associated morbidities before making this irreversible decision? (3) Who decides how much objective medical information is required to make an irreversible decision? (4) Is the mother's decision a reasonable decision?

In the early years of neonatology, antenatal diagnosis was infrequent and provisional at best. Physicians were trained to resuscitate and stabilize all infants at birth so there would be time to perform tests directly and adequately on the infant and arrive at more accurate diagnoses before making any irreversible decision about the infant's life.[76] With the advent of ultrasonography, fetal echocardiography, fetal chromosomal diagnosis, and myriad other tests with much higher degrees of specificity, the accuracy of prenatal diagnosis has made quantum leaps. Pediatricians, neonatologists, and obstetricians have recently begun to take a more flexible stance regarding resuscitation in the delivery area.[75,77] Although the American Academy of Pediatrics' most recent policy statement still favors a presumption in favor of treatment in the delivery area, both the academy and the American Medical Association support nonintervention at birth if appropriate accurate information is available before delivery.[4,77] There is no legal requirement that the health care provider intubate every infant at birth as part of the assessment.[6]

It should also be noted that there is no legal, ethical, or moral difference between withdrawing LSMT and failing to initiate LSMT.[77] A decision not to monitor a pregnancy, labor, or delivery is really a form of fetal withdrawal of life support and similarly depends not only on the accuracy of the prenatal diagnosis but on the sufficiency (breadth) of information given to the patient (parents) as well.[53] An antenatal consultation with the neonatologist (or pediatrician) who is to care for the infant at birth is most useful for several reasons.[53,75] Based on the maternal history and antenatal testing, the neonatologist can provide site-specific information about the fetal chances for survival and the incidence rates of any comorbidities as well. The neonatologist is also more likely qualified to address the very human parental concerns about any pain and suffering the infant may undergo. If the parents indicate a desire to place limits on the intervention, the neonatologist can help guide them in formulating this desire in the clinical context. For example, most infants can be bag-mask ventilated while the neonatologist does his or her initial assessment either to confirm or to repudiate any antenatal diagnosis in the resuscitation area. If the antenatal diagnosis is confirmed, the neonatologist can report this finding to the mother or father and they will feel much more supported about a decision to not intubate their child. Finally, since the majority of parents ultimately decide to do everything reasonably possible to benefit their infant, the antenatal consultation affords the parents and the neonatologist the opportunity to begin a relationship based on mutual trust.[53]

The third critical factor that must be addressed is usually posed as what quantity of objective factual information is required to support a course of action that is irrevocable once undertaken. The answer is provided not with some clinical measure of recorded facts, but with an understanding of who makes the determination of sufficiency and how they arrive at that determination.[53] Before the ascendancy of patient autonomy in decision making, the recommended ethical approach was to resuscitate the infant and then reassess patient interests and parental desires shortly after birth.[78] Unfortunately, this most often was replaced by the "wait until near-certainty approach"[78] because a health care provider (usually the physician) wanted one more head ultrasound, one more blood gas, one more ventilator change, or some other piece of technological information in an attempt to give the infant another chance before agreeing with an ethically correct but possibly fallible parental request to withdraw LSMT.[79,80] The result has been an outpouring of parental resentment for becoming disenfranchised in the decision-making process.[81] With the recent developments in legal and ethical patient autonomy, it is apparent that the patient who is 18 years of age (or a legally emancipated minor) is clearly empowered to determine solely when he or

she has heard sufficient information on which to make a medical decision.[11] Parents as surrogate decision makers are also legally entitled to make this same determination, but their authority is not as absolute as that of the patient of age.[35] Such parental decisions by law and ethics are always subject to a determination of reasonableness based on the child's best interests.[6,35]

The recognition that a particular mother or set of parents has made a reasonable decision in their individual fetus's or infant's best interests can be extremely difficult for physicians and other health care providers. In contrast, judges and lawyers are quite accustomed to using a conventional, objective, and usually predictable test of reasonability in tort and several other areas of law.[82] This standard simply measures human behavior and choices by what the majority of people would decide in the same or similar circumstances. The standard does not ask for a convincing majority: a simple majority greater than 50% suffices. Law has a much more difficult time making subjective evaluations. Since a portion of the parental decision is based on cultural, social, and other subjective familial values, the objective legal test of reasonability frequently fails application in this area of legal medicine. For this reason judges dislike hearing these cases and most often rely on a presumption that the parents know what is best for their child unless the physician can convincingly demonstrate the contrary.[35] This is the same issue a physician must face when deciding whether or not to comply with an informed parental request to withhold LSMT.[6] The situation is better handled by a physician who understands the family's value systems well and can, it is hoped, recognize when he or she is allowing his or her own values to be projected on the family's ("if this were my baby, I would . . . "). In judging such a parental request, the physician should consider the mortality rate associated with the condition or treatment, the possibility of associated morbidities, the likelihood of any morbidity's being temporary or permanent, and whether or not there is any objectively measured pain and suffering associated with either the condition itself, the treatment, or any morbidities.[33] The physician can reflect on his or her own experience as to whether or not other similarly situated parents have made similar decisions. At this point, if the physician is still having difficulty assessing the reasonableness of the parental request, he or she may ask (but not require[50]) an ethics committee consultation.[37]

The answers to the hypothetical questions posed in this section should now be more easily answered. If the antenatal diagnosis is statistically reliable, the parents have been adequately informed by someone with knowledge of the infant's treatment, and the obstetrician feels they have made a reasonable request in their fetus's best interests, then the request should be granted.

The one question left to be resolved is who should attend the delivery for the baby. Even if the parents request no intervention on behalf of the fetus, prudent physicians should arrange for the presence of someone skilled at neonatal assessment and resuscitation at all deliveries that may be remotely viable in the event that the antenatal diagnosis is wrong or the parents change their mind at delivery.[53,83] Physicians may feel that in certain obstetric emergencies there may not be time to ascertain a mother's wishes with respect to her fetus or infant. The time it takes to tell the person granting consent that you presume she wants everything done for the infant and would she please inform you if her wishes are otherwise is measured in seconds and not minutes. Physicians and ethicists will likely agree that such a limited conversation hardly constitutes informed consent, but lawyers and judges will certainly note that the physician has made the effort to obtain consent and that may be sufficient to protect the physician.[5] There is as yet no appellate case law that deals specifically with physician liability for resuscitating a newborn against express parental wishes to the contrary. However, the jury in *State v. Messenger* rather quickly acquitted a father of a homicide charge for removing his premature infant son from a ventilator after the child had been intubated against the parent's wishes.[53]

Organ Transplantation

Unless the physician is planning to perform surgery on the fetus and return it to the uterus, this discussion to transplant an organ must necessarily bridge the transition from fetus to infant. Presume a diagnosis of hypoplastic left heart syndrome has been made in a fetus at 27 weeks' gestation. The perinatologist who made the diagnosis has referred the parents to a colleague in another institution for a confirmatory opinion. Once the diagnosis has been independently confirmed, the treating physician assists the parents in making contact with numerous physicians at multiple children's centers with recognized expertise in both the Norwood procedure and neonatal cardiac transplantation. The parents request and are granted a consultation by the hospital ethics committee. The parents request and are granted a meeting with the entire Division of Neonatology (four physicians) for the purpose of ascertaining their collective experiences in dealing with these infants both medically and postoperatively. Before the onset of labor, the parents announce that they wish a neonatologist to stabilize the infant at birth and obtain an echocardiogram on the baby to confirm the antenatal diagnosis. If the diagnosis of hypoplastic left heart syndrome is indeed confirmed, then they wish only to feed and care for their infant like any other parents for such time as the baby lives. Have these parents made a reasonable decision in their infant's best interest? Have the surgi-

cal outcomes for either the Norwood procedure or neonatal cardiac transplantation progressed to become sufficiently good and predictable to outweigh a parental decision not to intervene surgically?

Surgical intervention for hypoplastic left heart syndrome requires the patient to achieve an adequate systemic perfusion quickly, a pulmonary blood flow in the normal range, and relief of pulmonary venous obstruction to flow; the ultimate goal is separation of the systemic and pulmonary circuits.[84] Although many procedures have been attempted in the past, the two operations currently being utilized with the most success are staged reconstruction[85,86] (the Norwood procedure) and orthotopic neonatal cardiac allotransplantation.[87] For the physician who is treating this infant to reach some conclusion about the reasonableness of the hypothetical parent's decision, the physician must ethically and legally be aware of current outcomes for the surgical interventions that these parents have declined.[6,25,80] Current results of each of the two surgical interventions can be discussed separately because of the major differences between each approach. Before this is done, it should be noted that the approaches share one common feature: it has proved difficult to ascertain the number of infants who die while being stabilized and transported to the various centers that have reported their outcomes. This preselection bias is worth noting not only for the fact that it tends to eliminate the worst surgical risks, but also because this unknown bias may theoretically be modified by arranging to have the birth of a fetus with a surgically correctable cardiac defect occur in a center with a neonatal cardiac surgical program.

The first procedure in staged reconstruction is designed to create a univentricular heart with a single great vessel and simultaneously a systemic to pulmonary artery shunt.[84–86] Infants who survive the medical and surgical (shunt or coarctation repairs) morbidities typically undergo a second-stage superior vena cava to pulmonary artery anastomosis (bidirectional Glenn or hemi-Fontan) at 6 to 18 months of age. Those who survive undergo a third-stage repair that consists of an inferior vena cava to pulmonary artery anastomosis with creation of an intraatrial baffle (Fontan procedure) at a later date—typically at 13 to 30 months of age. Bove and Lloyd recently reported on 158 consecutive patients undergoing first-stage reconstruction with the Norwood procedure.[85] They categorized 127 patients as standard risk and 31 patients as high risk. Hospital survival (alive at discharge) for the first stage in the standard-risk group was 86%, and it was 42% in the high-risk group, with an overall survival of 76%. Of the original 158 patients, 106 have met the clinical criteria for and have received a second-stage hemi-Fontan; this group's hospital survival rate has been 97%. Of these patients, 62 have lived long enough to meet the clinical criteria for the Fontan procedure; their postoperative hospital survival rate was 86%. This series reports significant or potentially significant morbidity in 25 of 120 hospital survivors (21%) following the first-stage repair. There was one late death and three complications that precluded consideration for the Fontan procedure following the hemi-Fontan surgery. One late death is reported in the group that underwent the Fontan procedure. The reported 5-year actuarial survival was 69 ± 8% for patients with typical anatomy and standard risk, 71 ± 17% for standard-risk patients with variant anatomy, and 58 ± 9% for the entire cohort. Bando et al.[86] have reported an overall first-stage survival of 50% in 34 patients but have identified a subgroup of more recent cases with a survival of 75%. In the group of 17 stage 1 survivors, there was one late death and two infants who underwent transplantation because of tricuspid regurgitation. Ten of the remaining 14 patients have progressed to requiring a stage 2 procedure. Three of these 10 patients underwent coarctation repair before the second-stage procedure; all 10 survived the second-stage repair. Seven of these 10 patients have met the criteria for a third-stage Fontan procedure; all 7 survived the surgery. The more frequently reported morbidities of staged repair include thromboembolic stroke, developmental delay, dysrhythmia requiring either permanent pacemaker or chronic medications, chronic pleural effusions, hemidiaphragm paralysis, and medical management of the balance between good ventricular function and low pulmonary vascular resistance.[85,86] Survival at 10 years in patients undergoing the Fontan procedure alone has been reported to be 60%; only 43% of these survivors have been able to exercise at their peer level.[88]

Cardiac transplantation requires only one surgical procedure but presents a markedly different postoperative medical management. Razzouk et al.[87] have reported on 190 infants registered for transplantation with hypoplastic left heart syndrome. Fourteen infants (7%) were unlisted because of medical contraindications or parental request. Of the remaining 176 patients, 34 (19%) died while waiting for a donor. In this group of 176 patients there were 13 early and 22 late deaths. The reported actuarial 7-year survival is 70%, but the actual survival for the entire study group can be calculated (107/176) to be 61%. This number would be lower if the 7 patients who were initially registered but became unlisted for medical reasons were counted (58%). Bando et al.[86] have reported a 1-year survival of 77% in 17 infants who underwent transplantation for hypoplastic left heart syndrome. There were two postoperative deaths and three late deaths, yielding a survival rate of 71% at the time of publication. Whereas some complications such as seizures, developmental delay, and renovascular complications may be related to the surgical procedure, a significant postsurgical problem is the management of rejection with immunosuppression and the techniques available to recognize rejection safely and accurately in an infant.[87,89,90] These patients are at risk of developing graft rejection and graft vasculopathy in the coronary arteries,[87,89,90] infection (50% in the first year[87]), lymphoproliferative disease (rare[87]), and altered renal function (hypertension in 18.7%[87]). Sudden death secondary to coronary artery disease has been reported.[87,89] Infants and children, in distinction from adults, must grow and develop. Although the effects of long-term immunosuppression on maturation are suggested,[87,91] they are not well quantified.

If the reasonableness of the hypothetical parental decision is to be measured solely by the objective criteria of survival with the previously described tort definition as the yardstick, then the parents have made an unreasonable decision that is not in their infant's best interests because short- to intermediate-term surgical intervention survival has apparently surpassed the 50% legal requirement. Physicians who are faced with a truly unreasonable parental decision get the chance to explain why it is unreasonable when they seek permission for surgery from a judge.[6] The reality is that survival is not the only measure to be taken. Parents are allowed and are arguably obligated to consider the various surgical and medical complications in the context of any familial value systems in their attempt to discern what is best for their child.[35,37] The pain and suffering that a child undergoes with either surgical procedure is real and must be weighed in the balance. Parents must be told that in contrast to some other surgical procedures, neither staged reconstruction or transplantation restores normal organ function.[91] Parents must be informed that their child will most likely have exercise intolerance, a less than normal life span, and the risk of significant but not as well quantified serious complications. Physicians who minimize these complications and outcomes in discussing options with parents run the very real risk of losing a suit for either failing to obtain adequate informed consent or for coercion of the consent.[25]

Fortunately, most physicians agree with judges that the law rarely has a place in these decisions. Based on these considerations and the knowledge that many parents in similar circumstances have chosen compassionate medical care as the surgical alternative, it cannot be said that the parents in the hypothetical case have made an unreasonable decision.[91] Finally, whereas the hypothetical case scenario was derived almost entirely from a real clinical experience, it must be noted that few parents go to the extremes to which this family did to reach their decision.

SUMMARY

Our legal system attempts to set the outer boundaries within which physicians and their patients are left to make ethically appropriate and medically intelligent choices. United States legal doctrines that govern informed consent, parents as guardians of their children's best interests, and real or perceived maternal–fetal conflicts in relation to maternal autonomy are first reviewed. They are then applied to clinical medicine in an attempt to solve issues that can arise in the areas of antenatal assessment, termination as an option, potential maternal–fetal conflicts, and neonatal treatment options regarding cardiac transplantation.

REFERENCES

1. Stoner JR: *Common Law and Liberal Theory: Coke, Hobbes, and the Origins of American Constitutionalism*. Lawrence, KA: University Press of Kansas; 1992.
2. Furrow BR, Greaney TL, Johnson SH, et al. (Eds.): *Health Law*. St. Paul, MN: West Publishing Company; 1995.
3. Beauchamp TL, Childress JF: *Principles of Biomedical Ethics*, 4th ed. New York: Oxford University Press; 1994.
4. Council on Ethical and Judicial Affairs, American Medical Association: *Code of Medical Ethics: Current Opinions*, 8th ed. Chicago: American Medical Association; 1994.
5. The liability of health care professionals. In: Furrow BR, Greaney TL, Johnson SH, et al., eds. *Health Law*. St. Paul, MN: West Publishing Company; 1995.
6. Clark FI: Withdrawal of life-support in the newborn: Whose baby is it? *Southwest Law Rev.* 23:1–46, 1993.
7. Potential fetal-maternal conflicts. In: Furrow BR, Greaney TL, Johnson SH, et al., eds. *Health Law*. St. Paul, MN: West Publishing Company; 1995.
8. Chervenak FA, McCullough LB: The fetus as patient: An essential ethical concept for maternal-fetal medicine. *J Matern Fetal Med.* 5:115, 1996.
9. *Schloendorff v. Society of the New York Hospital:* 105 N.E. 92 (1914).
10. President's Commission for the Study of Ethical Problems in Medicine and Biomedical and Behavioral Research: *Deciding To Forego Life-Sustaining Treatment*. Washington, DC: U.S. Government Printing Office; 1983.
11. *Cruzan v. Director:* 497 U.S. 261, 1990.
12. Clark FI: Informed consent in Missouri: Where has it taken us? *Missouri Med.* 91:72, 1994.
13. McNeil BJ, Paucker SG, Sox HC, et al.: On the elicitation of preferences for alternative therapies. *N Engl J Med.* 306:1259, 1982.
14. Brock DW, Wartman SA: When competent patients make irrational choices. *N Engl J Med.* 322:1595, 1990.
15. King NMP: Transparency in neonatal intensive care. *Hastings Cent Rep.* 22:18, 1992.
16. Jellinek MS, Catlin EA, Todres ID, et al.: Facing tragic decisions with parents in the neonatal intensive care unit: Clinical perspectives. *J Pediatr.* 89:119, 1992.
17. Making decisions about death and dying. In: Furrow BR, Greaney TL, Johnson SH, et al., eds. *Health Law*. St. Paul, MN: West Publishing Company; 1995.
18. Medical treatment of the child: Who speaks for the child? In Mnookin RH, Weisberg DK, eds. *Child, Family and State*, 2nd ed. Boston: Little, Brown; 1989.
19. *Canterbury v. Spence:* 454 F. 2d 772 (D.C. Cir. 1972) cert. denied, 409 U.S. 1064.
20. *Logan v. Greenwich Hospital Association:* 465 A. 2d 294 (Conn. 1983).
21. *Harbeson v. Parke Davis:* 746 F. 2d 517 (9th Cir. 1984).
22. *Moore v. Baker:* 989 F. 2d 1129 (11th Cir. 1993).
23. *Truman v. Thomas:* 611 P. 2d 902 (Cal. 1980).
24. *Phillips v. Hull:* 516 So. 2d 488 (Miss. 1987).
25. Bursztajn HJ, Saunders LS, Brodsky A: Medical negligence and informed consent in the managed care era. *Health Lawy.* 9(5):14, 1997.
26. *Moore v. Regents of the University of California:* 793 P.2d. 479 (Cal. 1990), cert. denied, 499 U.S. 936.
27. *Estrada v. Jaques:* 321 S.E.2d 240 (N.C. App. 1984).
28. Paris JJ, Schreiber MD. Physician's refusal to provide life-prolonging medical interventions. *Clin Perinatol.* 23(3):563, 1996.
29. *Bouvia v. Superior Court:* 225 Cal. Rptr. 297.
30. *In Re Wanglie:* No. PX-91-283 (Minn. D. Ct. June 28, 1991).
31. *In the Matter of Baby "K":* 16 F.3d 590 (4th Cir. 1994).
32. Paris JJ, Crone RK, Reardon FE: Physicians' refusal of requested treatment: The case of baby L. *N Engl J Med.* 322:1012–1015, 1990.
33. Clark FI: Intensive care treatment decisions: The roots of our confusion. *Pediatrics.* 94:98, 1994.
34. The child, the family and the state. In: Mnookin RH, Weisberg DK, eds. *Child, Family and State*, 2nd ed. Boston: Little, Brown; 1989.
35. *Bowen v. American Hospital Association:* 476 U.S. 610 (1986).
36. *Meyer v. Nebraska:* 262 U.S. 340 (1923).
37. Seriously ill newborns. In: President's Commission for the Study of Ethical Problems in Medicine and Biomedical and Behavioral Research, eds. *Deciding to Forego Life-Sustaining Treatment*. Washington, DC: U.S. Government Printing Office; 1983.
38. Discriminating against the handicapped by withholding treatment or nourishment; Notice to health care providers. *Fed Reg.* 47:26,027, 1982.
39. Nondiscrimination on the basis of handicap. *Fed Reg.* 48:9630, 1983.
40. *American Academy of Pediatrics v. Heckler,* F. [Suppl.] 561:395 (D.C. Cir. 1983).
41. Pub. L. No. 98–457, 98 Stat. 1749.
42. Child abuse and neglect prevention and treatment. 45 C.F.R. Part 1340 (1992).
43. Rhoden NK: Treatment dilemmas for imperiled newborns: Why quality of life counts. *S. Cal. Law Rev.* 58:1285, 1985.
44. Kopelman LM, Irons TG, Kopelman AE: Neonatologists judge the "Baby Doe" rules. *N Engl J Med.* 318:667, 1988.
45. *In re Barry:* 445 So.2d 365 (Fla. Dist. Ct. App. 1984).
46. *In re LHR:* 321 S.E.2d 716 (Sup. Ct. Ga. 1984).
47. *In re Crum:* 580 N.E.2d 876 (Prob. Ct. Franklin Co. 1991).
48. *Care and Protection of Beth:* 587 N.E.2d 1377 (Sup. Jud. Ct. Mass. 1992).
49. *In re CA:* 603 N.E.2d 1171 (Ill. App. 4d 1992).
50. *In re Joelle Rosebush:* 491 N.W.2d 633 (Mich. App. 1992).

51. *Velez v. Bethune*: 466 S.E.2d (Ga. App. 1995).
52. *Long Island Jewish Medical Center v. Baby Doe*, 641 N.Y.S.2d 989 (1996).
53. Clark FI: Making sense of *State v. Messenger. Pediatrics.* 97:579, 1996.
54. Chervenak FA, McCollough LB: The fetus as patient: Implications for directive versus nondirective counseling for fetal benefit. *Fetal Diagn Ther.* 6:93, 1991.
55. Flake AW, Harrison MR: Fetal therapy: Medical and surgical approaches. In: Creasy RK, Resnik R, eds. *Maternal Fetal Medicine: Principles and Practice*, 3rd ed. Philadelphia: WB Saunders; 1994.
56. Maxwell D, Allan L, Tynan MJ: Balloon dilitation of the aortic valve in the fetus; A report of two cases. *Br Heart J.* 65:256, 1991.
57. Allan LD, Maxwell DJ, Carminati M, et al.: Survival after fetal aortic balloon valvuloplasty. *Ultrasound Obstet Gynecol.* 5:90, 1995.
58. *In re A.C.*: 573 A.2d 1235 (D.C. App. 1990).
59. *In re Application of Jamaica Hospital*: 491 N.Y.S.2d 898, (N.Y. Sup. 1985).
60. *Jefferson v. Griffing Spalding County Hospital Authority:* 274 S.E.2d 457 (Ga. 1981).
61. *Matter of Fletcher*: 533 N.Y.S.2d 241 (N.Y. Fam. Ct. 1988).
62. *McFall v. Shimp*: 10 Pa.D. & C.3d 90 (Allegheny County Ct. 1978).
63. Fletcher J: Drawing moral lines in fetal therapy. *Clin Obstet Gynecol.* 29:595, 1986.
64. *Whitner v. State of South Carolina*: Op. No. 24468, 1996 (S.C. 1996) LEXIS 120.
65. *State of Wisconsin ex. rel. Angela M.W.*: 561 N.W.2d 729 (Wis. 1997).
66. *Roe v. Wade*: 410 U.S. 113 (1973).
67. *Planned Parenthood of Southeastern Pennsylvania v. Casey*, 505 U.S. 833 (1992).
68. *Shea v. Esensten*: 107 F.3d 625 (8th Cir. 1997).
69. Abortion. In: Furrow BR, Greaney TL, Johnson SH, et al., eds. *Health Law.* St. Paul, MN. West Publishing Company; 1995.
70. *Turpin v. Sortini*: 643 P.2d 954 (Cal. 1982).
71. *Becker v. Schwartz*: 386 N.E.2d 807 (N.Y. 1978).
72. *James G. v. Caserta*: 332 S.E.2d 872 (W.Va. 1985).
73. *Smith v. Cote*: 512 A.2d 341 (N.H. 1985).
74. Wrongful birth, wrongful life and wrongful conception. In: Furrow BR, Greaney TL, Johnson SH, et al., eds. *Health Law.* St. Paul, MN: West Publishing Company; 1995.
75. Committee on Fetus and Newborn, American Academy of Pediatrics and Committee on Obstetric Practice, American College of Obstetrics and Gynecology: Perinatal care at the threshold of viability. *Pediatrics.* 96:974, 1995.
76. Caplan A, Cohen CB (Eds.): Hastings Center project: Imperiled newborns. *Hastings Cent Rep.* 17:5, 1987.
77. Committee on Bioethics, American Academy of Pediatrics: Guidelines on foregoing life-sustaining medical treatment. *Pediatrics.* 93:532, 1994.
78. Phoden NK: Treating Baby Doe: The ethics of uncertainty. *Hastings Cent Rep.* 16:34, 1987.
79. Paris JJ, Kodish E: Ethical issues. In: Pomerance JJ, Richardson CJ, eds. *Neonatology for the Clinician.* Norwalk, CT: Appleton & Lange; 1993.
80. Paris JJ. Schreiber MD: Parental discretion in refusal of treatment for newborns. In: Freed GE, Hageman JR, eds. Ethical dilemmas in the prenatal, perinatal, and neonatal periods. *Clin Perinat.* 23:573, 1996.
81. Harrison H: The principles for family-centered care. *Pediatrics.* 92:643, 1993.
82. Negligence: Standard of conduct. In Keeton WP, Dobbs DB, Keeton RE, et al., eds. *Prosser and Keeton on the Law of Torts*, 5th ed. St. Paul, MN: West Publishing Company; 1984.
83. Fetus and Newborn Committee, Canadian Paediatric Society and Maternal-Fetal Medicine Committee, Society of Obstetricians and Gynaecologists of Canada: Management of the woman with threatened birth of an infant of extremely low gestational age. *Can Med Assoc J.* 151:547, 1994.
84. Beeman SK, Hammon JW: Neonatal left ventricular outflow tract surgery. In: Long WA, ed. *Fetal and Neonatal Cardiology.* Philadelphia: WB Saunders; 1990.
85. Bove EL, Lloyd TR: Staged reconstruction for hypoplastic left heart syndrome: Contemporary results. *Ann Surg.* 224:387, 1996.
86. Bando K, et al.: Surgical management of hypoplastic left heart syndrome. *Ann Thorac Surg.* 62:70, 1996.
87. Razzouk AJ, et al. Transplantation as a primary treatment for hypoplastic left heart syndrome: Intermediate term results. *Ann Thorac Surg.* 62:1, 1996.
88. Driscoll DJ, Offord KP, Feldt RH, et al.: Five to fifteen year follow-up after Fontan operation. *Circulation.* 85:469, 1992.
89. Pahl E, et al.: Coronary arteriosclerosis in pediatric heart transplant survivors: Limitation of long term survival. *J Pediatr.* 116:177, 1990.
90. Braunlin EA, et al.: Coronary artery disease in pediatric cardiac transplant recipients receiving triple-drug immunosuppression. *Circulation.* 84 (suppl III):303, 1991.
91. Zahka KG, Spector M, Hanisch D: Hypoplastic left-heart syndrome: Norwood operation, transplantation, or compassionate care. *Clin Perinatol.* 20:145, 1993.

CHAPTER TWENTY-FOUR

Ethical Issues in Diagnosis and Treatment of Fetal and Neonatal Cardiac Disease

John C. Fletcher, Michelle N. Meyer, and Howard P. Gutgesell

This chapter examines the ethical aspects of clinical decision making surrounding the fetus and neonate, especially as these decisions are related to cardiovascular diseases. Although ethical issues occur in patients of all ages, they tend to be most frequent in the care of the very young and the very old. In this chapter we discuss general ethical concepts with emphasis on how these are relevant in decisions about diagnosis and treatment to the fetus and newborn. Although hopes for treating the fetus with cardiac disease are more than a decade old, only modest attempts have been made in this direction. However, with the development of new techniques in endoscopy and fetal surgery, the prospects for fetal treatment appear to be very promising, thus heightening ethical concerns that have accompanied fetal diagnosis and therapy for several years.

In regard to the fetus, we review the question of when the fetus becomes a patient, the ethics of fetal diagnosis, informed consent for either diagnostic procedures or therapy, and ethical and public policy positions on abortion. In terms of the neonate, we discuss the situations in which parents and physicians have conflicts regarding intensive care for neonates with major cardiac or noncardiac conditions and we explore issues of resource allocation as it pertains to these infants.

FETAL DIAGNOSIS AND TREATMENT

How Does the Fetus Become a Patient?

All clinicians who do medical interventions in pregnancy aimed at aiding the fetus must confront this eth-

ical question: Is the fetus a "patient," thus obligating the respect and protection due to any individual in this role? It is self-evident that the pregnant woman is a patient who requires respect and protection in this role. However, moral argument is needed to explain how the fetus becomes a "patient" or, in fetal and perinatal cardiology research, a patient–subject in a study. Addressing this issue, in turn, begs questions about the moral status of the fetus, the woman's authority over her body, and the proper method of balancing these claims when they compete. Consequently, fetal cardiologists face situations in which the issues of abortion must be directly raised and addressed to the best of their ability. The ethical issues surrounding abortion are complex, and we discuss them more thoroughly in the section, Prenatal Diagnosis and Selective Abortion: Ethics and Public Policy. But because understanding how the fetus becomes a patient is so important to the ethics of fetal cardiology, we touch on this matter briefly at the outset.

Descriptively, the predominant moral tradition in obstetrics has been to recognize the fetus as a patient with moral status that could be independently grounded. A statement of this tradition appears on the opening page of the current edition of William's *Obstetrics:*

> Obstetrics is art and science combined and its practitioners must be concerned simultaneously with the lives of at least two intricately interwoven patients—the mother and her fetus(es). (Cunningham et al., reference 1, p. ix.)

This traditional stance has been challenged by others in the obstetrical field. McCullough and Chervenak,[2] for instance, argue that before viability, fetal moral status "can be established only by the pregnant woman's autonomous decision to confer the status of being a patient" upon the fetus. Our position, argued below, is similar but emphasizes fetal sentience rather than viability. Both arguments are sharply different from a third view, advanced by Squarcia et al.,[3] that the moral status of even the early fetus is equal to that of an independent, adult human being. Again, these differences are best discussed within the larger topic of the ethics of abortion, to which we return below.

Indications for Fetal Echocardiography

The first ethical issue regarding fetal echocardiography is whether to do it at all. The generally accepted indications for fetal echocardiography divide into two groups:

1. Indications based on signs or symptoms in the fetus itself (for example, irregular heart rhythm, polyhydramnios)
2. Indications based on perceived "risk factors" associated with a higher than average chance that the fetus has congenital heart disease (family history of congenital heart disease, maternal medications, etc.)

When performed because of signs of a fetal abnormality, echocardiography is somewhat analogous to diagnostic tests performed postnatally, with one important difference: In most instances, no immediate therapy is feasible. With the exception of antiarrhythmic therapy via the mother for fetal tachycardias, the options for the fetus found to have a cardiovascular disorder are primarily either termination of the pregnancy or delivery at a tertiary care center equipped for postnatal treatment of the abnormality.

When fetal echocardiography is performed because of maternal or other risk factors, the relevant issues are those which apply to screening tests in general: What will be done with the information? Is therapy available? Counseling? Clearly the fact that the study can be performed is not in itself an indication to perform it.

One fetal risk factor for congenital cardiac disease stands apart from all the others from a parental viewpoint: the presence of serious congenital heart disease in a previous sibling. Although maternal illness such as diabetes or systemic lupus erythematosus may be associated with an increased risk of fetal cardiac disease, this is generally not foremost in the parents' minds. However, if a previous sibling has had serious cardiac disease, especially if fatal, reassurance that the new baby's heart is normal is extremely important. In fact, assigning some monetary value to the prospective parents' peace of mind for the remainder of the pregnancy

was one of the few situations in which Danford et al.[4] were able to demonstrate that fetal echocardiography was cost effective.

Informed Consent to Fetal Diagnosis and Treatment

As noted above, fetal cardiac diagnosis and therapy may only be done with the voluntary and informed consent of the pregnant woman. Informed consent is not a one-time "event" of signing a form but a process that occurs over time with significant moral and legal dimensions.[5] An adequate consent process consists of two general elements: (1) information, and (2) consent. These two elements subdivide into: (a) disclosure of risks and benefits, (b) comprehension, (c) voluntariness, and (d) capacity to consent. In the context of a troubled pregnancy, each of these aspects of informed consent is difficult to facilitate, but the voluntariness of consent is perhaps the most vulnerable to anxiety and fear.

The consent process for fetal cardiology begins when information is given to the parents, especially to the woman, about possibilities of fetal diagnosis and treatment. Ideally, the woman's partner's understanding, support, and agreement should be forthcoming, but his consent is not ethically or legally required because of the woman's pivotal moral role: The fetus is growing in and dependent on her body. Assuming that she is a capable decision maker, therefore, diagnosis or treatment can proceed with the woman's voluntary consent alone.

The task of informing the parents and the voluntariness of consent may be more difficult to achieve in fetal therapy than in the situations described in McCullough and Chervenak's[2] excellent discussion of informed consent in general obstetrics and gynecology. The parents may be likely to hear information in a strongly biased way. Strong influences could prevent or weigh against a rational choice. They will have just received results from prenatal diagnosis that the fetus has a cardiac condition. Fetal therapy evokes powerful hopes that may be magnified or even distorted in the prenatal context. Maternal risk, especially to future pregnancies, may appear insignificant. The enthusiasm and metacommunication of the medical team may be influential.

Although a full and clear consent document needs to be developed for fetal diagnosis and treatment, clinicians should place a higher priority on creating and maintaining an optimal verbal process for informed consent. Table 24–1 displays the features of such a process with elements of informed consent. It combines guidelines developed by McCullough and Chervenak[2] with recommendations by Patterson.[6] It also draws on the experience of investigators with the consent process in fetal therapy.[7,8]

The privacy and confidentiality of the parents must be protected as in any other medical context.

TABLE 24–1. PROCESS AND ELEMENTS OF INFORMED CONSENT IN FETAL DIAGNOSIS AND TREATMENT

What Any Good Obstetrician Would Do[a]
To elicit from the pregnant woman what she knows about the fetus' diagnosis, available alternatives, and the prognosis without experimental therapy.
To correct factual errors and incompleteness in her fund of knowledge.
To explain the nature of the fetus' condition and all available alternatives to manage it, including the proposed intervention and doing nothing.
To help her identify her relevant values and beliefs.
To help her, in a nondirective manner, to evaluate the alternatives in terms of those values and beliefs.

Information Elements
Risks to mother and fetus of techniques of prenatal diagnosis and therapy.
Complications associated with diagnostic techniques and therapy.
Inconclusiveness of data to be obtained from fetal samples, if any, to assess condition or disease progression.
Continuation of the pregnancy posttherapy depends only on the woman's decision, within the limits of state law on midtrimester abortion.
The experimental status of particular therapies.
Fetal–maternal monitoring is necessary to detect early signs of maternal or fetal distress and for intervention.

Experience in Fetal Therapy[b]
Involvement of other family members, especially the father, in decision making.
An impartial physician, uninvolved in the fetal medicine team, who can "speak for" the fetus.
The mother's own physician, available, at least by telephone, to help her reflect on the risks to her, especially if surgery is involved.
Ethics consultation, on request, by physicians or parents.
Psychiatric consultation, on request by physician, if marital problems or other emotional issues complicate the decision making.
A genetic counselor to promote understanding of the pattern of inheritance and the risks of recurrence.

[a]Reprinted, with permission, from McCullough LB, Chervenack FA. Ethics in Obstetrics and Gynecology. *New York: Oxford University Press; 1994.*

[b]Adapted, with permission, from Harrison MR, et al. Fetal treatment. N Engl J Med: *1982; 307:1651; and Fletcher JC, Jonsen AR: Ethical considerations in fetal therapy. In Harrison MR, Golbus MS, Filly RA, eds.* Unborn Patient, *2nd ed. Orlando, FL: Grune & Stratton; 1990: 163–4.*

PRENATAL DIAGNOSIS AND SELECTIVE ABORTION: ETHICS AND PUBLIC POLICY

Discussing abortion in the context of the ethics of fetal cardiology is important for at least two reasons. First, as we noted at the opening of this chapter, moral argument is required to show when and why the fetus becomes a patient. Both this argument and any argument for or against abortion are species of a larger category of arguments about moral status and personhood. Second, as we mentioned in our discussion of indications for fetal echocardiography, with few exceptions, there is little that can be done for a fetus who shows signs of cardiac abnormality. Selective abortion thus becomes highlighted as a likely choice to be made by parents who opt for fetal diagnosis, so in answering the ethical questions of whether we should do fetal echocardiography at all, we must address the ethics of selective abortion. Selective abortion, in turn, is addressed within the wider context of elective abortion.

A Brief History of the Abortion Debate

Disagreements among fetal cardiologists, obstetricians, and other physicians over whether the fetus ought to

be considered a patient for the purposes of fetal cardiology reflect a much larger, more profound, and deeply embedded disagreement among people generally on the subject of fetal value. The "abortion issue" has divided professionals, families, communities, and the country as a whole for a number of reasons. Among the most influential of these reasons is that abortion tends to become a fertile and hotly contested battleground from which other political crusades are fought, such as the conservative crusade for family values and the liberal crusade for women's rights and, particularly, reproductive freedom. Moreover, various religious and philosophical traditions often take very strong, opposing stances on the issues of abortion. But what one religion or philosophy says about abortion is never enough to guide a pluralistic nation composed of members of various Western and non-Western religious and philosophical traditions, as well as individuals who do not view themselves as members of any tradition.

Bioethicists have engaged in a heated debate among themselves over the issue of abortion since at least the early 1970s. Perhaps in an attempt to shed some "objective" light on what appears to be a highly contentious, subjective area, some of them have engaged in a pursuit of a universal criterion for moral status. They began with the assumption that it was wrong to end the life of a human being and, asking why such killing was wrong, proceeded to propose various criteria for moral personhood that were supposed to have the effect of either supporting or rejecting abortion rights.

Conservative ethicists, including many of those working from religious traditions, tended to focus on criteria for moral personhood that the fetus possessed relatively early in gestation, including possession of a unique human genetic code.[9] Since the embryo and early fetus possessed such criteria, these ethicists and theologians argued that they ought to be considered morally equivalent to adult humans.

This genetic argument, however, is neither necessary nor sufficient for a criterion for moral value and protection. Two objections readily come to mind. First, human gametes are also alive and possess unique human genetic codes. Yet few, if any, would seriously claim that a sperm or egg is morally equivalent to a living person. Second, powerful arguments can be mounted against killing (at least for no serious reason) sophisticated creatures that lack a human genotype, such as dolphins, whales, and advanced primates.

More liberal thinkers who aimed to support abortion rights rejected conservative criteria for fetal moral status. They argued that criteria such as membership in the species *Homo sapiens*, or the fact that the conceptus has implanted in the woman's womb, or that an egg has been fertilized should not be considered morally relevant. Instead, they proposed various characteristics of "personhood" that adult humans possess but that most or all fetuses lack, including viability, the ability to communicate with other human beings through language, and the possession of certain intellectual faculties. Various liberal thinkers either selected one of these characteristics as the determining factor in moral status or relied on a group of characteristics to accomplish the same task.[10,11*] Additionally, many, including one of us,[12] have argued that as the fetus acquires these various characteristics, its moral status increases.

However, assigning moral relevance to such characteristics resulted in counterintuitive conclusions. For instance, in addition to showing that fetuses do not have full moral rights, the criterion of ability to reason and think rationally also demonstrates that infants and children, the mentally retarded, and perhaps the senile and those afflicted with Alzheimer's disease do not require full moral protection, either.

A second problem with the list of characteristics offered by liberal thinkers is that the arguments for moral protection and status which accompany these characteristics tend to commit what philosophers call the naturalistic fallacy—the error of deriving an "ought" from an "is." If we begin with the premise that a being possesses certain biologic and psychologic traits (the "is"), we cannot logically arrive at conclusions about what can and cannot be done to him or her (the "ought") without a further "bridge" premise that links the "ought" to the "is." For instance, the facts that a living person can think rationally or possesses a beating heart do not, by themselves, lead to any conclusions about the moral permissibility of killing that individual. Without further argument, these biologic and psychologic characteristics are just as arbitrary and irrelevant to moral status as those offered by conservative thinkers.

The lack of success in agreeing on one characteristic or group of characteristics to define personhood or moral status has led some bioethicists to move on to less contentious areas of study; the large volume of articles on abortion published in bioethics journals certainly appears to have subsided. Unfortunately, physicians in fetal–maternal medicine do not have the luxury of ignoring the abortion issue. One must either view the fetus as a patient or not; one must either treat or not. How, then, are clinicians, parents, and surrogates to make these decisions?

Sentience as a Criterion of Moral Status

We believe that despite the politicization of the abortion issue and the vehemence with which it is debated in our society, there is a coherent and pragmatic way of placing the issue of fetal status within a more general framework of moral status. Any theory of moral status should address all forms of matter that we encounter (or potentially could encounter), including not only "normal" adult human beings, but also nonliving matter, nonanimal life, nonhuman animals, and humans at all stages and of all qualities of life. In addition, a distinction must be made between those beings who merit moral consideration by moral agents and those beings who are themselves moral agents. A moral agent is, by definition, a person in the normative sense. However, one need not be a person in the normative sense to deserve moral consideration from those who are persons.

We believe that the possession of sentience—being capable of sensation and at least rudimentary consciousness—is relevant to deciding what one ought and ought not to do to a being. Morally speaking, it is a being's capacity to have interests of various kinds that requires us to take those interests into account during

---

*Mary Anne Warren listed five criteria for personhood—consciousness, self-consciousness, reasoning ability, self-motivated activity, and language use. Although she conceded that all five criteria are not necessarily required for personhood, she maintained that any being which lacks all of them is certainly not a person.[10] Joseph F. Fletcher was even more rigorous in his pursuit of personhood and listed no fewer than 15 criteria, including a minimum IQ, self-control, a sense of time, concern for others, and curiosity.[11]

moral deliberations, and one must be physiologically and psychologically sentient to have interests of any kind. The morally relevant criterion for basic moral status—i.e., the claim to have one's interests considered—is therefore not membership in a particular species or possession of a certain IQ, but the capacity to have interests of some kind. Nonsentient living beings and nonliving objects that have no interests regarding their treatment can have no claims on us as to how we are to behave toward them and, in fact, it is impossible for a moral agent to consider the interests of such a being in his or her moral deliberation, since that being would have no interests to be considered. No direct moral wrongdoing is therefore involved in destroying a tree, despite the fact that trees are often alive. Our treatment of trees and other nonsentient beings would only become good or bad in a moral sense if it related to beings who do require moral consideration, and the wronged party would never be the tree but rather the sentient being. For instance, if in destroying a forest, animals were displaced from their habitats, people were deprived of property, and esthetic beauty or medicinal resources and the environment were harmed, then the act of destroying the forest may well turn out to be gravely wrong. But if this is the case, then it must have to do with the harm done to animals and people by thwarting their interests, not with any harm or wrongdoing done to the trees. In spite of the way some ecologists talk, the environment itself cannot be wronged or harmed in a moral sense; the tragedy of the way we treat our environment concerns the damage we do to ourselves, to other animals, and perhaps to future generations.

Before the development of sentience, the fetus has no interests and, as such, cannot be a subject of harm.* Because the presentient fetus has no interests, and therefore no claims upon us, and because treating it necessarily involves invading the woman's body, the question of whether the presentient fetus is to be seen and treated as a person and patient must be answered by the woman alone. After the point of sentience, however, fetal treatment becomes a delicate balancing act between the interests of the fetus and those of the mother. It therefore becomes essential to determine when, during its development, the fetus becomes capable of having interests, as well as which interests related to its medical care it is capable of having.

---

*Actually, some philosophers would say that the presentient fetus who is "destined" (through the intentions of its mother) to become a sentient fetus and a person can be a subject of harm retroactively, in that damage done to the presentient fetus who lacks interests may later frustrate the interests of the sentient fetus- or neonate-to-be. We discuss the ethical consequences of this reality in the section, Additional Tools Used to Establish Fetal Moral Status: Potentiality and Maternal Value.

Sentience and Pain in the Fetus and Neonate

It seems very unlikely that even the late fetus possesses any of the more complex interests that normal adult human beings share—interests in being approved of by others, in achieving a positive self-image, or even in mere continued existence. The most obvious interest the sentient fetus is likely to have is in avoiding unpleasant sensations, especially pain. If fetuses were capable of perceiving pain, this revelation would have profound significance not only for the ethics of fetal cardiology, but also for the ethics of abortion and ethical issues arising from methods of childbirth.

In the late 1980s, embryologist Clifford Grobstein[13] wrote extensively on fetal development and selfhood. In addressing the question of whether a fetus is a person in the normative sense, Grobstein noted that

> [t]his question cannot be answered on scientific grounds alone. Human being, person, and human rights are not terms stemming from scientific definition. But one trained and accustomed to think as a scientist cannot fail to note significant disparity between the common meaning of these terms and a single cell. (C. Grobstein, reference 13, p. 5.)

The earliest detection of responsiveness to stimuli in embryos appears to occur at 7 to 8 weeks after conception, and at about 9 to 10 weeks, embryos begin to exhibit spontaneous movements apparently not related to any stimuli. Grobstein concluded, however, that these early embryonic responses were more automatic than they were intentional, purposive, or characteristic of selfhood. In fact, similar responses can be elicited in such organisms as protozoa, hydroids, and flatworms.[14] Yet based on the relative size and character of the organization of the fetus' cerebral cortex, Grobstein concluded that "the possibility of gradual emergence of a rudiment of self, or of at least diffuse sentience, certainly cannot be excluded during the second and certainly the third trimester" (from reference 14, p. 97). Given the biologic uncertainty of the neural development of the late fetus, however, Grobstein opted to draw a cautionary line at 26 weeks of gestation—"four weeks later than the earliest demonstrated thalamocortical connections in the developing brain but some four weeks prior to the first maturational change in the brain's electrical patterns and to extensive linkages among cortical neurons" (from reference 13, p. 145).[13,14]

In the last decade, experts on fetal development, human neurology, and the science of consciousness have not come much further than this in their investigations of fetal sentience. They disagree about whether the fetus is capable of experiencing pain and, if so, when in its development it acquires this capacity.

Nearly everyone acknowledges with Grobstein, however, that the earliest fetal movements (responses to stimuli at about 7.5 weeks and seemingly spontaneous movement beginning soon thereafter) are almost certainly not indications of rudimentary consciousness, much less the ability to feel pain, but are, instead, automatic spinal cord reactions.[15,16] The same reactions have been observed in anencephalic infants with only partial spinal cord functioning,[17] and in unconscious human adults and cats whose spinal cords have been severed above the level of stimulation and response.[14]

Experts also agree that the cortical, subcortical, and peripheral centers necessary for pain perception begin to develop early in the second trimester.[15,16,18] But merely having the structures necessary for pain perception (and even responding physiologically to certain potentially stressful stimuli) does not imply that pain perception occurs. There are two kinds of pain that must be kept clearly distinguished:

1. Conscious perceived pain—pain that is felt, feared, and remembered. The moral relevance of this aspect of pain is obvious.
2. The physical effects of pain on the body—major pain triggers a sequence of changes in body functions. These include increases in heart rate, breathing rate, and blood pressure; changes in blood flow to organs such as the lungs and brain; and release of hormones and other substances that have major effects on many body functions. There are three important characteristics of this sequence of events. First, it occurs whether or not pain is consciously perceived. Second, some of the events are harmful; they can lead to complications of the patient's illness, and even increase the risk of death. Third, they can be blunted or abolished by high doses of anesthetics or powerful analgesics.[19]

Thus, the fetus must be conscious to experience pain, and so moral status requires not merely the existence of brain structures or primitive brain function, as some have argued,[20]* but also the fairly sophisticated functioning of at least the cerebral cortex and perhaps the thalamus.[21]

The current disagreement among experts, then, is when after these structures are in place fetuses actually do experience pain and other sensations. The most conservative estimates place fetal capacity for pain percep-

tion at 23 weeks,[22] whereas others deny that any fetus can truly experience pain, since pain perception involves sophisticated sensory, emotional, and cognitive faculties not sufficiently developed in fetuses and even neonates.[15,23,24] Most experts, however, seem to take a middle road and are willing to concede that even if the experience of pain is different and less complex in sentient fetuses than it is in adults, it may nevertheless cause suffering; these moderates tend to place the possibility of suffering around 26 weeks, and note that it is more likely to occur significantly later than that.[13,14,16,25,26]

Our discussion of fetal pain gives rise to another ethical issue in fetal cardiology: whether to administer analgesics or anesthesia to late-term fetuses undergoing potentially painful or stressful cardiac therapy. Before the late 1980s, neonates were thought to be incapable of experiencing pain and, accordingly were not treated for pain during surgery. In the late 1980s, however, Anand and colleagues[18,27,28] reported research findings that neonates mounted hormonal stress responses to surgical interventions. Pain relief for neonates was quickly recommended,[29,30] and over the next 7 years it gradually became routine practice to treat both full-term neonates and premature infants in the Neonatal Intensive Care Unit (NICU) with analgesics and anesthesia. This practice was begun despite controversy regarding the conclusions that various experts thought should be drawn from the existence of neonatal stress responses. The feeling, however, was that since we do not have good data on when a developing human being begins to feel pain, we ought to err on the side of caution.

Interestingly, this same argument was not applied to late-term fetuses, who are often as old or older than their NICU counterparts. In light of the move toward managing the potential pain of neonates and premature infants, many have recently argued that, as a precautionary measure, we ought to treat late-term fetuses for their potential pain.[15,16,22] There is still disagreement, however, between those who maintain that the goal of analgesics and anesthesia is to prevent actual pain perception by fetuses,[16] and those who make the more conservative claim that they are needed merely to prevent potentially harmful physiologic stress responses on the developing nervous system.[15]

Given this latest assessment of fetal development, we would draw a cautionary line at 23 weeks in determining when fetal interests are likely to occur when they must be considered by clinicians, parents, and surrogates.

Additional Tools Used To Establish Fetal Moral Status: Potentiality and Maternal Value

The answer to the problem of moral status, however, is not quite so simple as determining where to draw a line,

---

*Baruch Brody argued that since people die when their brain function stops, they must begin to be persons when their brain functioning starts. Based on this criterion of personhood, Brody claimed that the 6-week fetus, which begins to evidence some primitive brain function, ought to be considered a person.[20]

especially when it comes to human fetuses. For the presentient fetus occupies a distinct position in the world of beings: whereas it has no interests or corresponding rights, it has the potential for having these and other interests and rights. The "argument from potential" is perhaps the strongest conservative position toward abortion.* It is not, we feel, invulnerable, however. American citizens of appropriate age and nationality are all potential Presidents of the United States. But no one but the actual president has the powers and rights of that office. Even a candidate running for president (who has much more presidential potential than most of us) does not have the powers of an actual president. No matter how close a presentient fetus comes to becoming a sentient fetus, the presentient fetus has no interests or corresponding rights; it merely has potential interests and rights, which are, when weighed against the real interests of actual persons, often less than compelling.

We must be careful to distinguish the morally relevant meaning of the word "interest," which we have been discussing, from another meaning of the word that bears no relevance to discussions of ethics. In this second sense of the word, a fetus has an "interest" in receiving (for instance) adequate nutrition, just as an acorn, to the extent that it is naturally to become an oak tree, has an "interest" in receiving the things that allow it to grow and develop. We might even say that adequate nutrition is "good" for both the acorn and the fetus. However, interests are only morally compelling, and complying with those interests is only morally good, when they are consciously experienced in the present (or, sometimes, when we know that they will be consciously held in the future). Strictly speaking, adequate prenatal nutrition can only serve the interests of the mother who hopes for a healthy baby—not the presentient fetus, who can have no conscious interest in its continued life or in avoiding the negative consequences of poor nutrition.

There is, however, one way in which the presentient fetus can be said to have an interest in receiving proper nutrition (among other things), and this is retroactively. Simply put, what is done to an embryo before it has interests has the potential if that embryo or early fetus is allowed to become a sentient fetus, child, or adult, to harm or benefit that future person. I have a retroactive interest in what occurred to my mother and "me" when "I" was in the womb, precisely because I now exist as a person with interests (this is the reasoning behind wrongful birth and wrongful life suits). In some sense, then, the fetus who is viewed as a future person by its mother can be thought already to

have interests that demand consideration. Although the retroactive causation of interests proves to be metaphysically troubling and is controversial among philosophers, pragmatically speaking, it seems clear that it is wrong, for instance, to perform highly experimental research on an embryo and then replace it in the mother's womb, allowing it to grow into a person who may one day suffer because of what was done to him or her when he or she was just an embryo, as yet without interests. It is critical to be clear that the mother, and the mother alone, has the authority to confer this retroactive status upon her fetus by allowing it to be gestated to term; it cannot be claimed that all embryos have such retroactive interests in (and thus *prima facie* rights to) their own continued existence, or anything else. To the extent that a fetus is considered a patient–person by its mother, then, and to the extent that she intends to allow it to gestate to full term, the fetus, *as a potential person with interests*, has a retroactive "interest" in what is done to it before it actually acquires these interests consciously. It is this potential for interests, combined with the already existing interests of the mother, that unite, in appropriate circumstances, to lend some moral status to even the presentient fetus.

Yet even when actual fetal interests exist, these do not automatically translate into absolute rights of the fetus; rather, they compel us only to *consider* the sentient fetus in our moral deliberation. Sentience is the criterion for minimal moral consideration, not for full moral personhood. It is quite possible that, upon deliberation, we may decide that the rights of the woman to bodily integrity, reproductive freedom, and personal autonomy outweigh those of the fetus. Whose interests "win out," and how the fetus is treated by the clinician, becomes in this case a delicate balancing act that inevitably invites controversy. The requirement to consider the interests of fetuses who have them therefore does not necessarily result in a prohibition of all post-sentience abortions or a requirement that all fetal treatments be administered after the point of sentience. If the mother views her presentient fetus as a patient and future person, then the appropriate position of the clinician is to view the fetus in the same manner. If the mother does not view the fetus as a patient, then there is no reason, before sentience, for the clinician either to view or to treat the fetus professionally as a patient, and in fact it would be unethical to do so contrary to the wishes of the mother. After sentience, there is reason for the clinician to be concerned with the care of the fetus, although this concern must be balanced against the clinician's concern for the adult mother whose interests may compete directly with those of the fetus. In short, there are four broad categories into which all potential recipients of fetal cardiology treatment fall, shown

---

*For a strong presentation of the argument from potential, see Marquis D: Why abortion is immoral. *J Phil.* 86:183, 1989.

	Sentient	Presentient
Mother views as patient	Patient	Patient
Mother does not view as patient	?	Not a Patient

Figure 24–1. When does a fetus become a patient?

in Figure 24–1, based on the sentience status of the fetus and the way in which the mother views the fetus.

Prenatal Diagnosis and Selective Abortion

Court cases that presumably reflect the moral views of the majority have consistently upheld a constitutional right to abortion, with some restrictions, in the United States.[31-35] These cases have all concerned elective abortion, the intent of which is to end a pregnancy altogether. In such cases, a woman chooses to abort because she does not want to be pregnant at all or at that time. The vast majority of abortion decisions are made in the context of pregnancies that are unwanted or unplanned. Some 60% of pregnancies are unwanted or mistimed, and half of those end in abortion.[36] In the context of prenatal diagnosis, however, Rothman[37] perceptively describes the woman's attitude toward her pregnancy as "tentative" rather than as unwanted or unplanned. This decision is focused on preventing the birth of a child with a particular genotype, syndrome, or malformation, rather than on terminating the pregnancy as a whole event. For this reason, selective abortion decisions have important moral, psychological, and social differences from choices about elective abortion. The review by Adler et al.[38] is the best summary of psychological issues in prenatal diagnosis.

We placed our discussion of the option of selective abortion within the broader ethical issue of elective abortion since, logically, the option of selective abortion depends on whether elective abortion can be morally and legally defended. Moreover, it is difficult to separate the issue of selective abortion for fetal conditions from abortion on social grounds or abortion on request, because in most nations there are no medical standards for hereditary disorders or fetal malformations that may warrant abortion. Instituting such standards in pluralistic societies could be oppressive, because different cultural groups may hold different views about the relative seriousness of different conditions. Setting medical standards for "seriousness" of hereditary disorders in the context of prenatal diagnosis and abortion would also place the balance of power in the hands of physicians, instead of women and families. The most ethically acceptable approach, therefore, is to leave selective abortion within the wider context of abortion on request, and to let women and families decide on the seriousness of a condition, in view of their personal and social situations.

Selective abortion attracts more public and written controversy than any other ethical problem in prenatal diagnosis and is controversial even among perinatal cardiologists.[3,39-41] However, in determining the actual moral magnitude of the problem of fetal diagnosis, far more people are harmed by lack of access to genetic services than they are adversely affected by selective abortion. This is so because, first, the incidence of selective abortions for genetic reasons is no more than 1% of all abortions,[42] vastly fewer than elective abortions resulting from social causes, failed contraception, or personal reasons, and second, because there is no harm to the aborted fetuses when done before sentience, and perhaps only minimal harm done to even sentient fetuses. In our view, a major factor that justifies selective abortion after prenatal diagnosis is that the option helps many more parents with genetic risks to have wanted children than in the past. Without this option, most parents at higher genetic risk would either electively abort each pregnancy, seek sterilization, or adopt a child. Some women and their partners do not choose abortion after hearing of genetic or physical abnormalities (e.g., in disorders such as cystic fibrosis[43]). Selective abortion choices are, however, a special source of emotional suffering and troubling moral deliberation, for the reasons shown in Table 24–2.

Bereavement and Selective Abortion

Most pregnancies that proceed as far as prenatal care and prenatal diagnosis are "wanted" pregnancies, even if they were not wanted or intended at the time of conception. There are different degrees of wantedness, but usually by the time a woman receives her prenatal test results she has started to think of herself as a mother. This is why many women who would not hesitate to abort an unwanted pregnancy for personal reasons feel emotional pain and guilt about aborting because there is something wrong with the unborn baby. The mother who receives unfavorable prenatal diagnostic findings must make her decision on the basis of the unborn baby's characteristics. She must also live with her decision. If she aborts, she may feel grief similar to that for loss of a child. If she carries to term, she and her family will be responsible for the child's care. It is important that she be fully aware of the long-term consequences of her choice, and, if a condition has a range of severity, that she know the full range. If she chooses abortion, she should be aware that, although most women recover emotionally and return to their usual activities within a month, many feel lingering grief and a few un-

TABLE 24–2. WHY ARE GENETIC ABORTION CHOICES SO DIFFICULT?

The choice usually involves a wanted pregnancy.

Many people attribute a higher moral status to the fetus at midtrimester and at viability.

There is a wide spectrum of severity in some chromosomal and genetic disorders.

Improved treatments for some disorders have led to longer life spans for affected persons.

There is concern that abortion may harm the mental health of living children (siblings of the fetus) who have the same genetic condition.

There is concern that selective abortion may set a precedent for neglect of genetically affected persons who survive, including a precedent for pediatric euthanasia.

There is concern that environment-based contributions to some genetic disorders may be underestimated and obscured.

Many parents who have already viewed the fetus on ultrasound will have endowed it with the qualities of a living child.

Reprinted, with permission, from World Health Organization, Hereditary Diseases Program: Guidelines on Ethical Issues in Medical Genetics and the Provision of Services. *Geneva: WHO; 1995. Used with permission.*

dergo clinically significant depression.[44,45] Follow-up is in order for all women who receive unfavorable prenatal diagnostic results, whatever their decision. Bereavement therapy or support groups should be available for those who decide on abortion. The standard of care is to provide emotional support and counseling before and after the procedure.[46,47]

NEONATAL DIAGNOSIS AND TREATMENT

The ethical issues in neonatal care include the delivery of high-technology care, quality-of-life considerations, the authority of parents, and conflict resolution when parents and health care professionals differ as to what constitutes reasonable care. Consideration of these issues is a fairly recent phenomenon, escalating sharply in the 1970s with the development of high-technology neonatal intensive care units, multisystem monitoring, and sophisticated mechanical ventilation. Although cardiac surgery has been successfully performed on progressively smaller infants since the 1960s, major neonatal procedures such as the arterial switch procedure for transposition of the great arteries and palliation for hypoplastic left heart syndrome have only been practiced widely since the early 1980s. Only two decades ago, surveys indicated that a majority of pediatricians did not recommend surgery for an infant with trisomy 21 and duodenal atresia,[48] an intervention that is almost taken for granted today.

The ethical conflicts in care of the neonate with cardiac disease are symbolized by two babies achieving widespread attention in the 1980s: Baby Doe and Baby Fae. In the Baby Doe regulations, President Reagan directed the Department of Health and Human Services to adopt regulations to prevent hospitals from withholding care from imperiled newborns, based on Section 504 of the 1973 Rehabilitation Act, which prohibited discrimination against the handicapped. The regulations seemed to require maximal treatment in all cases ex-

cept in those in which the infant was irreversibly and imminently dying. Although overturned, reissued, and gradually deemphasized, the regulations certainly heightened awareness of the ethical issues involved in neonatal care and probably elevated the intensity of care provided to infants with birth defects.[49]

If the Baby Doe case emphasized who should receive care, the Baby Fae case illustrated the extremes of care that might be attempted. An infant with hypoplastic left heart syndrome, Baby Fae was treated with a transplanted baboon heart.[50] Although she died shortly thereafter, this innovative therapy ignited considerable controversy regarding the competency of the mother to give truly informed consent, the adequacy of the scientific preparation for cross-species transplantation, and even the morality of sacrificing an animal in an attempt to save the child's life.[51]

Futile Treatment

There are two situations in which the opinion of medical personnel that further treatment of a neonate with congenital heart disease is futile may conflict with the wishes of the family: (1) the critically ill neonate, generally receiving assisted ventilation and other forms of life support, who appears to have little or no chance of recovery, and (2) the neonate with multiple congenital anomalies, especially those associated with a major chromosomal abnormality such as trisomy 13 or 18, who has congenital heart disease that in itself is amenable to surgical repair. Clearly a policy of nonconfrontation is best; in many instances the infant may die despite continued intensive care and in others the family ultimately comes to accept the futility of further care. If the family members strongly desire a procedure or level of care that the health care team considers inappropriate, it may be advisable to transfer the patient to an institution that agrees to provide the care desired by the family. From a legal standpoint, the courts have universally sided with the parents over the issue of withholding care from a child. The classic case occurred when two federal courts ordered "emergency treatment and ventilatory support" for an anencephalic infant, based on the mother's wishes, from 1993 to 1995.[52,53]

Withholding Treatment

In some instances, parents may not wish to pursue further therapy, especially surgical intervention, even though the physicians caring for the infant strongly advise such treatment. "I just couldn't put him through it" is a commonly stated reason for refusing such therapy; the actual reason may be religious, humanitarian, or purely selfish (the inconveniences and costs of caring for a handicapped child are by no means inconsequential). Whatever the reason for the refusal, the proposed therapy and its likelihood of success must be considered. For example, ligation of patent ductus arteriosus in a 1500-g premature infant with congestive heart failure is a relatively low-risk procedure that virtually cures the underlying cardiovascular abnormality and requires little subsequent cardiac follow-up. At the other extreme, cardiac transplantation and the Norwood procedure for an infant with hypoplastic left heart syndrome are expensive, high-risk procedures and the survivors require lifelong cardiovascular care, including multiple cardiac catheterizations and operations, and face an uncertain prognosis. A somewhat intermediate situation is the neonate with tetralogy of Fallot in need of a systemic-to-pulmonary shunt because of hypoxemia, probably to be followed by intracardiac repair later in childhood.

Decision making in these situations is best done by consensus building with involvement of all parties, taking into consideration medical data, anticipated quality of life, family beliefs, economic realities, and social support systems. For conflict resolution the following guidelines are suggested (Boyle and Spencer, p. 172)[49]:

- Decisions for children should be made by their parents unless they fall outside of societal mandates.
- The best interest of the patient should be the basis for these decisions.
- Clinical and ethical consultation should be strongly considered.

RESOURCE ALLOCATION

Caring for infants and children with congenital cardiac abnormalities is expensive, and costs add another dimension to decisions about medical practice. Economic issues are present at two distinct levels: the costs to an individual patient or family, and the costs to society. We argue that these costs should be considered separately.

To ignore the family resources totally when making recommendations for care of an individual patient with congenital heart disease is both naive and unrealistic. Physicians need to work with social workers, state and federal agencies, and third-party payors in an effort to ensure that, to the greatest extent possible, decisions about therapy are based on medical principles and the child's best interests rather than on monetary considerations. Nonetheless, there may be instances in which the family socioeconomic situation is such that a particularly expensive treatment (for example, cardiac transplantation in an infant with hypoplastic left heart syndrome) may not be in the child's best interests. However, the decision to forego the therapy in an individual patient should not be made on the grounds that "our society cannot afford to spend so much money on health care."

At the societal level, allocation of health care resources is an important issue. Should health care be rationed? Should we devote resources to saving expensive "miracle babies" or to preventing teenage pregnancy? Based on hospital charges for a large group of neonates with hypoplastic left heart syndrome treated with either transplantation or a Norwood procedure,[54] we estimate that it would cost about $90 million annually to pay for the initial hospitalization of the 800 infants born with this condition each year in the United States. These costs could be reduced if we adopted a rigorous program of prenatal screening fetal echocardiography, with subsequent abortion of fetuses with major cardiac abnormalities. Although such a policy has reduced the incidence of certain cardiac conditions in Great Britain,[55] it would face strong religious and political opposition in the United States.

CONCLUSION

This chapter has reviewed selected ethical aspects faced by clinicians and parents in the diagnosis and treatment of cardiovascular diseases in the fetus and newborn. We have provided recommendations regarding the process and content of decisions about (1) when the fetus becomes a patient, (2) obtaining informed consent for diagnosis and therapy, and (3) decision making regarding selective abortion. We have discussed selective abortion from within a larger perspective on the morality of elective abortion in this society. Although our position on this issue will obviously not be well received by those who hold differing views, we hope that we have been fair to them. We reaffirm the position that tolerance toward those who hold differing views on this divisive question is the most tangible achievement of our society with regard to this vexing and unsolved problem.

REFERENCES

1. Cunningham GF, et al.: *William's Obstetrics*, 19th ed. Norwalk, CT: Appleton & Lange; 1993.
2. McCullough LB, Chervenack FA: *Ethics in Obstetrics and Gynecology*. New York: Oxford University Press, 1994.
3. Squarcia U, et al.: Fetal diagnosis of congenital cardiac malformations—A challenge for physicians as well as parents. *Cardiol Young*. 6:256, 1996.
4. Danford DA, Latson LA, Cheatham JP: Fetal echocardiography—A cost-benefit analysis. *Am J Cardiol*. 66:520, 1990.
5. Beauchamp TL, Childress JF: *Principles of Biomedical Ethics*, 4th ed. New York: Oxford Unversity Press, 1994.
6. Patterson A: *In Utero Stem Cell Transplantation: Issues in Early Clinical Trial Development*. FDA Briefing Document, Feb. 13, 1996.
7. Harrison MR, et al.: Fetal treatment. *N Engl J Med*. 307:1651, 1982.
8. Fletcher JC, Jonsen AR: Ethical considerations of fetal therapy. In: Harrison MR, Golbus MS, Filly RA, eds. *Unborn Patient*, 2nd ed. Orlando, FL: Grune & Stratton, 1990.
9. Noonan JT: An almost absolute value in history. In: Noonan JT, ed: *The Morality of Abortion*. Cambridge, MA: Harvard University Press; 1970.
10. Warren MA: On the moral and legal status of abortion. *Monist*. 57:43, 1973.
11. Fletcher JF: *Humanhood: Essays in Biomedical Ethics*. Buffalo, NY: Prometheus Books; 1979.
12. Fletcher JF: On learning from mistakes. *Clin Ethics*. 6:264, 1995.
13. Grobstein C: *Science and the Unborn*. New York: Basic Books, 1988.
14. Grobstein C: *From Chance to Purpose: An Appraisal of External Human Fertilization*. Reading, MA: Addison-Wesley, 1981.
15. Lloyd-Thomas AR, Fitzgerald M: Reflex responses do not necessarily signify pain. *Br Med J*. 313:797, 1996.
16. Glover V, Fisk N: We don't know: better to err on the safe side from mid-gestation. *Br Med J*. 313:796, 1996.
17. Visser GHA, Laurini RN, de Vries JIP, et al.: Abnormal motor behavior in anencephalic fetuses. *Early Hum Devel*. 12:173, 1985.
18. Anand KJS, Hickey PR: Pain and its effects in the human neonate and the fetus. *N Engl J Med*. 317:1321, 1987.
19. Campbell N: Infants, pain and what health care professionals should want to know—A response to Cunningham Butler. *Bioethics*. 3:200, 1989.
20. Brody B: *Abortion and the Sanctity of Life*. Cambridge, MA: MIT Press; 1975.
21. Greenfield SA: *Journey to the Centres of the Mind: Towards a Science of Consciousness*. New York: Freeman; 1995.
22. Wyatt J: When do we begin to feel the pain? *Guardian*. Oct. 24, 1996, pS2.
23. Derbyshire SWG, Furedi A: "Fetal pain" is a misnomer. *Br Med J*. 313:795, 1996.
24. Szawarski Z: Probably no pain in the absence of "self." *Br Med J*. 313:796, 1996.
25. Grobstein, C: Human development from fertilization to birth. In: Reich, WT, ed. *Encyclopedia of Bioethics*, 2nd ed. New York: Simon & Schuster MacMillan; 1995.
26. Giannakoulopoulos X, Sepulveda W, Kourtis P, et al.: Fetal plasma cortisol and beta-endorphin response to intrauterine needling. *Lancet*. 344:77, 1994.
27. Anand KJS, Sippell WG, Aynsley-Green A: Randomized trial of fentanyl anaesthesia in preterm babies undergoing surgery: Effects of the stress response. *Lancet*. I:243, 1987.
28. Anand KJS, Hickey PR: Halthane-morphine compared with high-dose sufentanil for anesthesia and postoperative analgesia in neonatal cardiac surgery. *N Engl J Med*. 326:1, 1992.
29. Wolf AR: Treat the babies, not their stress responses. *Lancet*. 342:319, 1993.
30. Rogers MC: Do the right thing: Pain relief in infants and children. *N Engl J Med*. 326:55, 1992.
31. *Roe v. Wade*. 410 U.S. 113. 1973.
32. *Doe v. Bolton*. 93 S. Ct. 739. 1973.
33. *Planned Parenthood v. Casey*. 112 S. Ct. 2791. 1992.
34. *Webster v. Reproduction Services*. 109 S. Ct. 3040. 1989.
35. *Thornburgh v. American College of Obstetricians and Gynecologists*. 106 S. Ct. 2169. 1986.
36. Kulczycki A, Potts M., Rosenfield A: Abortion and fertility regulation. *Lancet*. 347:1663, 1996.
37. Rothman BK: *The Tentative Pregnancy: Prenatal Diagnosis and the Future of Motherhood*. New York: WW Norton, 1986.
38. Adler NE, Keyes S, Robertson P: Psychological issues in new reproductive technologies: Pregnancy-inducing technology and diagnostic screening. In: Rodin J, Collins A, eds. *Women and New Reproductive Technologies: Medical, Psychosocial, Legal, and Ethical Dilemmas*. Hillsdale, NJ: Lawrence Erlbaum; 1991.
39. Allan LD: Fetal diagnosis of congenital heart disease. *Cardiol Young*. 6:258, 1996.
40. Sandor GGS: Fetal diagnosis of congenital heart disease. *Cardiol Young*. 6:259, 1996.
41. Shinebourne EA, Carvalho JS: Ethics of fetal echocardiography. *Cardiol Young*. 6:261, 1996.
42. Wertz DC, Fletcher JC: *Ethics and Human Genetics: A Cross-Cultural Perspective*. Berlin: Springer-Verlag; 1989.
43. Wertz DC, Rosenfield JM, Janes SR, et al.: Attitudes toward abortion among parents of children with cystic fibrosis. *Am J Publ Health*. 81:992, 1991.
44. Beck Black R: Psychosocial issues in genetic testing and pregnancy loss. *Fetal Diagn Ther*. 8:164, 1993.
45. Tunis SL: Prenatal diagnosis of fetal abnormalities: Psychological impact. In: Simpson JL, Elias S, eds. *Essentials of Prenatal Diagnosis*. New York: Churchill Livingstone; 1992.
46. White-Van Mourik MCA, Connor HM, Ferguson-Smith MA: Patient care before and after termination of pregnancy for neural tube defects. *Prenat Diagn*. 10:497, 1990.
47. Elder SH, Laurence KM: The impact of supportive intervention after second trimester termination of pregnancy for fetal abnormality. *Prenat Diagn*. 11:47, 1991.
48. Todres ID, et al.: Life-saving therapy for newborns: A questionaire survey in the state of Massachusetts. *Pediatrics*. 81:643, 1988.

49. Boyle RJ, Spencer EM: Decisions about treatment in newborns, infants and children. In: Fletcher JC, et al., eds. *Introduction to Clinical Ethics*. Frederick, MD: University Publishing Group; 1995.

50. Bailey LL, Nehlsen-Cannarella SL, Concepcion W, et al.: Baboon-to-human cardiac xenotransplantation in a neonate. *JAMA*. 254:3321, 1985.

51. Caplan A: Is xenographting morally wrong? *Transplant Proc*. 24:722, 1992.

52. *In the Matter of Baby K*. 832 F. Suppl. 1022 (E.D. Va. 1993).

53. *In the Matter of Baby K*. 16 F. 3d 590 (4th Cir. 1994).

54. Gutgesell HP, Massaro TA: Management of hypoplastic left heart syndrome in a consortium of university hospitals. *Am J Cardiol*. 76:809, 1995.

55. Allan LD, Cook A, Sullivan I, et al.: Hypoplastic left heart syndrome: Effects of fetal echocardiography on birth prevalence. *Lancet*. 337:959, 1991.

CHAPTER TWENTY-FIVE

Digital Ultrasound Imaging: Current and Future Developments

Jacques Souquet and Jeff Powers

The past decade has seen dramatic improvements in ultrasound imaging performance. The introduction of color Doppler imaging has added a new dimension to blood flow measurement, displaying blood flow as a real-time map over a two-dimensional image rather than a spectrum from a single point of pulsed Doppler or the single line of continuous wave Doppler. The more recent refinement of power Doppler (also known as color power angiography) has increased color Doppler imaging's sensitivity significantly.

Until recently, ultrasound imaging systems have used analog signal processing in the beamformer, heart of the imaging system, relying on venerable analog components such as mixers and analog delay lines for signal delay and synchronization. The availability of high-speed digital processing electronics has refined the state of the art of beamformer performance, eliminating the bandwidth and distortion limitations imposed by analog delay lines and mixers. In the same way that digital audio recording with compact discs brought dramatic improvements to the fidelity of audio sound, digital broadband beamforming is bringing new diagnostic information to ultrasound images.

In this chapter, we first review the advantages of broadband digital beamforming technique; then we describe the characteristics of blood flow and tissue that allow the ultrasound system to be able to differentiate their echoes without the use of contrast agents. This leads to a description of the signal processing used to detect that particular flow signal and how it is optimized. Finally, we describe some future techniques being developed such as three-dimensional (3D) ultrasound and the use of ultrasound contrast agents.

TISSUE SIGNATURE AND BEAMFORMING

Each tissue within the body responds to ultrasound energy of different frequencies in a characteristic way, which is often referred as the *tissue signature* (Figure 25–1). The tissue signature information is carried within the spectrum of ultrasound frequencies returning from the tissue. This band of frequencies is referred to as the frequency spectrum bandwidth, or simply, *bandwidth*.

Together with the transducer, the beamformer determines the ultimate contrast resolution, spatial resolution, sensitivity, and accuracy of the system. If the acoustic information containing the tissue signature is reduced in quantity or distorted in the beamformer, there is no way of recovering it. The process of beamforming begins with pulsing the transducer elements to insonify the target. Sound waves reflected by the target return to the elements of the transducer, generating signals that are misaligned (unfocused) in time. The beamformer correctly aligns the signals (focusing) so when all the channels are properly summed together, the exact tissue signature is obtained (Figure 25–2).

The critical design requirements of the beamformer are:

- To preserve the entire bandwidth, which contains all the acoustic information
- To preserve without distortion the tissue signature during delay

This concept should be expanded to include specific signatures from ultrasound contrast agents, which appears to be a very promising development, especially as it relates to harmonics. This exciting new technique is an

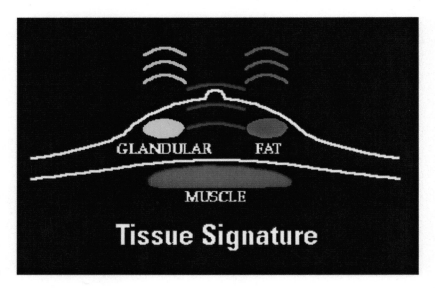

Figure 25–1. Tissue signature.

intrinsically large bandwidth phenomenon and therefore will fully benefit from the broadband beamforming technology of the new generation of ultrasound systems.

ANALOG BEAMFORMER TECHNOLOGY

The time delays required for beamforming can be accomplished by analog delay lines, a technology developed in the 1940s and introduced to ultrasound in the 1970s. These analog delay lines impose significant limitations on the beamformer performances, e.g., limited focusing accuracy and susceptibility to changes in value over time and temperature. Furthermore, some ultrasound systems implement additional compromises by approximating the time delay required for focusing with a phase shift:

$$\partial Phi = 2\pi F_0 \, \partial Tau$$

This mathematical expression establishes that a phase shift (∂Phi) is only an approximation of the true time delay required for precise focusing. The error in focusing increases with bandwidth and can reach up to 30% as one attempts to focus broadband signals. These analog approximations can be likened to optical imaging through a distorted lens (chromatic aberration), where different colors (different frequencies) are delayed by different amounts. The resulting artifact is a halo of false colors in the optical image similar to the smearing effect caused by time errors in ultrasound imaging. This old technology has no growth path, is becoming more expensive than digital implementation, and is not able to take advantage of new developments, such as harmonic imaging of contrast agents.

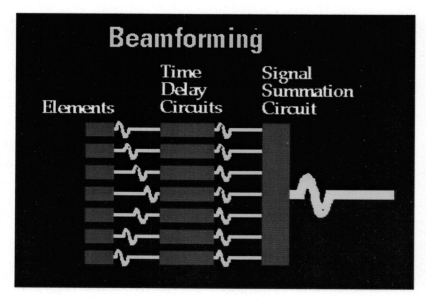

Figure 25–2. Beamformer concept.

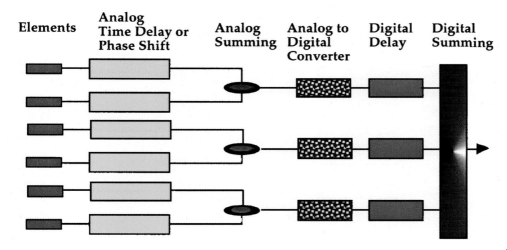

Figure 25–3. Hybrid analog–digital beamformer.

HYBRID DIGITAL BEAMFORMER SYSTEMS

One compromise approach used in some systems is to implement a section of the beamformer in analog and the rest in digital, leading to a hybrid solution. For instance, the number of true digital beamforming channels can be reduced by half if the signal from each element is delayed and then the pairs are summed in the analog domain. The summed signal is then digitized and subsequently delayed and summed (Figure 25–3). A further compromise is to approximate this element delay with a phase shift obtained by mixing with an intermediate frequency carrier.

Another approach to compromise the beamformer design in order to reduce the electronic complexity is to replace the digital time delay by digital phase shift (Figure 25–4). Obviously, this approach places performance limitations very similar to those of the analog implementation of phase shift, preventing the imaging

system from retaining all the tissue signature necessary for broadband imaging.

These hybrid systems still contain the focusing errors for broadband tissue imaging mentioned earlier, resulting in loss of information. Some systems have tried to compensate for these losses by adding beamforming channels, but this approach increases system complexity, size, and cost without providing a truly accurate tissue signature. It is clear that the only motivation for such compromises is the lack of mastering for the complex technology required to implement the true digital broadband solution.

TRUE BROADBAND DIGITAL BEAMFORMER

Similar to the compact disc, which preserves the original purity of music, the broadband digital beamformer preserves all the information content of the tissue signal. New ultrasound systems implement this ideal form

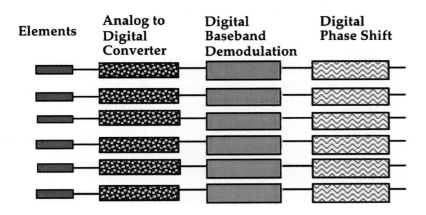

Figure 25–4. Digital beamformer with phase shift.

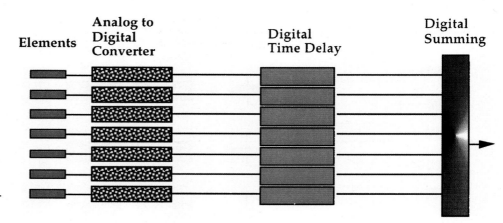

Figure 25–5. True digital beam-former.

of beamforming without any compromises, delivering all the tissue information (Figure 25–5). Products of this type deliver:

- True broadband time delay to preserve all the tissue signature information for optimum spatial and contrast resolution, as well as new developments such as harmonic imaging of contrast agents
- True dynamic focusing to provide optimum resolution at each point of the image

The undistorted quality of the broadband tissue signature can be utilized fully in the downstream processing of the beamformer. For instance, bandwidth may also be employed to reduce directly artifacts in the image, caused by phase cancellation (this causes a well-known noise on ultrasound images called "speckle"). Since the speckle patterns at different frequencies are independent, proper combination of information from several frequency bands results in reduced speckle and improved contrast resolution. The degree of this improvement depends on the total bandwidth available. This method is referred to as "frequency compounding."

CHARACTERISTIC SIGNATURE OF FLOWING BLOOD

The detection of blood flow raises a number of difficulties that can be overcome by careful analysis of the signature of the echo returned by red blood cells. The primary difficulty is the small amplitude of the signal returned from blood compared to the large amplitude (1000 times greater) of that returned from tissue. In blood flow detection what was considered signal for tissue imaging is now considered noise, or something to be eliminated. Therefore, for blood flow detection there are two noise sources that should be overcome: system noise, which is a low-amplitude, random noise signal spread across the entire frequency band, and clutter noise, which is typically a high-amplitude signal from stationary or slowly moving tissue.

Thus the blood flow signature is a signal the amplitude of which is greater than that of the system noise but that moves more rapidly than the surrounding tissue (Figure 25–6). What is the best method to detect it? It would be very difficult to identify the signature using a single pulse since the blood moves only a tiny amount

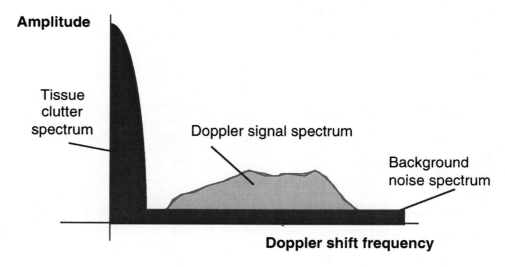

Figure 25–6. Doppler signal spectrum.

during the time it is being interrogated with a short burst of sound. By sending out multiple bursts and comparing the echoes received from consecutive bursts it is possible to identify the component that has moved and to separate it from the surrounding clutter. It is also possible to perform averaging, which reduces the effect of the random, low-amplitude system noise. These two steps are fundamental parts of any blood flow detection scheme, including all the variations of spectral Doppler, color flow, and Doppler power imaging. The differences between these flow imaging methods lie only in how many pulses are sent, how they are compared to eliminate clutter, how much they are averaged, and which attribute of the blood echo finally is displayed.

The simplest method of eliminating clutter simply subtracts consecutive pulses from each other and is known as moving target indication (MTI), from radar. Much more complex methods have been developed that combine several pulses simultaneously, but the basic principle is still the same. These techniques enhance the system's ability to separate the slowly moving clutter from the blood flow, doing a better job of detecting the specific signature of the blood, its motion. This part of the system is often called the wall filter, and it is present in all forms of Doppler flow detector, including power Doppler.

Once the clutter has been eliminated, some attribute of the signal must be displayed. Spectral Doppler displays a velocity spectrum, showing the different velocity components within a single sample volume. Color flow displays a single velocity value for every location on the screen. Power Doppler displays the amplitude of the signal from the moving blood. Each of these different attributes of the blood flow regime is useful for different clinical situations and each allows different tradeoffs in the number of pulses used and how they are averaged.

SPECTRAL DOPPLER

To gain the most velocity information from a single point in the image, the system must interrogate that location continuously. However, because of the pulse–echo nature of ultrasound, this continuous wave (CW) technique provides no *range resolution*, the ability to separate blood flow at one range from another. It also means that tissue signals coming from everywhere along the sound beam contribute to the clutter problem, making clutter elimination even more difficult. This requires the system to be able accurately to reproduce very small signals from the region of interest along with the huge clutter signals generated by shallow structure. The ability to maintain very small signals along with very large ones is referred to as *dynamic range* and is a key attribute of any blood flow detection system.

If some compromise can be allowed in the highest velocity that needs to be detected, the system can be pulsed in the direction of interest to provide range resolution. With pulsed wave (PW) Doppler, the position of the volume of red blood cell scatterers is only measured once every pulse repetition interval (PRI). Unfortunately if the volume of scatterers has moved more than one half of a wavelength of sound between pulses, there is no way to tell whether it has moved a long ways forward or a short ways backward. This artifact, illustrated in Figure 25–7, is known as *aliasing* and can lead to high-velocity flows appearing to go backward.

COLOR FLOW

Both PW and CW displays provide a spectral output showing all the different velocity components present at a one location, but they require an entire two-dimensional display because three variables—frequency, amplitude, and time—are being shown simultaneously. If blood flow information is required over the entire field of view, further compromises must be made in the amount of information displayed at each location. If only the mean velocity is displayed, rather than all velocity components present, then this can be encoded in color and displayed at the location in space where that velocity was detected, leading to a two-dimensional image of the flow. Color flow imaging uses one set of colors to depict flow moving toward the transducer and a different set to depict flow away from the transducer. A range of hues of those colors is chosen to characterize different velocities. This display is known as color flow.

With pulsed Doppler, the same location is interrogated with a steady stream of pulses. To detect flow throughout the entire image, the interrogating beam must be stepped from location to location rapidly, firing

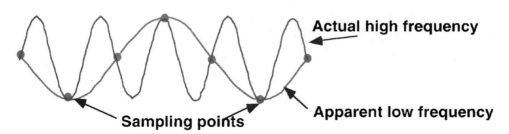

Figure 25–7. Aliasing.

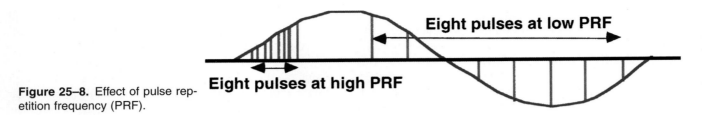

Figure 25–8. Effect of pulse repetition frequency (PRF).

just enough pulses in each direction to remove the clutter and obtain a satisfactory estimate of the mean velocity. How many pulses are fired and the rate at which they are fired have a big impact on the range of velocities that can be detected as well as on the frame rate. In general, the more pulses fired in one direction, the better the detection process, but the slower the frame rate.

The pulse repetition frequency (PRF) determines the highest velocity that can be unambiguously resolved without aliasing. The PRF, along with the number of pulses fired, or ensemble length, also helps determine the lowest frequency that can be detected. The longer the PRI and the more pulses that are fired (ensemble length), the longer the time interval over which the signal is actually being observed. Since low frequencies have longer wavelengths, they require longer periods of observation to either reject them as clutter or accept them as flow and estimate their frequency. This is illustrated in Figure 25–8. Therefore, knowing approximately the velocity or frequency range that is expected

from both the flow and the tissue enables the system to be better optimized for the particular flow regime.

One of the most critical aspects of a color flow system is the final decision making as to whether there is actually a flow signal detected in a given location or not. This is inherently a decision-making process, so a priori knowledge of the expected flow and clutter characteristics again helps in optimizing the final image. In other words, if the signal fits the expected signature, display it; if not, do not. For this detection process such characteristics as signal amplitude, frequency, and variance or randomness are all taken into account.

COLOR POWER DOPPLER

Suppose that we do not care how fast or in what direction blood is flowing, but instead are only interested in detecting the existence of flow with the greatest sensitivity. We still need to look at the signal for a component that is moving, that is stronger than the system noise, and that is smaller than tissue clutter signals, but we can discard all information about its actual velocity. By dis-

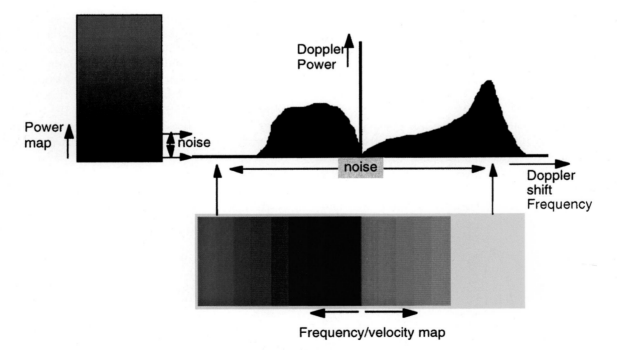

Figure 25–9. Color power Doppler.

playing only the power in the Doppler signal (Figure 25–9), we can indicate whether there is flow in that location and how much there is, not how fast it is moving. How does that change the situation?

It provides several advantages for flow detection. Since directional information is not displayed, all flow can be displayed with the same basic color hue so that aliasing is not shown. Since aliasing is no longer an issue, the PRF can be made very low to allow for the detection of very low velocities.

This provides an additional important benefit for low-level signal detection related to the background noise characteristics. Any location in the image has a frequency associated with it, even the low-level background noise. In fact, noise has random frequency content, leading to the typical red-blue mottled appearance seen when the gain is turned up too high on a color flow system. However, it typically has a low amplitude that is fairly uniform over the entire image. When the Doppler power signal is displayed, the noise characteristics then become a uniform low background level instead of random bright color dots. Clearly, this is much less distracting and allows the gain to be turned up significantly.

Another advantage is the amount of temporal smoothing that can be tolerated. With flow that is at all pulsatile, averaging more than a few frames for improved sensitivity detracts from the real-time feeling for the color flow. With power Doppler imaging, there is no attempt to image flow pulsatility, so the signals can be averaged over a longer period of time, allowing greater sensitivity.

THREE-DIMENSIONAL VASCULAR IMAGING

Color power is a technique that blends itself very well to the challenges of 3D visualization and representation of blood vasculature. Color Doppler provides increased signal sensitivity over any other Doppler technique and delivers high-resolution images of vascular structures independent of flow dynamics. The information processed is independent of the insonification angle and does not show ambiguous data (aliasing); furthermore, the image is smooth and provides natural segmentation (separation between tissue and flow) of the information for ease of 3D reconstruction. Thus, manually sweeping the transducer over the zone of interest, the user acquires a volume set of color Doppler data, enabling the system to reconstruct and visualize the 3D vascular data in under a minute (Figure 25–10). Such a technique is a true volumetric one that does not require performance of any type of surface rendering.

THE ADDITION OF A CONTRAST AGENT

The most obvious way to describe the effect of a contrast agent is that it simply increases the amplitude of the echo returned from blood. What contrast agents really do is

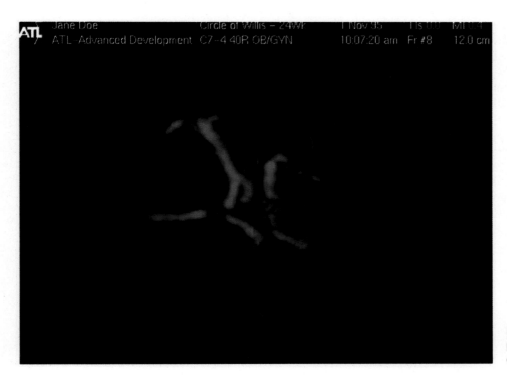

Figure 25–10. Color power Doppler of circle of Willis of 20-week-old fetus.

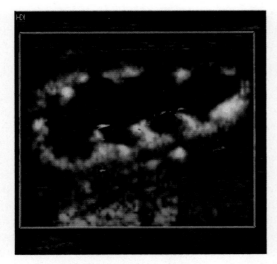

Before injection

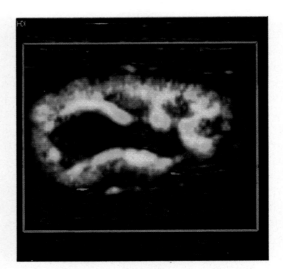

Harmonic contrast CPA

Figure 25–11. Harmonic contrast imaging of the kidney. CPA, color power angiography.

modify the characteristic signature of the echo from blood. Enhancements of the backscattered echo from arterial blood of between 10 and 30 dB have been measured. It therefore increases the detectability of weak flow states, but also it presents a problem when there is too great an echo amplitude, in which case the image is often filled with color, compromising detail resolution.

Recent work has focused on trying to find a unique signature for contrast, meaning a unique signal that can be displayed and that carries only information related to the contrast agent, independent of its surrounding. One such signature is based on the fact that, when insonified at certain power levels, the contrast agent (composed of microbubbles filled with gas) resonates and produces a signal at double the frequency of insonification, the harmonic frequency. When using a broadband ultrasound system, this signal can be captured and displayed, providing unique information from the agent since it is the only component in the body that responds at such frequency (Figure 25–11).

Application of this technique is showing great promise in radiology, with its capability to assess tumor vascularization, and also in cardiology, where myocardial perfusion can now be seen without the use of radionuclide agents. The next step, naturally, is to be able to quantify those new findings accurately.

CONCLUSION

As can be seen, the advent of broadband digital ultrasound imaging contributes greatly to new progress in clinical performance and efficacy. The digital revolution is also the central point for new means of managing images using the DICOM protocol to link the ultrasound unit with centralized file servers and/or printers. Leveraging Web technology is equally feasible with an all-digital architecture; using Internet or intranet structures, the physician, wherever he or she is located, will always be in touch with the patient.

SUGGESTED READINGS

1. Burns P, Powers J, et al.: Harmonic power mode Doppler using microbubble contrast agents: An improved method for small vessel flow imaging: Paper presented at the 1994 Ultrasonics Symposium,
2. O'Donnell M, et al.: Real time phased array imaging using digital beamforming and autonomous channel control. Paper presented at the 1990 Ultrasonics Symposium,
3. Burns P: Doppler artifacts. In: Taylor KJW, Burns PN, Wells PNT, eds. *Clinical Applications of Doppler Ultrasound*, Vol 2. New York: Raven Press, 1995:46–76.
4. Gehlbach S, Somer FG: Frequency diversity speckle processing. *Ultrasonic Imaging.* 9:1987.

Index

Page numbers in *italics* refer to illustrations; page numbers followed by t refer to tables.

C